Lecture Notes in Computer Science   10670

Commenced Publication in 1973
Founding and Former Series Editors:
Gerhard Goos, Juris Hartmanis, and Jan van Leeuwen

More information about this series at http://www.springer.com/series/7412

Alessandro Crimi · Spyridon Bakas
Hugo Kuijf · Bjoern Menze
Mauricio Reyes (Eds.)

Brainlesion: Glioma, Multiple Sclerosis, Stroke and Traumatic Brain Injuries

Third International Workshop, BrainLes 2017
Held in Conjunction with MICCAI 2017
Quebec City, QC, Canada, September 14, 2017
Revised Selected Papers

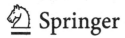 Springer

Editors
Alessandro Crimi
African Institute of Mathematical Sciences
Cape Town
Ghana

Bjoern Menze
Technical University Munich
Munich
Germany

Spyridon Bakas
University of Pennsylvania
Philadelphia, PA
USA

Mauricio Reyes
Universität Bern
Bern
Switzerland

Hugo Kuijf
University Medical Center Utrecht
Utrecht
The Netherlands

ISSN 0302-9743 ISSN 1611-3349 (electronic)
Lecture Notes in Computer Science
ISBN 978-3-319-75237-2 ISBN 978-3-319-75238-9 (eBook)
https://doi.org/10.1007/978-3-319-75238-9

Library of Congress Control Number: 2018934331

LNCS Sublibrary: SL6 – Image Processing, Computer Vision, Pattern Recognition, and Graphics

Printed on acid-free paper

This Springer imprint is published by the registered company Springer International Publishing AG
part of Springer Nature
The registered company address is: Gewerbestrasse 11, 6330 Cham, Switzerland

Preface

This volume contains articles from the Brain-Lesion Workshop (BrainLes) as well as the International Multimodal Brain Tumor Segmentation (BraTS) and White Matter Hyperintensities (WMH) Segmentation challenges, which were held jointly at the Medical Image Computing for Computer Assisted Intervention (MICCAI) Conference on September 14, 2017 in Quebec City, Canada.

The presented papers describe the research of computational scientists and clinical researchers working on glioma, multiple sclerosis, cerebral stroke, traumatic brain injuries, and white matter hyperintensities of presumed vascular origin. This compilation does not claim to provide a comprehensive understanding from all points of view; however, the authors present their latest advances in segmentation, disease prognosis, and other applications to the clinical context.

The volume is divided into four parts: The first part comprises two invited papers summarizing the presentations of the keynotes, the second includes the submissions to the BrainLes Workshop, the third contains a selection of papers regarding methods presented at the BraTS challenge 2017, and lastly a selection of papers on methods presented at the WMH challenge.

The two invited papers provide a review of the work done to date in detecting and segmenting multiple sclerosis, and propose performance scores for segmentation that go beyond the controversial Dice and Jaccard index.

The aim of the second part is to provide an overview of new advances of medical image analysis in all of the aforementioned brain pathologies, bringing together researchers from the medical image analysis domain, neurologists, and radiologists working on at least one of these diseases. The aim is to consider neuroimaging biomarkers used for one disease applied to the other diseases. This session did not have a specific dataset to be used.

The third part focuses on the papers from the BraTS challenge. In order to gauge the current state of the art in automated brain tumor segmentation using multiple magnetic resonance imaging (MRI) modalities and compare the different methods, a large dataset of brain scans was made available via www.med.upenn.edu/sbia/brats2017.html. The participants at the challenge compared the results obtained with their methods against manual segmentations.

The fourth part contains descriptions of a selection of the 20 algorithms participating in the WMH segmentation challenge. The purpose of this challenge was to directly compare methods for the automatic segmentation of white matter hyperintensities (WMH) of presumed vascular origin. A dataset consisting of 60 multimodal brain MR images from three different institutes/scanners was released for training. A secret test set of 110 cases from five different scanners was used for evaluation. The test data were not released, but participants had to submit their method to: http://wmh.isi.uu.nl/.

We heartily hope that this volume will promote further exiting research about brain lesions.

January 2018

Alessandro Crimi
Spyridon Bakas
Hugo Kuijf
Bjoern Menze
Mauricio Reyes
Heinz Handels

Organization

Main Organizing Committee

Spyridon Bakas	Center for Biomedical Image Computing and Analytics, University of Pennsylvania, USA
Alessandro Crimi	African Institute for Mathematical Sciences, Ghana
Hugo Kuijf	University Medical Center Utrecht, The Netherlands

Challenges Organizing Committee

Frederik Barkhof	Image Analysis Centre, VU Amsterdam, The Netherlands
Matthijs Biesbroek	Brain Center Rudolf Magnus, UMC Utrecht, The Netherlands
Geert Jan Biessels	Brain Center Rudolf Magnus, UMC Utrecht, The Netherlands
Christopher Chen	Memory Aging and Cognition Center, NUHS, Singapore
Christos Davatzikos	Center for Biomedical Image Computing and Analytics, University of Pennsylvania, USA
Jeroen de Bresser	Department of Radiology, UMC Utrecht, The Netherlands
Keyvan Farahani	National Institute of Health, USA
Heinz Handels	Universität zu Lübeck, Germany
Rutger Heinen	Brain Center Rudolf Magnus, UMC Utrecht, The Netherlands
Bjoern Menze	Technische Universität München, Germany
Mauricio Reyes	Universität Bern, Switzerland
Wiesje van der Flier	Alzheimer Center, VU Amsterdam, The Netherlands
Max Viergever	Image Sciences Institute, UMC Utrecht, The Netherlands

Program Committee

Meritxell Bach Cuadra	University of Lausanne, Switzerland
Ender Konukoglu	ETH-Zurich, Switzerland
Christine Tanner	ETH-Zurich, Switzerland
Oskar Maier	Universität zu Lübeck, Germany
Koen Van Leemput	Harvard Medical School, USA
Stefan Winzeck	University of Cambridge, UK

Sponsoring Institutions

Center for Biomedical Image Computing and Analytics, University of Pennsylvania, USA

Image Sciences Institute, University Medical Center Utrecht, The Netherlands

Contents

Ischemic Stroke Lesion Image Segmentation

Invited Talks

Dice Overlap Measures for Objects of Unknown Number: Application to Lesion Segmentation

Ipek Oguz[1(✉)], Aaron Carass[2,3], Dzung L. Pham[4], Snehashis Roy[4],
Nagesh Subbana[1], Peter A. Calabresi[5], Paul A. Yushkevich[1],
Russell T. Shinohara[6], and Jerry L. Prince[2,3]

[1] Department of Radiology, University of Pennsylvania,
Philadelphia, PA 19104, USA
ipekoguz@pennmedicine.upenn.edu
[2] Department of Electrical and Computer Engineering,
The Johns Hopkins University, Baltimore, MD 21218, USA
[3] Department of Computer Science, The Johns Hopkins University,
Baltimore, MD 21218, USA
[4] CNRM, The Henry M. Jackson Foundation for the Advancement
of Military Medicine, Bethesda, MD 20817, USA
[5] Department of Neurology, The Johns Hopkins University School of Medicine,
Baltimore, MD 21287, USA
[6] Department of Biostatistics and Epidemiology, University of Pennsylvania,
Philadelphia, PA 19104, USA

Abstract. The Dice overlap ratio is commonly used to evaluate the performance of image segmentation algorithms. While Dice overlap is very useful as a standardized quantitative measure of segmentation accuracy in many applications, it offers a very limited picture of segmentation quality in complex segmentation tasks where the number of target objects is not known *a priori*, such as the segmentation of white matter lesions or lung nodules. While Dice overlap can still be used in these applications, segmentation algorithms may perform quite differently in ways not reflected by differences in their Dice score. Here we propose a new set of evaluation techniques that offer new insights into the behavior of segmentation algorithms. We illustrate these techniques with a case study comparing two popular multiple sclerosis (MS) lesion segmentation algorithms: OASIS and LesionTOADS.

Keywords: Segmentation · Evaluation · MS · Lesion

1 Introduction

Segmentation is a broad and critical field of research in medical image analysis. The evaluation of segmentation algorithms is crucial both for assessing the performance of new algorithms and for choosing a particular algorithm for a

© Springer International Publishing AG, part of Springer Nature 2018
A. Crimi et al. (Eds.): BrainLes 2017, LNCS 10670, pp. 3–14, 2018.
https://doi.org/10.1007/978-3-319-75238-9_1

new task. In medical image segmentation, the Dice [6] and Jaccard [11] overlap ratios are the most popular evaluation measures [16,22]. The mean and maximum surface distances between 3D objects are also commonly used to evaluate segmentation algorithms [9], as are distances between segmentation results and manual landmarks. However, such measures are based on the implicit assumption that the number of segmentation targets is known *a priori*, e.g., whether it is one liver, two hippocampi, or five lung lobes. This is in contrast to a different but equally important class of segmentation tasks, such as the segmentation of white matter lesions or lung nodules, where the number of target objects can vary from zero to hundreds or more. In these scenarios, the object detection and segmentation tasks become intertwined and as such, performance evaluation needs to take both aspects into consideration. Although, it has been customary to use the image-wide Dice overlap in these combined detection and segmentation problems, this is an oversimplification and can often hide differences in algorithm behaviors (e.g., Fig. 1). Another popular criterion in these types of applications is the number of segmented objects, which attempts to evaluate the detection success. However, the object count alone is an ambiguous metric as it reflects not only the false positive and false negative detections but also larger objects that may be erroneously split into multiple smaller ones, or multiple small objects erroneously merged into a single, larger object. Furthermore, these commonly used metrics fail to relate the size of the object to the final score, which can be important: for many applications, an algorithm that misses large objects is considered less clinically relevant than an algorithm that misses small objects.

A prime example of an application domain with a variable number of objects is multiple sclerosis (MS) lesion segmentation from MRI scans of the brain. White matter lesions are the hallmark of MS and their segmentation and quantification are critical for clinical purposes. Many approaches to MS lesion segmentation have been proposed: artificial [10] and convolutional neural networks [1]; Bayesian models [7]; Gaussian mixture models [23]; graph cuts [8]; and random forests [12]. This field of research remains very active and several grand challenges (MICCAI 2008 [19], ISBI 2015 [2], MICCAI 2016 [13]) have been organized in recent years. The evaluation of new algorithms often relies on Dice and Jaccard overlaps and lesion counts, which limits our ability to fully assess other characteristics in performance difference.

We propose a new set of evaluation techniques to compare segmentations with a variable number of target objects, including a classification of segmentation results and statistics at object and category levels. We illustrate these techniques in an MS lesion segmentation study comparing two algorithms: Lesion-TOADS [17] which is an unsupervised clustering algorithm with topological constraints; and OASIS [21] is a supervised classifier based on multi-modal logistic regression.

2   Methods

2.1   Data and Compared Methods

As a case study, we used a set of T1w, T2w, PD, and FLAIR images from 70 MS patients acquired at 3T. The images of each subject were co-registered rigidly to the T1w space, which was also rigidly aligned to the MNI template. Lesions were manually segmented in each T1w-FLAIR pair by an expert with more than 15 years of experience. Two popular algorithms, OASIS [21] and Lesion-TOADS [17], were applied to this dataset. For OASIS, data from a disjoint set of 20 MS patients imaged with the same protocol were used for training. Lesion-TOADS was run with T1w and FLAIR inputs; the smoothing parameter was adjusted from 0.2 to 0.4 as we empirically found this to improve the quality of the segmentations and a different weight (0.7 vs. 1.0 vs. 1.2) was used for the FLAIR image in the multi-channel segmentation based on the lesion load (*Low* vs. *Med.* vs. *High*)—see Shiee et al. [18] for details.

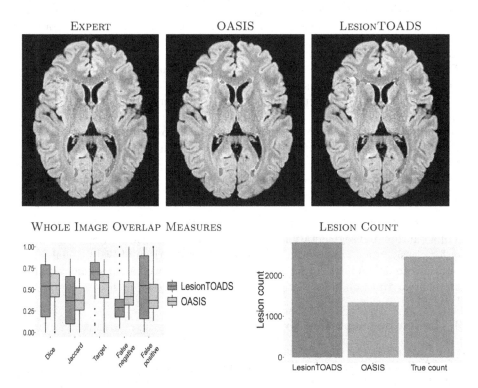

Fig. 1. The top row shows a typical example of segmentation results for the two algorithms and expert delineation. The second row shows image-wide overlap measures and the lesion count for both methods and the expert delineation (True count).

2.2 Object Correspondence Identification and Classification

Given a pair of segmentations S_{i1} and $S_{i2} \in \{0,1\}^V$ for a subject i, e.g., an automated and a manual segmentation, respectively, we begin by identifying the (6-) connected components in each segmentation as individual objects (i.e., lesions in our application). We name these two sets of objects C_{i1} and C_{i2}. Then, for each object in C_{i1}, we identify its corresponding objects by determining all objects in C_{i2} (if any) that it overlaps with. Formally, for an object $O_{ij1} \in C_{i1}$, the set of matching objects is $m(O_{ij1}) = \{O_{ik2}, \forall k : O_{ij1} \cap O_{ik2} \neq \emptyset\}$. Note that this means 0, 1, or multiple corresponding objects are possible. Similarly, for each object $O_{ij2} \in C_{i2}$, we identify its set of corresponding objects, $m(O_{ij2})$, by determining all objects in C_{i1} (if any) that it overlaps with.

Following correspondence identification, it is possible to determine the match configuration for each object by considering the number of forward and backward correspondences. For example, if an object $O_{ij1} \in C_{i1}$ corresponds to a single object $O_{ik2} \in C_{i2}$, and O_{ik2} corresponds to a single object (i.e., O_{ij1}), then we have a 1-1 match. In contrast, if an object $O_{ij1} \in C_{i1}$ corresponds to multiple objects O_{i12}-O_{iN2}, and each of the $O_{i\cdot2}$ correspond only to O_{ij1}, then we have a 1-N match. Following the nomenclature of [15], we have the following categories:

- **Correct detection:** 1-1 match.
- **False alarm:** 1-0 match. An object exists in C_{i1} that does not exist in C_{i2}, i.e., a false positive if C_{i2} is the truth.
- **Merge:** 1-N match. Multiple objects in C_{i2} are merged into a single object in C_{i1}.
- **Split:** N-1 match. A single object in C_{i2} is split into multiple objects in C_{i1}.
- **Split-merge:** N-N match. The conditions for both merge and split are satisfied.
- **Detection failure:** 0-1 match. An object exists in C_{i2} that does not exist in C_{i1}, i.e., a false negative if C_{i2} is the truth.

We note that while the results presented in this paper focus on the comparison of an automated segmentation S_{i1} and a manual segmentation S_{i2}, the same idea for classification can also be applied to the comparison of two manual segmentations to assess intra- or inter-rater variability, as well as to segmentations from different timepoints in a longitudinal study to assess the disease course.

2.3 Lesion Segmentation Evaluation

We propose a battery of statistics to compare two binary segmentations for a subject i, S_{i1} and S_{i2}, which will be illustrated in Sect. 3.

We begin by reporting the classical image-wide overlap measures. In particular, for each subject i, we report the Dice overlap ($\mathrm{DSC}_i = 2\frac{|S_{i1} \cap S_{i2}|}{|S_{i1}| + |S_{i2}|}$) [6], the Jaccard overlap ($2\frac{|S_{i1} \cap S_{i2}|}{|S_{i1} \cup S_{i2}|}$) [11], target overlap ($\frac{|S_{i1} \cap S_{i2}|}{|S_{i2}|}$), the false negative error ($\frac{|S_{i2} - S_{i1}|}{|S_{i2}|}$) and the false positive error ($\frac{|S_{i1} - S_{i2}|}{|S_{i1}|}$). We also report the number of connected objects ($|C_{i1}|$), which is another popular evaluation measure.

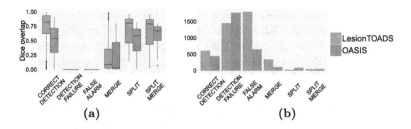

Fig. 2. For both LesionTOADS and OASIS, we show the **(a)** Dice overlap by lesion class and the **(b)** lesion count by class.

Next, we classify the object segmentation as described in Sect. 2.2 and report the number of objects n_{ik1} and n_{ik2}, defined by S_{i1} and S_{i2}, in each category k. We further report the average per-object Dice overlap, $\overline{DSC}_{ik1} = n_{ik1}^{-1}\sum_{j=1}^{n_{ik1}} DSC_{ijk}$, for each category k, where DSC_{ijk} is the Dice of an object j, defined as the Dice overlap between the segmentation of the jth object of type k in S_i1, O_{ijk1}, and the matching set $m(O_{ijk1})$.

Next, we analyze the mean per-object Dice overlap as a function of true object size, i.e., $f(s) = \mathbb{E}(DSC_{ijk} \mid |O_{ijk}| = s)$, where $|\cdot|$ denotes the volume of an object and $\mathbb{E}$ is the expectation operator. This is done both globally for all objects, as well as separately for each category of matches (which we denote by $f_k(s)$), using locally weighted scatterplot smoothing (LOESS) [3]. We use scatterplots of Dice vs. true object size to visualize this data. To estimate 95% confidence bands for the LOESS scatterplots, we use a nonparametric bootstrap. We resample by subject to respect the nested object-within-subject correlation structure. That is, for each $b \in [1, 10000]$, we resample subjects $i \in [1, n]$ with replacement to form a bootstrapped sample of pairs of segmentations $(S_{11}^{(b)}, S_{12}^{(b)}), \ldots, (S_{n1}^{(b)}, S_{n2}^{(b)})$ and re-estimate $f(s)$, and $f_k(s)$ and denote these estimates by $\hat{f}^{(b)}(s)$, and $\hat{f}_k^{(b)}(s)$. We then calculate the pointwise 2.5% and 97.5% quantiles of $\hat{f}^{(b)}$ and $\hat{f}_k^{(b)}$ to estimate the lower and upper limits of confidence bands. For the false alarm and correct detection classes, we use histograms of object size (since the Dice is always 0 for these classes). Additionally, for these two classes, we report the spatial distribution of the occurrences by registering all images into a common atlas space to construct a spatial occurrence frequency map.

3   Results

Figure 1 shows a summary of the whole-image overlap measures. LesionTOADS and OASIS have comparable Dice and Jaccard measures, which is important since these are two of the most commonly used measures for comparing segmentation algorithms. LesionTOADS has a smaller false negative ratio but a higher false positive ratio than OASIS. The number of distinct lesions as segmented by the expert manual rater was 2461; OASIS detected 1340 distinct lesions whereas LesionTOADS detected 2810. LesionTOADS reports more lesions than OASIS, but it is uncertain using these measures whether this is driven by a higher successful detection rate, more false alarms, more split lesions, or other reasons.

Figure 2(a) shows the per-lesion Dice overlap, summarized per class. Note that the Dice for the detection failures and false alarms is 0 by construction. The LesionTOADS algorithm has a higher Dice than OASIS in every category, which is rather surprising given that the whole-image Dice measures are nearly equal between the two methods (see Fig. 1). Figure 2(b) shows the number of lesions in each of the classes described in Sect. 2. Compared to overall lesion counts, this analysis provides further insight into the algorithm behavior: compared to OASIS, LesionTOADS has a larger number of correctly detected lesions (good), and fewer detection failures (good), but also more merges (bad), and many more false alarms (bad). As such, it is difficult to declare an overall "winner" but each algorithm is "winning" for different classes of lesions.

Figure 3(a) shows the per-lesion Dice overlap as a function of true lesion size. On average, LesionTOADS seems to perform better than OASIS for small and large lesions, whereas OASIS performs better for the more prevalent medium-sized lesions. It is also interesting that in this medium-size range, OASIS appears to have a tighter distribution of Dice scores whereas LesionTOADS performs either very well (Dice > 0.8) or very poorly (Dice < 0.2). Figures 3(c) and (d) provide additional insight by breaking down this data into individual classes.

Figure 4 takes this analysis one step further by directly comparing the algorithms' behaviors in each class. Figure 4(a) shows this comparison for the correctly detected lesions. We note that the average performance of the LesionTOADS algorithm increases steeply with size in this class, indicating the algorithm is highly accurate for all but the smallest lesions (which are notoriously difficult to segment correctly), for those lesions that it manages to detect correctly. In contrast, OASIS performance improves more slowly with lesion size. Figure 4(b) compares the two methods for merged lesions; while the performance of the two algorithms are roughly comparable and both improve with lesion size, there are overall fewer merged lesions for OASIS, which is desirable. Figures 4(c) and (d) provide the same comparison for split and split-merge classes, respectively.

For false alarms and detection failures, instead of scatterplots, we present spatial distribution maps and size histograms of lesions. Figure 5 shows the detection failures for the two algorithms. It is interesting that the distribution of these failures are remarkably similar between the two algorithms for smaller lesions, suggesting many of these smaller lesions may be generally difficult to detect. The spatial distributions of these detection failures concentrate on the septum area for both methods. OASIS has an additional hotspot for detection failures near the temporal horn of the ventricles.

Figure 6 compares the false alarms for the two algorithms. LesionTOADS appears to generate hardly any small false positive lesions, but many medium-to-large false positive lesions. This rather surprising finding explains the counterintuitive result that while LesionTOADS reports better Dice overlap for each lesion category (Fig. 2), the whole-image Dice scores are nearly identical between the two methods (see Fig. 1). We note that the large number of false alarms reported

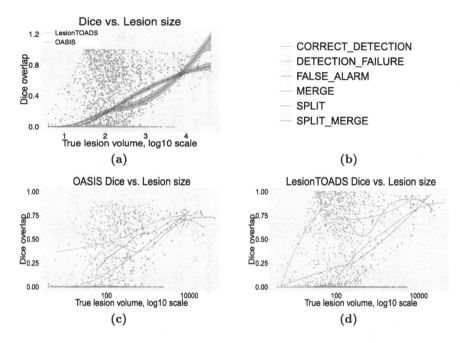

Fig. 3. (a) For both LesionTOADS and OASIS, we show per-lesion Dice overlap as a function of true lesion size, bootstrapped per subject. Per-lesion Dice overlap as a function of true lesion size, color-coded by classification (see legend in (b)), for both (c) OASIS and (d) LesionTOADS.

for LesionTOADS is likely due to the use of a limited range of parameters for this study for a fair comparison to OASIS. In other use scenarios, LesionTOADS could be run with different parameter settings for each patient. Furthermore, it is striking that two algorithms with such similar whole-image Dice scores can have such dramatically different performance in different types of lesions, which can go unnoticed in studies that only report the whole-image Dice score. The spatial distributions of false alarms concentrate around the ventricles as well as the inferior brain for both methods; the latter region is especially pronounced for LesionTOADS.

4 Discussion

We have presented a battery of new complementary measures to better evaluate the performance of segmentation algorithms. Detailed evaluations can also be useful for parameter tuning: algorithms typically require multiple parameters to be set and the effects of changing these parameters are not always clear based on image-wide Dice alone. While the current study focuses on the MS lesion segmentation task, the presented evaluation scheme is directly applicable to other segmentation tasks where the object of interest is of variable number,

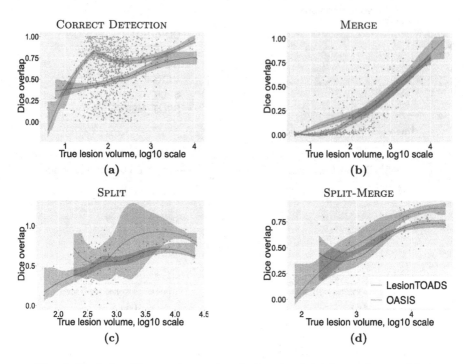

Fig. 4. Per-lesion Dice overlap vs. true lesion size, bootstrapped per subject.

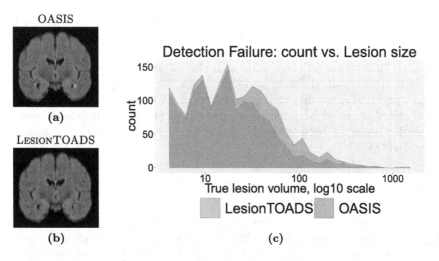

Fig. 5. Spatial distribution of detection failures on a coronal slice for **(a)** OASIS and **(b)** LesionTOADS, with both methods exhibiting failures around the septum. Size statistics of detection failures for **(c)** both OASIS and LesionTOADS.

such as lung nodule segmentation and cell counting. Additionally, even when the number of objects is known *a priori*, it has been argued [4] that reducing the segmentation quality to a single value represented by the Dice or Haussdorff score may be an oversimplification, and that a more detailed evaluation scheme may be beneficial.

The results in our case study highlight a common problem with the popular evaluation approach that relies only on Dice overlap: two algorithms with have nearly identical overall Dice overlap ratios, but digging deeper reveals that the behaviors of the algorithms are dramatically different. Additionally, in this particular study, the number of false alarms happens to be consistent with the image-wide false negative rate, and the number of detection failures happens to be consistent with the image-wide false positive rate. However, this does not have to be the case, as multiple small missed lesions and few large missed lesions are indistinguishable in the image-wide measures; similarly for multiple small false positive lesions and few large false positive lesions.

It is well known that the pathology of large lesions may often be different than that of smaller lesions; multiple small lesions are not equivalent to a single large lesion in terms of white matter damage, even if their overall size and location may be similar. Therefore, in addition to their relevance for shedding light onto the overall performance of segmentation algorithms, the Split, Merge, and Split-Merge categories are also potentially clinically relevant. Moreover, in longitudinal studies, it is often desired to "track" lesions over time [14, 20], and thus analysis of the merging behavior can also be highly relevant in such studies.

One potential weakness of the present study is that the identification of overlapping lesions is currently performed with no tolerance; i.e., if two lesions overlap by even a single voxel, they are considered to be in correspondence.

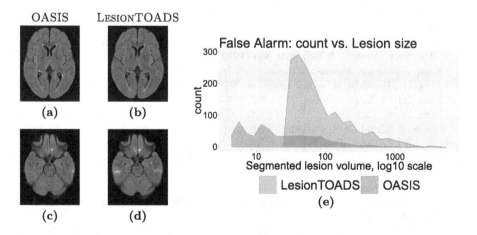

Fig. 6. False alarm category. Spatial distribution for **(a, c)** OASIS and **(b, d)** Lesion-TOADS, and **(e)** size statistics. LesionTOADS appears to generate hardly any small false positive lesions, but many medium-to-large false positive lesions.

While it would be straightforward to modify this to allow a threshold of tolerance (e.g., only consider it a match if X voxels or $Y\%$ of the true lesion volume are overlapping), this would add a layer of complexity to the interpretation of the results. The connectivity could also be extended beyond just 6-connectivity. These concerns can be taken into account similar to the multi-label evaluation approach in [5] that considers fuzzy segmentations. Further, while it would be straightforward to also report Jaccard, target overlap, false negative, and false positive errors at the per-lesion scale, here we focused on Dice for the sake of brevity. However, such metrics would likely provide additional insights into algorithm behavior. These additional analyses will be performed in future work.

Acknowledgments. This work was supported, in part, by NIH grants NINDS R01-NS094456, NINDS R01-NS085211, NINDS R21-NS093349, NIBIB R01-EB017255, NINDS R01-NS082347, NINDS R01-NS070906, as well as National MS Society grant RG-1507-05243.

References

1. Birenbaum, A., Greenspan, H.: Multi-view longitudinal CNN for multiple sclerosis lesion segmentation. Eng. Appl. Artif. Intell. **65**, 111–118 (2017)
2. Carass, A., Roy, S., Jog, A., Cuzzocreo, J.L., Magrath, E., Gherman, A., Button, J., Nguyen, J., Prados, F., Sudre, C.H., Cardoso, M.J., Cawley, N., Ciccarelli, O., Wheeler-Kingshott, C.A.M., Ourselin, S., Catanese, L., Deshpande, H., Maurel, P., Commowick, O., Barillot, C., Tomas-Fernandez, X., Warfield, S.K., Vaidya, S., Chunduru, A., Muthuganapathy, R., Krishnamurthi, G., Jesson, A., Arbel, T., Maier, O., Handels, H., Iheme, L.O., Unay, D., Jain, S., Sima, D.M., Smeets, D., Ghafoorian, M., Platel, B., Birenbaum, A., Greenspan, H., Bazin, P.L., Calabresi, P.A., Crainiceanu, C., Ellingsen, L.M., Reich, D.S., Prince, J.L., Pham, D.L.: Longitudinal multiple sclerosis lesion segmentation: resource & challenge. NeuroImage **148**, 77–102 (2017)
3. Cleveland, W.S.: Robust locally weighted regression and smoothing scatterplots. J. Am. Stat. Assoc. **74**(368), 829–836 (1979)
4. Crimi, A.: Brain lesions, introduction. In: Crimi, A., Menze, B., Maier, O., Reyes, M., Handels, H. (eds.) BrainLes 2015. LNCS, vol. 9556, pp. 1–5. Springer, Cham (2016). https://doi.org/10.1007/978-3-319-30858-6_1
5. Crum, W.R., Camara, O., Hill, D.L.G.: Generalized overlap measures for evaluation and validation in medical image analysis. IEEE Trans. Med. Imag. **25**(11), 1451–1461 (2006)
6. Dice, L.R.: Measures of the amount of ecologic association between species. Ecology **26**(3), 297–302 (1945)
7. Elliott, C., Arnold, D.L., Collins, D.L., Arbel, T.: Temporally consistent probabilistic detection of new multiple sclerosis lesions in brain MRI. IEEE Trans. Med. Imag. **32**(8), 1490–1503 (2013)
8. García-Lorenzo, D., Lecoeur, J., Arnold, D.L., Collins, D.L., Barillot, C.: Multiple sclerosis lesion segmentation using an automatic multimodal graph cuts. In: Yang, G.-Z., Hawkes, D., Rueckert, D., Noble, A., Taylor, C. (eds.) MICCAI 2009. LNCS, vol. 5762, pp. 584–591. Springer, Heidelberg (2009). https://doi.org/10.1007/978-3-642-04271-3_71

9. Gerig, G., Jomier, M., Chakos, M.: Valmet: a new validation tool for assessing and improving 3D object segmentation. In: Niessen, W.J., Viergever, M.A. (eds.) MICCAI 2001. LNCS, vol. 2208, pp. 516–523. Springer, Heidelberg (2001). https:// doi.org/10.1007/3-540-45468-3_62

10. Goldberg-Zimring, D., Achiron, A., Miron, S., Faibel, M., Azhari, H.: Automated detection and characterization of multiple sclerosis lesions in brain MR images. Mag. Reson. Imaging **16**(3), 311–318 (1998)

11. Jaccard, P.: The distribution of the flora in the alpine zone. New Phytol. **11**(2), 37–50 (1912)

12. Jog, A., Carass, A., Pham, D.L., Prince, J.L.: Multi-output decision trees for lesion segmentation in multiple sclerosis. In: Proceedings of SPIE Medical Imaging (SPIE-MI 2015), Orlando, FL, 21–26 February 2015, vol. 9413, pp. 94131C–94131C-6 (2015)

13. Maier, O., Menze, B.H., von der Gablentz, J., Häni, L., Heinrich, M.P., Liebrand, M., Winzeck, S., Basit, A., Bentley, P., Chen, L., Christiaens, D., Dutil, F., Egger, K., Feng, C., Glocker, B., Götz, M., Haeck, T., Halme, H.L., Havaei, M., Iftekharuddin, K.M., Jodoin, P.M., Kamnitsas, K., Kellner, E., Korvenoja, A., Larochelle, H., Ledig, C., Lee, J.H., Maes, F., Mahmood, Q., Maier-Hein, K.H., McKinley, R., Muschelli, J., Pal, C., Pei, L., Rangarajan, J.R., Reza, S.M.S., Robben, D., Rueckert, D., Salli, E., Suetens, P., Wang, C.W., Wilms, M., Kirschke, J.S., Krämer, U.M., Münte, T.F., Schramm, P., Wiest, R., Handels, H., Reyes, M.: ISLES 2015 - a public evaluation benchmark for ischemic stroke lesion segmentation from multispectral MRI. Med. Image Anal. **35**, 250–269 (2017)

14. Meier, D.S., Guttmann, C.R.G.: MRI time series modeling of MS lesion development. NeuroImage **32**(2), 531–537 (2006)

15. Nascimento, J.C., Marques, J.S.: Performance evaluation of object detection algorithms for video surveillance. IEEE Trans. Multimed. **8**(4), 761–774 (2006)

16. Rohlfing, T.: Image similarity and tissue overlaps as surrogates for image registration accuracy: widely used but unreliable. IEEE Trans. Med. Imaging **31**(2), 153–163 (2012)

17. Shiee, N., Bazin, P.L., Ozturk, A., Reich, D.S., Calabresi, P.A., Pham, D.L.: A topology-preserving approach to the segmentation of brain images with multiple sclerosis lesions. NeuroImage **49**(2), 1524–1535 (2010)

18. Shiee, N., Bazin, P.L., Zackowski, K., Farrell, S.K., Harrison, D.M., Newsome, S.D., Ratchford, J.N., Caffo, B.S., Calabresi, P.A., Pham, D.L., Reich, D.S.: Revisiting brain atrophy and its relationship to disability in multiple sclerosis. PLoS ONE **7**(5), e37049 (2012)

19. Styner, M., Lee, J., Chin, B., Chin, M.S., Commowick, O., Tran, H.H., Markovic-Plese, S., Jewells, V., Warfield, S.: 3D segmentation in the clinic: a grand challenge II: MS lesion segmentation. In: 11th International Conference on Medical Image Computing and Computer Assisted Intervention (MICCAI 2008) 3D Segmentation in the Clinic: A Grand Challenge II, pp. 1–6 (2008)

20. Sweeney, E.M., Shinohara, R.T., Dewey, B.E., Schindler, M.K., Muschelli, J., Reich, D.S., Crainiceanu, C.M., Eloyan, A.: Relating multi-sequence longitudinal intensity profiles and clinical covariates in incident multiple sclerosis lesions. NeuroImage Clin. **10**, 1–17 (2016)

21. Sweeney, E.M., Shinohara, R.T., Shiee, N., Mateen, F.J., Chudgar, A.A., Cuzzocreo, J.L., Calabresi, P.A., Pham, D.L., Reich, D.S., Crainiceanu, C.M.: OASIS is automated statistical inference for segmentation, with applications to multiple sclerosis lesion segmentation in MRI. NeuroImage Clin. **2**, 402–413 (2013)

22. Taha, A.A., Hanbury, A.: Metrics for evaluating 3D medical image segmentation: analysis, selection, and tool. BMC Med. Imaging **15**(1), 29 (2015)
23. Tomas-Fernandez, X., Warfield, S.K.: A model of population and subject (MOPS) intensities with application to multiple sclerosis lesion segmentation. IEEE Trans. Med. Imaging **34**(6), 1349–1361 (2015)

Lesion Detection, Segmentation and Prediction in Multiple Sclerosis Clinical Trials

Andrew Doyle[1], Colm Elliott[1], Zahra Karimaghaloo[1], Nagesh Subbanna[1],
Douglas L. Arnold[2], and Tal Arbel[1(✉)]

[1] Centre for Intelligent Machines, McGill University, Montréal, Canada
arbel@cim.mcgill.ca
[2] NeuroRx Research, Montréal, Canada

Abstract. A variety of automatic segmentation techniques have been successfully applied to the delineation of larger T2 lesions in patient MRI in the context of Multiple Sclerosis (MS), assisting in the estimation of lesion volume, a common clinical measure of disease activity and stage. In the context of clinical trials, however, a wider number of metrics are required to determine the "burden of disease" and activity in order to measure treatment efficacy. These include: (1) the number and volume of T2 lesions in MRI, (2) the number of *new* and *enlarging* T2 volumes in longitudinal MRI, and (3) the number of *gadolinium enhancing* lesions in T1 MRI, the portion of lesions that enhance in T1w MRI after injection with a contrast agent, often associated with active inflammations. In this context, accurate lesion *detection* must ensure that even small lesions (e.g. 3 to 10 voxels) are detected as they are prevalent in trials. Manual or semi-manual approaches are too time-consuming, inconsistent and expensive to be practical in large clinical trials. To this end, we present a series of fully-automatic, probabilistic machine learning frameworks to detect and segment all lesions in patient MRI, and show their accuracy and robustness in large multi-center, multi-scanner, clinical trial datasets. Several of these algorithms have been placed into a commercial software analysis pipeline, where they have assisted in improving the efficiency and precision of the development of most new MS treatments worldwide. Recent work has shown how a new *Bag-of-Lesions* brain representation can be used in the context of clinical trials to automatically predict the probability of future disease activity and potential treatment responders, leading to the possibility of personalized medicine.

1 Introduction

Multiple Sclerosis (MS) is an inflammatory and neuro-degenerative disease of the central nervous system (CNS) that usually onsets in young adulthood, and is characterized by a wide range of symptoms. The most common form is relapsing-remitting MS (RRMS), which presents with intermittent attacks or relapses followed by full or partial recovery. There is presently no known cure for MS, but treatments have been developed to mitigate symptoms, and to halt further disease development. Magnetic Resonance Imaging (MRI) has been used both as a

© Springer International Publishing AG, part of Springer Nature 2018
A. Crimi et al. (Eds.): BrainLes 2017, LNCS 10670, pp. 15–28, 2018.
https://doi.org/10.1007/978-3-319-75238-9_2

diagnostic and monitoring tool for MS. One of the hallmarks of MS on MRI is the appearance of hyper-intense lesions on T2-weighted MRI. T2 lesion volume has been used to assess "disease burden", to identify disease stage [10], and to aid in other MRI analysis such as healthy tissue segmentation and measurements of atrophy. Many automated techniques have been developed to accurately segment T2 lesion voxels in MRI [4, 11, 18, 22, 23]. This work has been focused on maximizing a global measure of segmentation accuracy (e.g. DICE), which prioritizes accuracy for large lesions over smaller lesions which are often dominant in MS.

For clinical trials, in addition to T2 lesion volume, a wider number of metrics are required to determine "burden of disease" and activity in order to measure treatment efficacy. These include: (1) The number and volume of T2 lesions in MRI, (2) the number of new and enlarging T2 lesions in longitudinal MRI, and (3) the number of gadolinium enhancing lesions, which is defined as the portion of lesions that enhance in T1w MRI after injection with a contrast agent, often associated with active inflammations. As accurate lesion counts are required, the problem is primarily one of lesion *detection* rather than traditional voxel-based segmentation. This is particularly challenging in the case of very small lesions (3–10 voxels) which are prevalent in MS.

Given the heterogeneity of clinical trial datasets, automated detection and segmentation are required to be accurate and robust across dozens or hundreds of different sites worldwide, across a range of scanners and field strengths, across different trials and robust to heterogeneity in patient demographics, disease stage and lesion burden. Finally, consistency over time is critical to precisely distinguish actual lesion changes from artifactual changes as well as from stable lesions. To meet these objectives, we present a series of fully-automatic, probabilistic machine learning frameworks to detect and segment all lesions in patient MRI. This includes: (1) an iterative, hierarchical graphical model (MRF) to detect and segment T2 lesions in MRI, (2) a Bayesian spatio-temporal model for the detection and segmentation of new and enlarging, as well as resolving, T2 lesions in longitudinal MRI, and (3) a temporal, hierarchical adaptive graphical model (CRF) for the automatic detection of gadolinium-enhancing lesions in MRI. The methods have been shown to be accurate and robust across large multi-center, multi-scanner clinical trial datasets, several of which have been placed into a commercial software analysis pipeline, where they have assisted in improving the efficiency and precision of the development of most new MS treatments worldwide.

Pharmaceutical companies conduct clinical trials to evaluate whether patients will respond to treatments by comparing population averages of biomarkers for MS activity across treatment arms. However, even if a trial fails to meet its clinical objectives, a subset of patients could potentially be responders to treatment. In this work, we describe a fully automatic, probabilistic framework for the prediction of future lesion activity in MS patients, based on a new Bag-of-Lesions (BoL) representation of baseline multi-modal MRI, and use it to identify potential responders to treatments.

The framework is trained and tested on a large, proprietary, multi-centre, multi-modal clinical trial dataset, where the automated identification of potential responders in two different treated treatment arms resulted in high sensitivities and specificities, leading to a promising approach towards personalized treatment for MS patients.

2   T2 Lesion Detection and Segmentation

In recent work [20], we describe a new iterative, multistage probabilistic graphical model for the automatic detection and segmentation of lesions, and healthy tissues, that encodes local, voxel-based information and regional context. Our model includes two levels of Markov Random Fields (MRFs). At the bottom level, an adapted voxel-based MRF identifies potential lesion voxels, as well as other tissue classes, using local and neighbourhood intensity and class priors. Contiguous voxels of a particular tissue type are then grouped into regions. A higher, non-lattice MRF is constructed, in which each node corresponds to a region. Edges between nodes are defined based on neighbourhood relationships between regions, where the effects of different surrounding tissues have been included in the edge weights by learning spatial tissue transition probabilities. The goal of the regional MRF is to examine the candidate lesions, and assess their plausibility probabilistically based on regional intensities, textures as well as neighbouring regions. The inferred information is then propagated to the voxel-level MRF. This process of iterative inference between the two levels then repeats as long as desired, working to suppress false positives and refine lesion boundaries. Figure 1 illustrates the framework. The method has been shown to be accurate and robust to variability when applied to real, multi-centre, multi-scanner clinical trial patient brain images, and generalizes well across trials. The method was trained on 1320 multi-channel MRI volumes at 1.5T and

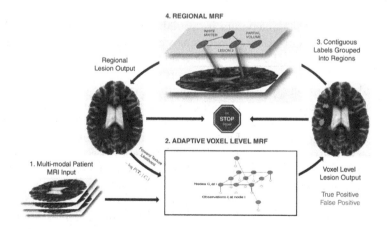

Fig. 1. Flowchart of the cross-sectional segmentation method [21].

208 volumes 3T, and tested on a different trial that included 535 volumes at 1.5T from 128 different centres and 62 volumes at 3T from 24 centres. When considering results on lesions of all sizes, the framework performed well overall with around 10% improvement over other methods. It significantly outperformed other approaches, however, in detecting small lesions, a result that is significant given that 40% of the lesions in the dataset were quite small (3–10 voxels). The performance of this method for the detection of small lesions is compared against other methods in Fig. 2.

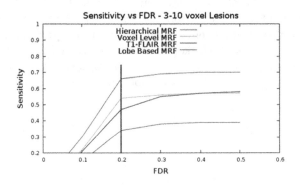

Fig. 2. Results of Hierarchical MRF classifier for detection of small lesions compared to other methods. An ROC-like curve of sensitivity vs. false detection ratio (FDR) shows that the hierarchical MRF outperforms competing methods. All methods were designed and tested in the operating range of 0.1–0.5 FDR, beyond which the detection metrics, which involve counting individual lesions becomes impossible because lesions begin to merge [21].

3   T2 Lesion Longitudinal Analysis

When scans from multiple timepoints are available for the same patient, it is desirable to detect changes in existing lesions as well detect the appearance of new T2 lesions over time. New T2 lesion counts and volume, as well as overall change in T2 lesion over time, are considered important surrogate markers of disease activity and progression [1]. A common paradigm used for detection of change in T2 lesions is that of subtraction imaging, which involves considering the difference image between two co-registered timepoints [16]. While subtraction imaging provides a more direct measure of change, many artifactual intensity differences will be observed, attributable to imperfect registration between scans, biological change not attributable to new lesions (such as atrophy), different manifestations of acquisition noise and distortion, as well as other imaging artifacts.

In recent work, we developed a method for automatic Bayesian spatio-temporal detection of new T2 lesions based on performing classification of both healthy and lesional tissue classes jointly across successive timepoints, where dependencies are modeled probabilistically across time (between co-registered voxels at reference and follow-up) as well as spatially [7,9]. The method favours temporally consistent classification, while remaining sensitive to real biological change, where intensity *differences* between reference and follow-up timepoints serve as indicators of change. Classification of both healthy tissue and lesion allows for differentiation of observed change due to biological change of interest (i.e. new lesion) and those arising from artifactual sources such as acquisition artifact or misregistration. Hierarchical classification is performed in two stages: (1) a voxelwise classification using generative Bayesian models and (2) a lesion-level classification using a random forest. The Bayesian model provides a classification of both healthy tissue and lesion based on local intensities, anatomical priors, and interactions between voxels in the same local spatial and temporal neighbourhood, while the lesion-level classification refines the detection of new lesions by taking into account lesion-level features and the larger anatomical context of new lesion candidates detected in the first voxel-level classification stage. This is depicted graphically in Fig. 3.

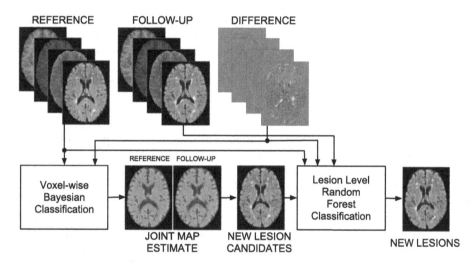

Fig. 3. Automatic detection of new MS lesions. Reference and difference images are input to the Joint Bayesian Classifier, while reference, follow-up and difference images are used for lesion-level classification using a random forest classifier. The image showing the final classification of new lesions shows candidates rejected by the lesion-level classification in blue (additionally shown with blue arrows) while those that are retained are shown in red [8]. (Color figure online)

The method for automatic detection of new T2 lesions was evaluated on a per-lesion basis by comparing to a rigorously created gold standard for new T2 lesions. The relative performance of the classifier as compared to a set of 9 manual raters who identified new T2 lesion using only the FLAIR images was also assessed. Even when considering only the FLAIR images as input, the method outperformed any single manual rater and had comparable performance to the consensus of the 9 raters. When all available MRI sequences (T1w, T2w, PDw, and FLAIR) were used as input, the method outperformed the consensus of the 9 manual raters by a wide margin. Results are summarized in Fig. 4 [8].

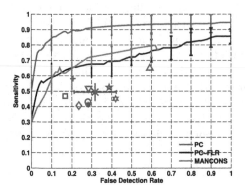

Fig. 4. PC = Proposed Classifier, PC-FLR = Proposed Classifier (FLAIR only), MAN-CONS = Consensus of expert raters. Each symbol represents an individual expert rater, while the X represents the mean expert rater. Individual points on the curve for PC and PC-FLR were generated by varying the random forest output threshold for acceptance as new lesion. Individual points on the MANCONS curve were generated by including increasing numbers of experts in the consensus [8].

The appearance of a new T2 lesion is generally followed by a period of repair or lesion *resolution*, during which time the lesion will shrink. Measuring the amount of lesion resolution may provide a marker of lesion repair and help identify lesion phenotypes that contribute differently to patient disability [17]. Our Bayesian method for automatic detection of lesion resolution embeds previous observations about the dynamics of lesion formation and resolution [17] as prior knowledge into a probabilistic Bayesian framework [9]. A generative model is used, where for all voxels that are lesion in the reference timepoint, *resolution status* is inferred at a follow-up timepoint, based on MRI intensities at the current timepoint and intensity differences between co-registered reference and follow-up timepoints. Additionally, the distance from lesion boundary is used to model a concentric pattern of resolution, and lesion size is used to model the increased relative rates of resolution of larger new lesions. Finally, the time from lesion peak (maximum lesion size during lesion formation) is considered, to model the fact that most resolution occurs soon after lesion onset.

Combining methods for automatic detection of new T2 lesions and automatic detection of resolving T2 lesions provides a direct and precise quantification of change in T2 lesion [7]. Direct quantification of lesion change was shown to provide a more consistent segmentation of T2 lesions over time. This added precision resulted in a more statistically powerful measure of lesion volume change as measured by ability to discriminate treatment arms in retrospective analysis

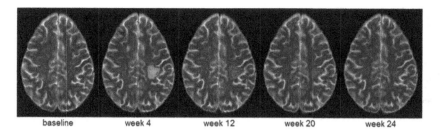

baseline   week 4   week 12   week 20   week 24

Fig. 5. Automatic 4-D segmentation of lesions. Lesion segmentation is categorized as stable (red), new (green) or resolving (blue) at each timepoint [7]. (Color figure online)

of clinical trial data [9]. Figure 5 shows an example of longitudinal segmentation of T2 lesion via direct quantification of change by explicit detection of new, resolving and stable lesions.

4 Gadolinium-Enhancing Lesion Detection and Segmentation

Gadolinium-enhancing lesions refer to the portion of lesion that are enhanced in T1w MRI after the administration of the contrast agent, and are associated with active inflammations. These lesions that take up the contrast agent provide an objective measure of disease activity at the time of the scan, which is a useful measure to evaluate new MS therapies. As a result, gadolinium-enhancing lesion frequency is routinely used in clinical trials to provide evidence of drug efficacy [19]. Gadolinium-enhancing lesion detection and segmentation is particularly challenging due their general small size and variability in location. Some gadolinium-enhancing lesions lack enough definition to be identified on the contrast image alone without comparison to a pre-contrast T1w image. Some are in the deep white matter while others are very close to the cortex. Furthermore, other healthy structures (e.g. blood vessels) enhance at similar intensities to the lesions. Intensity alone is insufficient to correctly distinguish gadolinium-enhancing lesions from other enhancements [14,15]. Examples of lesional and non-lesional enhancements are shown in Fig. 6.

We introduced a series of probabilistic multi-level Conditional Random Field (CRF) models for the automatic detection and segmentation of gadolinium-enhancing lesions in patient MRI. The Hierarchical Adaptive Texture Conditional Random Field (HAT-CRF) works by detecting candidate lesion voxels using a CRF-based classifier, where higher order cliques of sizes up to three are included to capture more complex interactions in the image. Once the candidate lesions are detected, higher order features modeling the texture of the lesion and surrounding tissue are calculated for the patches that contain the candidates. A higher level CRF model is designed by combining the higher order textures and voxel-wise interactions at candidate lesion voxels. The higher level is applied to the candidate lesions to remove falsely detected regions, and each

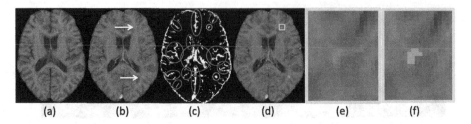

(a)   (b)   (c)   (d)   (e)   (f)

Fig. 6. An example of a brain MR image with MS gadolinium-enhancing lesions. (a) and (b) show the pre- and post-contrast T1w MR images. (c) shows voxels with sufficient enhancement to be considered enhancing lesion candidates. Based on common criteria for clinical trials, this binary mask includes voxels with 20% enhancement comparing T1w pre- and post-contrast images. True lesions shown in green while other non-lesional enhancements are shown with red. (d) shows the only two manually labeled active lesions marked in green. (e) and (f) show zoomed images of one of the enhanced lesions in the pink square in (d) without and with manual labels respectively. Note the small size and low contrast of the lesion [12].

iteration adapts to the new size and shape of candidate lesions modeled by the lower level. The Temporal Hierarchical Adaptive Texture Conditional Random Field (THAT-CRF) [13] extended the framework to include image information from a prior timepoint when available, and included differences in image intensities and features across the time points. An overview of the THAT-CRF method is shown in Fig. 7. The THAT-CRF was further tuned with optimal multi-scale textures and various optimization strategies to produce the Adaptive

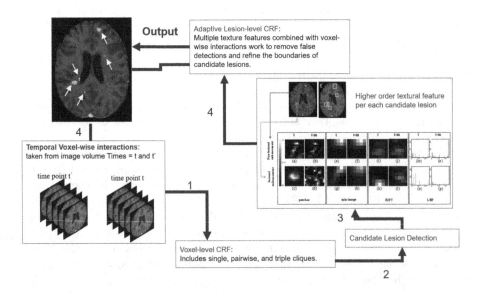

Fig. 7. THAT-CRF framework overview [12]

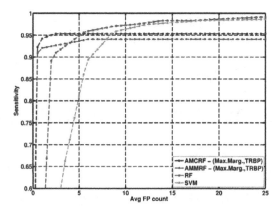

Fig. 8. Performance of the AMCRF model in terms of sensitivity vs. average false positive counts per scan. Comparing the performance of the AMCRF model to Adaptive Multi-level Markov Random Field (AMMRF), Random Forest (RF) and Support Vector Machine (SVM). AMMRF is similar to AMCRF except that the Ising model is adapted for the pairwise interactions. Maximum margin learning together with Tree-weighted belief propagation (Max.Marg, TRBP) are used for both AMCRF and AMMRF [12].

Multi-level Conditional Random Field (AMCRF) [12]. The AMCRF model was trained on a large multi-modal clinical trial dataset consisting of MRI from 1760 subjects acquired at 180 sites. Figure 8 shows results of experiments on an entirely separate clinical trial consisting of 120 subjects' MRI from 24 sites, where the AMCRF outperformed other methods, including a Random Forest (RF) and Support Vector Machine (SVM). At the target sensitivity of 90%, average false positive counts per scan ranged from 0.17 to 0 for very small lesions (3–5 voxels) to very large ones (over 50 voxels). Results on a second independent large trial consisting of 2770 patients led to a sensitivity of 91% for average false positive counts of 0.46.

5   Predicting Future Disease Activity and Potential Responders to Treatment

Although several methods have been proposed to predict the conversion of patients with preliminary symptoms to MS [2,3,24], predicting future lesion activity from current MS patient images could lead to a better understanding of the disease, as well as prediction of treatment efficacy. Automatic prediction is a challenge because of the wide variety in lesion presentation and the unknown effect of lesion characteristics on the course of the disease. In recent work, we developed the first fully automatic, probabilistic machine learning framework to model the variability of lesions in multi-modal MRI of patients with RRMS with the objectives of: (1) automatic identification of lesion types across the population, (2) probabilistic prediction of new lesion activity in patients two

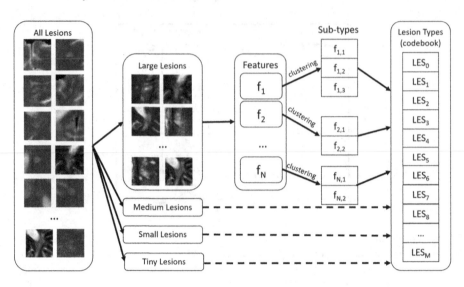

Fig. 9. Learning the Bag of Lesions. Lesions are first separated by size. Features (e.g. RIFT) are extracted from each lesion. Each feature is modelled as a separate GMM, with each component referred to as a feature-type. Each lesion codeword is the combination of sub-types of each feature being modeled [6].

years in the future based only on baseline multi-modal MRI and (3) automatic identification of responders to treatment using lesion activity prediction learned for untreated and treated groups [6]. Based on the success of the Bag-of-Words model in performing unsupervised categorization in computer vision, we develop a new unsupervised Bag-of-Lesions (BoL) model for brain image representation in the context of MS, patient images based on a variety of image-based features extracted from lesions, including lesion intensity, shape, texture and probabilistic tissue context. A probabilistic codebook of lesion types is created by clustering features using Gaussian mixture models (GMM). An overview of the method can be seen in Fig. 9, with examples of lesions drawn randomly from different automatically-learned lesion-types in Fig. 10. Patients are represented as a probabilistic histogram of lesion-types, permitting the automatic unsupervised grouping of images through histogram clustering. A supervised classifier can be trained to predict the probability of future MS lesion activity based on patients' Bag of Lesions representation at baseline. A backwards elimination method is used to select the most informative lesion types [5].

Ground truth information regarding which patients in a treatment group have definitively responded to treatment is rarely available. In this work, activity prediction models are learned for untreated and treated populations separately. Patients in the treated groups are labelled as *responders* if they are predicted, with high confidence, to have new or enlarging lesions two years from baseline if left untreated (on placebo), but instead have no lesion activity two years later. A new patient is considered to be a potential responder to treatment if the baseline

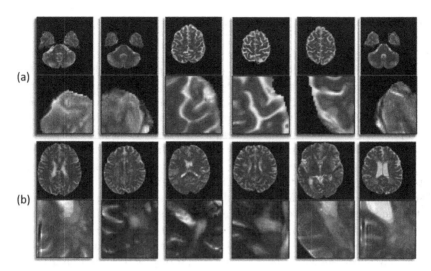

Fig. 10. Examples of lesions from two lesion types in different patients. (a) Small cortical lesions. (b) Large peri-ventricular lesions. Top: Lesions (red) over T2w images. Bottom: Zoomed in. (Color figure online)

images indicate a high probability of future activity using the "untreated" model, and low probability using the "treated" model. The probability thresholds are set very high, essentially stating that the two models disagree with high confidence.

Experiments were performed on a large multi-centre, multi-scanner clinical trial dataset comprised of RRMS patients with three treatment arms: 259 Untreated (placebo), 280 Drug A, 259 Drug B. Lesion labels were extracted semi-manually. The trial did not achieve its primary endpoint due to insufficient evidence of effectiveness across the entire cohort, but there was a clear trend towards a treatment response for some patients in the trial. A 50-fold cross-validation experiment comparing a variety of automatic classifiers and distance metrics showed that random forests outperformed other models when estimating deterministic activity outcomes. When a probability threshold of 0.8 was chosen, 25 responders to Drug A and 24 responders to Drug B were identified. Table 1 illustrates the automated responder prediction results for the two different treated groups of patients, showing sensitivities of 92% and 94% and specificities of 82% and 84% respectively. This indicates the promise of the approach towards personalized treatment for MS patients.

Table 1. Potential responder prediction results for treatments A & B, with probability thresholds 0.8.

	Sensitivity	Specificity
Drug A	92%	82%
Drug B	94%	84%

6   Conclusion

In this paper, we describe a series of probabilistic machine learning frameworks designed for the specific requirements of clinical trial analysis for new treatments of MS. The methods are optimized to achieve high accuracy for a series of clinically-derived measures of disease burden and activity in order to determine treatment efficacy. In this context, accurate lesion-level *detection* is shown to be more important than voxel-based segmentation, as all lesions must be accurately counted - even small ones as they are prevalent in trials - and as the delineation of lesion boundaries has been found to be unreliable and unstable. We therefore presented: (1) an iterative, hierarchical graphical model (MRF) to detect and segment T2 lesions in MRI, (2) a Bayesian spatio-temporal model for the detection and segmentation of new and enlarging, as well as resolving, T2 lesions in longitudinal MRI, and (3) a temporal, hierarchical adaptive graphical model (CRF) for the automatic detection of gadolinium-enhancing lesions in MRI. The methods have been shown to be accurate and robust across large multi-center, multi-scanner clinical trial datasets. As a result, several of the segmentation and detection algorithms presented have been integrated into the commercial software analysis pipeline of our industrial collaborator to further automate the analysis of treatment efficacy for new drugs under development, leading to an estimated 5X speed and monetary savings for the company, speeding up the evaluation of new drugs and reducing the time to market. Most new MS treatments developed in recent years have benefited or are benefiting from the improved efficiency and precision of these measurements.

We then present the first, fully automatic, probabilistic framework for the prediction of future lesion activity in MS patients, based on a new Bag-of-Lesions (BoL) representation of baseline multi-modal MRI. Activity prediction is then used to automatically identify potential responders to two treatments in the context of a multi-centre, multi-scanner clinical trial for MS patients, showing sensitivities of 92% and 94% and specificities of 82% and 84% respectively. This suggests the possibility of a tool for personalized treatment for new MS patients, and for assessing treatment efficacy.

Acknowledgements. This work was supported by a Canadian Natural Science and Engineering Research Council collaborative Research and Development Grant (CRDPJ 411455-10), and an International Progressive MS Alliance Collaborative Network Award (PA-1603-08175).

References

1. Bakshi, R., et al.: MRI in Multiple Sclerosis: current status and future prospects. Lancet Neurol. **7**(7), 615–625 (2008)
2. Barkhof, F., et al.: Comparison of MRI criteria at first presentation to predict conversion to clinically definite Multiple Sclerosis. Brain **120**(11), 2059–2069 (1997)

3. Brosch, T., Yoo, Y., Li, D.K.B., Traboulsee, A., Tam, R.: Modeling the variability in brain morphology and lesion distribution in multiple sclerosis by deep learning. In: Golland, P., Hata, N., Barillot, C., Hornegger, J., Howe, R. (eds.) MICCAI 2014. LNCS, vol. 8674, pp. 462–469. Springer, Cham (2014). https://doi.org/10.1007/978-3-319-10470-6_58

4. Cabezas, M., et al.: A review of atlas-based segmentation for magnetic resonance brain images. Comput. Methods Programs Biomed. **104**(3), e158–177 (2011)

5. Díaz-Uriarte, R., De Andres, S.A.: Gene selection and classification of microarray data using random forest. BMC Bioinform. **7**(1), 3 (2006)

6. Doyle, A., Precup, D., Arnold, D.L., Arbel, T.: Predicting future disease activity and treatment responders for multiple sclerosis patients using a bag-of-lesions brain representation. In: Descoteaux, M., Maier-Hein, L., Franz, A., Jannin, P., Collins, D.L., Duchesne, S. (eds.) MICCAI 2017. LNCS, vol. 10435, pp. 186–194. Springer, Cham (2017). https://doi.org/10.1007/978-3-319-66179-7_22

7. Elliott, C.: A Bayesian framework for 4-D segmentation of Multiple Sclerosis lesions in serial MRI in the brain. Ph.D. thesis, McGill University Libraries (2016)

8. Elliott, C., et al.: Temporally consistent probabilistic detection of new Multiple Sclerosis lesions in brain MRI. IEEE TMI **32**(8), 1490–1503 (2013)

9. Elliott, C., et al.: A generative model for automatic detection of resolving Multiple Sclerosis lesions. In: BAMBI (2014)

10. Filippi, M., et al.: Association between pathological and MRI findings in Multiple Sclerosis. Lancet Neurol. **11**(4), 349–360 (2012)

11. Fischl, B., et al.: Whole brain segmentation: automated labeling of neuroanatomical structures in the human brain. Neuron **33**(3), 341–355 (2002)

12. Karimaghaloo, Z., et al.: Adaptive multi-level conditional random fields for detection and segmentation of small enhanced pathology in medical images. MIA **27**, 17–30 (2016)

13. Karimaghaloo, Z., et al.: Temporal hierarchical adaptive texture CRF for automatic detection of gadolinium-enhancing Multiple Sclerosis lesions in brain MRI. IEEE TMI **34**(6), 1227–1241 (2015)

14. Karimaghaloo, Z., Shah, M., Francis, S.J., Arnold, D.L., Collins, D.L., Arbel, T.: Detection of gad-enhancing lesions in multiple sclerosis using conditional random fields. In: Jiang, T., Navab, N., Pluim, J.P.W., Viergever, M.A. (eds.) MICCAI 2010. LNCS, vol. 6363, pp. 41–48. Springer, Heidelberg (2010). https://doi.org/10.1007/978-3-642-15711-0_6

15. Karimaghaloo, Z., et al.: Automatic detection of gadolinium-enhancing Multiple Sclerosis lesions in brain MRI using conditional random fields. IEEE TMI **31**(6), 1181–1194 (2012)

16. Lee, M., et al.: Defining Multiple Sclerosis disease activity using MRI T2-weighted difference imaging. Brain **121**(11), 2095–2102 (1998)

17. Meier, D., et al.: MR imaging intensity modeling of damage and repair in Multiple Sclerosis: relationship of short-term lesion recovery to progression and disability. Am. J. Neuroradiol. **28**(10), 1956–1963 (2007)

18. Milletari, F., et al.: V-Net: fully convolutional neural networks for volumetric medical image segmentation. In: 3D Vision, pp. 565–571. IEEE (2016)

19. Sormani, M.P., et al.: Magnetic resonance active lesions as individual-level surrogate for relapses in Multiple Sclerosis. Mult. Scler. J. **17**(5), 541–549 (2011)

20. Subbanna, N., Precup, D., Arnold, D., Arbel, T.: IMaGe: iterative multilevel probabilistic graphical model for detection and segmentation of Multiple Sclerosis lesions in Brain MRI. In: Ourselin, S., Alexander, D.C., Westin, C.-F., Cardoso, M.J. (eds.) IPMI 2015. LNCS, vol. 9123, pp. 514–526. Springer, Cham (2015). https://doi.org/10.1007/978-3-319-19992-4_40

21. Subbanna, N.: Iterative Multilevel Probabilistic Graphical Model for Detection and Segmentation of Tumours and Lesions in Brain MRI. Ph.D. thesis, McGill University (2016)

22. Wang, H., et al.: Multi-atlas segmentation with joint label fusion. IEEE TPAMI **35**(3), 611–623 (2013)

23. Warfield, S.K., et al.: Adaptive, template moderated, spatially varying statistical classification. MIA **4**(1), 43–55 (2000)

24. Yoo, Y., Tang, L.W., Brosch, T., Li, D.K.B., Metz, L., Traboulsee, A., Tam, R.: Deep learning of brain lesion patterns for predicting future disease activity in patients with early symptoms of multiple sclerosis. In: Carneiro, G., et al. (eds.) LABELS/DLMIA -2016. LNCS, vol. 10008, pp. 86–94. Springer, Cham (2016). https://doi.org/10.1007/978-3-319-46976-8_10

Brain Lesion Image Analysis

Automated Segmentation of Multiple Sclerosis Lesions Using Multi-dimensional Gated Recurrent Units

Simon Andermatt$^{(\boxtimes)}$, Simon Pezold, and Philippe C. Cattin

Department of Biomedical Engineering, University of Basel, Allschwil, Switzerland
simon.andermatt@unibas.ch

Abstract. We analyze the performance of multi-dimensional gated recurrent units on automated lesion segmentation in multiple sclerosis. The segmentation of these pathologic structures is not trivial, since location, shape and size can be arbitrary. Furthermore, the inherent class imbalance of about 1 lesion voxel to 10 000 healthy voxels further exacerbates the correct segmentation. We introduce a new MD-GRU setup, using established techniques from the deep learning community as well as our own adaptations. We evaluate these modifications by comparing them to a standard MD-GRU network. We demonstrate that using data augmentation, selective sampling, residual learning and/or DropConnect on the RNN state can produce better segmentation results. Reaching rank #1 in the ISBI 2015 longitudinal multiple sclerosis lesion segmentation challenge, we show that a setup which combines these techniques can outperform the state of the art in automated lesion segmentation.

Keywords: MD-GRU · MDGRU · Automatic MS lesion segmentation

1 Introduction

Multiple sclerosis (MS) is a frequent disease of the central nervous system, which prevalently occurs in young adults, especially in women. The evaluation of lesions in the brain is part of the clinical diagnostic procedure and is important when evaluating medical trials for new treatments. The manual segmentation of lesions, especially on high-resolution 3d scans, is very time consuming as well as prone to errors due to inter- and intra-rater variability [5]. Recently, recurrent neural networks (RNN) have shown the capability to match the state of the art in brain segmentation. In the brain segmentation benchmark used in [1,10], three of the top six methods are based on RNN. Not only their performance, but also the elegant way of describing data with tied weights do speak for them, since fewer parameters have to be used for the model. We take a closer look at the multi-dimensional gated recurrent unit (MD-GRU) [1] due to its high ranking on the MRBrains challenge. Lesions, as any pathology, are hard to model. We hence treat lesion segmentation independently from anatomy segmentation and

© Springer International Publishing AG, part of Springer Nature 2018
A. Crimi et al. (Eds.): BrainLes 2017, LNCS 10670, pp. 31–42, 2018.
https://doi.org/10.1007/978-3-319-75238-9_3

consider to reevaluate some findings in [1, 10] in the context of lesion segmentation. In the following, we explore different extensions to the MD-GRU with the focus on improvements on lesion segmentation. We investigate some design choices made in the original publication of the MD-GRU [1] and apply emerging deep learning techniques which proved to be effective. We investigate our adaptations on the training data of a publicly available challenge dataset. We then use the best performing combination of our modifications and apply it on the full dataset. Our implementation can be found at https://github.com/zubata88/mdgru.

2   Materials and Methods

2.1   Longitudinal MS Lesion Segmentation Challenge (ISBI 2015)

The longitudinal MS lesion segmentation challenge [2] was held in conjunction with ISBI 2015, but the data and challenge is still available online for further use. The data consists of 5 training patients and 15 test patients, with 4 to 6 screenings each, consisting of an MPRAGE, a T2, a PD and a FLAIR sequence. In all of our experiments, we only incorporate the provided preprocessed MR data and their high-pass filtered counterparts (see Sect. 2.3), as shown in Fig. 1. The remaining screenings for the first patient in the training data are shown in Fig. 2. For the training data, each screening of each patient holds two segmentation masks. Segmentation masks for the test data are not available, but binary predictions can be evaluated automatically on the challenge website.

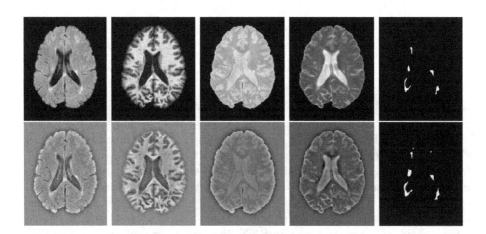

Fig. 1. Slice 90 of the baseline scan of the first training sample. *Top row (left to right):* FLAIR, MPRAGE, PD, T2 scan and label mask of rater 1. *Bottom row:* respective high-pass filtered versions and label mask of rater 2.

2.2   Original MD-GRU Setup

In the following, we define the peculiarities of MD-GRU [1] that are relevant for the evaluation of our modifications to the model. Equation (1) denotes channel j of output H, which consists of the sum of all outputs of the $N \cdot D$ individual convolutional gated recurrent units (C-GRUs) it is made of. Each C-GRU computes the data along either the forward or backward direction n of dimension d:

$$H^j(x) = \sum_{n \in \{1,-1\}} \sum_d^D h^{j,n,d}. \tag{1}$$

The following are the original C-GRU equations [1]. Index t denotes the timestep and iterates over the slices along d in direction n. Since the computations of each C-GRU are independent, we omit the indices for n, d for better readability in the following:

$$r^j = \sigma \left(\sum_i^I (x^i * w_r^{i,j}) + \sum_k^J (h_{t-1}^k * u_r^{k,j}) + b_r^j \right), \tag{2}$$

$$z^j = \sigma \left(\sum_i^I (x^i * w_z^{i,j}) + \sum_k^J (h_{t-1}^k * u_z^{k,j}) + b_z^j \right), \tag{3}$$

$$\tilde{h}_t^j = \phi \left(\sum_i^I (x^i * w^{i,j}) + r^j \odot \sum_k^J (h_{t-1}^k * u^{k,j}) + b^j \right), \tag{4}$$

$$h_t^j = z^j \odot h_{t-1}^j + (1 - z^j) \odot \tilde{h}_t^j. \tag{5}$$

The indices i and j, k denote the respective input and output channels. Variables u, w and b are trainable weights. We refer to Eqs. (2) and (3) as *reset* and *update gate*, Eq. (4) as *proposal* and Eq. (5) as *output* or *state*.

To analyze the influence of different adjustments, we will use a standard network, similar to the one published in [1]. It consists of 3 layers of MD-GRUs of 16, 32 and 64 channels, which are connected with voxelwise fully connected layers with biases consisting of 25 and 45 channels followed by a tanh activation function. The last MD-GRU is connected to a voxelwise fully connected layer of c channels, one for each class. Finally, a softmax layer is applied and the network is trained minimizing the negative log likelihood. Equation (6) summarizes the setup, where superscript numbers denote the number of channels at each layer and subscripts enumerate the independent layers of the same type:

$$h = \text{softMax}(\text{conv111}_3^c(H_3^{64}(\tanh(\text{conv111}_2^{45}(H_2^{32}(\tanh(\text{conv111}_1^{25}(H_1^{16}(x))))))))). \tag{6}$$

2.3   Evaluated Design Choices

The MD-GRU showed promising results with a relatively simple architecture. In the following we motivate and evaluate modifications to the original architecture.

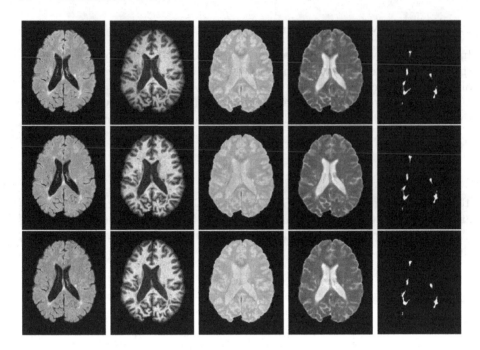

Fig. 2. Slice 90 of each followup scan of first training sample. *From left to right:* FLAIR, MPRAGE, PD, T2 scan and combined rater mask.

High-Pass Filtering. A high-pass filter was applied to the images by subtracting a Gaussian filtered version of the image volumes from the original volumes. Especially in situations with almost piecewise constant functions, such as MR images of the brain, this preprocessing step can help "announcing" a change of tissue before it actually happens, as can be seen for instance around the masked brains in Fig. 1. In Fig. 3, we inspect the voxel values along one anteroposterior line through the volume. In our experiments, we investigate, how much high-pass filtered data can help detract the influence of low frequency intensity changes in the data.

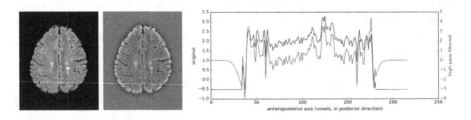

Fig. 3. Impact of high-pass filtering on the fourth screening of the sixth training sample. *Left:* Slice 110 of original and high-pass filtered FLAIR scan. *Right:* Plot of marked red and blue lines on the left for both images after normalization. (Color figure online)

Reset Gate Location. Compared to the original formulation of the GRU [3], the C-GRU applies the reset gate at a slightly different position, as depicted in Fig. 4a. In the GRU, the reset gate r is directly multiplied to the previous output h_{t-1}:

$$\tilde{h}_t^j = \phi([Wx]^j + [U(r \odot h_{t-1})]^j) \tag{7}$$

In the C-GRU however, it is multiplied to the result of the convolution of the previous output h_{t-1} with u, as shown in Eq. (4).

The provided motive for this decision is, that r is the result of convolutions and already contains information of its neighbors. This effectively means that the reset gate of channel j only directly affects the proposal of channel j instead of all proposals. We evaluate this decision by comparing to a modified C-GRU, which more closely follows the original formulation:

$$\hat{\tilde{h}}_t^j = \phi\left(\sum_i^I (x^i * w^{i,j}) + \sum_k^J ((r^{k,j} \odot h_{t-1}^k) * u^{k,j}) + b^j\right). \tag{8}$$

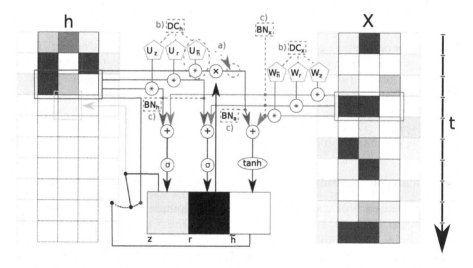

Fig. 4. Schematic and computational graph of a C-GRU with one-dimensional filters. *The proposed changes are marked with dashed red lines:* (a) the order of the reset gate application, (b) DropConnect at state and input weights and (c) batch normalization at input, gate states and proposal activation states. (Color figure online)

Contribution Weights for Individual C-GRU Outputs. In the original MD-GRU formulation, the individual C-GRU outputs are simply summed to gather the result H. As already implemented in the first bidirectional RNN [9], the states for each direction could be weighted independently, resulting in a

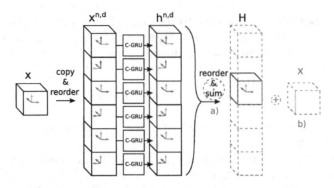

Fig. 5. Composition of an MD-GRU. *The proposed changes are marked with dashed red lines:* (a) leaving out the sum of the individual directional states or (b) adding residual learning at the MD-GRU level. (Color figure online)

more complex model. We investigate the potential benefit of concatenating the C-GRU outputs, thereby in our case of 3d volumes increasing the number of output channels sixfold. Figure 5a shows this on the example of MD-GRUs that handle volumetric data.

DropConnect. Instead of dropout, a similar method called DropConnect (DC) [11] is used at a constant rate of 0.5, which drops weights instead of outputs. In the original formulation [1], we decided to implement DC on the input weights in MD-GRU and to use a fixed drop rate of 0.5. Dropout has been reported to not work well on MD-LSTM [10] and applying it on the state in RNN has been advised against [12]. We analyze the effect of applying DC on input, state or both using different drop rates (Fig. 4b).

2.4   Techniques to Improve Accuracy and Shorten Training Time

Batch/Instance Normalization. The first technique we investigate is batch normalization (BN) [7]. BN allows for higher learning rates and faster convergence, thereby drastically reducing the training time. By normalizing the input to activations, the so-called covariate shift is reduced. This enables a layer further down the network to learn more independently from the layers before it. We build on the results on BN in one-dimensional RNN in [4] and define BN as

$$BN(x, \gamma) = \gamma \frac{x - \hat{\mu}}{\sqrt{\hat{\sigma} + \epsilon}} + \beta, \tag{9}$$

where we set β to 0 at any place, due to the biases that are already in place [4]. Due to our inherent mini-batch of one (we can only process one subvolume at a time per training iteration), we calculate the statistics for mean $\hat{\mu}$ and standard deviation $\hat{\sigma}$ on the whole data per channel. Since the data in the subvolumes

is heavily correlated, we calculate our training statistics for each training itera-
tion k from the m most recent training samples with $\hat{\mu}^{(k)} = \frac{1}{m}\sum_{q=k-m+1}^{k}\mu^{(q)}$
and $\hat{\sigma}^{(k)} = \frac{1}{m}\sum_{q=k-m+1}^{k}\sigma^{(q)}$. We keep a separate exponential moving average
for both mean and standard deviation over all training samples to be used for
testing. We apply the following BN:

$$r^j = \sigma(BN_x(\sum_i^I(x^i * w_r^{i,j}), \gamma_x) + BN_h(\sum_k^J(h_{t-1}^k * u_r^{k,j}), \gamma_h) + b_r^j), \quad (10)$$

$$z^j = \sigma(BN_x(\sum_i^I(x^i * w_z^{i,j}), \gamma_x) + BN_h(\sum_k^J(h_{t-1}^k * u_z^{k,j}), \gamma_h) + b_z^j), \quad (11)$$

$$\tilde{h}_t^j = \phi(BN_x(\sum_i^I(x^i * w^{i,j}), \gamma_x) + BN_a(r^j \odot \sum_k^J(h_{t-1}^k * u^{k,j}), \gamma_a) + b^j), \quad (12)$$

where we keep individual statistics for the input convolutions, the gate state convolutions and the state convolution of the proposal. Figure 4c shows the different
locations we apply BN at.

Residual Learning. Using skip connections allowed ResNet [6] to ascend on
top of a number of ILSVRC & COCO 2015 competitions, as it reportedly allows
for deeper networks and faster convergence. We introduce skip connections linking input and output of each MD-GRU (Fig. 5b), allowing the network to choose
between learning a residual or ignoring the previous input. We evaluate the
following adjustment in between individual MD-GRU layers:

$$H_{res}(x) = \overset{c}{\text{conv}111}(x) + \overset{c}{H}(x), \quad (13)$$

where c denotes the number of output channels of H and the additional convolution increases the input channels to c. We refrain from applying additional

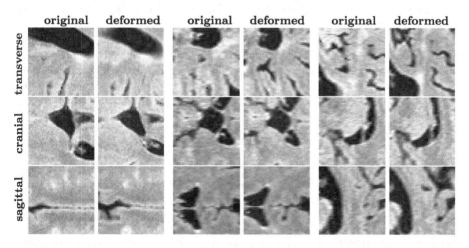

Fig. 6. Examples of random deformations performed on 48^3 subvolumes. *Rows:* transverse, coronal and sagittal planes of the original *(left)* and deformed *(right)* sample.
Columns: individual random samples.

residual learning inside the MD-GRU, as it has been shown that residual networks with shared weights can be reformulated as plain RNN [8].

Data Augmentation. Data augmentation can have beneficial effects on networks which are trained with little data [1]. On a low resolution grid of spacing f voxels, we draw three values from a normal distribution $\mathcal{N}(0, 5)$. Using cubic interpolation, we create a smooth deformation field, which we apply on the voxelwise sampling of the subvolumes used for training (Fig. 6).

3   Experiments and Results

We train each model for 3000 iterations, which will not produce competitive results, but should give an indicator of how much an adjustment affects the method. We only included the first 4 baseline scans during training and evaluate all combinations on the baseline scan of the 5th training patient. Using only 4 samples, we remove any redundancy in the data and decrease the search space, allowing for faster convergence. For all experiments, we train on 48^3 random samples and create a full volume during the test phase by stitching patches of 32^3 with a padding of 8 together .

Data Sampling Techniques and MD-GRU Design Evaluation. We considered the following different data sampling techniques. To quantify the impact of the high-pass filtered data, we trained networks with only the original data, only the high-pass filtered data and both. We further analyzed the impact of data augmentation through random deformation, varying the size f of the deformations. We evaluate the impact of forcing every second random training sample to contain lesions (selective sampling). We also evaluate potentially not summing the individual C-GRU results and the misplacement of the reset gate as defined in Eq. (12). The respective results are listed in Table 1A.

Table 1. Summary of the different combinations which were trained on the first four and evaluated on the fifth training sample of the ISBI challenge data. Dice coefficients are provided in percent and bold face denotes results that were better than those of the baseline architecture (A, top row). The two provided masks we compare ourselves to are denoted as M1 and M2.

A	Dice		B	Dice		C		Dice		
	M1	M2		M1	M2			M1		M2
Baseline [1]	38.18	37.70	DC(0.5,h,x)	29.39	26.35		m=16	m=1	m=16	m=1
Only original	0.00	0.00	DC(0.5,h)	**44.06**	**41.55**	BNx	31.77	30.58	26.60	24.94
Only filtered	28.30	25.65	No DC	27.85	23.54	BNx+DC(x)	37.53	20.92	32.19	18.45
Def($f = 24$)	**43.74**	36.94	DC(0.75,x)	21.27	17.24	BNh	31.78	29.42	30.03	31.98
Def($f = 48$)	**48.43**	**49.12**	DC(0.75,x,h)	15.79	13.63	BNh+DC(x)	28.95	30.13	26.03	27.74
			DC(0.75,h)	23.27	20.13					
Selective samples	**44.95**	**40.70**	DC(0.875,x)	21.82	19.33	BNa	3.05	3.04	2.50	2.49
No MD-GRU sum	17.79	15.39	DC(0.875,h)	19.87	17.29	BNa+DC(x)	9.70	10.20	8.59	9.02
Misplaced r	24.75	21.20	RL	**41.51**	35.71					

Table 2. Mean and standard deviation of the crossvalidation with the Dice coefficient in percent, the Hausdorff distance (HD) as well as the average volume distance (AVD) with best scores and lowest standard deviations in bold face.

	Dice		HD		AVD	
	M1	M2	M1	M2	M1	M2
Baseline [1]	20.03 ± 14.13	19.86 ± 13.17	39.82 ± 7.62	39.15 ± 6.69	7.34 ± 7.89	6.79 ± 6.52
DC(h)	33.47 ± 8.57	32.93 ± 8.82	35.84 ± 5.87	$36.64 \pm \mathbf{4.40}$	5.78 ± 6.16	5.64 ± 5.58
Residual learning	35.95 ± 13.78	35.10 ± 10.19	40.61 ± 9.45	36.29 ± 6.65	7.27 ± 6.90	6.61 ± 5.48
Selective sampling	$44.10 \pm \mathbf{4.55}$	$40.54 \pm \mathbf{4.64}$	$41.32 \pm \mathbf{3.15}$	40.31 ± 4.57	5.07 ± 5.42	4.87 ± 4.75
Def ($f = 48$)	38.29 ± 21.51	34.70 ± 19.82	37.27 ± 8.89	38.57 ± 8.09	2.91 ± 3.35	2.64 ± 2.43
All of the above	$\mathbf{62.85} \pm 15.31$	$\mathbf{55.24} \pm 13.66$	$\mathbf{32.60} \pm 8.58$	$\mathbf{29.82} \pm 4.72$	$\mathbf{1.83} \pm \mathbf{1.22}$	$\mathbf{2.18} \pm \mathbf{1.73}$

DropConnect, Batch Normalization and Residual Learning. Since both DC and BN act as regularization, we evaluated them both jointly and individually. In Table 1B, we list Dice coefficients obtained using different DC settings on input x and/or state h with the designated drop rate. At the bottom, we list the result obtained by applying residual learning (RL) in between MD-GRU layers. In Table 1C, the Dice coefficients resulting from different BNs both with and without simultaneous DC with a drop rate of 0.5 on the input are shown.

Putting it All Together. In a last experiment, we performed leave-one-out crossvalidation with the modifications which performed better than the standard network (Table 1) and the sum of those modifications. Using the Dice as performance measure, the selected techniques were random deformation with a grid spacing of 48, selective sampling, residual learning and DC on the state instead of the input. The crossvalidation results can be found in Table 2.

3.1   Improved Network

So far, we restricted ourselves to a subset of the data and only 3 000 training iterations. For the final evaluation on the challenge website, we considered the complete training data, instead of just using the first scan of each patient. We decided to use a combination of data augmentation through random deformation ($f = 75$) and subvolumes of 80^3 together with DC on the state h, residual learning and selective sampling. We merged rater masks by creating 4 classes, one for each label combination during training and assumed a lesion voxel during inference, when its probability for background was below 0.5. We trained the network for 10 000 iterations and managed to achieve first place in the ISBI challenge. Figure 7 shows slice 80 of the best and worst segmentation, judging from the challenge score computed on both raters. The first five entries of the challenge are listed in Table 3 with the mean of each metric that contributes to the challenge score. The fifth entry was created using the MD-GRU as described in its original publication [1] and 40 000 training iterations. Unfortunately, none of the other competing entries have been published yet, which makes a comparison of the methods impossible.

Table 3. The five best scoring methods of the longitudinal MS lesion segmentation challenge with challenge score, volume correlation (VC), Dice coefficient, positive predictive value (PPV), lesion false positive rate (LFPR), lesion true positive rate (LTPR). Dice, PPV, LFPR and LTPR are denoted in percent and best values out of five are printed in bold. In brackets we denote the relative weight of each metric on the final score.

	Score	VC ($^1/_4$)	Dice ($^1/_8$)	PPV ($^1/_8$)	LFPR ($^1/_4$)	LTPR ($^1/_4$)
asmsl (proposed)	**92.076**	0.862	62.98	**84.46**	20.13	48.71
nic_vicorob_test	91.440	0.840	64.29	79.25	15.46	38.72
VIC_TF_FULL	91.331	0.866	63.05	78.67	**15.29**	36.40
MIPLAB_v3	91.267	0.823	62.74	79.97	23.17	45.40
miac_results [1]	91.011	**0.867**	**66.78**	74.05	40.73	**58.29**

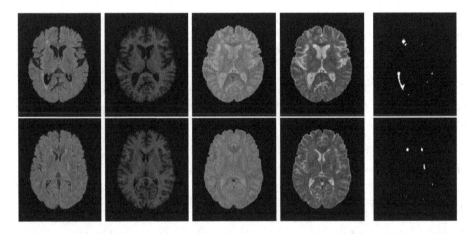

Fig. 7. Main challenge results. *Columns, left to right:* FLAIR, MPRAGE, PD and T2 scan together with the computed segmentation at Slice 80. *Rows:* best *(top)* and worst *(bottom)* segmentation (baseline scan of patient 4 and 7 respectively), with respect to the challenge score computed on both raters' segmentations.

4   Discussion

We encountered expected as well as odd behavior in our exploratory study. Contrary to what has been advised for in the literature [12], dropping information from the state weights results in better regularization, as the Dice coefficients in Table 1B indicate. This behavior could be due to the fact that we only ignore part of the previous state per iteration and channel. Interestingly though, a combination of DC on both input and state produces worse results, even with a reduced drop rate. As dropout tends to prolong training, further experiments with longer training times might shed light on this effect. Another surprising result is the inability of BN to surpass baseline Dice scores in our preliminary tests in Table 1, in all variations we tested. Due to the correlation in our mini-batch of one and the varying weights in the case of the running average, the assumption does not hold that the statistics of our mini-batch are similar to the global statistics. Residual learning between MD-GRU layers seems to contribute to the overall improvement. Surprisingly, neither concatenating the C-GRU nor placing the reset gate as in the original GRU did result in an improved Dice.

The high pass filtering as preprocessing step proved to be fruitful, especially in the setting where we only trained for 3000 iterations, where leaving it out resulted in no segmentation at all. Using only original data, a visible tendency towards lesions could be found, but with probabilities well below 0.5. The main reason why this step is so important can be seen in Fig. 3, where values of the filtered image lie mostly around zero and in the original scan around two. All the weights of our network are initialized to handle data from a standard normal distribution. Inside the brain, filtering the original image would result in sums far away from zero. Using a hyperbolic tangent or sigmoid function on such a result will return a value close to 1 and hence a very flat gradient, which will not be able to help adjust the weights to correct for this in a fast manner.

Selective sampling and random deformation succeeded to be the most important improvements, which is easily explainable with the huge class imbalance present in our data and the low amount of training data. As the crossvalidation shows, all of the selected techniques resulted in overall better scores except for the HD in selective sampling, which is likely due to a higher probability of producing outliers when oversampling the lesion class.

By achieving rank 1 in the actual challenge, we show that our proposed method is at the state of the art. Unfortunately, none of the listed results in Table 3 have been published yet, as already mentioned. The highest Dice score in the top 5 was achieved using exactly the same MD-GRU network as in its original publication [1] and training it for 40 000 iterations. Since we only trained our network for 10 000 iterations and showed superior performance over the original setup in our evaluation, we believe that an even higher score is possible by training for a longer time.

MD-GRUs allow for any number of dimensions in the data, hence it would also be possible to use the actual 4d data from the challenge, with the new dimension being the screening number. Using 4d data could pose a number of problems though, for instance the reduced spatial resolution that can be fed to the network per training iteration due to the memory constraints and the low number of screenings that are available. Further research might be necessary to determine, if a suitable trade-off between spatial resolution and temporal information exists.

In conclusion, the following four modifications can drastically improve the accuracy of lesion segmentation in terms of Dice, HD and AVD with the

MD-GRU: Selective sampling speeds up training drastically, since most of the data can be labeled safely as background. DC on the state does a better job in regularization than on the input. Random deformation prevents the model from overfitting. Finally, residual learning in between MD-GRUs might shorten training time by simplifying the estimation task.

References

1. Andermatt, S., Pezold, S., Cattin, P.: Multi-dimensional gated recurrent units for the segmentation of biomedical 3D-data. In: Carneiro, G., et al. (eds.) LABELS/DLMIA-2016. LNCS, vol. 10008, pp. 142–151. Springer, Cham (2016). https://doi.org/10.1007/978-3-319-46976-8_15
2. Carass, A., Roy, S., Jog, A., Cuzzocreo, J.L., Magrath, E., Gherman, A., Button, J., Nguyen, J., Prados, F., Sudre, C.H., Jorge Cardoso, M., Cawley, N., Ciccarelli, O., Wheeler-Kingshott, C.A.M., Ourselin, S., Catanese, L., Deshpande, H., Maurel, P., Commowick, O., Barillot, C., Tomas-Fernandez, X., Warfield, S.K., Vaidya, S., Chunduru, A., Muthuganapathy, R., Krishnamurthi, G., Jesson, A., Arbel, T., Maier, O., Handels, H., Iheme, L.O., Unay, D., Jain, S., Sima, D.M., Smeets, D., Ghafoorian, M., Platel, B., Birenbaum, A., Greenspan, H., Bazin, P.L., Calabresi, P.A., Crainiceanu, C.M., Ellingsen, L.M., Reich, D.S., Prince, J.L., Pham, D.L.: Longitudinal multiple sclerosis lesion segmentation: resource and challenge. NeuroImage **148**, 77–102 (2017)
3. Cho, K., van Merrienboer, B., Gulcehre, C., Bahdanau, D., Bougares, F., Schwenk, H., Bengio, Y.: Learning phrase representations using RNN encoder-decoder for statistical machine translation. arXiv:1406.1078 [cs, stat], June 2014
4. Cooijmans, T., Ballas, N., Laurent, C., Gülçehre, Ç., Courville, A.: Recurrent batch normalization. arXiv:1603.09025 [cs], March 2016
5. Filippi, M., Horsfield, M.A., Bressi, S., Martinelli, V., Baratti, C., Reganati, P., Campi, A., Miller, D.H., Comi, G.: Intra- and inter-observer agreement of brain MRI lesion volume measurements in multiple sclerosis. Brain **118**(6), 1593–1600 (1995)
6. He, K., Zhang, X., Ren, S., Sun, J.: Deep residual learning for image recognition. arXiv:1512.03385 [cs], December 2015
7. Ioffe, S., Szegedy, C.: Batch normalization: accelerating deep network training by reducing internal covariate shift. arXiv:1502.03167 [cs], February 2015
8. Liao, Q., Poggio, T.: Bridging the gaps between residual learning, recurrent neural networks and visual cortex. arXiv:1604.03640 [cs], April 2016
9. Schuster, M., Paliwal, K.K.: Bidirectional recurrent neural networks. IEEE Trans. Signal Process. **45**(11), 2673–2681 (1997)
10. Stollenga, M.F., Byeon, W., Liwicki, M., Schmidhuber, J.: Parallel multi-dimensional LSTM, with application to fast biomedical volumetric image segmentation. In: Cortes, C., Lawrence, N.D., Lee, D.D., Sugiyama, M., Garnett, R. (eds.) Advances in Neural Information Processing Systems, vol. 28, pp. 2998–3006. Curran Associates, Inc. (2015)
11. Wan, L., Zeiler, M., Zhang, S., Cun, Y.L., Fergus, R.: Regularization of neural networks using dropconnect. In: Proceedings of the 30th International Conference on Machine Learning (ICML-2013), pp. 1058–1066 (2013)
12. Zaremba, W., Sutskever, I., Vinyals, O.: Recurrent neural network regularization. arXiv:1409.2329 [cs], September 2014

Joint Intensity Fusion Image Synthesis Applied to Multiple Sclerosis Lesion Segmentation

Greg M. Fleishman[1]([✉])([iD]), Alessandra Valcarcel[2], Dzung L. Pham[3],
Snehashis Roy[3], Peter A. Calabresi[4], Paul Yushkevich[1],
Russell T. Shinohara[2], and Ipek Oguz[1]

[1] Department of Radiology, University of Pennsylvania, Philadelphia, PA 19104, USA
gflei@mail.med.upenn.edu
[2] Department of Biostatistics and Epidemiology, University of Pennsylvania,
Philadelphia, PA 19104, USA
[3] CNRM, The Henry M. Jackson Foundation for the Advancement of Military
Medicine, Bethesda, MD 20817, USA
[4] Department of Neurology, The Johns Hopkins University School of Medicine,
Baltimore, MD 21287, USA

Abstract. We propose a new approach to Multiple Sclerosis lesion segmentation that utilizes synthesized images. A new method of image synthesis is considered: joint intensity fusion (JIF). JIF synthesizes an image from a library of deformably registered and intensity normalized atlases. Each location in the synthesized image is a weighted average of the registered atlases; atlas weights vary spatially. The weights are determined using the joint label fusion (JLF) framework. The primary methodological contribution is the application of JLF to MRI signal directly rather than labels. Synthesized images are then used as additional features in a lesion segmentation task using the OASIS classifier, a logistic regression model on intensities from multiple modalities. The addition of JIF synthesized images improved the Dice-Sorensen coefficient (relative to manually drawn gold standards) of lesion segmentations over the standard model segmentations by 0.0462 ± 0.0050 (mean $\pm$ standard deviation) at optimal threshold over all subjects and 10 separate training/testing folds.

1 Introduction

Multiple Sclerosis (MS) is a chronic, inflammatory, autoimmune disease of the central nervous system (CNS) wherein myelin sheaths which surround and insulate CNS nerves are damaged [7]. Regions of active inflammation and/or prior damage are visible in various magnetic resonance imaging (MRI) modalities as lesions. MS lesion segmentation has been an active area of research with many contributions including LesionTOADs [17], S3DL [15], IMaGe [19], and QuEEN [13,20], with many others recently reviewed [8] and evaluated [3]. However, no existing tool is a complete solution and improved lesion segmentation in MS could lead to better characterization of disease trajectory and/or enable the

© Springer International Publishing AG, part of Springer Nature 2018
A. Crimi et al. (Eds.): BrainLes 2017, LNCS 10670, pp. 43–54, 2018.
https://doi.org/10.1007/978-3-319-75238-9_4

observation of effective new therapies, either of which could improve patient outcomes.

Our aim is to improve MS lesion segmentation through image synthesis. Image synthesis is the process of artificially generating an image with geometry and appearance similar to those of a desired target [10]. Among the many approaches to image synthesis is the general idea of combining patches from real image acquisitions to synthesize an image with realistic contrast [16]. Image synthesis has been proposed as a means of assisting MS lesion segmentation, wherein for a given MS subject whose actual images contain lesions, an image is synthesized without lesions but with comparable features elsewhere [5].

Another method in which patches from different sources are fused to synthesize a final product is multi-atlas label fusion (MALF) [9]. In MALF, a library of atlases with associated segmentations are deformably registered to a target image. The segmentations for all atlases are resampled to the space of the target and fused according to a procedure that varies between methods to produce a final segmentation of the target. Another method which fuses patches is non-local means (NLM) filtering: non-local patches from within the same image are found and fused to reduce noise locally without blurring edges [1,2,22,23].

This work is inspired by the intersection of MALF and NLM, wherein corresponding patches from warped control atlases are fused rather than labels or patches from within the same image. These patches are local spatially, but non-local in that they derive from independent images. As a result, we synthesize images whose characteristics we can constrain by the choice of atlases. We refer to our proposed method as joint intensity fusion (JIF). The synthesized images are then utilized in MS lesion segmentation as additional features to a classifier. To summarize, our goal is to synthesize lesion-free images of MS subjects and test the hypothesis that the addition of such images to a lesion classifier would improve performance.

2   Methods

Our complete pipeline is summarized in Fig. 1. A library of healthy control atlases is registered and subsequently histogram matched to a target. The registered/histogram matched atlases and target are input to the Joint Label Fusion (JLF) algorithm, which produces a spatially varying weight map for each atlas. The atlases are combined according to these spatially varying weights to yield a synthesized image. Synthesized images are then treated as additional modalities to the OASIS multi-modality MS lesion classifier; we investigate whether their inclusion improves classification of lesions.

2.1   Data and Preprocessing

Our data set consists of 98 MS subjects (whose images we refer to as targets) and 29 healthy controls (whose images we refer to as atlases). Each subject has one scan from each of four modalities: T1-weighted (T1w), T2-weighted (T2w),

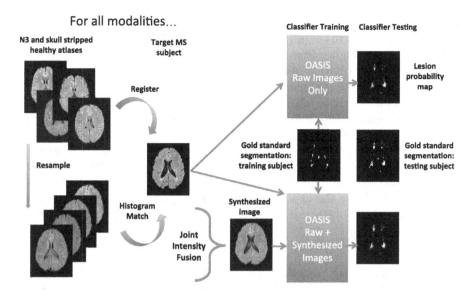

Fig. 1. Joint Intensity Fusion Image Synthesis for MS lesion segmentation. Manual segmentations were used when training the OASIS models; for test subjects, they were used for evaluation only.

proton density weighted (PD), and fluid attenuation inversion recovery (FLAIR). All scans were acquired on the same 3T MRI scanner (a Phillips scanner at the Johns Hopkins Hospital). Each MS subject also has a gold standard lesion mask segmented manually by a neuroscientific researcher.

For all subjects, all images were rigidly aligned to the Montreal Neurological Institute (MNI) standard space (voxel resolution 1 mm^3) [12]. We also applied the N3 inhomogeneity correction algorithm [18] to all images and removed extracerebral voxels using SPECTRE, a skull-stripping procedure [4].

2.2   Registration and Intensity Normalization

For each modality in parallel, all preprocessed atlases were registered to each preprocessed target. Registration included three steps: a 6 parameter rigid alignment, a 12 parameter affine alignment, and a deformable registration. Registrations were done with the package *greedy* which is described in Yushkevich et al. [25]. We normalize the non-standardized image intensity histograms by histogram matching each registered atlas to its corresponding target.

2.3   Joint Intensity Fusion

Our image synthesis approach is inspired by the multi-atlas label fusion (MALF) method for image segmentation. In MALF, a target image is segmented by registering to it a library of segmented atlases. All atlas labels are resampled to the space of the target; producing a sampling of labels at each voxel. This sampling is fused into a consensus segmentation with fusion strategies that often involve spatially varying weights based on image similarity metrics [9]. The primary methodological contribution of this work is to use a MALF-like strategy to fuse MRI signal directly rather than labels.

In particular, we chose to apply the joint label fusion (JLF) MALF strategy which has proven a successful means to achieve MALF segmentation, rated the best of nearly 25 methods in the 2012 MICCAI Grand Challenge and Workshop on Multi-Atlas Labeling [11]. JLF fuses labels by weighted averaging, the distribution of weights over atlases varies with position. However the definition of the weights accounts for correlations between atlases in the library [24]. JLF chooses weights that minimize the expected squared difference between the (unknown) ground truth label and the estimated label. To do so, JLF requires a matrix:

$$M_x(i, j) = p(\delta^i(x)\delta^j(x) = 1|I_T, A_1, ..., A_n) \tag{1}$$

whose ij^{th} entry is the probability that both atlases A_i and A_j mislabel location x in the target image I_T; $\delta^i(x) \in \{0, 1\}$ is the label error, 0 if $A_i(x)$ gives the correct label and 1 otherwise. M_x captures the correlations between atlases in the library. However, M_x is unknown and must be approximated. Let $\mathcal{N}(x)$ be a neighborhood around voxel x; JLF approximates this matrix as:

$$
\begin{aligned}
&p(\delta^i(x)\delta^j(x) = 1 \mid I_T(y), A_i(y), A_j(y) \mid y \in \mathcal{N}(x)) \\
&= \left[\sum_{y \in \mathcal{N}(x)} |I_T(y) - A_i(y)||I_T(y) - A_j(y)| \right]^{\beta}
\end{aligned}
\tag{2}
$$

We apply the JLF technique to the set of registered healthy control atlases and MS targets, but use the resultant weights to fuse the atlases themselves rather than labels. That is, we synthesize an image where each location is the weighted average of the warped healthy control atlases, with the weights given by JLF. Recall, JLF weights vary spatially. We call this method of image synthesis Joint Intensity Fusion (JIF). Examples of JIF synthesized images are shown in the second column of Fig. 4.

2.4   MS Lesion Classification and Evaluation

We trained two versions of OASIS MS lesion classifiers [21]: one using only the four target MS subject modalities (FLAIR, T1w, T2w, and PD) and another using those same modalities and their JIF synthesized versions. OASIS is a logistic regression model for the probability that any voxel V is in a lesion $P(V = \text{lesion})$. The logit function of the model is:

$$
\begin{aligned}
\text{logit}\big(P(V = \text{lesion})\big) &= \beta_0 + \beta_1 FLAIR + \beta_2 T1 + \beta_3 T2 + \beta_4 PD \\
&+ \beta_5 FLAIR \times FLAIR_{\sigma 1} + \beta_6 T1 \times T1_{\sigma 1} + \beta_7 T2 \times T2_{\sigma 1} + \beta_8 PD \times PD_{\sigma 1} \\
&+ \beta_9 FLAIR \times FLAIR_{\sigma 2} + \beta_{10} T1 \times T1_{\sigma 2} + \beta_{11} T2 \times T2_{\sigma 2} + \beta_{12} PD \times PD_{\sigma 2}
\end{aligned}
\tag{3}
$$

where each modality is represented by its name, $X_{\sigma 1}$ and $X_{\sigma 2}$ are versions of modality X smoothed with isotropic Gaussians of standard deviations $\sigma 1$ and $\sigma 2$ respectively, and the β_i are regression coefficients. We augment this function to include the JIF synthesized images as if they were four new modalities:

$$
\begin{aligned}
\text{logit}\big(P(V = \text{lesion})\big) = {} & \beta_0 + \beta_1 FLAIR + \beta_2 T1 + \beta_3 T2 + \beta_4 PD \\
& + \boldsymbol{\beta_5 FLAIR^s} + \boldsymbol{\beta_6 T1^s} + \boldsymbol{\beta_7 T2^s} + \boldsymbol{\beta_8 PD^s} \\
& + \beta_9 FLAIR \times FLAIR_{\sigma 1} + \beta_{10} T1 \times T1_{\sigma 1} + \beta_{11} T2 \times T2_{\sigma 1} + \beta_{12} PD \times PD_{\sigma 1} \\
& + \beta_{13} FLAIR \times FLAIR_{\sigma 2} + \beta_{14} T1 \times T1_{\sigma 2} + \beta_{15} T2 \times T2_{\sigma 2} + \beta_{16} PD \times PD_{\sigma 2} \\
& + \boldsymbol{\beta_{17} FLAIR^s \times FLAIR^s_{\sigma 1}} + \boldsymbol{\beta_{18} T1^s \times T1^s_{\sigma 1}} + \boldsymbol{\beta_{19} T2^s \times T2^s_{\sigma 1}} + \boldsymbol{\beta_{20} PD^s \times PD^s_{\sigma 1}} \\
& + \boldsymbol{\beta_{21} FLAIR^s \times FLAIR^s_{\sigma 2}} + \boldsymbol{\beta_{22} T1^s \times T1^s_{\sigma 2}} + \boldsymbol{\beta_{23} T2^s \times T2^s_{\sigma 2}} + \boldsymbol{\beta_{24} PD^s \times PD^s_{\sigma 2}}
\end{aligned}
$$

$$(4)$$

where X^s is the synthesized version of modality X; new terms are bolded. We refer to the control model (3) as OASIS(raw) and the experimental model (4) as OASIS(raw+synth).

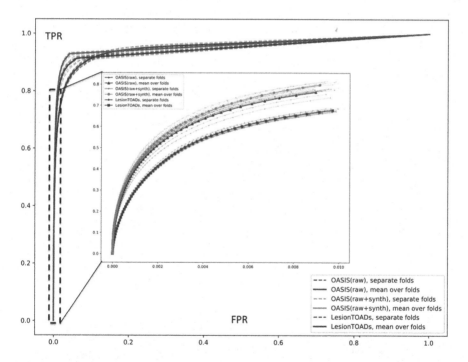

Fig. 2. ROC and pROC curves for OASIS(raw+synth), OASIS(raw), and Lesion-TOADs classifier models. All 10 folds and their average are depicted. The OASIS(raw+synth) curves dominate the OASIS(raw) curves. The LesionTOADs curve only exceeds OASIS(raw) and OASIS(raw+synth) for very high false positive rates that have limited value in practice. The inset shows that OASIS(raw+synth) performance exceeds both alternatives within the clinically relevant range.

48   G. M. Fleishman et al.

2.5   Experiments and Evaluation

We compare OASIS(raw) and OASIS(raw+synth) with ten-fold cross validation.
Each fold consists of 20 randomly selected training subjects. The remaining 78
subjects are tested. For each test subject, OASIS provides a probability map
(p-map), i.e. each voxel is assigned a probability $p \in [0, 1]$ where $p = 0$ implies
certainty of non-lesion and $p = 1$ implies certainty of lesion. We threshold the
p-maps at all values in $\{0, 0.01, ..., 1.0\}$ and report the Dice-Sorensen coefficient
(DSC) and the receiver operating characteristic (ROC) curve to evaluate performance. The significance of the difference between OASIS(raw+synth) and
OASIS(raw) curves from corresponding cross validation folds was assessed with
the DeLong test [6]. A balanced and random sub-selection of true positive and
true negative voxels were selected from each subject to satisfy consistency with
the DeLong test assumption of independent samples.

Additionally, we include results on the same 10 testing folds computed with
the LesionTOADS method [17]. LesionTOADS is an unsupervised algorithm to
segment brain tissues and lesions simultaneously. Unlike OASIS which requires
training data for lesion segmentation, LesionTOADS uses fuzzy c-means to segment the T1w and FLAIR image intensities into multiple tissue classes such

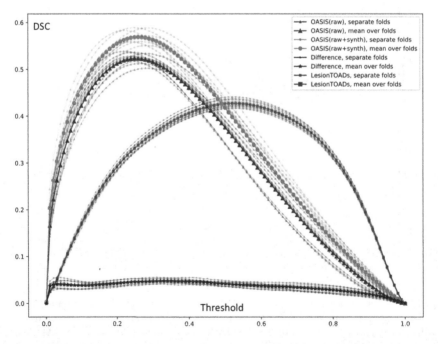

Fig. 3. DSC over probability map threshold for OASIS(raw), OASIS(raw+synth), and
LesionTOADs classifier models. All 10 folds and their average are depicted. The differ-
ence curves are OASIS(raw+synth) - OASIS(raw) and are non-negative, indicating the
OASIS(raw+synth) curves are everywhere greater than their OASIS(raw) counterparts.
Both OASIS(raw+synth) and OASIS(raw) have higher peak DSC than LesionTOADs.

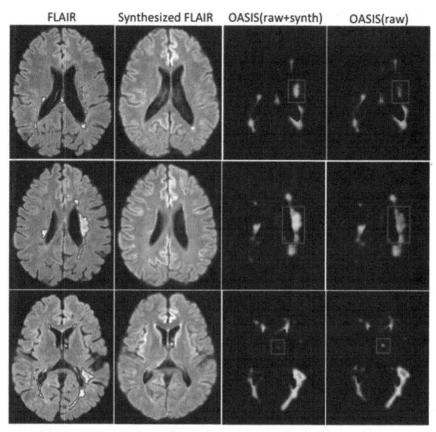

Pink outline: gold standard boundary. **Red:** gold standard segmentation
Probability map values: 0 ▬▬▬▬▬ 1

Fig. 4. Acquired FLAIRs with manual segmentation boundary, corresponding synthesized FLAIRs, and manual segmentation masks overlaid with lesion probability maps for OASIS(raw+synth) and OASIS(raw). **First row:** true positive where OASIS(raw+synth) gives high probability, but OASIS(raw) does not. **Second row:** true positive where OASIS(raw+synth) has higher probability than OASIS(raw). **Third row:** true negative where OASIS(raw+synth) has lower probability than OASIS(raw).

as grey matter, white matter, cerebrospinal fluid, and lesions. Further, Lesion-TOADS enforces topology checks so that the resultant segmentation is topologically similar to a template. LesionTOADS produces fuzzy memberships of lesions, which are thresholded at $\{0, 0.01, ..., 1.00\}$ to produce binary lesion segmentations. Although LesionTOADS can be tuned with different parameters [14] for different expected lesion load present in a subject, we processed all subjects with the default parameter set for uniform comparison with OASIS.

Table 1. Mean and median DSC for all models at peak threshold for each fold.

MEAN of Fold:	1	2	3	4	5	6	7	8	9	10	Mean (Std. dev.)
OASIS(raw+synth)	**0.56**	**0.58**	**0.59**	**0.56**	**0.56**	**0.57**	**0.57**	**0.55**	**0.59**	**0.57**	**0.57 (0.01)**
OASIS(raw)	0.53	0.53	0.54	0.51	0.52	0.53	0.53	0.50	0.53	0.52	0.52 (0.01)
LesionTOADs	0.42	0.44	0.44	0.43	0.42	0.43	0.42	0.42	0.44	0.42	0.43 (0.01)
OASIS(raw+unlm)	0.54	0.54	0.55	0.53	0.53	0.54	0.54	0.52	0.54	0.53	0.53 (0.01)
MEDIAN of Fold:	1	2	3	4	5	6	7	8	9	10	Median (IQR)
OASIS(raw+synth)	**0.64**	**0.63**	**0.63**	**0.64**	**0.62**	**0.64**	**0.63**	**0.61**	**0.64**	**0.64**	**0.64 (0.63, 0.64)**
OASIS(raw)	0.60	0.58	0.58	0.58	0.59	0.59	0.60	0.57	0.59	0.60	0.59 (0.58, 0.60)
LesionTOADs	0.46	0.48	0.50	0.50	0.48	0.50	0.46	0.48	0.50	0.48	0.48 (0.48, 0.50)
OASIS(raw+unlm)	0.61	0.58	0.59	0.60	0.59	0.61	0.62	0.61	0.61	0.62	0.61 (0.60, 0.61)

Because they are averages of multiple acquisitions, the synthetic images have higher signal to noise ratio (SNR) than the raw acquisitions. Thus, it is necessary to investigate whether any differences in lesion segmentation are solely due to the higher SNR, or some other property of the synthetic images. We test this by using Unbiased Non-Local Means (UNLM) [22], which averages non-local neighborhoods that are similar in appearance to the current patch, as an alternative

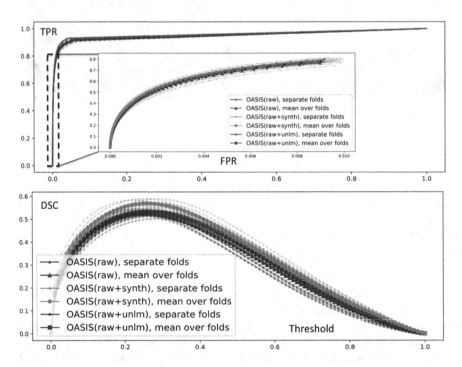

Fig. 5. UNLM: Unbiased Non-Local Means smoothing. For ROC, pROC, and DSC, OASIS(raw+unlm) appears to perform only slightly better than OASIS(raw) and visibly worse than OASIS(raw+synth); see Table 1 also.

smoothing method. For every target MS image, we generated a smoothed version with UNLM. We then trained OASIS models using the target images and their UNLM smoothed counterparts; we refer to these models as OASIS(raw+unlm). We compare the performance of OASIS(raw+synth) and OASIS(raw+unlm).

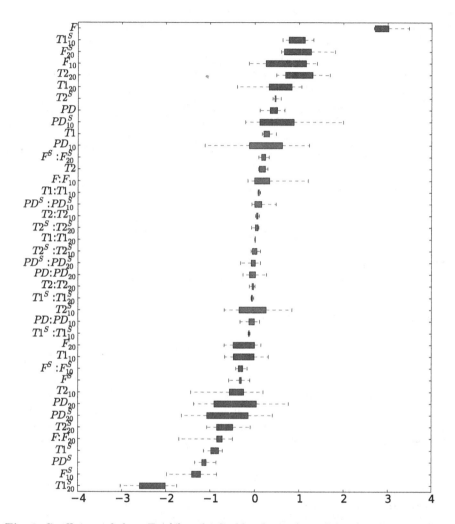

Fig. 6. Coefficients β_i from Eq. (4) multiplied by the median of their corresponding feature; boxplot is over all 10 training folds. If the median is between ± 0.2 then the box is red; blue and green depict positive and negative contributors respectively. Noticeably, the interaction features tend to be the least predictive, whereas FLAIR and T1w features (both raw and synthetic) tend to be the most predictive. (Color figure online)

3   Results

The ROC and partial ROC (pROC) curves (up to false positive rates of 0.01) are shown in Fig. 2. False positive rates above 0.01 are not clinically useful for MS lesion segmentation; consider, 1% of the volume of a healthy control subject is on the order of $10\,cm^3$, which is commensurate with the average lesion load of an MS subject. The ROC and pROC curves show that OASIS(raw+synth) has higher true positive rates for any given false positive rate including those in the clinically relevant range. The DeLong test showed that the improvement in the OASIS(raw+synth) model was significant with $p < 2.2 \times 10^{-16}$ in all 10 folds.

DSC as a function of threshold is shown in Fig. 3. The differences between corresponding OASIS(raw+synth) folds and OASIS(raw) folds are non-negative, indicating that including the JIF synthesized images results in higher DSC for any threshold. Table 1 shows the mean and median (over subjects) DSC obtained at optimal threshold for each fold by OASIS(raw+synth), OASIS(raw), and the LesionTOADs package [17]. For each fold, OASIS(raw+synth) obtains the highest mean and median DSC. Figure 4 shows 3 qualitative results illustrating the behavior of the two models.

Figure 5 contrasts OASIS(raw), OASIS(raw+unlm), and OASIS(raw+synth) and is analogous to Figs. 2 and 3. It shows that the addition of UNLM smoothed images to OASIS is not sufficient to recover the improvements gained by the OASIS(raw+synth) model, i.e. the improvements gained in OASIS(raw+synth) are not likely due solely to the increased SNR in the synthetic images.

4   Discussion and Conclusions

The results indicate that including the JIF synthesized images in the OASIS model improves lesion segmentation relative to the standard OASIS model. Inspection of Eq. (4) illuminates the improvement. Only features present in the library of atlases can be reconstructed in a synthesized image. As the atlas library is composed of only healthy controls, it is unlikely to synthesize a region with appearance similar to a lesion. Equation (4) contains linear combinations of the MS target images and their synthesized counterparts. Hence, what is present in the target images but missing in the synthesized images can be accentuated.

We investigated which of the input features were most useful to the model. The magnitude of the coefficients β_i in Eq. (4) are an indicator of the importance of their corresponding feature. However, these coefficients must be normalized to the scale of their features. Figure 6 shows boxplots (over the 10 cross-validation folds) of the coefficients of the OASIS(raw+synth) model, where each coefficient is multiplied by the median value of its corresponding feature. Those coefficients furthest from zero (either close to the top or bottom of the plot) were the most discriminatory between lesion and non-lesion voxels. Noticeably, many of the interaction terms are in the center, and are the weakest contributors. FLAIR and T1w modalities, both raw and synthetic, are the most discriminatory.

The proposed method involves multiple registrations, histogram matching, JIF computation of weights, fusion, and subsequent training and testing of a classifier model; we report approximate runtimes for those steps: **registration:** 300s per image pair, **HM:** 5s per image pair, **JIF:** 540s total for 29 atlases, **fusion:** 10s per synthetic image, and **OASIS:** 60s per image.

The registration package *greedy* [25] is, compared to other publicly available packages, a very fast implementation of diffeomorphic image registration. The time reported above represents rigid, affine, and deformable registrations done in sequence. As with any gradient descent based optimization, run time will depend on the quality of the initialization, i.e., how well matched the input images are initially. For JIF, the run time is a function of the number of atlases; the reported time was computed using 29 atlases.

OASIS training fits a logistic regression model and OASIS testing evaluates that model; the time for both computations is constant given a fixed number of inputs. However, OASIS does feature selection prior to training and testing, the most computationally expensive portion of which is smoothing the input images multiple times. We thus only report the time required to perform feature selection for one image. When training using N input modalities and M subjects, the total training time is approximated by $N \times M \times R$ where R is the number reported above.

In closing, inclusion of JIF synthetic images significantly improves lesion classification of the OASIS mode and with the inclusion of synthetic images, OASIS outperformed other state-of-the-art methods. Future work will investigate alternative classifier models and additional applications for JIF synthesized images.

Acknowledgements. This work supported by the National Institutes of Health grants: R01-NS094456, R01-EB017255, R01-NS085211, R21-NS093349, R01-NS082347, R01-NS070906 and by the National Multiple Sclerosis Society grant: RG-1507-05243.

References

1. Awate, S., Whitaker, R.: Unsupervised, information-theoretic, adaptive image filtering for image restoration. IEEE Trans. PAMI **28**, 364–376 (2006)
2. Buades, A., Coll, B., Morel, J.M.: Nonlocal image and movie denoising. Int. J. Comput. Vis. **76**(2), 123–139 (2008)
3. Carass, A., et al.: Longitudinal multiple sclerosis lesion segmentation: resource and challenge. NeuroImage **148**, 77–102 (2017)
4. Carass, A., Cuzzocreo, J., Wheeler, M.B., Bazin, P.L., Resnick, S.M., Prince, J.L.: Simple paradigm for extra-cerebral tissue removal: algorithm and analysis. NeuroImage **56**(4), 1982–1992 (2011)
5. Cardoso, M.J., Sudre, C.H., Modat, M., Ourselin, S.: Template-based multimodal joint generative model of brain data. In: IPMI, pp. 17–29 (2015)
6. DeLong, E.R., DeLong, D.M., Clarke-Pearson, D.L.: Comparing the areas under two or more correlated receiver operating characteristic curves: a nonparametric approach. Biometrics **44**, 837–845 (1988)
7. Dendrou, C.A., Fugger, L., Friese, M.A.: Immunopathology of multiple sclerosis. Nat. Rev. Immunol. **15**(9), 545–558 (2015)
8. Garcia-Lorenzo, D., Francis, S., Narayanan, S., Arnold, D.L., Collins, D.L.: Review of automatic segmentation methods of multiple sclerosis white matter lesions on conventional magnetic resonance imaging. Med. Image Anal. **17**(1), 1–18 (2013)

9. Iglesias, J.E., Sabuncu, M.R.: Multi-atlas segmentation of biomedical images: a survey. Med. Image Anal. **24**(1), 205–219 (2015)
10. Jog, A., Roy, S., Carass, A., Prince, J.L.: Magnetic resonance image synthesis through patch regression. In: Proceedings of IEEE ISBI 2013, pp. 350–353 (2013)
11. Landman, B.A., Warfield, S.K.: MICCAI 2012 workshop on multi-atlas labeling. In: MICCAI 2012 Grand Challenge and Workshop on Multi-Atlas Labeling Challenge Results (2012)
12. Mazziotta, J.C., Toga, A.W., Evans, A., Fox, P., Lancaster, J.: A probabilistic atlas of the human brain: theory and rationale for its development. NeuroImage **2**(2), 89–101 (1995)
13. Mejia, A.F., Sweeney, E.M., Dewey, B., Nair, G., Sati, P., Shea, C., Reich, D.S., Shinohara, R.T.: Statistical estimation of T1 relaxation times using conventional magnetic resonance imaging. NeuroImage **133**, 176–188 (2016)
14. Roy, S., Agarwal, H., Carass, A., Bai, Y., Pham, D.L., Prince, J.L.: Fuzzy c-means with variable compactness. In: IEEE International Symposium on Biomedical Imaging (2008)
15. Roy, S., Carass, A., Prince, J.L., Pham, D.L.: Subject specific sparse dictionary learning for atlas based brain MRI segmentation. In: Wu, G., Zhang, D., Zhou, L. (eds.) MLMI 2014. LNCS, vol. 8679, pp. 248–255. Springer, Cham (2014). https://doi.org/10.1007/978-3-319-10581-9_31
16. Tsaftaris, S.A., Gooya, A., Frangi, A.F., Prince, J.L. (eds.): SASHIMI 2016. LNCS, vol. 9968. Springer, Cham (2016). https://doi.org/10.1007/978-3-319-46630-9
17. Shiee, N., Bazin, P.L., Ozturk, A., Reich, D.S., Calabresi, P.A., Pham, D.L.: A topology-preserving approach to the segmentation of brain images with multiple sclerosis lesions. NeuroImage **49**(2), 1524–1535 (2010)
18. Sled, J.G., Zijdenbos, A.P., Evans, A.C.: A nonparametric method for automatic correction of intensity nonuniformity in MRI data. IEEE Trans. Med. Imaging **17**(1), 87–97 (1998)
19. Subbanna, N., Precup, D., Arnold, D., Arbel, T.: Image: iterative multilevel probabilistic graphical model for detection and segmentation of multiple sclerosis lesions in brain MRI. In: IPMI, pp. 514–526 (2015)
20. Suttner, L., Mejia, A., Dewey, B., Sati, P., Reich, D., Shinohara, R.: Statistical estimation of white matter microstructure from conventional MRI. NeuroImage: Clinical **12**, 615–623 (2016)
21. Sweeney, E.M., Shinohara, R.T., Shiee, N., Mateen, F.J., Chudgar, A.A., Cuzzocreo, J.L., Calabresi, P.A., Pham, D.L., Reich, D.S., Crainiceanu, C.M.: OASIS is automated statistical inference for segmentation, with applications to multiple sclerosis lesion segmentation in MRI. NeuroImage: Clinical **2**, 402–413 (2013)
22. Tristán-Vega, A., García-Pérez, V., Aja-Fernández, S., Westin, C.F.: Efficient and robust nonlocal means denoising of MR data based on salient features matching. Comput. Methods Programs Biomed. **105**(2), 131–144 (2011)
23. Tustison, N., Avants, B., Wang, H., Xie, L., Coupe, P., Yushkevich, P., Manjon, J.: A patch-based framework for new ITK functionality: Joint fusion, denoising, and non-local super-resolution. Insight Journal (2017)
24. Wang, H., Suh, J.W., Das, S.R., Pluta, J.B., Craige, C., Yushkevich, P.A.: Multi-atlas segmentation with joint label fusion. IEEE Trans. PAMI **35**(3), 611–623 (2013)
25. Yushkevich, P.A., et al.: Fast automatic segmentation of hippocampal subfields and medial temporal lobe subregions in 3 Tesla and 7 Tesla T2-weighted MRI. Alzheimer's & Dement. J. Alzheimer's Assoc. **12**(7), P126–P127 (2016)

MARCEL (Inter-Modality Affine Registration with CorrELation Ratio): An Application for Brain Shift Correction in Ultrasound-Guided Brain Tumor Resection

Nima Masoumi[1,2(✉)], Yiming Xiao[1,2], and Hassan Rivaz[1,2]

[1] PERFORM Centre, Concordia University, Montreal, Canada
n_masoum@encs.concordia.ca
[2] Department of Electrical and Computer Engineering,
Concordia University, Montreal, Canada

Abstract. Tissue deformation during brain tumor removal often renders the original surgical plan invalid. This can greatly affect the quality of resection, and thus threaten the patient's survival rate. Therefore, correction of such deformation is needed, which can be achieved through image registration between pre- and intra-operative images. We proposed a novel automatic inter-modal affine registration technique based on the correlation ratio (CR) similarity metric. The technique was demonstrated through registering intra-operative ultrasound (US) scans with magnetic resonance (MR) images of patients, who underwent brain gliomas resection. By using landmark-based mean target registration errors (TRE) for evaluation, our technique has achieved a result of 2.32 ± 0.68 mm from the initial 5.13 ± 2.78 mm.

1 Introduction

Gliomas are tumors in glial cells occurring either in brain or spine, and are currently the most common types of brain tumors in adults [1]. According the world health organization (WHO), brain gliomas can be classified into four different grades: low grade (Grade I and II) and high-grade (Grade III and IV). Low-grade gliomas (LGG) have a slower tumor growth rate, but will eventually progress to the deadlier high-grade tumors. Thus, early tumor removal can increase patient's survival rate [2].

During brain surgery, brain deforms to some extent, which is called brain shift and is caused by multiple reasons such as physiological factors [3]. Therefore, image guided neurosurgery systems (IGNS) that do not take brain shift into account can often render the pre-surgical plans invalid and can lead to incomplete or unnecessary resection.

Acquiring Magnetic Resonance Imaging (MRI) intra-operatively is difficult and requires special surgical tools and setups. Therefore, intra-operative ultrasound (US) has become popular due to its portability and non-invasiveness in recent years. The drawbacks with US are the low image quality and difficulty

© Springer International Publishing AG, part of Springer Nature 2018
A. Crimi et al. (Eds.): BrainLes 2017, LNCS 10670, pp. 55–63, 2018.
https://doi.org/10.1007/978-3-319-75238-9_5

in interpreting the image contents. In order to track the surgical progress and brain shift, US images can be registered to pre-operative MRI to help recover the tissue deformation during operation [4]. Both T1-weighted MRI and T2-FLAIR MRI are rountinely acquired for planning brain tumor resection procedures. However, low-grade gliomas are often more distinguishable in T2-FLAIR than in T1-weighted MRI [5].

Intensity based registration techniques need a similarity metric to evaluate similarities between two images. In these techniques, the goal of the registration is maximization of the similarity metric. Among popular similarity metrics, mutual information (MI) is the most general one and assumes statistical relationship between images. On the contrary, normalized cross-correlation (NCC) and sum of squared differences (SSD) assume linear relationship between images and are more restrictive. Correlation ratio (CR) assumes functional relationship between images, and provides enough generality to be used as a similarity metric between US and MRI [6–8]. In [7] automatic multimodal deformable registration performed with utilization of a modified version of CR. They also proposed a robust method for dealing with resected tumor [9].

Deformable registration problems, usually have much more parameters than affine and rigid registration, which respectively have twelve and six parameters. As a result, they usually have more accurate registration. However, in practice, affine registration has a lower chance of failure and is generally less computationally intensive.

In this paper, we introduced an automatic affine registration method using Robust paTch based cOrrelation Ration (RaPTOR) [7] to help recover brain shift using intra-operative US and pre-operative MRI scans. We used REtroSpective Evaluation of Cerebral Tumors (RESECT) database [5] to validate our method.

2   Materials and Methods

2.1   Registration Overview

Let I_f and I_m be respectively fixed and moving images. In the context of IGNS, we set I_f to the pre-operative MRI, and deform the intra-operative US image I_m towards the pre-operative MRI. We formulate the registration process as an optimization problem. Our cost C is defined in Eq. 1:

$$C = D(I_f(\mathbf{x}), I_m(\mathbf{T}(\mathbf{x}))) \tag{1}$$

where D is our objective function that should be minimized, I_f is the fixed image, I_m is the moving image, $\mathbf{x}$ is the point of interest in space, and $\mathbf{T}$ is the affine transformation matrix. The affine transformation matrix is defined in Eq. 2:

$$\mathbf{T} = \begin{bmatrix} a_1 & a_2 & a_3 & a_4 \\ a_5 & a_6 & a_7 & a_8 \\ a_9 & a_{10} & a_{11} & a_{12} \\ 0 & 0 & 0 & 1 \end{bmatrix} \tag{2}$$

where a_i, $1 \leq i \leq 12$ denotes the twelve affine transformation parameters. If $\mathbf{x} = [x_i, \ x_j, \ x_k]$ denotes the position of a point in Cartesian coordinates, we employ the transformation as in Eq. 3:

$$
\begin{bmatrix} y_i \\ y_j \\ y_k \\ 1 \end{bmatrix} = \boldsymbol{T}(\boldsymbol{x}) = \boldsymbol{T} \times \begin{bmatrix} x_i \\ x_j \\ x_k \\ 1 \end{bmatrix} \tag{3}
$$

where $\mathbf{y} = [y_i, \ y_j, \ y_k]$ specifies the transformed point. We define the objective function D as a dissimilarity metric in Eq. 4. The dissimilarity metric is RaP-TOR (Robust PaTch based cOrrelation Ratio), which is modified version of CR (Correlation Ratio) [7].

$$
D(Y, X) = RaPTOR(X, Y) = \frac{1}{N_p} \sum_{i=1}^{N_p} (1 - \eta(Y|X; \boldsymbol{\Omega_i})) \tag{4}
$$

In Eq. 4, N_P is the number of patches, $\boldsymbol{\Omega_i}$ is the set of all voxels included in patch i, and η is CR. D varies between 0 and 1. In higher similarity, D is closer to 0 and in lower similarity D is closer to 1.

The definition of CR in Eq. 4 is as following:

$$
1 - \eta(Y|X) = \frac{1}{N\sigma^2} \left(\sum_{t=1}^{N} i_t^2 - \sum_{j=1}^{N_b} N_j \mu_j^2 \right) \tag{5}
$$

$$
\mu_j = \frac{\sum_{t=1}^{N} \lambda_{t,j} i_t}{N_j}, N_j = \sum_t \lambda_{t,j} \tag{6}
$$

where N is total number of samples in Y, $\sigma^2 = Var[Y]$, i_t is the intensity of voxel number t in Y, N_b is the total number of bins, and $\lambda_{t,j}$ is the contribution of sample t in bin j as explained in [7].

2.2 Optimization and Outlier Suppression

We calculated the derivation of objective function analytically in order to speed up the registration procedure. We used derivative of the cost function in two distinct part. First in outlier suppression part. Second in updating equation of the optimization part.

Derivative of the cost function with respect to affine transformation parameters is as following:

$$
\frac{\partial D}{\partial \mathbf{a}} = \begin{bmatrix} \frac{\partial D}{\partial a_1} & \frac{\partial D}{\partial a_2} & \cdots & \frac{\partial D}{\partial a_{12}} \end{bmatrix}^T \tag{7}
$$

In Eq. 7, $\mathbf{a}$ is a vector consisting of affine transformation parameters. Now the derivative with respect to each of the parameters is:

$$
\frac{\partial D}{\partial a_k} = \frac{1}{N_p} \sum_{i=1}^{N_p} \frac{\partial (1 - \eta(Y|X; \boldsymbol{\Omega_i}))}{\partial a_k} \tag{8}
$$

where a_k, $1 \leq k \leq 12$ declares affine transformation parameters. Utilizing the chain rule, we have:

$$\frac{\partial(1 - \eta(Y|X; \boldsymbol{\Omega}_i))}{\partial a_k} = \frac{\partial(1 - \eta)}{\partial a_k} = \frac{\partial(1 - \eta)}{\partial I_m(\mathbf{T(x)})} \cdot \frac{I_m(\mathbf{T(x)})}{\partial \mathbf{d}} \cdot \frac{\partial \mathbf{d}}{\partial a_k} \tag{9}$$

where $\mathbf{d} = [d_x, d_y, d_z]$ in Eq. 9 is the displacement vector in Cartesian coordinates. Right hand side of Eq. 9 has three terms. The first term was calculated in [7]. In order to comply with our equations, we bring up the calculation in following equations. Note that the first term in Eq. 9 is the size of transformed moving image and we consider each element of this term as in Eq. 10 using Eq. 5.

$$\begin{aligned}
\frac{\partial(1-\eta)}{\partial i_t} &= \frac{\partial}{\partial i_t}\left(\frac{1}{N\sigma^2}\left(\sum_{k=1}^{N} i_k^2 - \sum_{j=1}^{N_b} N_j \mu_j^2\right)\right) \\
&= \frac{-2(N-1)}{N^3\sigma^4}(i_t - \mu)\left(\sum_{k=1}^{N} i_k^2 - \sum_{j=1}^{N_b} N_j \mu_j^2\right) \\
&\quad + 2(i_t - \sum_{j=1}^{N_b} \mu_j \lambda_{t,j})(\frac{1}{N\sigma^2})
\end{aligned} \tag{10}$$

In Eq. 10 μ is mean of Y. Second term in right hand side of Eq. 9 is simply the gradient of transformed moving image and third term is Jacobian of transformation.

Mini-Batch Gradient Descent Optimization: While batch gradient descent is time consuming and stochastic gradient descent (SGD) doesn't have required accuracy, choice of mini-batch gradient descent gives a trade-off between implementation time and result accuracy. For a certain resolution of input images, we select a set of random patches from the images in every iteration.

We employ Gaussian pyramid in the optimization. There are three pyramid levels in our analysis excluding the original size of images. In order to enable the dissimilarity metric to have a better perception of similarities between two input images, we select the set size of patches proportional to the resolution and size of input images in each level. Note that increasing the set size of patches will increase the computation time. Thus selecting the set size of patches in each pyramid level is a compromise between accuracy and computation time. The update equation for mini-batch gradient descent is as Eq. 11:

$$a_n = a_{n-1} - \alpha_n \frac{\partial D}{\partial a_{n-1}} \tag{11}$$

where a_n is the vector consisting of affine transformation parameters in n-th iteration, $\frac{\partial D}{\partial a_n}$ can be achieved by Eq. 7, and α_n is step size. Step size is a function of iteration number and is defined in Eq. 12.

$$\alpha_n = \frac{a}{(A + n)^\tau} \tag{12}$$

In Eq. 12 $a > 0$, $A \geq 0$, $0 < \tau \leq 1$ are constants. Klein et al. [8] suggested approximate values for these parameters. According to [8], we set $a = 0.001$, $A = 0.3 \times MaxIterations$, and $\tau = 0.65$.

In comparison to the MRI, US has quite unique image features and its own challenges. The inherent properties of the ultrasound images can have a major effect on performance of the dissimilarity metric. Since we select patches in each iteration randomly, before any operation on the selected patches, we should pre-select the patches that have potent image features (e.g., consistent and strong lines). We used outlier suppression proposed in [7]. We discard patches that are greater than a threshold T in Eq. 13.

$$r.r_g > T \tag{13}$$

Heuristically, $T = 1$ gives acceptable results for us. Parameter r is defined in Eq. 14.

$$r = min \left\{ \frac{Var(\frac{\partial D}{\partial d_x})}{\langle \frac{\partial D}{\partial d_x} \rangle^2}, \frac{Var(\frac{\partial D}{\partial d_y})}{\langle \frac{\partial D}{\partial d_y} \rangle^2}, \frac{Var(\frac{\partial D}{\partial d_z})}{\langle \frac{\partial D}{\partial d_z} \rangle^2} \right\} \tag{14}$$

where $\frac{\partial D}{\partial d_x}$, $\frac{\partial D}{\partial d_y}$, and $\frac{\partial D}{\partial d_z}$ are derivatives in x, y, and z direction respectively and $\langle . \rangle$ is mean operator. The denominators are low at relatively uniform regions, but are high in textured regions (i.e., with high gradients). Definition of r_g in Eq. 13 can be found in Eq. 15.

$$r_g = \frac{\|\nabla I_f\| * B}{\|\nabla I_m\| * B} \tag{15}$$

Here ∇ is gradient operator, $\|.\|$ indicates magnitude of the gradient, $*$ is convolution, and B is a kernel of size of the image with all ones in the selected patch and zeros the rest. The nominator and denominator represent summation of gradient values of fixed and moving image respectively.

2.3 Patient Data

To validate the proposed technique, we employed the MRI and intra-operative US scans of five patients, who underwent brain tumor resection procedures. All patients' data were randomly selected from the publicly available RESECT (REtroSpective Evaluation of Cerebral Tumors) database [5], which includes both pre-operative MRI and intra-operative US scans of patients with low-grade gliomas, as well as homologous anatomical landmarks for validating registration algorithms. For registration, we employed T2w FLAIR MR images, which better visualize the boundaries of the brain tumors than the T1w MR scans, and intra-operative US scans obtained before resection. The T2w FLAIR images (TE = 388 ms, TR = 5000 ms, flip angle = 120°, voxel size = $1 \times 1 \times 1 \, mm^3$, sagittal acqusition) were obtained one day before surgery on a 3T Magnetom Skyra (Siemens, Erlangen). The MRI volumes have been rigidly registered to the patient's anatomy on the surgical table. The spatially tracked US images were obtained with a sonowand Invite neuronavigation system (Sonowand AS, Trondheim, Norway), and then reconstructed as 3D volumes with resolutions range from $0.14 \times 0.14 \times 0.14 \, mm^3$ to $0.24 \times 0.24 \times 0.24 \, mm^3$ depending on the transducer types and imaging depths. All US volumes have full coverage of the tumors. Since the US volumes were spatially tracked during surgeries, the positions of the tissues truthfully reflect the tissue formation during the procedures. Corresponding anatomical landmarks between the MRI and US volumes were provided in the dataset for registration validation.

2.4   Registration Procedure

For each patient, we first up-sampled the MR image to the image space (and resolution) of the corresponding US images. Then, the US volumes were registered to the re-sampled MRI volumes using the technique introduced earlier. For our registration, we used a hierarchical approach, which facilitate the optimization efficiency. The registration results are reported as mean target registration errors (mTREs) for all patients under study.

2.5   Validation

In order to assess the accuracy of our method, we used the landmarks which were provided in RESECT database for each patient. Supplied landmarks can be used to calculate mean target registration error (mTRE) [10]. mTRE for a patient is defined as Eq. 16.

$$mTRE = \frac{1}{N} \sum_{i=1}^{N} \|T(x_i) - x_i'\| \tag{16}$$

where x_i and x_i' are two corresponding landmarks in moving image (US in our case) and fixed image respectively. In Eq. 16, N is the total number of landmarks.

3   Results

After image registration, we have observed an improvement in terms of image feature correspondence. From Figs. 1 and 2, we can see that borders of tumors (blue arrows) and sulci (green arrows) have been visibly re-aligned between the MR and US images. The detailed mTRE evaluation for each patient is shown in Table 1. Figure 3 depicts mTRE values before and after registration as well. Both in Table 1 and Fig. 3, we observe that mTRE values decreased after registration. Moreover, it is instructive to compare mean and standard deviation of mTRE values before registration with ones after registration. In Table 1, we can see not only the mean value but also the standard deviation decreased.

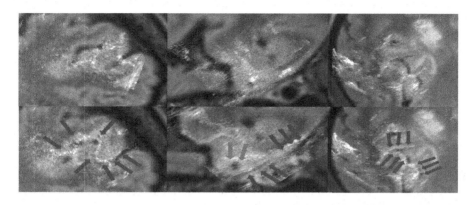

Fig. 1. Overlay of MR and US before and after registration for patient one, two, and three. First row is before registration and second row is after registration. Patient one, two, and three are first, second, and third column respectively. Green arrows correspond to sulcus and blue arrows correspond to tumor borders. (Color figure online)

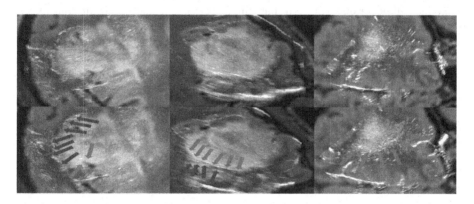

Fig. 2. Overlay of MR and US before and after registration for another view of patient three, four, and five. First row is before registration and second row is after registration. Patient three, four, and five are first, second, and third column respectively. Green arrows correspond to sulcus and blue arrows correspond to tumor borders. (Color figure online)

Table 1. mTRE (mm) before and after registration

Patients no	Initial mTRE	Final mTRE	No. of landmarks
1	5.72	2.86	15
2	9.58	3.21	15
3	2.65	1.79	15
4	4.70	2.14	15
5	2.99	1.62	15
Mean	5.13	2.32	
Std	2.78	0.68	

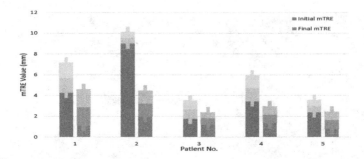

Fig. 3. Mean Target Registration Error (mTRE) Before and After Registration. Yellow and green bars indicate standard deviation before and after registration respectively. (Color figure online)

4 Discussion and Future Work

Although affine transformation has much fewer parameters than non-linear deformation, and thus may not fully represent the underlying soft tissue deformation, a few reasons justify the use of affine transformation for the demonstrated application. First, as important factors in the clinic, affine registration is often faster and less prone to failure than nonlinear registration. Second, the US volumes used mainly cover the tumorous tissues, and thus the deformation can be approximated sufficiently well locally with affine transformation. Lastly, the tissue deformation before resection is not severe, and affine registration is often sufficient for the surgeons to navigate the surgical plans. Here, we have preliminarily demonstrated the proposed technique using five brain cancer patients, in the future, we will validate the method on more subjects from the RESECT database, as well as inter-modality registration tasks in other applications.

5 Conclusion

We have proposed an automatic affine registration method based on correlation ratio. The technique has been demonstrated retrospectively for MRI-US registration in the context of brain shift correction during low-grade brain gliomas resection. From both quantitative and qualitative assessments, our proposed method has shown to successfully realigned the intra-operative US with the preoperative MRI scans.

Acknowledgement. This work is funded by Natural Science Engineering Council of Canada (NSERC) grant RGPIN-2015-04136. The authors would like to thank anonymous reviewers for their valuable feedback.

References

1. Holland, E.C.: Progenitor cells and glioma formation. Curr. Opin. Neurol. **14**(6), 683–688 (2001)
2. Dolecek, T.A., et al.: CBTRUS statistical report: primary brain and central nervous system tumors diagnosed in the United States in 2005–2009. Neuro-Oncol. **14**(suppl 5), v1–v49 (2012)
3. Gerard, I.J., et al.: Brain shift in neuronavigation of brain tumors: a review. Med. Image Anal. **35**, 403–420 (2017)
4. De Nigris, D., Collins, D.L., Arbel, T.: Multi-modal image registration based on gradient orientations of minimal uncertainty. IEEE Trans. Med. Imaging **31**(12), 2343–2354 (2012)
5. Xiao, Y., et al.: REtroSpective Evaluation of Cerebral Tumors (RESECT): a clinical database of pre-operative MRI and intra-operative ultrasound in low-grade glioma surgeries. Med. Phys. **44**, 3875–3882 (2017)
6. Roche, A., et al.: Multimodal image registration by maximization of the correlation ratio. Ph.D. thesis. INRIA (1998)
7. Rivaz, H., Chen, S.J.S., Collins, D.L.: Automatic deformable MR-ultrasound registration for image-guided neurosurgery. IEEE Trans. Med. Imaging **34**(2), 366–380 (2015)
8. Klein, S., Staring, M., Pluim, J.P.W.: Evaluation of optimization methods for nonrigid medical image registration using mutual information and B-splines. IEEE Trans. Image Process. **16**(12), 2879–2890 (2007)
9. Rivaz, H., Collins, D.L.: Near real-time robust non-rigid registration of volumetric ultrasound images for neurosurgery. Ultrasound Med. Biol. **41**(2), 574–587 (2015)
10. Daga, P., et al.: Accurate localization of optic radiation during neurosurgery in an interventional MRI suite. IEEE Trans. Med. Imaging **31**(4), 882–891 (2012)

Generalised Wasserstein Dice Score for Imbalanced Multi-class Segmentation Using Holistic Convolutional Networks

Lucas Fidon[1]([✉]), Wenqi Li[1], Luis C. Garcia-Peraza-Herrera[1],
Jinendra Ekanayake[2,3], Neil Kitchen[2], Sébastien Ourselin[1,3],
and Tom Vercauteren[1,3]

[1] TIG, CMIC, University College London, London, UK
`l.fidon@cs.ucl.ac.uk`
[2] NHNN, University College London Hospitals, London, UK
[3] Wellcome/EPSRC Centre for Interventional and Surgical Sciences,
UCL, London, UK

Abstract. The Dice score is widely used for binary segmentation due to its robustness to class imbalance. Soft generalisations of the Dice score allow it to be used as a loss function for training convolutional neural networks (CNN). Although CNNs trained using mean-class Dice score achieve state-of-the-art results on multi-class segmentation, this loss function does neither take advantage of inter-class relationships nor multi-scale information. We argue that an improved loss function should balance misclassifications to favour predictions that are semantically meaningful. This paper investigates these issues in the context of multi-class brain tumour segmentation. Our contribution is threefold. (1) We propose a semantically-informed generalisation of the Dice score for multi-class segmentation based on the Wasserstein distance on the probabilistic label space. (2) We propose a holistic CNN that embeds spatial information at multiple scales with deep supervision. (3) We show that the joint use of holistic CNNs and generalised Wasserstein Dice score achieves segmentations that are more semantically meaningful for brain tumour segmentation.

1 Introduction

Automatic brain tumour segmentation is an active research area. Learning-based methods using convolutional neural networks (CNNs) have recently emerged as the state of the art [9,11]. One of the challenges is the severe class imbalance. Two complementary ways have traditionally been used when training CNNs to tackle imbalance: (1) using a sampling strategy that imposes constraints on the selection of image patches; and (2) using pixel-wise weighting to balance the contribution of each class in the objective function. For CNN-based segmentation, samples should ideally be entire subject volumes to support the use of fully convolutional network and maximise the computational efficiency of convolution operations within GPUs. As a result, weighted loss functions appear more

© Springer International Publishing AG, part of Springer Nature 2018
A. Crimi et al. (Eds.): BrainLes 2017, LNCS 10670, pp. 64–76, 2018.
https://doi.org/10.1007/978-3-319-75238-9_6

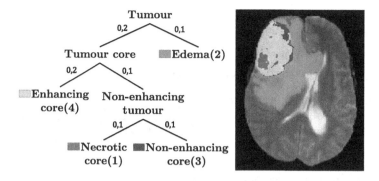

Fig. 1. Left: tree on BraTS label space. Edge weights have been manually selected to reflect the distance between labels. Right: illustration on a T2 scan from BraTS'15 [14].

promising to improve CNN-based automatic brain tumour segmentation. Using soft generalisations of the Dice score (a popular overlap measure for binary segmentation) directly as a loss function has recently been proposed [15,18]. By introducing global spatial information into the loss function, the Dice loss has been shown to be more robust to class imbalance. However at least two sources of information are not fully utilised in this formulation: (1) the structure of the label space; and (2) the spatial information across scales. Considering the class imbalance and the hierarchical label structure illustrated in Fig. 1, both of them are likely to play an important role for multi-class brain tumour segmentation.

In this paper, we propose two complementary contributions that leverage prior knowledge about brain tumour structure. First, we exploit the Wasserstein distance [7,17], which can naturally embed semantic relationships between classes for the comparison of label probability vectors, to generalise the Dice score for multi-class segmentation. Second, we propose a new holistic CNN architecture inspired by [8,19] that embeds spatial information at different scales and introduces deep supervision during the CNN training. We show that the combination of the proposed generalised Wasserstein Dice score and our Holistic CNN achieves better generalisation compared to both mean soft Dice score training and classic CNN architectures for multi-class brain tumour segmentation.

2   A Wasserstein Approach for Multi-class Soft Dice Score

2.1   Dice Score for Crisp Binary Segmentation

The Dice score is a widely used overlap measure for pairwise comparison of binary segmentations S and G. It can be expressed both in terms of set operations or statistical measures as:

$$D = \frac{2|S \cap G|}{|S| + |G|} = \frac{2\Theta_{TP}}{2\Theta_{TP} + \Theta_{FP} + \Theta_{FN}} = \frac{2\Theta_{TP}}{2\Theta_{TP} + \Theta_{AE}} \tag{1}$$

with Θ_{TP} the number of true positives, Θ_{FP}/Θ_{FN} the number of false positives/false negatives, and $\Theta_{AE} \doteq \Theta_{FP} + \Theta_{FN}$ the number of all errors.

2.2   Dice Score for Soft Binary Segmentation

Extensions to soft binary segmentations [1,2] rely on the concept of disagreement for pairs of probabilistic classifications. The classes S_i and G_i of each voxel $i \in \mathbf{X}$ can be defined as random variables on the label space $\mathbf{L} = \{0,1\}$ and the probabilistic segmentations can be represented as label probability maps: $p = \{p^i := P(S_i = 1)\}_{i \in \mathbf{X}}$ and $g = \{g^i := P(G_i = 1)\}_{i \in \mathbf{X}}$. We denote $P(\mathbf{L})$ the set of label probability vectors. We can now generalise Θ_{TP} and Θ_{AE} to soft segmentations:

$$\Theta_{AE} = \sum_{i \in \mathbf{X}} |p^i - g^i|, \quad \Theta_{TP} = \sum_{i \in \mathbf{X}} g^i(1 - |p^i - g^i|) \tag{2}$$

In the common case of a crisp segmentation g (i.e. $\forall i \in \mathbf{X}, g^i \in \{0,1\}$), the associated soft Dice score can be expressed as:

$$D(p,g) = \frac{2\sum_i g^i p^i}{\sum_i (g^i + p^i)} \tag{3}$$

A second variant has been used in [15], with a quadratic term in the denominator.

2.3   Previous Work on Multi-class Dice Score

The easiest way to derive a unique criterion from the soft binary Dice score for multi-class segmentation is to consider the mean Dice score:

$$D_{mean}(p,g) = \frac{1}{|\mathbf{L}|} \sum_{l \in \mathbf{L}} \frac{2\sum_i g_l^i p_l^i}{\sum_i (g_l^i + p_l^i)} \tag{4}$$

where $\{g_l^i\}_{i \in \mathbf{X}, l \in \mathbf{L}}$, $\{p_l^i\}_{i \in \mathbf{X}, l \in \mathbf{L}}$ are the set label probability vectors for all voxels for the ground truth and the prediction.

A generalised soft multi-class Dice score has also been proposed in [4,18] by generalising the set theory definition of the Dice score (1):

$$D_{FM}(p,g) = \frac{2\sum_l \alpha_l \sum_i \min(p_l^i, g_l^i)}{\sum_l \alpha_l \sum_i (p_l^i + g_l^i)} \tag{5}$$

where $\{\alpha_l\}_{l \in \mathbf{L}}$ allows to weight the contribution of each class. However, those definitions are still based only on pairwise comparisons of probabilities associated with the same label and don't take into account inter-class relationships.

2.4   Wasserstein Distance Between Label Probability Vectors

The Wasserstein distance (also sometimes called the *Earth Mover's Distance*) represents the minimal cost to transform a probability vector p into another one q when for all $l, l' \in \mathbf{L}$, the cost to move a unit from l to l' is defined as the distance $M_{l,l'}$ between l and l'. This is a way to map a distance matrix M (often referred to as the *ground distance matrix*) on $\mathbf{L}$, into a distance on $P(\mathbf{L})$ that leverages prior knowledges about $\mathbf{L}$. In the case of a finite set $\mathbf{L}$, for $p, q \in P(\mathbf{L})$, the Wasserstein distance between p and q derived from M can be defined as the solution of a linear programming problem [17]:

$$W^M(p,q) = \min_{T_{l,l'}} \sum_{l,l' \in \mathbf{L}} T_{l,l'} M_{l,l'},$$

$$\text{subject to} \quad \forall l \in \mathbf{L}, \sum_{l' \in \mathbf{L}} T_{l,l'} = p_l, \text{ and } \quad \forall l' \in \mathbf{L}, \sum_{l \in \mathbf{L}} T_{l,l'} = q_{l'}. \tag{6}$$

where $T = (T_{l,l'})_{l,l' \in \mathbf{L}}$ is a joint probability distribution for (p, q) with marginal distributions p and q. A value $\hat{T}$ that minimises (6) is called an *optimal transport* between p and q for the distance matrix M.

2.5   Soft Multi-class Wasserstein Dice Score

The Wasserstein distance W^M in (6) yields a natural way to compare two label probability vectors in a semantically meaningful manner by supplying a distance matrix M on $\mathbf{L}$. Hence we propose using it to generalise the measure of disagreement between a pair of label probability vectors and provide the following generalisations:

$$\Theta_{AE} = \sum_{i \in \mathbf{X}} W^M(p^i, g^i) \tag{7}$$

$$\Theta_{TP}^l = \sum_{i \in \mathbf{X}} g_l^i (W^M(l, b) - W^M(p^i, g^i)), \quad \forall l \in \mathbf{L} \setminus \{b\} \tag{8}$$

where $W^M(l, b)$ is shorthand for $M_{l,b}$ and M is chosen such that the background class b is always the furthest away from the other classes. To generalise Θ_{TP}, we propose to weight the contribution of the classes similarly to (5):

$$\Theta_{TP} = \sum_{l \in \mathbf{L}} \alpha_l \Theta_{TP}^l \tag{9}$$

We chose $\alpha_l = W^M(l, b)$ to make sure that background voxels do not contribute to Θ_{TP}. The Wasserstein Dice score with respect to M can then be defined as:

$$D^M(p,g) = \frac{2 \sum_l W^M(l, b) \sum_i g_l^i (W^M(l, b) - W^M(p^i, g^i))}{2 \sum_l [W^M(l, b) \sum_i g_l^i (W^M(l, b) - W^M(p^i, g^i))] + \sum_i W^M(p^i, g^i)} \tag{10}$$

In the binary case, setting $M = \left[\begin{smallmatrix} 0 & 1 \\ 1 & 0 \end{smallmatrix}\right]$ leads to $W^M(p^i, g^i) = |p^i - g^i|$ and reduces the proposed Wasserstein Dice score to the soft binary Dice score (2).

2.6   Wasserstein Dice Loss with Crisp Ground Truth

Previous work on Wasserstein distance-based loss functions for deep learning have been limited because of the computational burden [17]. However, in the case of a crisp ground-truth $\{g^i\}_i$, and for any prediction $\{p^i\}_i$, a closed-form solution exists for (6). An optimal transport is $\forall l, l' \in \mathbf{L}, T_{l,l'}^i = p_l^i g_{l'}^i$ and the Wasserstein distance becomes:

$$W^M(p^i, g^i) = \sum_{l,l' \in \mathbf{L}} M_{l,l'} p_l^i g_{l'}^i \tag{11}$$

We define the Wasserstein Dice loss derived from M as $\mathcal{L}_{D^M} := 1 - D^M$.

3   Holistic Convolutional Networks for Multi-scale Fusion

We now describe a holistically-nested convolutional neural network (HCNN) for imbalanced multi-class brain tumour segmentation inspired by the holistically-nested edge detection (HED) introduced in [19]. HCNN has been used successfully for some imbalanced learning tasks such as edge detection in natural images [19] and surgical tool segmentation [8]. The HCNN features multi-scale prediction and intermediate supervision. It can produce a unified output using a fusion layer while implicitly embedding spatial information in the loss. We further improve on the ability of HCNNs to deal with imbalanced datasets by leveraging the proposed generalised Wasserstein Dice loss. To keep up with state-of-the-art CNNs, we also employ ELU as activation function [3] and use residual connections [10]. Residual blocks include a pair of 3^3 convolutional filters and Batch Normalisation [20]. The proposed architecture is illustrated in Fig. 2.

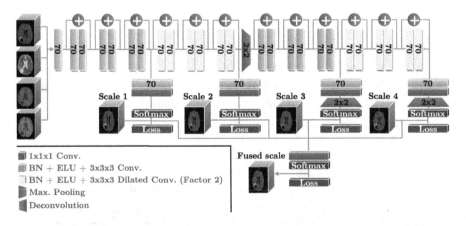

Fig. 2. Proposed holistically-nested CNN for multi-class labelling of brain tumours.

3.1 Multi-scale Prediction to Leverage Spatial Consistency in the Loss

As the receptive field increases across successive layers, predictions computed at different layers embed spatial information at different scales. Especially for imbalanced multi-class segmentation, different scales can contain complementary information. In this paper, to increase the receptive field and avoid redundancy between successive scale predictions, max pooling and dilated convolutions (with a factor of 2 similar to [13]) have been used. As predictions are computed regularly at intermediate scales along the network (Fig. 2), we chose to increase the number of features before the first prediction is made. For simplicity reasons, we then selected the same value for all hidden layers (fixed to 70 given memory constraints).

3.2 Multi-scale Fusion and Deep Supervision for Multi-class Segmentation

While classic CNNs provide only one output, HCNNs provide outputs $\hat{y}^s$ at S different layers of the network, and combine them to provide a final output $\hat{y}^{fuse}$:

$$(\hat{y}_l^{fuse})_{l \in \mathbf{L}} = \text{Softmax}\Big(\big(\sum_{s=1}^{S} w_{l,s}\hat{y}_l^s\big)_{l \in \mathbf{L}}\Big).$$

As different scales can be of different importance for different classes we learn class-specific fusion weights $w_{l,s}$. This transformation can also be represented by a convolution layer with kernels of size 1^3 where the multi-scale predictions are fused in separated branches for each class, as illustrated in Fig. 2 similarly to the scalable layers introduced in [5]. In addition to applying the loss function $\mathcal{L}$ to the fused prediction, $\mathcal{L}$ is also applied to each scale-specific prediction thereby providing deep supervision (coefficients $\bar{\lambda}$ and λ_s are set to $1/(S+1)$ for simplicity):

$$\mathcal{L}_{Total}((\hat{y}^s)_{s=1}^S, \hat{y}^{fuse}, y) = \bar{\lambda}\mathcal{L}(\hat{y}^{fuse}, y) + \sum_{s=1}^{S} \lambda_s \mathcal{L}(\hat{y}^s, y)$$

4 Implementation Details

4.1 Brain Tumour Segmentation

We evaluate our HCNN model and Wasserstein Dice loss functions on the task of brain tumour segmentation using BraTS'15 training set that provides multimodal images (T1, T1c, T2 and Flair) for 220 high-grade gliomas subjects and 54 low-grade gliomas subjects. We divide it randomly into 80% for training, 10% for validation and 10% for testing so that the proportion of high-grade and low-grade gliomas subjects is the same in each fold. The scans are labelled with five classes (Fig. 1): (0) background, (1) necrotic core, (2) edema, (3) non-enhancing core and (4) enhancing tumour. The most common evaluation criteria for BraTS is to use the Dice scores for the whole tumour (labels $1, 2, 3, 4$), the core tumour (labels $1, 3, 4$) and the enhanced tumour (label 4). All the scans of BraTS dataset are skull stripped, resampled to a 1 mm isotropic grid and co-registered to the T1-weighted volume of each patient. Additionally, we applied histogram standardisation to each imaging modality independently [16].

4.2   Implementation Details

We train the networks using ADAM [12] with a learning rate $lr = 0.01$, $\beta_1 = 0.9$ and $\beta_2 = 0.999$. To regularise the network, we use early stopping on the validation set and dropout in all residual blocks before the last activation (as proposed in [20]), with a probability of 0.6. We use multi-modal volumes of size 80^3 from one subject concatenated as input during training and a sampling strategy to maximise the number of classes in each patch. Experiments have been performed using Tensorflow 1.1[1] and a Nvidia GeForce GTX Titan X GPU.

5   Results

We evaluate the usefulness of the proposed soft multi-class Wasserstein Dice loss and the proposed HCNN with deep supervision. We compare the soft multi-class Wasserstein Dice loss to the state-of-the-art mean Dice score [5,13] for the training of our HCNN in Tables 1 and 2. We also evaluate the segmentation at the different scales of the HCNN in Table 3.

Table 1. Evaluation of different multi-class Dice scores for training and testing. $\mathcal{L}_{D^{M_{tree}} - PT}$ stands for pre-training the HCNN with mean Dice score (4 epochs) and retraining it with $\mathcal{L}_{D^{M_{tree}}}$ (85 epochs).

Loss function	Evaluation: Mean(std) Dice scores (%)					
	Whole	Core	Enh.	Mean Dice	$D^{M_{0-1}}$	$D^{M_{tree}}$
Mean Dice	83(13)	70(21)	68(26)	**60**(12)	77(11)	80(12)
$\mathcal{L}_{D^{M_{0-1}}}$	86(12)	59(29)	69(23)	48(5)	82(6)	85(5)
$\mathcal{L}_{D^{M_{tree}}}$	88(8)	**73**(23)	70(25)	54(7)	84(5)	86(5)
$\mathcal{L}_{D^{M_{tree}} - PT}$	**89**(6)	**73**(22)	**74**(23)	59(10)	**84**(4)	**87**(4)

5.1   Examples of Distance Metrics on BraTS Label Space

To illustrate the flexibility of the proposed generalised Wasserstein Dice score, we evaluate two semantically driven choices for the distance matrix M on **L**:

---

[1] The code is publicly available as part of NiftyNet (http://niftynet.io) [21].

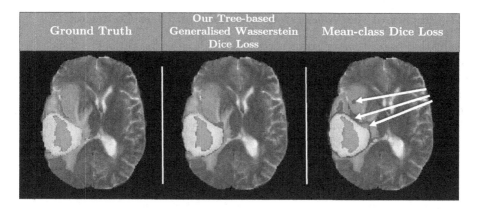

Fig. 3. Qualitative comparison of HCNN predictions at testing after training with the proposed Generalised Wasserstein Dice loss ($\mathcal{L}_{D^{M_{tree}}-PT}$) or mean-class Dice loss. Training with $\mathcal{L}_{D^{M_{tree}}-PT}$ allows avoiding implausible misclassifications encountered in predictions after training with mean-class Dice loss (emphasized by white arrows).

$$M_{0-1} = \begin{pmatrix} 0 & 1 & 1 & 1 & 1 \\ 1 & 0 & 1 & 1 & 1 \\ 1 & 1 & 0 & 1 & 1 \\ 1 & 1 & 1 & 0 & 1 \\ 1 & 1 & 1 & 1 & 0 \end{pmatrix}, \quad \text{and} \quad M_{tree} = \begin{pmatrix} 0 & 1 & 1 & 1 & 1 \\ 1 & 0 & 0.6 & 0.2 & 0.5 \\ 1 & 0.6 & 0 & 0.6 & 0.7 \\ 1 & 0.2 & 0.6 & 0 & 0.5 \\ 1 & 0.5 & 0.7 & 0.5 & 0 \end{pmatrix}.$$

M_{0-1} is associated with the discrete distance on $\mathbf{L}$ with no inter-class relationship. M_{tree} is derived from the tree structure of $\mathbf{L}$ illustrated in Fig. 1. This tree is based on the tumour hierarchical structure: whole, core and enhancing tumour. We set branch weights to 0.1 for contiguous nodes and 0.2 otherwise.

5.2 Evaluation and Training with Multi-class Dice Score

The mean Dice corresponds to the mean of soft Dice scores for each class as used in [5,13]. Results in Table 1 confirm that training with mean Dice score, $D^{M_{0-1}}$ or $D^{M_{tree}}$ allow maximising results for the associated multi-class Dice score during inference.

While $D^{M_{tree}}$ takes advantage of prior information about the hierarchical structure of the tumour classes it makes the optimisation more complex by adding more constraints. To relax those constraints, we propose to pretrain the network using the mean Dice score during a few epochs (4 in our experiment) and then retrain it using $D^{M_{tree}}$. This approach leads to the best results for all criteria, as illustrated in the last line of Table 1. Moreover, it produces segmentations that are more semantically plausible compared to the HCNN trained with mean Dice only as illustrated by Fig. 3.

5.3 Impact of the Wasserstein Dice Loss on Class Confusion

Evaluating brain tumour segmentation using Dice scores of label subsets like whole, core and enhancing tumour doesn't allow measuring the ability of a model to learn inter-class relationships and to favour voxel classifications, be it correct or not, that are semantically as close as possible to the ground truth. We propose to measure class confusion using pairwise comparisons of all labels pair between the predicted segmentation and the ground truth (Table 2). Mathematically, for all $l, l' \in \mathbf{L}$, the quantity in row l and colomn l' stands for the soft binary Dice score:

$$D_{l,l'} = \frac{2 \sum_i g_l^i p_{l'}^i}{\sum_i (g_l^i + p_{l'}^i)} \tag{12}$$

Table 2. Dice score evaluation of the confusion after training the HCNN using different loss functions. Each line (resp. column) corresponds to the mean(standard deviation) Dice scores (%) of a region of the ground truth (resp. prediction) with all regions of the prediction (resp. ground truth) computed on the testing set.

Mean Dice	Prediction				
Ground truth	Background	Necrotic core	Edema	Non-enh.	Enh.
Background	99.6(0)	0(0)	0.8(0)	0.1(0)	0.1(0)
Necrotic core	0.(0)	36.8(30)	1.2(3)	8.3(9)	1(1)
Edema	0.3(0)	0.9(1)	62.9(18)	21.7(13)	4.3(6)
Non-enh.	0.1(0)	8.7(9)	6.5(8)	33(15)	14.8(11)
Enh.	0(0)	0.9(1)	0.3(0)	6.9(7)	67.6(25)
$\mathcal{L}_{DM_{tree}}$	**Prediction**				
Ground truth	Background	Necrotic core	Edema	Non-enh.	Enh.
Background	99.7(0)	0(0)	0.3(0)	0(0)	0(0)
Necrotic core	0(0)	0(0)	2.4(5)	28.2(22)	1.4(1)
Edema	0.6(0)	0(0)	71.3(12)	8.5(7)	3.5(5)
Non-enh.	0.1(0)	0(0)	15.4(13)	28.9(14)	14.2(10)
Enh.	0(0)	0(0)	1.7(1)	6.9(7)	70.5(25)
$\mathcal{L}_{DM_{tree}-PT}$	**Prediction**				
Ground truth	Background	Necrotic core	Edema	Non-enh.	Enh.
Background	99.7(0)	0(0)	0.2(0)	0(0)	0(0)
Necrotic core	0(0)	20.2(27)	2.3(5)	23.2(18)	1(1)
Edema	0.6(0)	0.3(0)	73.3(11)	5.7(5)	3.1(4)
Non-enh.	0.1(0)	2.1(7)	16.1(13)	30(17)	13(8)
Enh.	0(0)	0(0)	2.4(2)	3.8(4)	73.5(22)

Table 3. Evaluation of scale-specific and fused predictions of the HCNN with Dice score of whole, core, enhancing tumour and D^{Mtree} after being pre-trained with mean Dice score (4 epochs) and retrained with $\mathcal{L}_{D^{Mtree}}$ (85 epochs).

Prediction	Mean(Std) Dice score (%)			
	Whole tumour	Core tumour	Enh. tumour	D^{Mtree}
Scale 1	84(8)	68(23)	70(25)	84(5)
Scale 2	**89**(5)	**73**(22)	**74**(23)	**87**(4)
Scale 3	88(6)	72(23)	71(22)	86(4)
Scale 4	**89**(5)	72(22)	71(21)	86(3)
Fused	89(6)	**73**(22)	**74**(23)	**87**(4)

Results in Table 2 compare class confusion of the proposed HCNN after being trained either using mean Dice loss, tree-based Wasserstein Dice loss ($\mathcal{L}_{D^{Mtree}}$) or tree-based Wasserstein Dice loss pre-trained with mean Dice loss($\mathcal{L}_{D^{Mtree}-PT}$). The first one aims only at maximising the true positives (diagonal) while the two other additionally aim at balancing the misclassifications to produce semnatically meaningful segmentations.

The network trained with mean Dice loss segments correctly most of the voxels (diagonal in Table 2) but makes misclassifications that are not semantically meaningful. For example, it makes poor differentiation between the edema and the core tumour as can be seen in the line corresponding to edema in Table 2 and in Fig. 3.

In contrast, the network trained with $\mathcal{L}_{D^{Mtree}}$ makes more meaningful confusion but it is not able to differentiate necrotic core and non-enhancing tumour at all (columns 2 and 4). It illustrates the difficulty to train the network with $\mathcal{L}_{D^{Mtree}}$ starting from a random initialisation because $\mathcal{L}_{D^{Mtree}}$ embeds more constraints than the mean Dice loss.

$\mathcal{L}_{D^{Mtree}-PT}$ allows combining advantages of both loss function: pre-training the network using the mean Dice loss allows initialising it so that it produces quickly an approximation of the segmentation, and retraining it with $\mathcal{L}_{D^{Mtree}}$ allows reaching a model which provides semantically meaningful segmentations (Fig. 3) with a higher rate of true positives compared to training with $\mathcal{L}_{D^{Mtree}}$ or mean Dice loss alone (Table 2).

5.4   Evaluation of Deep Supervision

Results in Table 3 are obtained after pre-training HCNN with mean Dice score during 4 epochs and then training it with $\mathcal{L}_{D^{Mtree}}$ during 85 additional epochs. Scales 2 to 4 and fused achieve similar Dice scores for whole, core tumour and the objective function D^{Mtree} while scale 1 obtains lower Dice scores. Holes in tumour segmentations produced by scale 1, as illustrated in Fig. 4, suggest an unsufficient receptive field could account for those lower Dice scores. The best

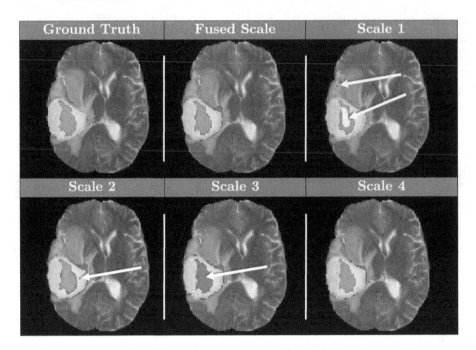

Fig. 4. Qualitative comparison of fused and scales predictions at testing after training our HCNN with the proposed Generalised Wasserstein Dice loss ($\mathcal{L}_{DM_{tree}-PT}$). White arrows emphasize implausible misclassifications.

result for the enhancing tumour is achievied by both scale 2 and fused, which was expected as this is the smallest region of interest and the full resolution is maintained until scale 2. Moreover, as illustrated in Fig. 4, scales 3 and 4 fail at segmenting the thinest regions of the tumour because of their lower resolution contrary to scales 1 and 2 and fused. However, scales 1 to 3 contained implausible segmentation regions contrary to scale 4 and fused. This suggests trade-offs between high receptive field and high resolution that are class specific. It confirms the usefulness of the multi-scale holistic approach for the multi-class brain tumour segmentation task.

6   Conclusion and Future Work

We proposed a semantically driven generalisation of the Dice score for soft multi-class segmentation based on the Wasserstein distance. This embeds prior knowledge about inter-class relationships represented by a distance matrix on the label space. Additionally, we proposed a holistic convolutional network that uses multi-scale predictions and deep supervision to make use of multi-scale information. We successfully used the proposed Wasserstein Dice score as a loss function to train our holistic networks and show the importance of multi-scale and inter-class relationships for the imbalanced task of multi-class brain tumour segmentation.

The proposed distance matrix based on the label space tree structure leads to higher Dice scores compared to the discrete distance. Because the tree-based distance matrix used was heuristically chosen we think that better heuristics or a method to directly learn the matrix from the data could lead to further improvements.

As the memory capacity of GPUs increases, entire multi-modal volumes could be used as input of CNN-based segmentation. However, it will also increase the class imbalance in the patches used as input. We expect this to increase the impact of our contributions. Future work includes extending the use of Wasserstein distance by defining a matrix distance on the entire output space $\mathbf{X} \times \mathbf{L}$ similarly to [6]. This would allow embedding spatial information directly in the loss, but the computation burden of the Wasserstein distance, in that case, remains a challenge [17].

Acknowledgement. This work was supported by the Wellcome Trust (WT101957, 203145Z/16/Z, HICF-T4-275, WT 97914), EPSRC (NS/A000027/1, EP/H046410/1, EP/J020990/1, EP/K005278, NS/A000050/1), the NIHR BRC UCLH/UCL, a UCL ORS/GRS Scholarship and a hardware donation from NVidia.

References

1. Anbeek, P., Vincken, K.L., van Bochove, G.S., van Osch, M.J., van der Grond, J.: Probabilistic segmentation of brain tissue in MR imaging. NeuroImage **27**(4), 795–804 (2005)
2. Chang, H.H., Zhuang, A.H., Valentino, D.J., Chu, W.C.: Performance measure characterization for evaluating neuroimage segmentation algorithms. Neuroimage **47**(1), 122–135 (2009)
3. Clevert, D.A., Unterthiner, T., Hochreiter, S.: Fast and accurate deep network learning by exponential linear units (elus). arXiv:1511.07289 (2015)
4. Crum, W.R., Camara, O., Hill, D.L.: Generalized overlap measures for evaluation and validation in medical image analysis. IEEE TMI **25**(11), 1451–1461 (2006)
5. Fidon, L., Li, W., Garcia-Peraza-Herrera, L.C., Ekanayake, J., Kitchen, N., Ourselin, S., Vercauteren, T.: Scalable multimodal convolutional networks for brain tumour segmentation. In: Descoteaux, M., Maier-Hein, L., Franz, A., Jannin, P., Collins, D.L., Duchesne, S. (eds.) MICCAI 2017, Part III. LNCS, vol. 10435, pp. 285–293. Springer, Cham (2017). https://doi.org/10.1007/978-3-319-66179-7_33
6. Fitschen, J.H., Laus, F., Schmitzer, B.: Optimal transport for manifold-valued images. In: Lauze, F., Dong, Y., Dahl, A.B. (eds.) SSVM 2017. LNCS, vol. 10302, pp. 460–472. Springer, Cham (2017). https://doi.org/10.1007/978-3-319-58771-4_37
7. Frogner, C., Zhang, C., Mobahi, H., Araya, M., Poggio, T.A.: Learning with a wasserstein loss. In: NIPS, pp. 2053–2061 (2015)
8. Garcia-Peraza-Herrera, L.C., Li, W., Fidon, L., Gruijthuijsen, C., Devreker, A., Attilakos, G., Deprest, J., Vander Poorten, E., Stoyanov, D., Vercauteren, T., Ourselin, S.: ToolNet: holistically-nested real-time segmentation of robotic surgical tools. In: IROS (2017)
9. Havaei, M., Davy, A., Warde-Farley, D., Biard, A., Courville, A., Bengio, Y., Pal, C., Jodoin, P.M., Larochelle, H.: Brain tumor segmentation with deep neural networks. Med. Image Anal. **35**, 18–31 (2017)

10. He, K., Zhang, X., Ren, S., Sun, J.: Deep residual learning for image recognition. In: IEEE CVPR (2016)

11. Kamnitsas, K., Ledig, C., Newcombe, V.F., Simpson, J.P., Kane, A.D., Menon, D.K., Rueckert, D., Glocker, B.: Efficient multi-scale 3D CNN with fully connected CRF for accurate brain lesion segmentation. Med. Image Anal. **36**, 61–78 (2017)

12. Kingma, D., Ba, J.: Adam: A method for stochastic optimization. arXiv:1412.6980 (2014)

13. Li, W., Wang, G., Fidon, L., Ourselin, S., Cardoso, M.J., Vercauteren, T.: On the compactness, efficiency, and representation of 3D convolutional networks: brain parcellation as a pretext task. In: Niethammer, M., Styner, M., Aylward, S., Zhu, H., Oguz, I., Yap, P.-T., Shen, D. (eds.) IPMI 2017. LNCS, vol. 10265, pp. 348–360. Springer, Cham (2017). https://doi.org/10.1007/978-3-319-59050-9_28

14. Menze, B.H., Jakab, A., Bauer, S., Kalpathy-Cramer, J., Farahani, K., Kirby, J., Burren, Y., Porz, N., Slotboom, J., Wiest, R., et al.: The multimodal brain tumor image segmentation benchmark (BraTS). IEEE TMI **34**(10), 1993–2024 (2015)

15. Milletari, F., Navab, N., Ahmadi, S.A.: V-Net: fully convolutional neural networks for volumetric medical image segmentation. In: Proceedings of 3DV 2016, pp. 565–571 (2016)

16. Nyul, L.G., Udupa, J.K., Zhang, X.: New variants of a method of MRI scale standardization. IEEE TMI **19**(2), 143–150 (2000)

17. Pele, O., Werman, M.: Fast and robust earth mover's distances. In: ICCV (2009)

18. Sudre, C.H., Li, W., Vercauteren, T., Ourselin, S., Cardoso, M.J.: Generalised Dice overlap as a deep learning loss function for highly unbalanced segmentations. In: Deep Learning in Medical Image Analysis and Multimodal Learning for Clinical Decision Support, pp. 240–248. Springer (2017)

19. Xie, S., Tu, Z.: Holistically-nested edge detection. In: ICCV (2015)

20. Zagoruyko, S., Komodakis, N.: Wide residual networks. arXiv:1605.07146 (2016)

21. Gibson, E., Li, W., Sudre, C., Fidon, L., Shakir, D., Wang, G., Eaton-Rosen, Z., Gray, R., Doel, T., Hu, Y., Whyntie, T.: NiftyNet: a deep-learning platform for medical imaging. arXiv preprint arXiv:1709.03485 (2017)

Overall Survival Time Prediction for High Grade Gliomas Based on Sparse Representation Framework

Guoqing Wu[1], Yuanyuan Wang[1(✉)], and Jinhua Yu[1,2(✉)]

[1] Department of Electronic Engineering, Fudan University, Shanghai, China
{yywang, jhyu}@fudan.edu.cn
[2] The Key Laboratory of Medical Imaging Computing and Computer Assisted Intervention of Shanghai, Shanghai, China

Abstract. Accurate prognosis for high grade glioma (HGG) is of great clinical value since it would provide optimized guidelines for treatment planning. Previous imaging-based survival prediction generally relies on some features guided by clinical experiences, which limits the full utilization of biomedical image. In this paper, we propose a sparse representation-based radiomics framework to predict overall survival (OS) time of HGG. Firstly, we develop a patch-based sparse representation method to extract the high-throughput tumor texture features. Then, we propose to combine locality preserving projection and sparse representation to select discriminating features. Finally, we treat the OS time prediction as a classification task and apply sparse representation to classification. Experiment results show that, with 10-fold cross-validation, the proposed method achieves the accuracy of 94.83% and 95.69% by using T1 contrast-enhanced and T2 weighted magnetic resonance images, respectively.

Keywords: High grade gliomas · Survival time prediction
Sparse representation

1 Introduction

High grade gliomas (HGG), the World Health Organization (WHO) grade III and IV, not only exhibit a very poor prognosis but also have significant difference in terms of overall survival (OS) time. An accurate preoperative prediction of HGG is highly desired by clinicians since it helps the treatment planning.

WHO histopathologic grading, imaging characteristics, and some basic clinical information have been widely used to investigate their relationship to OS time [1–5]. Pope et al. [1] analyzed 15 T1 MRI features and found that non-enhancing tumor, edema, and multifocality/satellites were statistically significant predictors of OS. In [3], about 60 features including imaging characteristics and clinical information were used to derive imaging predictors of patient survival via machine learning algorithm. Tumors growth may change both the structural and the functional brain connectivities. Therefore, authors in [4, 5] extracted features from diffusion tensor imaging (DTI) and functional magnetic resonance imaging (fMRI) images, respectively, to study the OS time of glioblastoma patients. Most of these methods used the handcrafted and

© Springer International Publishing AG, part of Springer Nature 2018
A. Crimi et al. (Eds.): BrainLes 2017, LNCS 10670, pp. 77–87, 2018.
https://doi.org/10.1007/978-3-319-75238-9_7

engineered features guided by the previous clinical experiences, which often limits the ability to take full advantage of all the underlying pathophysiologic information in biomedical images.

Recently, radiomics has been successfully used in clinical diagnosis and prognosis [6]. By converting medical images into mineable high-throughput features, radiomics provides a more comprehensive quantification of the entire tumor, and subsequently makes effective decision on these data. In [7], 402 radiomic features extracted from the peritumoral brain zone (PBZ) were used to evaluate the efficacy of PBZ features in predicting survival in glioblastoma. Zhang et al. [8] exploited the combination of 255 radiomics features and 15 clinical features to predict OS and progression-free survival via four machine learning models, and achieved promising prediction performance. Multi-modality radiomics features were combined in [9] to predict the OS time for HGG. Among these applications of radiomics, extracting and selecting effective features for specific problem is very crucial, since good features lead directly to accurate classification.

Sparse representation (SR) has demonstrated great advantages in image restoration, feature selection and pattern recognition. In image processing, SR generally exploits adaptive learning dictionaries rather than the traditional analytically-designed dictionaries with fixed basis, such as wavelet, to represent images. Therefore it gave rise to the ability to extract or represent some small textures and details [10] which usually play a critical role in image classification. In addition, SR considers that natural signals can be represented linearly by a small number of atoms in dictionary. These atoms represent the essential features of target data and can be selected by the lp-norm regularizer of sparse model [11]. Based on this principle, SR is successfully used for feature selection [12], canonical correlation analysis [13] and multi-output linear regression [14].

Based on the advantages of SR in extracting image texture information and selecting the essential features of data, we propose a SR-based radiomics framework to predict the OS time for HGG. Specifically, first, we develop a SR-based method to convert the statistical distribution of tumor texture into high-throughput texture features. Second, we propose a novel model combining locality preserving projection (LPP) and SR to select the most discriminative features. Particularly, a new structure preservation regularizer is introduced in feature selection model for considering the structures of within-class samples and between-class samples. Meanwhile, SR-based effective distance is used to measure the structural relationships among samples. Finally, we use sparse representation classification (SRC) [15] to predict the OS time.

2 Data Acquisition and Preprocessing

We use the dataset provided by the *Medical Image Computing and Computer Assisted Intervention (MICCAI)* 'BraTS 2017' to validate the proposed method [16–18]. The provided data are distributed after their pre-processing, i.e. co-registered to the same anatomical template, interpolated to the resolution and skull-stripped. The size and voxel resolution of the provided images are 240 * 240 * 155 and 1 * 1 * 1 mm^3, respectively. Tumor segmentation results based on the benchmark proposed by [19] have also been included in the dataset. According to 'BraTS 2017', we cast the OS time prediction problem as a multi-classification task and divide the data into three categories based on survival, i.e. long-survivors (e.g., >18 months), mid-survivors (e.g. between 6 and 18 months) and short-survivors (e.g., <6 months). Finally, our data set consists of 37 long-survivors, 39 mid-survivors and 40 short-survivors. By following the suggestions of doctors, we choose T1 contrast-enhanced and T2-weighted MRI images for the study of the OS time prediction.

We perform some automatic pretreatment on the provided segmentation results prior to the following analysis. Specifically, first, remove some regions with less than 50 voxels. Second, select the maximal connected region. Finally, fill segmentation regions. Figure 1(a) and (b) show the segmentation results before and after pretreatment, respectively. As shown in Fig. 1(c), the provided segmentation results include 4 categories: the necrotic and non-enhancing tumor (NCR/NET), peritumoral edema (ED), the GD-enhancing tumor (ET), and everything else. ED is usually smoother and has less texture information than NCR/NET and ET, while the proposed method exploits the texture feature to classify images. Therefore we only use the image information in NCR/NET and ET (region outlined in green and red) to predict the OS time.

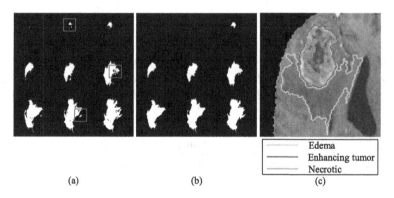

Edema
Enhancing tumor
Necrotic

(a)   (b)   (c)

Fig. 1. Illustrations of the pretreatment and the target region we will study. (Color figure online)

3 The Proposed Method

3.1 Sparse Representation-Based Feature Extraction

Tumor phenotypic information, especially some texture information, is found to be highly correlated with prognosis. In this paper, based on the concept of bag-of-feature (BoF), we propose a SR-based texture feature extraction which first perform sparse coding for the local image texture information, then use the histogram of the coding coefficient to represent the global texture features. Figure 2 shows the flow chart of the SR-based feature extraction. First, we extract image patch sets from the segmented tumor images. Specifically, multiply the 3D image matrix by the segmentation label matrix to obtain the segmented tumor image, then extract image patches form each layer of tumor images with the sliding distance of 5 pixels. We denote by $\mathbf{Y}_L \in \mathbf{R}^{n \times d}$,

$\mathbf{Y}_M \in \mathbf{R}^{n \times d}$ and $\mathbf{Y}_S \in \mathbf{R}^{n \times d}$ the extracted image patch sets corresponding to long-survivors, mid-survivors and short-survivors, respectively. Where n and d denote the size and number of image patches, respectively. Second, we learn three dictionaries $\mathbf{D}_L \in \mathbf{R}^{n \times k}$, $\mathbf{D}_M \in \mathbf{R}^{n \times k}$ and $\mathbf{D}_S \in \mathbf{R}^{n \times k}$ from $\mathbf{Y}_L \in \mathbf{R}^{n \times d}$, $\mathbf{Y}_M \in \mathbf{R}^{n \times d}$ and $\mathbf{Y}_S \in \mathbf{R}^{n \times d}$, respectively, by using the K-singular value decomposition algorithm [20]. Last, we put the three learning dictionaries together for constructing the final feature extraction dictionary $\mathbf{D} = [\mathbf{D}_L, \mathbf{D}_M, \mathbf{D}_S] \in \mathbf{R}^{n \times 3k}$.

Note that, since the three sub-dictionaries are learned from images of the corresponding classes, respectively. They contain some exclusive texture features of each class of images. Hence, using $\mathbf{D}$ to sparsely represent the test image, the statistical distribution of the representation coefficients can naturally reflect the correlation between the testing image and these three classes of images. Suppose $\mathbf{Y} = [\mathbf{y}_1, \cdots \mathbf{y}_i, \cdots \mathbf{y}_m]$ represents the image patch set extracted from a testing image, where $\mathbf{y}_i$ denotes the i-th image patch, m denotes the number of image patches. The proposed feature extraction model is formulated as:

$$
\begin{cases}
\hat{\Lambda} = \sum_{i=1}^{m} \arg\min_{\alpha_i} \|\mathbf{y}_i - \mathbf{D}\alpha_i\|_2^2 + \phi\|\alpha_i\|_0 \\
f = \frac{1}{m}\sum_{i=1}^{m} |\alpha_i|
\end{cases}
, \tag{1}
$$

where $\hat{\Lambda} = [\alpha_1, \cdots \alpha_i, \cdots \alpha_m]$, $\alpha_i \in R^{3k}$ is the SR coefficients corresponding to $\mathbf{y}_i$, ϕ is a regularization parameter. $f \in R^{3k}$ is the final obtained texture feature. Orthogonal matching pursuit (OMP) algorithm could be used to solve the SR model in Eq. (1).

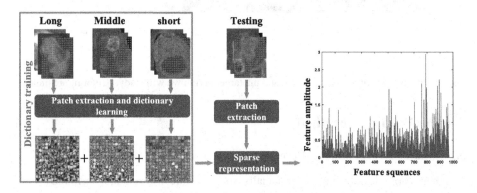

Fig. 2. Sparse representation-based feature extraction.

3.2   Sparse Representation-Based Feature Selection

The extracted high-dimensional feature contains lots of redundant information which not only increases the computational complexity, but also has negative effects on classification. Hence, we propose a SR-based feature selection method to select the discriminative features for classification. Feature selection method combined LPP and SR demonstrates promising performance [21], whose model is formulated as:

$$\min_{\mathbf{w}} \frac{1}{2}\left\|\hat{\mathbf{X}} - \mathbf{w}^T\mathbf{F}\right\|_F^2 + \lambda_1 tr(\mathbf{w}^T\mathbf{F}\mathbf{L}\mathbf{F}^T\mathbf{w}) + \lambda_2\|\mathbf{w}\|_{2,1}, \qquad (2)$$

where $\hat{\mathbf{X}} \in \mathbf{R}^{C \times N}$ denotes a coding matrix of class labels, $\mathbf{F} = [\boldsymbol{f}_1 \cdots \boldsymbol{f}_i \cdots \boldsymbol{f}_N] \in \mathbf{R}^{d \times N}$ denotes high-dimensional feature data, d, N and C are respectively the number of feature variables, subjects and classes. $\mathbf{w} \in \mathbf{R}^{d \times C}$ is a coefficient matrix whose zero rows correspond to the redundant features. $\mathbf{L} \in \mathbf{R}^{N \times N}$ is the graph laplacian matrix that keeps the structure information between samples. $tr(\mathbf{w}^T\mathbf{F}\mathbf{L}\mathbf{F}^T\mathbf{w})$ and $\|\mathbf{w}\|_{2,1}$ are the structure preservation and sparse regularization terms, respectively. λ_1 and λ_2 are the tuning parameters. For model (2), theoretically, the structural information reflected in $\mathbf{L}$ should be that the similarity of within-class samples are higher than that of between-class samples. But in practice, unexpected noise and redundant information may lead to opposite results in the process of calculating $\mathbf{L}$. As a result, the undesired structural information stored in $\mathbf{L}$ may not guarantee the class-discriminative power of selected features. For this end, we construct within-class and between-class structure preservation regularization terms to preserve the structure information of samples, respectively. Meanwhile we exploit SR-based effective distance [22] to measure the structure information.

Specifically, first, we compute similarity matrix $\mathbf{S} = \{S_{i,j}\}_{i,j=1}^N$ based on effective distance [22], where $S_{i,j}$ denotes the similarity between $\boldsymbol{f}_i$ and $\boldsymbol{f}_j$. Then according to $\mathbf{S}$ and class information of samples, we construct two disjoint sets for each sample:

$$\begin{cases} knn_w(i) = \{\boldsymbol{f}_i^j | \boldsymbol{f}_i^j \text{ and } \boldsymbol{f}_i \text{ are in the same class, } 1 \leq j \leq k\} \\ knn_b(i) = \{\boldsymbol{f}_i^j | \boldsymbol{f}_i^j \text{ and } \boldsymbol{f}_i \text{ are in different class, } 1 \leq j \leq k\} \end{cases}, \qquad (3)$$

where $\boldsymbol{f}_i^j$ is the j-nearest sample to $\boldsymbol{f}_i$, k is a constant. Based on (3), we define two weight matrices $\mathbf{S}^w = \{S_{i,j}^w\}_{i,j=1}^N$ and $\mathbf{S}^b = \{S_{i,j}^b\}_{i,j=1}^N$ to restore the within-class and between-class structure information, respectively:

$$S_{i,j}^w = \begin{cases} 1, & \boldsymbol{f}_i \in knn_w(j) \text{ or } \boldsymbol{f}_j \in knn_w(i) \\ 0, & \text{otherwise} \end{cases}, \qquad (4)$$

$$S_{i,j}^b = \begin{cases} 1, & \boldsymbol{f}_i \in knn_b(j) \text{ or } \boldsymbol{f}_j \in knn_b(i) \\ 0, & \text{otherwise} \end{cases}. \qquad (5)$$

In order to effectively keep the structural information of samples in feature selection, we define the following regularization term:

$$R(\mathbf{w}) = \beta \sum_{i=1}^N \sum_{j=1}^k \left\|\mathbf{w}^T\boldsymbol{f}_i - \mathbf{w}^T\boldsymbol{f}_j\right\|_2^2 S_{i,j}^w - (1-\beta) \sum_{i=1}^N \sum_{j=1}^k \left\|\mathbf{w}^T\boldsymbol{f}_i - \mathbf{w}^T\boldsymbol{f}_j\right\|_2^2 S_{i,j}^b, \qquad (6)$$

where the first and the second terms in Eq. (6) are used to measure the compactness of within-class samples and the separation of between-class samples, respectively. $0 \leq \beta \leq 1$ is the tuning parameter. Hence, in the process of feature selection, minimizing Eq. (6) will keep the within-class samples closer while between-class samples far away in the dimension-reduced feature space, leading to an easier classification of samples. Let $\mathbf{D}^w$ and $\mathbf{D}^b$ denote two diagonal matrices, where $D^w_{i,i} = \sum_{j=1}^{N} S^w_{i,j}$ and $D^b_{i,i} = \sum_{j=1}^{N} S^b_{i,j}$, then the regularization term Eq. (6) can be rewritten as:

$$R(\mathbf{w}) = \beta tr(\mathbf{w}^T \mathbf{FL}^w \mathbf{F}^T \mathbf{w}) - (1 - \beta) tr(\mathbf{w}^T \mathbf{FL}^b \mathbf{F}^T \mathbf{w}), \tag{7}$$

where $\mathbf{L}^w = \mathbf{D}^w - \mathbf{S}^w$ and $\mathbf{L}^b = \mathbf{D}^b - \mathbf{S}^b$ are the two graph Laplacian matrices, $\mathbf{F} = [\mathbf{f}_1 \cdots \mathbf{f}_i \cdots \mathbf{f}_N]$. Finally, we formulate our SR-based feature selection model as:

$$\min_{\mathbf{w}} \frac{1}{2} \left\| \hat{\mathbf{X}} - \mathbf{w}^T \mathbf{F} \right\|_F^2 + \mu_1 [\beta tr(\mathbf{w}^T \mathbf{FL}^w \mathbf{F}^T \mathbf{w}) - (1 - \beta) tr(\mathbf{w}^T \mathbf{FL}^b \mathbf{F}^T \mathbf{w})] + \mu_2 \|\mathbf{w}\|_{2,1}, \tag{8}$$

where regularization parameters μ_1 and μ_2 are used to balance the tradeoff between the three regularization terms. Objective function (8) can be solved by the accelerated proximal gradient method [21]. Once we obtain the sparse matrix $\mathbf{w}$, we rank the l_2-norm value of each row of $\mathbf{w}$ in the descending order, then select features corresponding to the top-ranked rows.

3.3   Sparse Representation Classification

SRC proposed in [15] has achieved much success in pattern classification due to its good properties in handling errors and avoiding over-fitting. Hence, we apply SRC to predict the OS time based on the selected features. Suppose $f_t \in \mathbf{R}^q$ represents a testing sample feature, q is the number of the selected features. Suppose $\mathbf{A} = [\mathbf{A}_1, \cdots \mathbf{A}_c, \cdots \mathbf{A}_C]$ represents the feature set of training samples, C is the number of classes, $\mathbf{A}_c$ is the training feature set from class c. The SRC can be described as the following two steps.

1. Sparsely code f_t over $\mathbf{A}$ by solving:

$$\hat{\chi} = \arg\min_{\chi} \|f_t - \mathbf{A}\chi\|_2^2 + \gamma\|\chi\|_1 \tag{9}$$

   where $\hat{\chi}$ is the sparse representation coefficient to be calculated. γ is a regularization parameter.
2. Identify the class label of f_t via:

$$ID(f_t) = \arg\min_{c} \|f_t - \mathbf{A}\delta_c(\hat{\chi})\|_2^2 \tag{10}$$

   where $\delta_c(\cdot)$ is used to select the coefficients associated with the c-th class.

4   Experimental Results

4.1   Classification Accuracy

For each subject in the data set, we first extract 1452 texture features from T1 contrast-enhanced and T2-weighted MRI images, respectively, by using the method described in Sect. 3.1. Then we use the SR-based feature selection method to remove the redundant features. Finally, the selected features are fed into SRC to predict OS time. We use leave-one-out cross validation (LOOCV) and 10-fold cross validation (Tenth) to validate the proposed model, respectively. Particularly, we average the feature selection results of the training set of every cross validation to get the final feature selection result. In the proposed method, the size of patch is set to 11×11. Dictionaries are trained with four-fold redundancy. The sparsity of the OMP algorithm for solving (1) is set to $3/1452$, μ_1, μ_2 and β in (8) are set to 0.1, 1 and 0.9. γ is set to 1e -5. We calculate the classification accuracy of the overall subjects and each class of subjects, respectively, to evaluate the prediction performance. The prediction results of the proposed framework is reported in Table 1. For 'T1-Loocv', 'T1-Tenth', 'T2-Loocv' and 'T2-Tenth', the parts before and behind dash represent the used image modality and cross validation method, respectively.

We can see from Table 1 that the texture feature of T1 contrast-enhanced image achieves the promising prediction result, with the highest accuracy of 96.55% in terms of LOOCV, and the corresponding accuracy of each class of subjects reach 91.89%, 97.44% and 100%, respectively. For the two modalities, the gaps between the results of two validation methods are less than 3%. This demonstrates that the proposed method has high robustness in terms of the proportion of training samples to testing samples. In addition, the prediction performance of these two modalities is close to each other.

Table 1. Prediction accuracy of different features and validation methods (%).

Method	ACC	ACC-long	ACC-middle	ACC-short
T1-Loocv	**96.55**	91.89	97.44	100.0
T1-Tenth	94.83	94.59	89.74	100.0
T2-Loocv	93.10	97.30	92.31	90.00
T2-Tenth	95.69	91.89	97.44	97.50

Figure 3 shows the curves of classification accuracy versus different numbers of selected T1 contrast-enhanced features. Where [21] refers to that we use model (2) to select features. We can see that, in the case of the same extracted features and classifier, the proposed feature selection method achieves the overall better performances than [21]. Particularly, our method obtains the improvement of accuracy more than 3% over [21] in terms of the highest and the lowest classification accuracy. In addition, using the same number of selected features, the proposed method achieves higher classification accuracies than [21] in most cases.

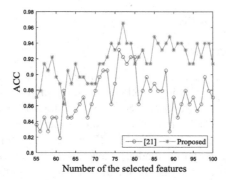

Fig. 3. Classification accuracies versus different numbers of selected features.

4.2 Effects of Parameters on Classification Accuracy

Figure 4 shows the classification performance versus the patch size $\sqrt{n}$ (T1 contrast image features, LOOCV). As could be seen, the classification performances of $\sqrt{n} = 11$ and $\sqrt{n} = 13$ are close to each other, while are obviously superior to that of $\sqrt{n} = 9$. Generally, the smaller the size of image patch, the lower the texture resolution of image patch. In terms of our OS time classification task, when the patch size is lower than 11, the effect of the texture information in image patch on tumor image classification decrease obviously. Considering the computational complexity, we set the patch size to 11 in our method. Figure 5 presents the parameters' sensitivity by changing values μ_1 and μ_2 in Eq. (8) (T1 contrast image features, LOOCV). We can clearly see that, when $\mu_2 \leq 1$, the accuracy slightly fluctuate with the change of the two parameters and all accuracies are higher than 90%. The best parameter combination is found to be $\mu_1 = 0.1$ and $\mu_2 = 1$. Figure 6 shows the classification performance versus γ (T1 contrast image features, LOOCV). As could be seen, the accuracies corresponding to 1e–5 and 1e–4 are very close and higher than that corresponding to 1e–3 and 1e–2 in most cases. We set $\gamma = 1e–5$ in Eq. (6).

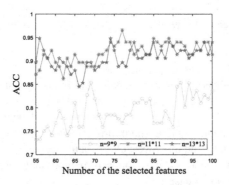

Fig. 4. Classification accuracies with respect to the size of image patch.

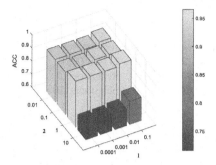

Fig. 5. Classification accuracies versus parameters μ_1 and μ_2.

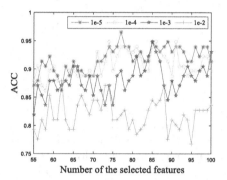

Fig. 6. Classification accuracies versus γ.

5   Conclusions

In this paper, we proposed a novel sparse representation framework to predict the (long, middle or short) OS time for HGG patients. Based on the assumption that tumors with different OS time demonstrate different texture features, we first learned a dictionary containing these discriminative features through dictionary training, and quantified the texture feature of testing images by sparsely representing these images over the training dictionary. Then we designed a feature selection method combining sparse representation and LPP to select the most discriminative features. Finally, the selected features were fed into SRC classifier for OS time prediction. Experimental results shown that our extracted features significantly improved the predictive accuracy of OS time. This further demonstrates that there is a close relationship between image texture and the OS time, even though these relationship is still poorly understood in clinical, the proposed method will help to understand it.

Acknowledgments. This work was supported by the National Basic Research Program of China (2015CB755500), the National Natural Science Foundation of China (61471125, 11474071).

References

1. Pope, W.B., et al.: MR imaging correlates of survival in patients with high-grade gliomas. AJNR Am. J. Neuroradiol. **26**(10), 2466–2474 (2005)
2. Gutman, D.A., et al.: MR imaging predictors of molecular profile and survival: multi-institutional study of the TCGA glioblastoma data set. Radiology **267**(2), 560–569 (2013)
3. Macyszyn, L., et al.: Imaging patterns predict patient survival and molecular subtype in glioblastoma via machine learning techniques. Neuro-Oncology **18**(3), 417–425 (2016)
4. Zacharaki, E.I., et al.: Survival analysis of patients with high-grade gliomas based on data mining of imaging variables. Am. J. Neuroradiol. **33**(6), 1065–1071 (2012)
5. Pillai, J.J., Zacá, D.: Clinical utility of cerebrovascular reactivity mapping in patients with low grade gliomas (2011)
6. Aerts, H.J.: The potential of radiomic-based phenotyping in precision medicine: a review. JAMA Oncol. **2**(12), 1636–1642 (2016)
7. Prasanna, P., et al.: Radiomic features from the peritumoral brain parenchyma on treatment-naïve multi-parametric MR imaging predict long versus short-term survival in glioblastoma multiforme: preliminary findings. Eur. Radiol., 1–10 (2016)
8. Zhang, H., et al.: SU-F-R-04: radiomics for survival prediction in glioblastoma (GBM). Med. Phys. **43**(6), 3373 (2016)
9. Liu, L., Zhang, H., Rekik, I., Chen, X., Wang, Q., Shen, D.: Outcome prediction for patient with high-grade gliomas from brain functional and structural networks. In: Ourselin, S., Joskowicz, L., Sabuncu, M.R., Unal, G., Wells, W. (eds.) MICCAI 2016. LNCS, vol. 9901, pp. 26–34. Springer, Cham (2016). https://doi.org/10.1007/978-3-319-46723-8_4
10. Dong, W., et al.: Image reconstruction with locally adaptive sparsity and nonlocal robust regularization. Signal Process-Image. Commun. **27**(10), 1109–1122 (2012)
11. Zhu, X., et al.: Robust joint graph sparse coding for unsupervised spectral feature selection. IEEE Trans. Neural Netw. Learn. Syst. **28**(6), 1263–1275 (2017)
12. Lin, D., et al.: Sparse models for correlative and integrative analysis of imaging and genetic data. J. Neurosci. Meth. **237**, 69–78 (2014)
13. Lin, D., et al.: Correspondence between fMRI and SNP data by group sparse canonical correlation analysis. Med. Image Anal. **18**(6), 891–902 (2016)
14. Vounou, M., et al.: Discovering genetic associations with high-dimensional neuroimaging phenotypes: a sparse reduced-rank regression approach. Neuroimage **53**(3), 1147–1159 (2010)
15. Wright, J., et al.: Robust face recognition via sparse representation. IEEE Trans. Pattern Anal. Mach. Intell. **31**(2), 210–227 (2009)
16. Bakas, S., et al.: Advancing the cancer genome atlas glioma MRI collections with expert segmentation labels and radiomic features. Nat. Sci. Data (2017, in press)
17. Bakas, S., et al.: Segmentation labels and radiomic features for the pre-operative scans of the TCGA-GBM collection. The Cancer Imaging Archive (2017). https://doi.org/10.7937/K9/TCIA.2017.KLXWJJ1Q
18. Bakas, S., et al.: Segmentation labels and radiomic features for the pre-operative scans of the TCGA-GBM collection. The Cancer Imaging Archive (2017). https://doi.org/10.7937/K9/TCIA.2017.GJQ7R0EF
19. Menze, B.H., et al.: The multimodal brain tumor image segmentation benchmark (BRATS). IEEE Trans. Med. Imaging **34**(10), 1993–2024 (2015)

20. Elad, M., Aharon, M.: Image denoising via sparse and redundant representations over learned dictionaries. IEEE Trans. Image Process. **15**(12), 3736–3745 (2006)
21. Zhu, X., et al.: Subspace regularized sparse multi-task learning for multi-class neurodegenerative disease identification. IEEE Trans. Biomed. Eng. **63**(3), 607–618 (2016)
22. Liu, M., Zhang, D.: Feature selection with effective distance. Neurocomputing **215**, 100–109 (2016)

Traumatic Brain Lesion Quantification Based on Mean Diffusivity Changes

Christophe Maggia[1,2,3], Thomas Mistral[1,2,3], Senan Doyle[4], Florence Forbes[2,5], Alexandre Krainik[1,2,3], Damien Galanaud[6], Emmanuelle Schmitt[7], Stéphane Kremer[8], Irène Troprès[2,3,9,10], Emmanuel L. Barbier[1,2], Jean-François Payen[1,2,3], and Michel Dojat[1,2(✉)] (iD)

[1] INSERM, U1216, 38000 Grenoble, France
michel.dojat@univ-grenoble-alpes.fr
[2] Université Grenoble Alpes, GIN, 38000 Grenoble, France
[3] CHUGA, 38000 Grenoble, France
[4] Pixyl, 38000 Grenoble, France
[5] Inria, MISTIS, 38330 Montbonnot, France
[6] APHP, Hopital Pitié Salpétrière, 75000 Paris, France
[7] CHU, Hopital Central, 54000 Nancy, France
[8] CHU de Strasbourg, 67000 Strasbourg, France
[9] CNRS, UMR 3552, 38000 Grenoble, France
[10] INSERM, U17, 38000 Grenoble, France

Abstract. We report the evaluation of an automated method for quantification of brain tissue damage, caused by a severe traumatic brain injury, using mean diffusivity computed from MR diffusion images. Our automatic results obtained on realistic phantoms and real patient images 10 days post-event provided by nine different centers were coherent with four expert manually identified lesions. For realistic phantoms automated method scores were equal to 0.77, 0.77 and 0.83 for Dice, Precision and Sensibility respectively compared to 0.78, 0.72 and 0.86 for the experts. The inter correlation class (ICC) was 0.79. For 7/9 real cases 0.57, 0.50 and 0.70 were respectively obtained for automated method compared to 0.60, 0.52 and 0.78 for experts with ICC = 0.71. Additionally, we detail the quality control module used to pool data from various image provider centers. This study clearly demonstrates the validity of the proposed automated method to eventually compute in a multi-centre project, the lesional load following brain trauma based on MD changes.

1 Introduction

In Europe, the incidence of hospitalization in intensive care units (ICUs) for fatal traumatic brain injury (TBI) is about 235 per 100,000 inhabitants [14]. Despite substantial efforts made over the past decades, the mortality rate following severe TBI, as defined by an initial Glasgow Coma Scale (GCS) score of less than 9, ranges between 30% and 50%, and only 20% of these patients will not have lasting disabilities [15]. Timely evacuation of mass lesions and strict

© Springer International Publishing AG, part of Springer Nature 2018
A. Crimi et al. (Eds.): BrainLes 2017, LNCS 10670, pp. 88–99, 2018.
https://doi.org/10.1007/978-3-319-75238-9_8

avoidance of conditions known to aggravate primary brain injury, such as arterial hypotension, systemic hypoxia, or severe hypocapnia form the mainstays of current management of severe TBI patients hospitalized in ICUs. OxyTC, a randomized controlled multi-centre trial (22 centers, objective of 400 patients), was initiated in 2016 to assess the impact of a new therapeutic strategy for severe TBI patients. The study continuously monitors brain tissue oxygenation using brain tissue O_2 pressure probes (PbtO_2) surgically inserted into the parenchyma to facilitate the detection of brain ischemic/hypoxic episodes and adapt consequently the therapy. Brain lesion volume is considered to be a clinically relevant criterion [1], and its evolution was analyzed to determine the efficacy of the therapeutic strategy. MRI is an excellent modality for estimating global and regional alterations in TBI and for following their longitudinal evolution [2]. Mean Diffusivity (MD) or Apparent Diffusion Coefficient (ADC) have been widely used to determine the volume of ischemic tissue [12]. A reduction of MD is related to cytotoxic edema while an increase of MD indicates a vasogenic edema [13]. A few papers address the quantification of brain damage following severe TBI [6] especially in acute phase i.e. less than ten days post-injury [13]. No evaluation of automatic quantification methods compared to manual delineation was reported. In this paper, we report the extensive evaluation of an existing automated method for quantification of brain tissue damage based on MD values [9]. We used both ground truth images (realistic phantoms) and real patient images 10 days post-event. Automated and manual delineations from 4 senior neuroradiologists (AK, DG, SK and ES) were then compared. Ultimately, our goal is to use the validated automated method for processing the large set of images provided by the OxyTC multi-centre study. A specific quality control pipeline was then designed to deal with the artefacts that may be present in the MR images coming from various scanners (3 different constructors, 9 different models). The quality pipeline coupled with our automatic segmentation method defines a valid methodology for our on-going multi-centre study.

2   Materials and Methods

The study was approved by the Institutional Review Board at the Hospital of Grenoble and informed consents were obtained prior to participation directly from the participants (controls) or next of kin (patients).

2.1   Datasets

Two types of datasets were used for an appropriate evaluation noted hereafter denoted by DS1 and DS2.

DS1: Realistic Phantoms. To overcome the absence of a gold standard, synthetic realistic lesions were manually inserted by a neuroradiologist (TM) in five healthy DTI acquired on a Philips Achieva 3.0T TX at the IRMaGe MRI facility (Grenoble, France; sequence parameters are indicated below). The range of multiplying coefficients applied to normal MD values was between 0.45 and 2.2, simulating cytotoxic (low MD) and vasogenic (high MD) edemas. Gaussian filtering was applied to increase realism. These five cases constituted our gold standard (see Fig. 2). Normative values were calculated on seven different control DTIs acquired in the same conditions.

DS2. Patients. Nine patients with a diagnosis of severe trauma were considered (GCS < 9). FLAIR, 3D-T1w, T2* and DTI images were acquired in 9 centers (one per patient) on different scanners (3T and 1.5T) with a standardized acquisition protocol including slight differences depending on the scanner (main 3T parameters FLAIR: TR/TE/TI:5000/390/1800 ms, 27 contiguous slices, 1 mm^3; 3D T1-weighted sequence: MPRAGE,TR/TE/TI: 2300/2/900 ms, $1 \times 1 \times 1$ mm^3; T2*: TR/TE:2200/16 ms, flip angle: 16°, $1 \times 1 \times 2$ mm^3; and axial DTI: TR/TE: 9800/80, 2 mm^3, 32 directions with a value of 1000 mT/m). A series without the diffusion gradient (the B-zero image) and a series with a phase encoding direction inversion were acquired for correction of spatial distortion. For each center, normative values were calculated on three control DTIs acquired in the same conditions.

2.2   Image Processing

Quality Control. To maximize data quality we adopted the same types of MR images in each center and harmonized MR acquisition protocols across sites. However, several factors were site-dependent such as magnetic field strength (1.5T or 3T), equipment manufacturers and models. Consequently, acquisition protocols had to be adapted depending on the scanner characteristics. All these factors may impact the MD measurement across scanners. Moreover, DTI is very sensitive to a number of imaging artefacts, in particular spatial distorTions that vary depending on the acquisition conditions. A specific pipeline (see Fig. 1) was therefore developed to check for the quality of the images coming from different centers. All DICOM tags were compared to a center-specific reference validated by a MR physicist (IT). Any change in a crucial sequence parameter (e.g. Echo Time for DTI) led to exam rejection. DTI were denoised [11] and hypo or hyper-intense slices were automatically detected. A visual check was performed to detect unusual artifacts. When necessary, artifacted slices were corrected by interpolating adjacent slices. If too many artifacted slices were present, the corresponding exam was rejected. DTI were then preprocessed using FSL[1] for geometric distortion correction. Two DWI images with opposite phase encoding directions were acquired to compute a fieldmap and correct the susceptibility artifacts. For the automated method, T1-weighted, FLAIR and T2* images were realigned to the corresponding corrected DTI image. The two former sequences were then processed using P-LOCUS, a Bayesian Markovian approach for tissue and CSF segmentation [3].

---

[1] http://www.fmrib.ox.ac.uk/fsl/.

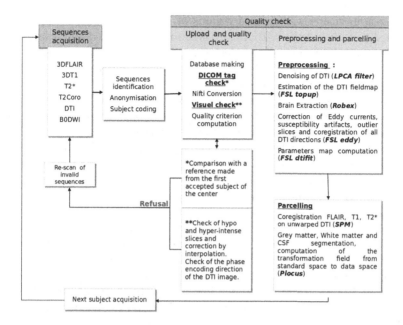

Fig. 1. Scheme describing all the quality control steps.

Processing. The diffusion tensor was estimated, and the local diffusion parameter MD was calculated for the entire brain for each patient and control using FSL. This parameter was computed from the three estimated eigenvalues that quantify the parameters of water diffusion in three orthogonal directions. Brain extraction was performed by the Robex software[2] using T1-weighed images. During segmentation process, P-LOCUS estimated the deformation field to register the atlas in standard space to patient's brain in individual space. Coupling ROBEX extraction with P-LOCUS deformation estimation allowing the handling of cases exhibiting large skull deformations as observed in severe TBI.

Automatic Approach (AA). The automated lesion segmentation technique (see [9] for details) was based on an outlier detection, inspired from the Pothole and Molehills method [17], using a multi-atlas technique to detect outliers as voxels departing from normative values. Given the variability in the spatial extent and the magnitude of the injury in case of severe TBI, the use of values averaged from large regions of White Matter (WM) would not allow the accurate detection of 'abnormal' values. Indeed, if the lesions are focal, the detection power is hampered by the averaging with healthy tissue values. The standard way is to use an atlas-based approach where MD at each voxel is compared with normative values computed from homogeneous regions of interest (ROIs) of a healthy volunteer's brain acting as a reference. We assume MD values to

---

[2] https://sites.google.com/site/jeiglesias/ROBEX.

be homogenous inside well defined regions of interest (ROIs) that are used to define local normative values. To divide the brain we combined four atlases found in the literature: Neuromorphometrics atlas[3], HarvardOxford atlas provided by FSL and Desikan provided by FreeSurfer[4] to identify cortical and sub-cortical regions (mainly grey matter, GM), and ICBM DTI81 atlas to subdivide WM. In case of multiple labels for one voxel, ICBM labels were always selected. In ICBM, mainly used in tractography studies, only tracks, a tiny part of the WM volume, are labeled. We automatically divided the remaining WM volume into small ROIs. Likewise, for the Neuromorphometrics atlas, large GM parcels were also subdivided. At the end we considered six parcellisations leading to 1402 different ROIs (see Fig. 2). Given that MD value distribution is not gaussian we used two different thresholds for outliers (lesions) detection: percentile-based and size-based. By fixing percentile thresholds $\alpha1$ for minimal and $\alpha2$ for maximal values, we identified clusters of extreme values. The skewness of the distribution is directed toward high values of MD and knowing these values are a marker of cell death and vasogenic edema, which are very frequent in severe TBI, we used a more lenient threshold for $\alpha2$. We considered lesions as clusters with a size higher than a threshold $\beta1$ for low MD and $\beta2$ for high MD based on differences we observed between vasogenic and cytotoxic edema. Voxels labeled as CSF, ventricles and hemorrhagic lesion were automatically excluded. Hemorrhagic lesions were detected using T2* images. Partial volume effect observed in MD may generate an incomplete CSF detection and a large number of false positives. Then, using a distance map, voxels close to CSF ($\leq 4\,\mathrm{mm}$) were not considered for segmentation. The parameters were empirically set on control data: $\alpha1$ was fixed at the 2nd percentile, $\alpha2$ at the 94.8th percentile, $\beta1$ and $\beta2$ at 20 and 15 contiguous voxels respectively (i.e. 160 and 120 mm^3). Because we introduced six parcellisations, each voxel belonged to six different ROIs, each with a corresponding MD values distribution. A voxel was considered as outlier (with low or high MD) when labelled as abnormal based at least on four atlases.

Manual Approach (MA). To quantify the volume of lesions, four neuroradiologists (AK, DG, SK and ES) with extensive experience in lesion assessment, manually segmented the lesion area for DS1 dataset. Three of them (AK, DG and SK) manually segmented DS2 dataset. They followed the same delineation protocol and used the ITK-SNAP software[5]. Focal lesions included any local regions of abnormal signal in the MD map. Low and high MD values were separately labeled.

Statistical Analysis. Spatial agreement was quantified with the Dice Metric (DM), Average Symmetrical Surface Distance (ASSD), the Hausdorff Distance (HD) and precision and recall (sensitivity) (see the corresponding formulas

---

[3] http://www.neuromorphometrics.com/.

[4] https://surfer.nmr.mgh.harvard.edu/.

[5] http://www.itk.org.

here[6]). Note that the standard HD is set by the maximum of the minimum distance values between two volume's surface points. A few outliers may greatly perturb the distance measure even though the two volumes may appear very close. A way to limit this effect is to introduce a modified HD based on a ranked distance [4]. We computed such a modified HD distance based on the 95th percentile. We computed using Staple (ST) [16] an estimation of the manual segmentation based on the four rater's results. We quantified volumetric association between manual and automated lesion delineation by computing the Pearson correlation [5]. Intra Class Correlation (ICC) was computed on volumes to assess consistency between raters and, between raters and the automated method.

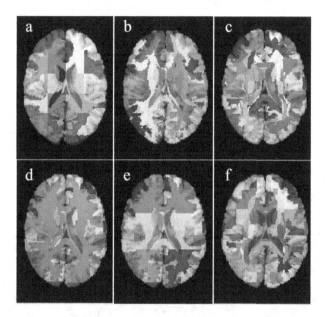

Fig. 2. Six parcellisations based on four atlases. a: HavardOxford + WM parcels size $\leq 32\,cm^3$.185 ROIs. b: Desikan atlas. 181 ROIs. c: Neuromorphometrics atlas + ICBM DTI181 + WM parcels size $\leq 12\,cm^3$. 244 ROIs. d: Neuromorphometrics atlas + GM parcels size $\leq 5\,cm^3$. 292 ROIs. e: Neuromorphometrics atlas + WM parcels size $\leq 124\,cm^3$. 248 ROIs. f: Neuromorphometrics atlas + ICBM DTI181 + WM parcels size $\leq 32\,cm^3$. 248 ROIs.

3 Results

DS1: For the realistic phantoms (five cases), Table 1 indicates the mean scores for the automated method, the four raters and their corresponding Staple values. Additionally we computed the same scores considering Staple as the ground truth for the automated method and for each rater. For the latter, Staple was

---

[6] http://www.isles-challenge.org/ISLES2015/.

computed on the 3 others raters. The mean of inter-rater scores is displayed in Table 1. The Inter Correlation Class (ICC) between raters was 0.80 and 0.79 when we included the automated approach. More coherence was obtained for low MD lesions segmentation with ICC = 0.98 for both manual and automated methods compared to ICC = 0.73 for manual and ICC = 0.71 for automated methods for high MD lesion segmentation.

Table 1. Mean scores and confidence interval (95%) for the five gold standard cases. Auto: automated method. Staple was computed on four raters.

	DM[0,1]	HD (mm)	ASSD (mm)	Prec. [0,1]	Sens. [0,1]
Rater1	0.76 ± 0.04	11.7 ± 6.09	0.82 ± 0.25	0.68 ± 0.04	0.86 ± 0.05
Rater2	0.75 ± 0.04	11.95 ± 4.63	0.85 ± 0.25	0.76 ± 0.05	0.74 ± 0.03
Rater3	0.78 ± 0.06	15.97 ± 9.29	0.85 ± 0.35	0.77 ± 0.05	0.79 ± 0.09
Rater4	0.69 ± 0.05	15.45 ± 4.01	1.24 ± 0.29	0.66 ± 0.04	0.73 ± 0.08
Staple	0.78 ± 0.05	11.28 ± 4.75	0.76 ± 0.29	0.72 ± 0.05	0.86 ± 0.06
Auto	0.77 ± 0.04	18.2 ± 10.7	1.09 ± 0.67	0.77 ± 0.08	0.83 ± 0.06
Auto vs Staple	0.75 ± 0.05	17.29 ± 11.31	1.21 ± 0.62	0.82 ± 0.08	0.71 ± 0.08

Figure 3 illustrated lesion segmentation for a synthetic case (case 5) including low and high MD.

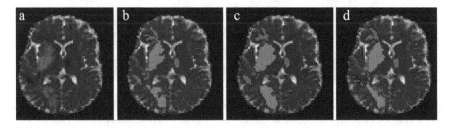

Fig. 3. Results on a synthetic lesion. a: MD image; b: Realistic phantom; c: Staple (4 raters); d: Automated method. Green: Low MD. Red: High MD. (Color figure online)

DS2: Table 2 indicates the mean scores for the five real cases. Results for Case 3 and for failed cases (Case 8 and Case 9) are respectively shown in Figs. 4, 6 and 7.

For both DS1 and DS2, volume agreements are shown in Fig. 5 with the corresponding Pearson coefficient.

Table 2. Mean scores for the automated method for the nine real cases using Staple (3 raters) as the reference.

	DM [0,1]	HD (mm)	ASSD (mm)	Prec. [0,1]	Sens. [0,1]
Case1	0.58	14.73	2.21	0.57	0.58
Case 2	0.76	20.93	1.73	0.65	0.90
Case 3	0.47	33.12	5.62	0.36	0.69
Case 4	0.35	44.19	6.07	0.30	0.44
Case 5	0.63	28.30	4.38	0.55	0.75
Case 6	0.56	15.29	5.00	0.50	0.62
Case 7	0.68	26.59	3.44	0.56	0.88
Case 8	0.01	29.13	12.66	0.004	0.17
Case 9	0.02	80.97	19.80	0.012	0.51

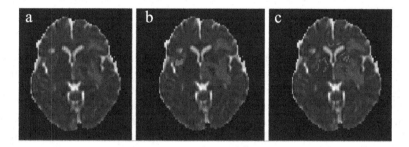

Fig. 4. Results on a real lesion (Case 5). a: MD image; b: Staple (3 raters); c: Automated method. Green: Low MD. Red: High MD. (Color figure online)

4 Discussion

Very few studies have investigated brain alterations due to severe trauma in acute phase, i.e. less than 10 days post-injury [6,13]. The methodological difficulties in performing MRI at this stage explain the rarity of studies. Moreover, currently proposed MR segmentation methods lack sufficient robustness to capture TBI-related changes without excessive user input [7], hampering large cohort studies. In this paper, we report our experiments comparing four manual delineations and one automated method on realistic phantoms (RP) and real images for MD lesion segmentation in severe brain trauma. The method focuses on detection of abnormal values in MD. The additional modalities, T1-weighted and FLAIR images, were used for brain extraction, atlas realignment (i.e. T1-weighted image) and CSF segmentation (T1+FLAIR images).

For RP, represented by synthetic images with low and high MD inserted by an expert, we found a good coherence between manual and automated results (see in Fig. 3 the similarity between manual and automated results for low and high MD). The high value of ICC (0.80) shows a good degree of agreement between the raters. When we considered the automated segmentation in the ICC calculation, the ICC value was very slightly decreased (0.79). This demonstrates that

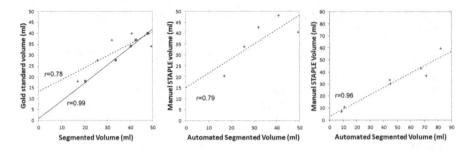

Fig. 5. Volume agreement. Left: For DS1, manual (Staple, four raters) and automated segmented volume vs gold standard. Center: For DS1, automated segmented volume vs Staple volume (four raters). Right: For DS2, automated segmented volume vs Staple volume (three raters). r: Pearson coefficient. Dash line: automated method. Black line: Staple method (four raters).

automated and manual segmentation provide very similar results. This was confirmed with the coherence between inter-observer scores, each rater vs RP (mean 0.74, 0.72 and 0.78 for DM, Precision and Sensibility respectively), and scores obtained for the automated method vs RP (0.77, 0.77 and 0.83) (see Table 1). We computed the automated method performances using RP or Staple as a reference (see Table 1, two last rows). This gives an idea of the potential effects on the performances using Staple when ground truth (here RP) is unknown (real case conditions). In these experimental conditions the reference change had a slight impact. The agreement (see Fig. 5, left) between the volume measurement was excellent between manual raters (Pearson coefficient = 0.99) and good for the automated technique versus RP or the Staple values (Pearson coefficient = 0.78 and 0.79 respectively). This again indicates that using Staple instead of RP is valid. There were some limitations to the automated approach on synthetic cases segmentation (see in Fig. 3 some differences for low MD between Staple and automated method). Indeed, when MD values were very close to normative values they were undetected by the automated approach, whereas experts used other cues such as texture or structural knowledge in addition to luminance to truly detect abnormalities.

For 7/9 real cases we obtained coherent results (see Table 2 & Fig. 4) with mean scores of DM = 0.57 ± 0.09, HD = 26.16 ± 7.74, ASSD = 4.07 ± 1.51, Precision = 0.50 ± 0.10 and Sensibility = 0.70 ± 0.12 respectively for the automated method vs Staple method compared to DM = 0.59 ± 0.06, HD = 19.94 ± 6.3, ASSD = 2.75 ± 0.9, Precision = 0.52 ± 0.12 and Sensibility = 0.78 ± 0.08 for inter-raters (each rater versus Staple computed on the two other). ICC was improved when considering the automated method (0.71) in addition to the three raters (0.66). The agreement between volume delineation was good with a Pearson coefficient equal to 0.96 (see Fig. 5, right). Altogether, these results clearly demonstrate the nice coherence between the automated method and the manual delineation. However, some discrepancies exist between the manual and automated methods. Clearly, for 2/9 cases the automated method failed (see Cases 8 and 9 in Table 2 and Figs. 6 and 7). For Case 8, our automatic method could not detect small diffuse axonal lesions and for Case 9 images were noisy and not sufficiently corrected by the QC module.

Dice and precision for both methods were quite low (0.57 and 0.59 for automated and manual methods respectively excluding the two failed cases) indicating the difficulty of the task even for experts. To our knowledge no fully automated alternative methods are available for a comparative evaluation with the method we propose and no evaluation results for traumatic brain lesion segmentation are reported in the literature. For comparison for ischemic stroke a Dice = 0.73 with Precision = 0.84 can be achieved by the best automated techniques [10]. Note that the use of a modified HD(95 percentile) may better describe the results (for RP, automated HD = 3.65 ± 3.9 and Staple HD = 1.66 ± 0.73 and for real cases, automated HD = 14.88 ± 6.70 and Staple HD = 8.11 ± 2.39). However, we kept standard HD values in Tables 1 and 2 for comparison with the literature.

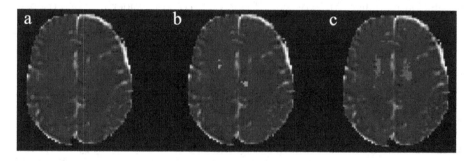

Fig. 6. Failed cases. Case 8. a: MD image; b: Staple (3 raters); c: Automated method. Green: Low MD. Red: High MD. (Color figure online)

These results were obtained on data coming from nine different scanners (3 × 3T Siemens, 2 × 1.5T GE, 2 × 3T Philips and 2 × 1.5 Philips with different models). The quality check and preprocessing steps were essential for improving the quality of DTI and removing CSF false positives and ensure the quality of the final results. A poor estimation of the normative mean in each ROI of the control group biases the detection of aberrant values [8]. Currently, for real cases, only three control DTI were available at each center for the normative values computation. In comparison for GT, seven controls were available from a single provider, the Grenoble center. This could explain the observed differences between synthetic data and real data performances. Then, we may expect substantial improvements in our results with the inclusion of 9 healthy controls in each center as planned. The involvement of more experts would allow the definition using Staple of a more accurate reference for real cases.

Finally, we observed that lesions were particularly difficult to segment manually due to low contrast and low spatial resolution in diffusion images. It took

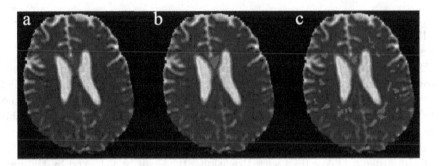

Fig. 7. Failed cases. Case 9. a: MD image; b: Staple (3 raters); c: Automated method.

approximative 30 min per case for each trained expert vs 10 min for the automated technique. Because we were interested in the detection of low and high MD values compared to normative values our method only relies on voxel intensities in diffusion modality. An extension of this work could consider new descriptors in multimodal images to capture brain modifications induced by trauma.

In conclusion, our results show that the proposed pipeline, including quality control and segmentation modules, allows the identification of severe TBI lesions based on mean diffusivity in coherence with the manual delineation by four experts. Its use on a large data cohort is ongoing. Nevertheless, a visual control by an expert is still required at two levels to control the quality of the images and validate the final automated segmentation produced.

Acknowledgments. Grenoble MRI facility IRMaGe was partly funded by the French program Investissement d'avenir run by the Agence Nationale pour la Recherche; grant Infrastructure d'avenir en Biologie Santé - ANR-11-INBS-0006. Research funded by French ministry of research and education under the Projet Hospitalier de Recherche Clinique grant OXY-TC to JFP.

References

1. Cunningham, A.S., Salvador, R., Coles, J.P., et al.: Physiological thresholds for irreversible tissue damage in contusional regions following traumatic brain injury. Brain **128**(Pt 8), 1931–42 (2005)
2. Davenport, N.D., Lim, K.O., Armstrong, M.T., Sponheim, S.R.: Diffuse and spatially variable white matter disruptions are associated with blast-related mild traumatic brain injury. Neuroimage **59**(3), 2017–24 (2012)
3. Doyle, S., Forbes, F., Dojat, M.: P-locus, a complete suite for brain scan segmentation. In: 9h IEEE International Symposium on Biomedical Imaging (ISBI) (2012)
4. Dubuisson, M., Jain, A.: A modified hausdorff distance for object-matching. In: 12th International Conference on Pattern Recognition (IPAR), pp. 566–568 (1994)
5. Fiez, J.A., Damasio, H., Grabowski, T.J.: Lesion segmentation and manual warping to a reference brain: intra- and interobserver reliability. Hum. Brain Mapp. **9**(4), 192–211 (2000)

6. Galanaud, D., Perlbarg, V., Gupta, R., et al.: Assessment of white matter injury and outcome in severe brain trauma: a prospective multicenter cohort. Anesthesiology **117**(6), 1300–10 (2012)
7. Irimia, A., Chambers, M.C., Alger, J.R., et al.: Comparison of acute and chronic traumatic brain injury using semi-automatic multimodal segmentation of MR volumes. J. Neurotrauma **28**(11), 2287–306 (2011)
8. Kim, N., Branch, C.A., Kim, M., Lipton, M.L.: Whole brain approaches for identification of microstructural abnormalities in individual patients: comparison of techniques applied to mild traumatic brain injury. PLoS One **8**(3), e59382 (2013)
9. Maggia, C., Doyle, S., Forbes, F., Heck, O., Troprès, I., Berthet, C., Teyssier, Y., Velly, L., Payen, J.-F., Dojat, M.: Assessment of tissue injury in severe brain trauma. In: Crimi, A., Menze, B., Maier, O., Reyes, M., Handels, H. (eds.) BrainLes 2015. LNCS, vol. 9556, pp. 57–68. Springer, Cham (2016). https://doi.org/10.1007/978-3-319-30858-6_6
10. Maier, O., Schroder, C., Forkert, N.D., Martinetz, T., Handels, H.: Classifiers for ischemic stroke lesion segmentation: a comparison study. PLoS One **10**(12), e0145118 (2015)
11. Manjon, J.V., Coupe, P., Concha, L., Buades, A., Collins, D.L., Robles, M.: Diffusion weighted image denoising using overcomplete local PCA. PLoS One **8**(9), e73021 (2013)
12. Narayana, P.A., Yu, X., Hasan, K.M., et al.: Multi-modal mri of mild traumatic brain injury. Neuroimage Clin. **7**, 87–97 (2015)
13. Pasco, A., Ter Minassian, A., Chapon, C., et al.: Dynamics of cerebral edema and the apparent diffusion coefficient of water changes in patients with severe traumatic brain injury. A prospective MRI study. Eur. Radiol. **16**(7), 1501–8 (2006)
14. Tagliaferri, F., Compagnone, C., Korsic, M., et al.: A systematic review of brain injury epidemiology in Europe. Acta Neurochir. **148**(3), 255–268 (2006). discussion 268
15. Thornhill, S., Teasdale, G.M., Murray, G.D., et al.: Disability in young people and adults one year after head injury: prospective cohort study. BMJ **320**(7250), 1631–5 (2000)
16. Warfield, S.K., Zou, K.H., Wells, W.M.: Simultaneous truth and performance level estimation (staple): an algorithm for the validation of image segmentation. IEEE Trans. Med. Imaging **23**(7), 903–21 (2004)
17. Watts, R., Thomas, A., Filippi, C.G., Nickerson, J.P., Freeman, K.: Potholes and molehills: bias in the diagnostic performance of diffusion-tensor imaging in concussion. Radiology **272**(1), 217–23 (2014)

Pairwise, Ordinal Outlier Detection of Traumatic Brain Injuries

Matt Higger$^{(\boxtimes)}$ ⓘ, Martha Shenton ⓘ, and Sylvain Bouix ⓘ

Psychiatry Neuroimaging Laboratory,
1249 Boylston Street, Boston, MA 02215, USA
Matt.Higger@gmail.com

Abstract. Because mild Traumatic Brain Injuries (mTBI) are heterogeneous, classification methods perform outlier detection from a model of healthy tissue. Such a model is challenging to construct. Instead, we utilize region-specific pairwise (person-to-person) comparisons. Each person-region is characterized by a distribution of Fractional Anisotropy and comparisons are made via Median, Mean, Bhattacharya and Kullback-Liebler distances. Additionally, we examine an ordinal decision rule which compares a subject's n^{th} most atypical region to a healthy control's. Ordinal comparison is motivated by mTBI's heterogeneity; each mTBI has some set of damaged tissue which is not necessarily spatially consistent. These improvements correctly distinguish Persistent Post-Concussive Symptoms in a small dataset but achieve only a .74 AUC in identifying mTBI subjects with milder symptoms. Finally, we perform subject-specific simulations which characterize which injuries are detected and which are missed.

1 Introduction

Mild Traumatic Brain Injuries (mTBI) affect upwards of 1.6 million individuals each year [6]. While symptoms often stop within weeks, some people experience Persistent Post-Concussive Symptoms (PPCS) including dizziness, fatigue, and sleep problems, which last months or years after the injury [4,16]. Those exposed to multiple mTBIs are at higher risk to develop Chronic Traumatic Encephalography (CTE) which continues to degrade brain tissue long after injuries are sustained [11]. The exact progression of mTBI symptoms or CTE etiology is not well known. There is value in developing methods which distinguish mTBI pathology as early as possible, doing so offers insight into the treatment of current injuries or prevention of future ones.

Diffusion Tensor Imaging can identify microstructural changes in brain tissue, a promising vantage point from which to characterize mTBI [1,2,9]. A central challenge in identifying mTBI is its heterogeneity, the location and severity of tissue damage are not spatially consistent [8,14]. For this reason, mTBI detection often uses outlier style classification methods; mTBIs may not look similar to each other but we can leverage the fact that they rarely appear as

© Springer International Publishing AG, part of Springer Nature 2018
A. Crimi et al. (Eds.): BrainLes 2017, LNCS 10670, pp. 100–110, 2018.
https://doi.org/10.1007/978-3-319-75238-9_9

healthy tissue. Earlier work has estimated the distribution of mean Fractional Anisotropy (FA) in each healthy region to produce z-scores which describe how atypical an observed region is [5,12]. Extensions to this method model the covariance of neighboring regions by imposing sparsity constraints on the precision matrix of the joint distribution [15].

Person-to-group mTBI outlier detection compares a candidate physiology to a model of healthy tissue across every region in the brain. Construction of this model is challenging given the variance due to demographics, different MRI scanners, and measurement noise. In this work, **we avoid modeling this distribution of features across the entire healthy population and instead focus on statistics from a set of pairwise (person-to-person) comparisons.** Doing so allows us to avoid assumptions about the distribution of healthy brain tissue where previous work required it follow a known distribution.

mTBI spatial location and severity is unique to each person. Previous work uses a spatially homologous classification rule. Doing so makes it difficult to simultaneously capture both the number of regions affected and how significantly tissue is damaged within each region. We propose comparing ordinally, equating each subject's n^{th} most abnormal region, to explicitly model both spatial size and severity of an mTBI.

Our algorithm, like many others, is not perfect. It misses mTBI cases and produces false positives and missed detections. It is unclear if its performance is due to the challenges inherent in the datasets we operate on or the procedure itself. Because of this, we develop a simple model of brain injury to allow us to contrast our performance with traditional z-score analysis in a controlled setting. Additionally, this simulation highlights differing sensitivities between the feature sets presented (Mean, Median, Kullback-Liebler and Bhattacharya distances applied to distributions of Fractional Anisotropy).

This simulation serves another purpose as well. So long as mTBI classification remains imperfect it can be challenging to derive clinical meaning from the output of a detection scheme. Alongside simulations, a positive detection is understood to be at-least-as-severe-as the demonstrated minimum threshold of detectability. Similarly, a 'no mTBI' classification can be interpreted as not-so-severe-as the same threshold. While classifiers make mistakes clinical value depends on a characterization of which injuries are likely to be detected and which may be missed.

2   Methods

Freesurfer's Desikan atlas [7] is registered to raw diffusion data. A single tensor is fit to the observed gradient directions via the Weighted Least Squares method from the Dipy toolbox [3,10]. In this way for each region (r) subject (x) pair we obtain a set of FA observations $\{f\}_{r,x}$. From these, we estimate the distribution of FA as a Gaussian Mixture Model:

$$\hat{P}_{F|X,R}(f|x,r) = \sum_i w_i \mathcal{N}(f|\mu_i, \sigma_i^2) \tag{1}$$

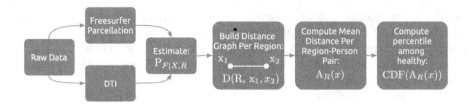

Fig. 1. Processing pipeline

where w_i, μ_i and σ_i^2 are the mixing weight, mean and variance of component i respectively. We regularize the number of components by penalizing via the Bayesian Information Criterion. Distributions are renormalized within the valid FA range $[0, 1]$ (Fig. 1).

Within each region a distance graph is constructed between each pair of subjects. This distance attempts to encapsulate the similarity between FA observations across the same region in two subjects. We explore four such distances, median, mean, Kullback-Liebler and Bhattacharya:

$$D_{\text{Median}}(r, x_1, x_2) = |\text{Med}(\{f\}_{r,x_1}) - \text{Med}(\{f\}_{r,x_2})| \tag{2}$$

$$D_{\text{Mean}}(r, x_1, x_2) = |\text{Mean}(\{f\}_{r,x_1}) - \text{Mean}(\{f\}_{r,x_2})| \tag{3}$$

$$D_{\text{KL}}(r, x_1, x_2) = \int_0^1 \hat{P}_{F|X,R}(f|x_1, r) \log \frac{\hat{P}_{F|X,R}(f|x_1, r)}{\hat{P}_{F|X,R}(f|x_2, r)} df$$
$$+ \int_0^1 \hat{P}_{F|X,R}(f|x_2, r) \log \frac{\hat{P}_{F|X,R}(f|x_2, r)}{\hat{P}_{F|X,R}(f|x_1, r)} df \tag{4}$$

$$D_{\text{Bhat}}(r, x_1, x_2) = \int_0^1 \sqrt{\hat{P}_{F|X,R}(f|x_1, r)\hat{P}_{F|X,R}(f|x_2, r)} df \tag{5}$$

where Med and Mean are functions which return the median and mean of a set. Note that we use a symmetric Kullback-Liebler such that $D_{\text{KL}}(r, x_1, x_2) = D_{\text{KL}}(r, x_2, x_1)$.

Median FA is included as a comparison metric. Mean FA will be more sensitive than median FA in reacting to small (relative to the size of the region) lesions which shift the FA dramatically. However, both of these metrics may not be sensitive enough. Consider two brain injuries, one which increases the FA of 10 voxels .05 and another which increases the FA of 1 voxel .5; the mean and median distances described above are largely ignorant of these size-severity differences among shifts in FA. To remedy this we introduce the second two distances which operate on the FA distributions themselves. Kullback-Liebler, in particular, may be very sensitive to small lesions which exhibit strongly atypical FA values. The ratio of likelihoods is reactive to observing even a few voxels whose FA is distinct from observations of other healthy tissue samples. This sensitivity comes at a cost; Kullback-Liebler may be equally reactive to distribution estimation errors which, unfortunately, are prevalent in sparsely sampled areas of the domain (e.g. the range of atypically observed FA values in healthy tissue). We include Bhattacharya as well with the hypothesis that it offers full distribution comparison and may be less sensitive to distribution estimation error than Kullback-Liebler.

We compute the 'Mean Distance to the Healthy Observations' per subject-region pair:

$$A_r(x) = \frac{1}{|H| - 1} \sum_{H \setminus \{x\}} D(r, x, x_i) \tag{6}$$

where H is the set of all healthy subjects. Intuitively, low values of $A_r(x)$ suggest that FA observations of region r for subject x are typical among all healthy subjects.

Even if a subject has a confirmed mTBI, $A_r(x)$ may be low as region r is unaffected. Because of this heterogeneity, we are motivated to produce a statistic which allows us to compare across regions. $A_r(x)$, by itself, is not suitable as its computation depends heavily on the statistics of the region itself. For example, consider a large, homogeneous region with a narrow range of observed healthy FA. While the A_r associated with this region is sensitive to small changes in FA, other regions may not enjoy the same benefit. To allow for cross-region comparisons we estimate the distribution of A_r for each region across all healthy subjects via a Guassian Kernel Density Estimate:

$$\hat{P}_{A_r}(a) = \frac{1}{N_H} \sum_{x_i : T_{x_i} = 0} \mathcal{N}(a | A_r(x_i), \sigma_r^2) \tag{7}$$

where σ_r^2 is chosen to maximize a cross-validated likelihood score. From this distribution we can compute the percentile, $CDF(A_r(x))$, which is suitable for cross-region comparison. Intuitively, **this percentile represents the percentage of healthy subjects whose observed FA values are more typical than x's.**

We are interested in aggregating the evidence, $CDF(A_r(x))$, of every region for one subject to determine if they have a mTBI. A first approach might compare spatially homologous regions to classify as:

$$P_{T|A_r}(t | A_r(x)) \propto \hat{P}_{A_r|T}(A_r(x)|t) P_T(t) \tag{8}$$

where T is a binary mTBI indicator and $\hat{P}_{A_r|T}(A_r(x)|t)$ is given in (7). This distribution of atypicality acts as a pre-processing fail-safe: in a worst case scenario where artifacts (e.g. head motions) are prevalent throughout the dataset our distribution of healthy atypicality (7) will vary more. mTBI would be more easily hidden resulting in lower detection rates but at least the false-positive rates will be minimally affected so that one is prevented from drawing dubious artifact-induced conclusions.

Finally, by assuming that each region's atypicality is independent of the next we may aggregate evidence across all a subject's regions as:

$$P_{T|X}(t|x) = \prod_r P_{T|A_r}(t | A_r(x)) \tag{9}$$

Homologous comparisons struggle to capture the heterogeneity of mTBI; **regions are affected differently per individual**. Consider that homologous fusion gives equal scores to a whole brain of slightly atypical regions and a small set of regions which are strongly atypical. Instead, **we propose ordinal comparison, equating each subject's n^{th} most abnormal region**. Doing so allows us to model the number of regions mTBIs affect. Homologous comparisons are incapable of identifying that only the first m most atypical regions are affected by mTBI. We define r_1^* to be each subject's most atypical region so that the ordinal fusion rule is given by (8) where r is replaced by r^*.

3 Dataset

We perform this analysis on two datasets. The first is 11 subjects who were scanned while experiencing Persistent Post-Concussive Symptoms (PPCS) resulting from an mTBI, and 11 matched controls previously used in [5]. The second dataset is part of the INTRUST study[1] and contains self-reported mTBI (exposure within the past few years and may not currently be experiencing symptoms) (Table 1):

Table 1. INTRUST dataset by collection site

	Healthy controls	mTBI
UCSD	10	6
Cincinnati	47	45
Dartmouth	27	12
Duke	25	10
MUSC	26	2
Brigham and Women's & Spaulding	28	41

Because the INTRUST dataset was collected across multiple sites and scanners, it is first harmonized via the method given in [13]. Remember that PPCS is associated with more severe, long lasting symptoms as compared to the self-reported mTBI group of INTRUST. We expect PPCS is easier to detect than self-reported mTBI.

We conducted a quality check of the data. This included a visual and semi-automated quality checks, including the detection of signal dropout or venetian blind artifacts, as well as head motion, ghosting, interslice and intra-slice intensity artifact, and checkerboard artifact. Further, we applied head motion and eddy current correction scripts. No datasets were excluded due to the presence of excessively poor quality, which we defined as at least five instances of the above-noted compromises of quality per individual volume.

---

[1] http://intrust.sdsc.edu/.

4   Simulation

To characterize the sensitivity of our algorithm we simulate an mTBI as a constant FA offset of some ratio of the total region volume. We choose arbitrary white and gray matter regions and identify the most typical healthy subject in the INTRUST dataset (the person with minimal $A_R(x)$ for that region). From the associated distribution of FA, $P_{F|R,X}$, we bootstrap sample to a total region size. Next, some ratio of 'healthy' tissue is given a constant FA offset and clipped to the appropriate domain ($[0, 1]$). We repeat this process while varying the total region size, the magnitude of the injury effect (ΔFA), and the ratio of voxels injured to total region size. Each experiment has 30 healthy controls and 30 simulated TBIs. Results are given in Fig. 2.

Unsurprisingly, larger ΔFA and injury ratio increase $A_R(x)$. Region size has a thresholding effect, degrading detection sensitivity below some volume. The region specific distribution of FA was significant in determining sensitivity. Intuitively, more homogeneous tissue makes for greater statistical contrast with abnormalities. In our example the smaller variance in FA of the Right Amygdala (Figs. 2a and b) yields higher $A_R(x)$ for equivalent mTBI injury profiles (see Figs. 2g and h). In other words, an injury's ΔFA can move tissue from one healthy mode to another to mask the damage more easily in higher variance distribution of FA (Figs. 2d and f vs Figs. 2c and e).

This first simulation (Fig. 2) only uses the Bhattacharya metric, to understand the varying performance of the different feature sets (Median FA, Mean FA, Kullback-Liebler and Bhattacharya) we repeat the simulation for each. Figure 3 gives the result. Figure 3a shows the median function's ability to ignore outliers makes it particularly insensitive to mTBI detection, requiring far greater injury severity before a detection is achieved. Some improvement is gained by using the Mean FA instead (Fig. 3b). Full distribution distances are the most successful as they explicitly penalize a single voxel which appears in a rarely observed domain of the healthy FA distribution (Figs. 3c and d). Kullback-Liebler seems to enjoy a slightly advantage over Bhattacharya for this experiment. Note that an algorithm's ability to detect outliers depends on how strongly it can characterize what typical (i.e. 'healthy') tissue looks like; it may be the case that the relative sensitives change as the population of observed 'healthy' brain regions increases. In this experiment we attempt to detect an injured brain region from among 30 other healthy observations.

5   Results

We report AUC derived from the likelihood scores given by $\hat{P}_{A_r|T}(A_r(x)|t)$ and $\hat{P}_{A_r|T}(A_{r^*}(x)|t)$ for region based and ordinal region based fusion (see discussion near (8)). PPCS was distinguished correctly via D_{Mean} under ordinal region fusion (Table 2). PPCS is characterized by a few brain regions, unique to each subject, which are strongly atypical Fig. 4a. Given the difference in symptom severity, it is unsurprising that PPCS classification performance exceeds

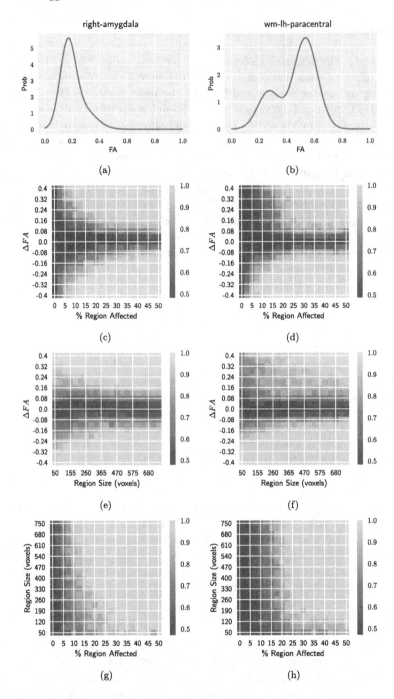

Fig. 2. Monte Carlo simulation of mTBI of varying severity under Bhattacharya feature set (see (5)). Color indicates average $CDF(A_R(x))$ across 30 simulated injuries. When not explicitly varied $\Delta FA = .2$, $\alpha = .2$ (percentage of region affected) and $N = 300$ (region size). (Color figure online)

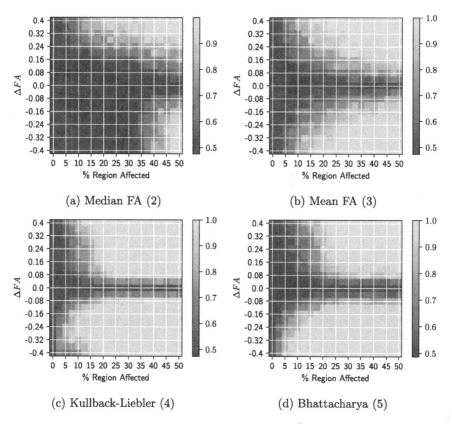

(a) Median FA (2) (b) Mean FA (3)

(c) Kullback-Liebler (4) (d) Bhattacharya (5)

Fig. 3. Monte Carlo simulation of mTBI in the Right Amygdala (see Fig. 2a) across different feature sets. Color indicates average $CDF(A_R(x))$ across 30 simulated injuries. (Color figure online)

INTRUST. Note that INTRUST's most atypical healthy regions are more atypical than the PPCS dataset's (see Figs. 4a and b). This larger range of healthy tissue can be attributed to INTRUST's larger sample size or the effect of multiple MRI scanners. There doesn't seem to be a strong relationship between the best D among the two datasets.

While the INTRUST dataset was challenging to classify the sensitivity simulation can be used to suggest that no lesions exist beyond a particular magnitude. If an undetected injury is present it is unlikely to exist in any of the detectable (i.e. yellow) regions of Fig. 2. Remember that the distribution of FA observed and region size affect sensitivity so simulations should be recomputed using a subject-specific FA distribution and region size.

No spatial patterns were noticed in either datasets injury locations.

Table 2. AUC values for each dataset, distance function and comparison method used to classify.

	Fusion	D_{Mean}	D_{Median}	D_{Bhat}	D_{KL}	Z-score
INTRUST	Homologous	0.652	0.665	0.521	0.741	0.567
	Ordinal	0.651	0.663	0.509	0.732	0.560
PPCS	Homologous	0.752	0.562	0.694	0.562	0.595
	Ordinal	1.000	0.711	0.860	0.678	0.554

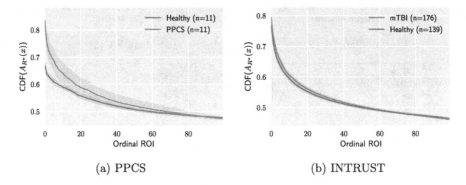

(a) PPCS   (b) INTRUST

Fig. 4. Distribution of $A_{R^*}(x)$ per illness class for D_{Mean}. Shaded area indicates one standard deviation. We use R^* to emphasize that this comparison is across ordinal ROI.

6   Conclusion

We present a method which identifies mTBIs as outliers in healthy regions of the brain. The algorithm honors the heterogeneity of mTBI by comparing each subjects n^{th} most atypical region; there is no guarantee that mTBI affects identical brain regions in all people. Further, we avoid modeling the considerable variation of healthy tissue across the brain by performing person-to-person comparisons rather than person-to-group. Our method does not make errors in identifying PPCS within a small dataset while in a larger, multi-scanner dataset of subjects with milder symptoms AUC was .74. We suspect that this performance drop is due to the more accepting definition of mTBI in the larger dataset; INTRUST's mTBI definition is any self-reported mTBI in the past few years while the other data requires a subject to be experiencing PPCS symptoms at the time of data collection. We suspect that explaining away as much variance in the healthy tissue as possible, potentially by learning dependencies on demographic variables (e.g. Age, Sex, IQ), will yield greater statistical contrast with mTBI outliers.

To explain these performance differences we perform Monte Carlo simulations which generate mTBI of varying severity in a typical white and gray matter region. The simulation shows that mTBI detection depends both on the physiological severity of the injury as well as the consistency of the healthy tissue. In other words, it is easier to hide an mTBI in a brain region whose healthy tissue varies more.

Acknowledgements. This work is supported by the INTRUST Posttraumatic Stress Disorder and Traumatic Brain Injury Clinical Consortium funded by the Department of Defense Psychological Health/Traumatic Brain Injury Research Program [X81XWH-07-CC-CSDoD], National Institute of Mental Health [T32 MH 016259-29] and the National Institute of Health [R01HD090641].

References

1. Aoki, Y., Inokuchi, R., Gunshin, M., Yahagi, N., Suwa, H.: Diffusion tensor imaging studies of mild traumatic brain injury: a meta-analysis. J. Neurol. Neurosurg. Psychiatry **83**(9), 870–876 (2012)
2. Basser, P.J., Pierpaoli, C.: Microstructural and physiological features of tissues elucidated by quantitative-diffusion-tensor MRI. J. Magn. Resonance **213**(2), 560–570 (2011)
3. Basser, P., Mattiello, J., Lebihan, D.: Estimation of the effective self-diffusion tensor from the NMR spin echo. J. Magn. Resonance Ser. B **103**(3), 247–254 (1994). http://linkinghub.elsevier.com/retrieve/pii/S1064186684710375
4. Bigler, E.D.: Neuropsychology and clinical neuroscience of persistent post-concussive syndrome. J. Int. Neuropsychol. Soc. **14**(1), 1–22 (2008)
5. Bouix, S., Pasternak, O., Rathi, Y., Pelavin, P.E., Zafonte, R., Shenton, M.E.: Increased gray matter diffusion anisotropy in patients with persistent post-concussive symptoms following mild traumatic brain injury. PLoS One **8**(6), e66205 (2013)
6. Coronado, V.G., Mcguire, L.C., Sarmiento, K., Bell, J., Lionbarger, M.R., Jones, C.D., Geller, A.I., Khoury, N., Xu, L.: Corrigendum to trends in traumatic brain injury in the U.S. and the and the public health response: 1995–2009. J. Safety Res. **48**, 117 (2014). http://dx.doi.org/10.1016/j.jsr.2013.12.006
7. Desikan, R.S., Ségonne, F., Fischl, B., Quinn, B.T., Dickerson, B.C., Blacker, D., Buckner, R.L., Dale, A.M., Maguire, R.P., Hyman, B.T., Albert, M.S., Killiany, R.J.: An automated labeling system for subdividing the human cerebral cortex on MRI scans into gyral based regions of interest. NeuroImage **31**(3), 968–980 (2006). http://www.sciencedirect.com/science/article/B6WNP-4JFHF4P-1/2/0ec667d4c17eafb0a7c52fa3fd5aef1c
8. Feng, Y., Abney, T.M., Okamoto, R.J., Pless, R.B., Genin, G.M., Bayly, P.V.: Relative brain displacement and deformation during constrained mild frontal head impact. J. R. Soc. Interface **7**(53), 1677–1688 (2010)
9. Gardner, A., Kay-Lambkin, F., Stanwell, P., Donnelly, J., Williams, W.H., Hiles, A., Schofield, P., Levi, C., Jones, D.K.: A systematic review of diffusion tensor imaging findings in sports-related concussion. J. Neurotrauma **29**(16), 2521–2538 (2012)
10. Garyfallidis, E., Brett, M., Amirbekian, B., Rokem, A., Van Der Walt, S., Descoteaux, M., Nimmo-Smith, I.: Dipy, a library for the analysis of diffusion MRI data. Front. Neuroinform. **8**, 8 (2014). http://journal.frontiersin.org/article/10.3389/fninf.2014.00008
11. Koerte, I.K., Lin, A.P., Willems, A., Muehlmann, M., Hufschmidt, J., Coleman, M.J., Green, I., Liao, H., Tate, D.F., Wilde, E.A., Pasternak, O., Bouix, S., Rathi, Y., Bigler, E.D., Stern, R.A., Shenton, M.E.: A review of neuroimaging findings in repetitive brain trauma. Brain Pathol. **25**, 318–349 (2015)

12. Lipton, M.L., Gellella, E., Lo, C., Gold, T., Ardekani, B.A., Shifteh, K., Bello, J.A., Branch, C.A.: Multifocal white matter ultrastructural abnormalities in mild traumatic brain injury with cognitive disability: a voxel-wise analysis of diffusion tensor imaging. J. Neurotrauma **25**(11), 1335–1342 (2008)
13. Mirzaalian, H., Ning, L., Savadjiev, P., Pasternak, O., Bouix, S., Michailovich, O., Grant, G., Marx, C.E., Morey, R.A., Flashman, L.A., George, M.S., McAllister, T.W., Andaluz, N., Shutter, L., Coimbra, R., Zafonte, R.D., Coleman, M.J., Kubicki, M., Westin, C.F., Stein, M.B., Shenton, M.E., Rathi, Y.: Inter-site and inter-scanner diffusion MRI data harmonization. NeuroImage **135**, 311–323 (2016). http://dx.doi.org/10.1016/j.neuroimage.2016.04.041
14. Rosenbaum, S.B., Lipton, M.L.: Embracing chaos: the scope and importance of clinical and pathological heterogeneity in mTBI. Brain Imaging Behav. **6**(2), 255–282 (2012)
15. Shaker, M., Erdogmus, D., Dy, J., Bouix, S.: Subject-specific abnormal region detection in traumatic brain injury using sparse model selection on high dimensional diffusion data. Med. Image Anal. **37**, 56–65 (2017). https://doi.org/10.1016/j.media.2017.01.005
16. Shenton, M.E., Hamoda, H.M., Schneiderman, J.S., Boulx, S., Pasternak, O., Rathi, Y., Vu, M.-A., Purohit, M.P., Helmer, K., Koerte, I., Lin, A.P., Westin, C.-F., Kikinis, R., Kubicki, M., Stern, R.A., Zafonte, R.: A review of magnetic resonance imaging and diffusion tensor imaging findings in mild traumatic brain injury. Brain Imaging Behav. **6**(2), 137–192 (2012)

Sub-acute and Chronic Ischemic Stroke Lesion MRI Segmentation

Senan Doyle[1(✉)], Florence Forbes[2,3], Assia Jaillard[4], Olivier Heck[4],
Olivier Detante[3,4,5], and Michel Dojat[3,5]

[1] Pixyl, 38000 Grenoble, France
senan.doyle@pixyl.io
[2] INRIA, Mistis, 38334 Montbonnot, France
[3] Université Grenoble Alpes, GIN, 38000 Grenoble, France
[4] CHUGA, 38000 Grenoble, France
[5] INSERM, U1216, 38000 Grenoble, France

Abstract. Automatic segmentation of chronic stroke lesion from magnetic resonance images (MRI) is motivated by the increasing need for reproducible and repeatable endpoints in clinical trials. The task is nontrivial, due to a number of confounding factors, including heterogeneous lesion intensity, irregular shape, and large deformations that render the conventional use of prior probabilistic atlases challenging. In this paper, we introduce a hidden Markov random field model that avails of a novel prior probabilistic vascular territory atlas to describe the natural vascular constraints in the brain. The vascular territory atlas is deformed in a joint registration-segmentation framework to overcome subject-specific morphological variability. T1-w and Flair sequences are used to populate our model, and a variational approach is implemented to find a solution. The performance of our model is demonstrated on two datasets, and compared to manual delineations by expert raters.

1 Introduction

Stroke is a global epidemic with levels of mortality and disability that entail a high societal cost. Approximately 70% of stroke survivors have significant sensorimotor, language and cognitive dysfunction requiring long-term special care and rehabilitation [8].

The measurement of ischemic stroke lesion volume is an important end-point in clinical studies, and can be used to improve diagnosis, prognosis, and guide therapeutic intervention. The currently accepted gold standard for lesion quantification is manual delineation by a medical expert [25]. However, manual delineation is subjective, tedious, time-consuming, costly, and suffers from inter-rater and intra-rater variability that can lead to unclear study conclusions [3,10,19]. Manual delineation does not, therefore, scale well to large population studies. Automatic segmentation methods are motivated by the increasing demand for large-scale multi-center clinical research studies that require an objective, reproducible and cost-efficient solution.

© Springer International Publishing AG, part of Springer Nature 2018
A. Crimi et al. (Eds.): BrainLes 2017, LNCS 10670, pp. 111–122, 2018.
https://doi.org/10.1007/978-3-319-75238-9_10

Automatic segmentation of sub-acute and chronic stroke lesions is challenging due to the heterogeneous appearance of stroke lesion in MRI, widely accepted as the most informative imaging modality [2]. A number of MRI sequences are used to gain insight into the state and evolution of brain tissue post-accident. DWI, T1w and Flair are common in routine examination, with Flair being particularly informative at the sub-acute and chronic phase [10,19]. In an automatic segmentation framework, multiple sequences increase the discriminative capacity of the model to identify tissues, structures and lesions independently of the age of the stroke.

Stroke lesion segmentation methods can be broadly divided into supervised (e.g. [13,15,18]) and unsupervised (e.g. [6,21,25]) approaches. Supervised approaches avail of a learning dataset to train a classifier, which is subsequently applied to new data in a testing phase. Supervised methods have performed well in recent publications and segmentation competitions. In [12], Maier *et al.* compare the performance of nine different classification methods. The study highlights the relative strength of Extra Tree Forest (ET), Random Decision Forest (RDF) and Convolutional Neural Network (CNN) methods. The poor performance of a Generalized Linear Model (GLM) classifier demonstrates the non-linear nature of the ischemic stroke classification task. The favorable performance of supervised methods was confirmed during the ISLES 2015 challenge [11]. The overall best method was Deep Medic, a 3D CNN approach [9].

However, unsupervised computational statistics and machine learning approaches remain competitive. For instance, the recent work by Menze *et al.* [14] extended the generative model to include non-local information with biological constraints. Indeed, incorporating additional knowledge *a priori* in the classification task is a Bayesian concept that can be appealing in medical applications. The segmentation result can be explained by decomposing the model into it's constituant parts. The prior information usually has anatomical or physiological significance, and can be designed, queried and controlled by medical experts.

In this paper, we develop an unsupervised method that builds on the generative model approach of Forbes *et al.* [4]. In [4], the authors adopt a two-stage approach, whereby candidate lesions are identified as outliers to a normal tissue segmentation in a first stage, and then used to parameterize a weighted distribution that explicitly models the lesions in a second stage. The proposed statistical model is an implementation of a hidden Markov random field (HMRF) with a number of innovations to address the challenges posed by sub-acute and chronic ischemic stroke MR scans. A general HMRF formulation is employed that encodes complex interactions between neighboring voxels, in particular, the fact that certain tissue combinations in the neighborhood are penalized more than others, whereas the standard Potts model penalizes dissimilar neighboring classes equally, regardless of the tissues they represent.

In the following section, we outline the segmentation model, before briefly describing the two datasets obtained in Sect. 3. The results obtained on these datasets is presented in Sect. 4. We describe the challenges encountered and future developments to overcome these challenges in Sect. 5.

2 A Hierarchical Bayesian Model for Stroke Lesion Segmentation

Hierarchical Bayesian models are very flexible in image analysis. We provide below the specification of our model adapted to stroke lesion segmentation. In particular we design a model, denoted here VBStroke, that enables the identification of, not only the total lesion volume, but also sub-regions of clinical interest, such as necrotic tissue. In its Bayesian formulation the model involves three sets of random quantities: the observed intensity values at each voxel, their respective assignments to a tissue class, and the model parameters that are also considered as random. This last assumption acts as a regularization of the solution that incorporates prior knowledge. The set of voxels is denoted by V. It contains N voxels on a regular 3D grid equipped with a neighborhood system. The observed intensity values are denoted by $\mathbf{y} = \{\mathbf{y}_1, \ldots, \mathbf{y}_N\}$ where $\mathbf{y}_i = \{y_{i1}, \ldots, y_{iM}\}$ is itself a vector of M intensity values corresponding to M different MR sequences. For the segmentation task, each voxel i is assigned to one class among K classes depending on its intensity values $\mathbf{y}_i$. The unknown classes are denoted by $\mathbf{z} = \{\mathbf{z}_1, \ldots, \mathbf{z}_N\}$ where $\mathbf{z}_i$ takes its values in $\{e_1, \ldots, e_K\}$, with e_k a K-dimensional binary vector whose k^{th} component is 1, all other components being 0. The model parameters are denoted by $\psi = \{\beta, \phi\}$. Their interpretation is specified below.

The joint distribution $p(\mathbf{y}, \mathbf{z}, \psi) = p(\mathbf{y}|\mathbf{z}, \psi)\, p(\mathbf{z}|\psi)\, p(\psi)$ is decomposed into three parts. The likelihood or data term is $p(\mathbf{y}|\mathbf{z}, \psi) = \prod_{i \in V} g(\mathbf{y}_i|\mathbf{z}_i; \phi)$, where the $g(\mathbf{y}_i|\mathbf{z}_i; \phi)$'s are probability density functions on $\mathbf{y}_i$ and are here defined as Gaussian distributions, $g(\mathbf{y}_i|\mathbf{z}_i = e_k; \phi) = \mathcal{N}(\mathbf{y}_i; \mu_k, \Sigma_k)$. The missing data term $p(\mathbf{z}|\psi)$ allows to encode spatial dependencies via a discrete Markov Random Field (MRF) modelling, $p(\mathbf{z}|\psi) \propto \exp(H_{\mathbf{Z}}(\mathbf{z}; \beta))$ with

$$H_{\mathbf{Z}}(\mathbf{z}; \beta) = -\sum_{i \in V} \mathbf{z}_i^t \alpha - \sum_{\substack{i,j \\ i \sim j}} \mathbf{z}_i^t \mathbb{B} \mathbf{z}_j,$$

where we write $\mathbf{z}_i^t$ for the transpose of vector $\mathbf{z}_i$ and $i \sim j$ when i and j are neighbors. The set of parameters includes therefore $\phi = \{\mu_k, \Sigma_k, k = 1 : K\}$ and β decomposed into $\beta = (\alpha, \mathbb{B})$ where α is a K−dimensional vector which acts as weights for the different values of $\mathbf{z}_i$ and $\mathbb{B}$ is a $K \times K$ matrix that encodes interactions between the different classes. If, in addition to a null α, $\mathbb{B} = b \times I_K$ where b is a real scalar and I_K is the $K \times K$ identity matrix, parameters β reduce to a single scalar interaction parameter b and we get the Potts model traditionally used for image segmentation. We adopt a model comprising of 4 normal tissue classes; *cerebrospinal fluid, white matter, grey matter*, and *other*. The lesion is modeled by a further six classes representing abnormal tissue states. In the absence of sufficient data to robustly and accurately estimate a full free $\mathbb{B}$ with $K = 10$, further constraints are imposed on the MRF interaction matrix.

The six lesion classes are considered sub-classes of a single *structure*, whose interaction with the normal tissue classes is not dependent on the specific lesion sub-class. Letting τ be the set of classes comprising the lesion structure, $\mathbb{B}$ is a matrix defined by:

$$\mathbb{B}(k, k') = b_t \quad \forall k, k' \in \tau$$
$$\mathbb{B}(k, k') = b_{\{k,k'\}} \quad \text{otherwise.} \tag{1}$$

Prior knowledge on the expected neighborhoods can be encoded in $\mathbb{B}$. For example, given two classes that are likely to be adjacent, the matrix entries for this pair can be initialized at, or even fixed to, a higher value. Conversely, when there is enough information in the data, a full free $\mathbb{B}$ matrix can be estimated and will reflect the class structure (*i.e.* which class is next to which as indicated by the data) and will then mainly serve as a regularizing term to encode additional spatial information. The α term can be used to encode atlas information, as in [20, 23]. We introduce a probabilistic vascular territory atlas to model the potential progression and delimitation of vascular accidents, and therefore overcome misclassification due to artefacts. The atlas is discrete, and so Gaussian blur is applied to express uncertainty inherent to patient-specific analysis. In effect, the territory prior does not prohibit the realization of lesion labels at any location in the image, but expresses the lower probability of solutions that contain lesions in multiple vascular territories. The vascular territory structure prior is subject to an affine transformation as the iterative segmentation-registration framework executes. This also helps to overcome patient-specific bias, and variability in lesion shape. The discrete vascular territory atlas is shown in Figs. 3a and b alongside an example of the Gaussian blurred territory for use in the joint segmentation & registration step (Fig. 3c). The final territory (Fig. 3d) is produced by the transformation of the initial territory in the joint model, and shows how the territory is adapted to the individual patient data.

In this study, no further prior is assumed on β which is estimated as a non random parameter although exponential priors would be possible if desired. In contrast, priors are assumed for the intensity distribution parameters ϕ. The conjugate Normal-inverse-Wishart priors [5] are used for (μ_k, Σ_k), $p(\mu_k | \Sigma_k) = \mathcal{N}(\mu_k; m_k^0, \Sigma_k / \eta_k^0)$ and $p(\Sigma_k) = invW(\Sigma_k; W_k^0, \nu_k^0)$. The hyperparameters $\{m_k^0, \eta_k^0, W_k^0, \nu_k^0, k = 1 : K\}$ must be specified. Typically, for the normal tissues classes, m_k^0 is fixed to a median value while for the lesion classes larger values are useful to favor hyperintensities. Similarly, η_k^0 acts on the variance and can be fixed to large values for the lesion classes to be more informative and favor values around m_k^0. Weakly informative values are preferred for $\{W_k^0, \nu_k^0\}$.

As regards inference, maximum a posteriori estimation of both parameters and class assignments can be derived using an adaptation of the variational EM algorithm [1] (Fig. 1).

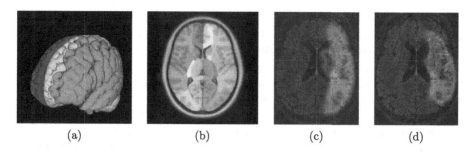

(a)   (b)   (c)   (d)

Fig. 1. Prior vascular territory atlas: (a) 3D view (b) Transverse view (c) Initial MCA probabilistic territory and (d) Post-processing individual MCA territory.

3   Materials and Methods

Sub-acute and chronic stroke analysis is of interest in this study. Two such datasets, DSA and DSB, were analysed to evaluate our approach and demonstrate the robustness of the method to multicenter data. The images were intensity normalized with respect to a reference image (not included in test dataset). The hyperparameters m_k^0 were set according to the expected intensity of each class in the reference image, and the hyperparameters dictating the variance of the mean, η_k^0, were set sufficiently small to avoid overfitting.

3.1   Dataset A (DSA)

The authors of [12] have kindly released their MRI images and manual delineations to promote open research in the domain[1]. The dataset consists of 37 cases deriving from two clinical studies on spatial neglect. Detailed information on the patients, lesion characteristics, imaging protocol and preprocessing pipeline can be found in [13]. T1-weighted and Flair sequences are available for 21 subjects, and the data has been preprocessed and and resampled to $3\,\text{mm}^3$. A number of the cases were used as part of the 2015 ISLES Challenge [11]. Manual delineation was performed by two raters (GTG & GTL) experienced in stroke imaging. DSA provides us an unique opportunity to compare our unsupervised method with the nine supervised segmentation approaches surveyed in the review [12].

3.2   Dataset B (DSB)

A high-quality sub-acute and chronic stroke dataset was supplied by the clinical study, HERMES, the ancillary MRI study of the clinical trial ISIS[2]. The MRIs

---

[1] The pre-processed data, ground truth and segmentation results are available at http://dx.doi.org/10.6084/m9.figshare.1585018.

[2] https://clinicaltrials.gov/show/NCT00875654.

were acquired on a Philips Achieva 3.0T TX at the IRMaGe MRI facility (Grenoble, France). The data was obtained from 27 ischemic stroke patients (5 weeks post-accident) with MCA infarct (right or left carotid ischemic stroke). A total of 47 cases with high resolution (1 mm^3) standard T1-weighted and 3D-Flair sequences were available for analysis. Manual delineation was performed by an expert rater with extensive stroke experience, using the Flair sequence that is particularly suitable for acute and chronic stroke manual tracing [19] and insensitive to individual strategy [17]. The dataset contains 20 patients with T1 and Flair sequences at two time points. All subjects were scanned at 2 months post-accident, two subjects were subsequently scanned at 4 months post-accident, and the remaining eighteen were subsequently scanned at 6 months. The evolution of lesion volume in time is of interest in clinical studies to establish therapeutic effect. DSB allows us to automatically assess the lesion evolution between two temporal points and test our method on images acquired with MR sequences that will be used in a European multicenter study, RESSTORE[3], involving 23 clinical centers and 400 stroke patients.

3.3   Processing Pipeline

The MR images are first preprocessed. The images are corrected for intensity inhomogeneities using the N4 algorithm [22]. The deformable transform that describes the mapping between the MNI template and the data space is calculated using Insight Segmentation and Registration Toolkit (ITK) libraries. The transform is used to register both the probabilistic tissue atlases and the vascular territory atlas, to the MR sequences. An initial preprocessing step identifies the vascular territory to be used in the subsequent segmentation step. Outlier intensities are quantified in each vascular territory grouping based on the Flair images, and the most affected territory group is selected as an *initial* region-of-interest. Adopting Bayesian principles, the algorithm performs joint segmentation and registration of the *a priori* probabilistic vascular territory structure, as described in [20]. Bias caused by commitment to the initial registration is thus alleviated by refining the registration as the algorithm executes. A postprocessing step removes potential false positives, such as Flair hyperintensities presenting symmetrically, in and around the ventricles, as well as proximal to the posterior horns.

3.4   Evaluation Metrics

In order to evaluate our method, the segmentation result obtained was compared to a ground truth i.e. the manual delination. The limited number of manual delineations for each subject prohibited the calculation of a probabilistic ground truth [24]. A number of different measurements were observed to give a comprehensive understanding of the segmentation performance. Classic segmentation-performance measures, such as Dice similarity coefficient (DSC), Haussdorf distance, ASSD, Precision and Sensitivity (or Recall) were computed for DSA and

---

[3] http://www.resstore.eu/.

DSB (see[4] for corresponding formulas). For DSB, we also computed the volumetric index PVD (percent volume difference) to compare automatic and manual delineation [3] and report the evolution of the lesion volume in time [16].

$$PVD(A, B) = 100 \times \frac{2 \times abs(A - B)}{A + B}$$

4 Results

4.1 DSA

Comparison with Ground Truth and Alternative Methods. DSA was manually delineated by two raters, GTL and GTG. The database contains detailed segmentation performance results for the nine methods described in [12]. We consider here only the highest-performing methods, including CNN, Random Decision Forest, Extra Trees and tuned-Extra Trees. We extracted the performance data of these methods for each of the 21 cases that contain both T1 and Flair sequences, to compare directly with our method. Our performance compared to each rater and 4 methods is shown in Table 1. An example of segmentation is shown in Fig. 2.

Table 1. Comparison of leading scores obtained by Maier et al. [12], and the approach outlined in this work. The ground truth for two raters, GTG and GTL, is shown.

Index	VBStroke		CNN		Tuned ET		ET		RDF	
	GTL	GTG	GTL	GTG	GTL	GTG	GTL	GTG	GTL	GTG
DC	0.75 ± 0.08	0.73 ± 0.10	0.71 ± 0.10	0.73 ± 0.10	0.69 ± 0.16	0.67 ± 0.17	0.68 ± 0.17	0.66 ± 0.17	0.70 ± 0.14	0.68 ± 0.15
HD (mm)	35.49 ± 17.62	33.77 ± 15.71	28.70 ± 26.73	28.73 ± 25.88	25.54 ± 14.51	28.91 ± 13.85	25.17 ± 14.48	28.44 ± 13.77	26.05 ± 20.86	29.45 ± 19.90
ASSD (mm)	2.62 ± 1.60	3.01 ± 1.66	4.82 ± 6.05	4.74 ± 5.98	4.38 ± 2.63	4.98 ± 2.70	4.36 ± 2.60	4.98 ± 2.69	4.39 ± 3.18	4.87 ± 3.16
Prec	0.75 ± 0.14	0.81 ± 0.15	0.68 ± 0.16	0.76 ± 0.16	0.78 ± 0.17	0.85 ± 0.17	0.79 ± 0.17	0.85 ± 0.17	0.75 ± 0.17	0.82 ± 0.18
Recall	0.79 ± 0.13	0.70 ± 0.15	0.78 ± 0.12	0.73 ± 0.12	0.67 ± 0.22	0.60 ± 0.21	0.66 ± 0.23	0.59 ± 0.22	0.71 ± 0.20	0.64 ± 0.20

4.2 DSB

Comparison with Ground Truth. The segmentation results are summarized in Table 2. We achieve a high performance compared to the results in the literature [11,12], although we acknowledge that directly comparing results obtained with different datasets is not ideal. An example of segmentation is shown on Fig. 4.

Lesion Volume Evolution. The lesion volume difference (PVD) between the two timepoints available was measured for both the manual delineation and the automatic segmentation (see Fig. 3a). Some discrepancies exist between the differences measured manually or automatically (3b).

---

[4] http://dx.doi.org/10.6084/m9.figshare.1585018.

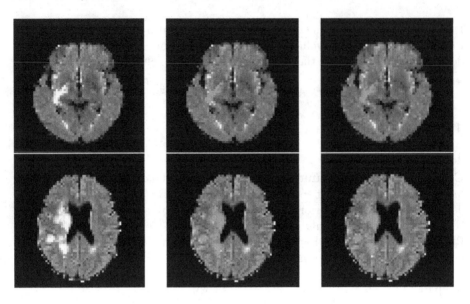

Fig. 2. Dataset A: Flair, groundtruth (GTG) and automatic segmentation shown for subject 9 (slice 24) and subject 11 (slice 29).

Table 2. Dataset B Segmentation Results

	DSC	ASSD	HD	Precision	Recall
Mean	0.720	3.508	43.357	0.674	0.799
Std. Dev.	0.147	2.648	16.543	0.168	0.146

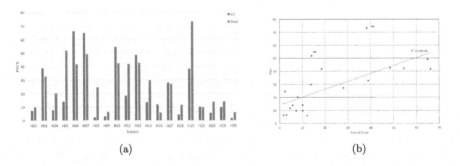

(a)   (b)

Fig. 3. Volume analysis: (a) PVD between two consecutive visits. (b) PVD correlation between automatic vs manual methods.

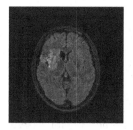 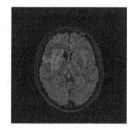 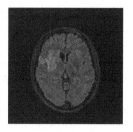

Fig. 4. Dataset A: case H19 Flair (top), Groundtruth (middle), and Automatic Segmentation (bottom)

5   Discussion and Conclusion

Recently, due to the impressive results obtained in lesion segmentation, attention has focused on supervised methods. However, their practical drawbacks are that they require a large collection of control datasets of good quality for training, including consistent manual tracings, and can be applied with success only on patient datasets with the same modality and quality as the control datasets. This dependence on the MR contrasts used for training (four in [15], one in [13] or [18]) hamper their versatility. Thus, the interesting results produced by LINDA for chronic stroke with T1-weighted images [18] cannot be successfully applied to sub-acute or chronic stroke due to different lesion appearance and modality used (i.e. FLAIR). Here we propose an unsupervised method with the hypothesis that such a class of method is less dependent of image quality and then more flexible to tackle the diversity images obtained with different sequence parameters and scanners; a particularly sensitive point for multi-center studies. The complex task of quantifying sub-acute and chronic stroke lesion volume is addressed by introducing prior information on the vascular territory in a Bayesian framework. The model parameters are instead estimated using a variational EM algorithm with MRF constraints and the inclusion of a priori probabilistic maps to provide a stable parameter trajectory during optimization. Vascular information is included via the use of a prior vascular territory atlas, that is adapted to the patient-specific data in a joint segmentation & registration framework. The performance of our method is comparable to the best supervised methods in [13]. As an illustration Fig. 2 shows case 21 for comparison with results obtained by nine methods (see Fig. 2 in [14]). Our method achieved good performance overall, with a number of challenging cases in which the lesion volume was overestimated (see Fig. 3b). In [17] a median inter-rater agreement for DSC was 0.78 with HD 23.4 mm (14 subjects and 9 raters) and in [3] a volume difference 18 ± 16 is reported; [21] reported a DSC equal to 0.64. For PVD [6] and [15] report respectively a mean of 29 (sd = 24) with a Pearson correlation r equal to 0.97 (30 cases) and 32 (sd = 22) with r = 0.76 (34 cases). In [10] a PVD of 79 (sd = 62) was found between two raters on 29 chronic FLAIR. These results should be compared to 24 and r = 98 we obtained on 47 cases (DSB).

The fusion of different methods, an approach demonstrated by [14] to have benefit in tumor and stroke segmentation, also shows potential and we are actively exploring techniques to remove these false positives.

To conclude, our method produces results that rival a manual delineation in most subjects. As an unsupervised technique, our method does not require a learning phase that can be intensive, impractical or sensitive, for most supervised methods. Despite its imperfection our automatic method can be interestingly coupled with a manual edition by the trained user who, in some difficult cases, corrects the initial automated demarcation in order to significantly speed up lesion delineation while keeping high precision [7]. Interestingly, this approach will be used in the RESSTORE cohort.

Acknowledgments. This work was partly supported by 'RESSTORE' project that has received funding from the European Union's Horizon 2020 research and innovation programme under grant agreement No 681044. Grenoble MRI facility IRMaGe was partly funded by the French program Investissement d'avenir run by the Agence Nationale pour la Recherche; grant Infrastructure d'avenir en Biologie Santé - ANR-11-INBS-0006.

The authors would also like to thank Oskar Maier and his colleagues for supplying dataset A.

References

1. Bishop, C.M.: Pattern Recognition and Machine Learning (Information Science and Statistics). Springer, New York (2006)
2. Chalela, J.A., Kidwell, C.S., Nentwich, L.M., Luby, M., Butman, J.A., Demchuk, A.M., Hill, M.D., Patronas, N., Latour, L., Warach, S.: Magnetic resonance imaging and computed tomography in emergency assessment of patients with suspected acute stroke: a prospective comparison. Lancet **369**(9558), 293–298 (2007)
3. Fiez, J.A., Damasio, H., Grabowski, T.J.: Lesion segmentation and manual warping to a reference brain: intra- and interobserver reliability. Hum. Brain Mapp. **9**(4), 192–211 (2000)
4. Forbes, F., Doyle, S., Garcia-Lorenzo, D., Barillot, C., Dojat, M.: A weighted multi-sequence markov model for brain lesion segmentation. In: Whye Teh, Y., Titterington, M. (eds.) Thirteenth International Conference on Artificial Intelligence and Statistics (AISTATS 2010) (2010)
5. Gelman, A., Carlin, J.B., Stern, H.S., Rubin, D.B.: Bayesian Data Analysis, 2nd edn. Chapman and Hall/CRC, Boca Raton (2004)
6. Griffis, J.C., Allendorfer, J.B., Szaflarski, J.P.: Voxel-based gaussian naive bayes classification of ischemic stroke lesions in individual t1-weighted MRI scans. J. Neurosci. Methods **257**, 97–108 (2016). https://www.ncbi.nlm.nih.gov/pubmed/26432931
7. de Haan, B., Clas, P., Juenger, H., Wilke, M., Karnath, H.O.: Fast semi-automated lesion demarcation in stroke. Neuroimage Clin. **9**, 69–74 (2015). https://www.ncbi.nlm.nih.gov/pubmed/26413473
8. Hommel, M., Miguel, S.T., Naegele, B., Gonnet, N., Jaillard, A.: Cognitive determinants of social functioning after a first ever mild to moderate stroke at vocational age. J. Neurol. Neurosurg. Psychiatry **80**(8), 876–880 (2009), Epub 8 Apr 2009. https://doi.org/10.1136/jnnp.2008.169672

9. Kamnitsas, K., Ledig, C., Newcombe, V.F., Simpson, J.P., Kane, A.D., Menon, D.K., Rueckert, D., Glocker, B.: Efficient multi-scale 3D CNN with fully connected CRF for accurate brain lesion segmentation. Med. Image Anal. **36**, 61–78 (2017)

10. Luby, M., Bykowski, J.L., Schellinger, P.D., Merino, J.G., Warach, S.: Intra- and interrater reliability of ischemic lesion volume measurements on diffusion-weighted, mean transit time and fluid-attenuated inversion recovery MRI. Stroke **37**(12), 2951–2956 (2006). https://www.ncbi.nlm.nih.gov/pubmed/17082470

11. Maier, O., Menze, B.H., von der Gablentz, J., Hani, L., Heinrich, M.P., Liebrand, M., Winzeck, S., Basit, A., Bentley, P., Chen, L., Christiaens, D., Dutil, F., Egger, K., Feng, C., Glocker, B., Gotz, M., Haeck, T., Halme, H.L., Havaei, M., Iftekharuddin, K.M., Jodoin, P.M., Kamnitsas, K., Kellner, E., Korvenoja, A., Larochelle, H., Ledig, C., Lee, J.H., Maes, F., Mahmood, Q., Maier-Hein, K.H., McKinley, R., Muschelli, J., Pal, C., Pei, L., Rangarajan, J.R., Reza, S.M., Robben, D., Rueckert, D., Salli, E., Suetens, P., Wang, C.W., Wilms, M., Kirschke, J.S., Kramer, U.M., Munte, T.F., Schramm, P., Wiest, R., Handels, H., Reyes, M.: Isles 2015 - a public evaluation benchmark for ischemic stroke lesion segmentation from multispectral MRI. Med. Image Anal. **35**, 250–269 (2017)

12. Maier, O., Schroder, C., Forkert, N.D., Martinetz, T., Handels, H.: Classifiers for ischemic stroke lesion segmentation: a comparison study. PLoS ONE **10**(12), e0145118 (2015)

13. Maier, O., Wilms, M., von der Gablentz, J., Kramer, U.M., Munte, T.F., Handels, H.: Extra tree forests for sub-acute ischemic stroke lesion segmentation in MR sequences. J. Neurosci. Methods **240**, 89–100 (2015)

14. Menze, B.H., Van Leemput, K., Lashkari, D., Riklin-Raviv, T., Geremia, E., Alberts, E., Gruber, P., Wegener, S., Weber, M.A., Szekely, G., Ayache, N., Golland, P.: A generative probabilistic model and discriminative extensions for brain lesion segmentation-with application to tumor and stroke. IEEE Trans. Med. Imaging **35**(4), 933–946 (2016)

15. Mitra, J., Bourgeat, P., Fripp, J., Ghose, S., Rose, S., Salvado, O., Connelly, A., Campbell, B., Palmer, S., Sharma, G., Christensen, S., Carey, L.: Lesion segmentation from multimodal MRI using random forest following ischemic stroke. Neuroimage **98**, 324–335 (2014)

16. Morey, R.A., Selgrade, E.S., Wagner, H. R., n., Huettel, S.A., Wang, L., McCarthy, G.: Scan-rescan reliability of subcortical brain volumes derived from automated segmentation. Hum. Brain Mapp. **31**(11), 1751–1762 (2010)

17. Neumann, A.B., Jonsdottir, K.Y., Mouridsen, K., Hjort, N., Gyldensted, C., Bizzi, A., Fiehler, J., Gasparotti, R., Gillard, J.H., Hermier, M., Kucinski, T., Larsson, E.M., Sorensen, L., Ostergaard, L.: Interrater agreement for final infarct MRI lesion delineation. Stroke **40**(12), 3768–3771 (2009)

18. Pustina, D., Coslett, H.B., Turkeltaub, P.E., Tustison, N., Schwartz, M.F., Avants, B.: Automated segmentation of chronic stroke lesions using linda: lesion identification with neighborhood data analysis. Hum. Brain Mapp. **37**(4), 1405–1421 (2016). https://www.ncbi.nlm.nih.gov/pubmed/26756101

19. Ritzl, A., Meisel, S., Wittsack, H.J., Fink, G.R., Siebler, M., Modder, U., Seitz, R.J.: Development of brain infarct volume as assessed by magnetic resonance imaging (MRI): follow-up of diffusion-weighted MRI lesions. J. Magn. Reson. Imaging **20**(2), 201–207 (2004). https://www.ncbi.nlm.nih.gov/pubmed/15269944

20. Scherrer, B., Forbes, F., Garbay, C., Dojat, M.: A joint Bayesian framework for MR brain scan tissue and structure segmentation based on distributed Markovian agents. In: Bichindaritz, I., Vaidya, S., Jain, A., Jain, L.C. (eds.) Computational Intelligence in Healthcare 4. SCI, vol. 309, pp. 81–101. Springer, Heidelberg (2010). https://doi.org/10.1007/978-3-642-14464-6_5

21. Seghier, M.L., Ramlackhansingh, A., Crinion, J., Leff, A.P., Price, C.J.: Lesion identification using unified segmentation-normalisation models and fuzzy clustering. Neuroimage 41(4), 1253–1266 (2008)

22. Tustison, N.J., Avants, B.B., Cook, P.A., Zheng, Y., Egan, A., Yushkevich, P.A., Gee, J.C.: N4itk: improved N3 bias correction. IEEE Trans. Med. Imaging. 29(6), 1310–1320. https://doi.org/10.1109/TMI.2010.2046908. Epub 8 Apr 2010 (2010)

23. Van Leemput, K., Maes, F., Vandermeulen, D., Suetens, P.: Automated model-based bias field correction in MR images of the brain. IEEE Trans. Med. Imag. 18(10), 885–896 (1999)

24. Warfield, S.K., Zou, K.H., Wells, W.M.: Simultaneous truth and performance level estimation (staple): an algorithm for the validation of image segmentation. IEEE Trans. Med. Imaging 23(7), 903–921 (2004)

25. Wilke, M., de Haan, B., Juenger, H., Karnath, H.O.: Manual, semi-automated, and automated delineation of chronic brain lesions: a comparison of methods. Neuroimage 56(4), 2038–2046 (2011)

Brain Tumor Segmentation Using an Adversarial Network

Zeju Li[1], Yuanyuan Wang[1,2($\boxtimes$)], and Jinhua Yu[1,2($\boxtimes$)]

[1] Department of Electronic Engineering, Fudan University, Shanghai, China
{yywang, jhyu}@fudan.edu.cn
[2] Key Laboratory of Medical Imaging Computing and Computer Assisted Intervention of Shanghai, Shanghai, China

Abstract. Recently, the convolutional neural network (CNN) has been successfully applied to the task of brain tumor segmentation. However, the effectiveness of a CNN-based method is limited by the small receptive field, and the segmentation results don't perform well in the spatial contiguity. Therefore, many attempts have been made to strengthen the spatial contiguity of the network output. In this paper, we proposed an adversarial training approach to train the CNN network. A discriminator network is trained along with a generator network which produces the synthetic segmentation results. The discriminator network is encouraged to discriminate the synthetic labels from the ground truth labels. Adversarial adjustments provided by the discriminator network are fed back to the generator network to help reduce the differences between the synthetic labels and the ground truth labels and reinforce the spatial contiguity with high-order loss terms. The presented method is evaluated on the Brats2017 training dataset. The experiment results demonstrate that the presented method could enhance the spatial contiguity of the segmentation results and improve the segmentation accuracy.

Keywords: Brain tumor segmentation · Adversarial network · Deep learning

1 Introduction

Automatic segmentation of brain tumors in magnetic resonance (MR) images is of great clinical value. Nevertheless, the task is technically challenging because tumor regions vary a lot in the shape and location [1]. Among the existing segmentation methods, the convolutional neural network (CNN) provides very outstanding results and attracts increasing attentions [2]. A CNN obtains stacked features and produces segmentation results by classifying image voxels based on these features. One defect of a CNN-based segmentation method is that the receptive field is always limited by the size of convolutional kernels [3]. In other words, each pixel in the image is predicted almost independently with each other. This problem could become more apparent in brain tumor segmentation because the appearance of brain tumors is unpredictable and MR images are inhomogeneous in the intensity. Therefore, the segmentation results of CNN-based methods always have rough boundaries and perform poorly on details of tumor sub-regions.

© Springer International Publishing AG, part of Springer Nature 2018
A. Crimi et al. (Eds.): BrainLes 2017, LNCS 10670, pp. 123–132, 2018.
https://doi.org/10.1007/978-3-319-75238-9_11

Actually, many efforts have been made to reinforce the spatial contiguity of the segmentation results. One solution is to add another CNN pathway with a larger receptive field [4]. The multiple pathway CNN structure could take advantage of both the visual details and larger context of the region around a certain pixel. However, the long-range connection would make the network more complex and bring a huge increase in the network computation. The conditional Markov random field (CRF) is another common approach to enhance the spatial contiguity of the output labels [5, 6]. A fully connected CRF is usually taken as the post-processing procedure of the CNN and takes the feature maps of the CNN as unary potentials to build the global probabilistic models. By the inference of graphical models, the CRF makes it possible to recover fine details in the output maps. Nevertheless, in practical applications, the global optimal parameters of the CRF are hard to find for the multiple classification problem. Refinement of different tumor sub-regions require different parameters of the CRF model, thus a CRF model with fixed parameters is only applicable to a specific kind of tumor sub-regions [6]. Instead of adding the context information or CRF, we want to strength the spatial contiguity by using an auxiliary high-order loss term, which can make the network more perceptive towards spatial-connected tumor regions. This idea is inspired by the generative adversarial network (GAN) [7]. The GAN, through the use of adversarial loss, has successfully been applied to the generation of real-life images in an unsupervised way [8].

In this paper, we present a novel CNN-based brain tumor segmentation method by using an adversarial network. A fully connected CNN is firstly applied to provide the segmentation results. A discriminator network, also taking advantage of the original images, is designed to discriminate the synthetic labels from the ground truth labels. The adversarial loss provided by the discriminator network encourages the generator network to correct the segmentation mistakes and produce more accurate and space continuous results. The presented method was evaluated on the Brats2017 training dataset. Experiment results demonstrated the effectiveness of adversarial network and showed that the presented method could provide competitive segmentation results.

2   Method

The proposed method consists of two CNN networks, named the generator network and the discriminator network. These two networks are tightly connected. The detailed structure is described in Fig. 1.

The generator network is similar to a regular CNN which is a feedforward neural network architecture. Patches of MR images are set as the input of the generator network. Ground truth labels of smaller patches with the same center are set as the targets. The backpropagation procedure helps the generator network learn to produce segmentation results.

The discriminator network is another separate CNN network. MR images and segmentation results are input to the discriminator network and then concatenated together in the network. The discriminator network is trained to distinguish between the synthetic labels and ground truth labels. The derivatives of the synthetic labels are computed by the backpropagation from the output at the top where the network takes the synthetic labels as real.

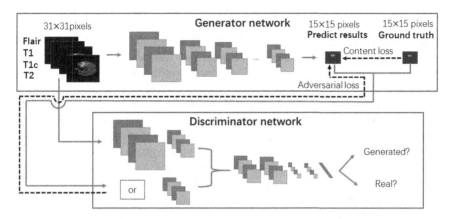

Fig. 1. Schematic diagram of the proposed framework. Forward propagations are depicted using blue lines and backward propagations are depicted using black dotted lines. (Color figure online)

The derivatives of synthetic labels are fed back to the generator network to provide external adjustments. The adversarial loss is added up with the pixel-wise content loss in the output layer of the generator network. These two networks are trained in an iterative way. Specifically, a single batch of images is input to the generator network to create the synthetic labels with fixed network parameters. Then, the synthetic labels together with the ground truth labels are input to the discriminator network. Along with the training process of the discriminator network, the gradient is propagated through all the way to the bottom and forms the adversarial loss. Lastly, the adversarial loss is delivered to the generator network and participates in the training of the generator network. The detailed network structures were demonstrated in Fig. 2. Implement details of the presented method are described in the following paragraphs.

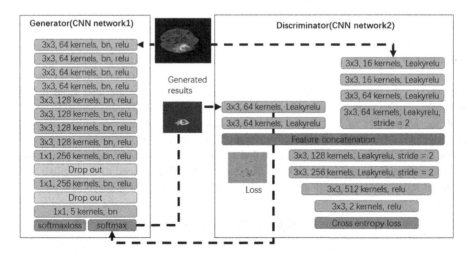

Fig. 2. The network structures of the two CNN networks used in this work.

2.1   Generator Network

Taking into account that the portion of tumor regions is quite small in the brain MR images, the network training process is carried out with image patches, instead of taking the full-size image as the input. The selection of the patches is uneven for the better recognition of tumor regions. Patches with tumor regions are more likely to be selected. During the training phase, image patches I with the size of 31×31 pixels are input to the network. The generator network consists of 11 layers. All first eight layers include three stages of convolutional layers with 3×3 kernels, relu layers and batch normalization layers. The convolutional layers are built without padding, therefore the output features maps have the size of 15×15 pixels $(31 - 2 \times 8)$. The last three layers are taken as dense layers, where convolutional kernels with the size of 1×1 are utilized. Two dropout layers are added before the last two layers.

The lost function of the generator network consists of two parts, called the content loss and the adversarial loss. Specifically, the loss function is calculated as:

$$L^G = L_{softmax}(G(I), label_{GT}) + L_{Ad}^G \tag{1}$$

The first term $L_{softmax}$, namely the content loss, is the pixel-wise derivatives. The content loss is calculated based on the softmax-loss between the prediction and ground truth of four given labels. I represent the patches of four modalities MR images. $label_{GT}$ represent the given ground truth labels which are corresponding to I. In order to take advantage of more context information, the size of the predicted label is small than the input images. Specifically, $label_{GT}$ are the ground truth labels with the size of 15×15 pixels around the same image center of I. The second term, L_{Ad}^G namely the adversarial loss, is produced simultaneously by the adversarial network and is discussed in the next section. It is worth being mentioned that only the generator network is utilized during the test phase. Therefore, the presented method would not increase the complexity of the CNN network.

2.2   Discriminator Network

Adversarial Training. The discriminator network is a core of the presented method. The synthetic labels and the ground truth labels, with the form of the one-hot coding, are input to the discriminator network. The original MR images are also input to the network as references. The discriminator network consists of 10 convolutional layers with the kernel size of 3×3 and full padding. Leaky relu layers are utilized but no pooling layers are included in the discriminator network, as suggested by a previous GAN study [9]. Images are down sampled to the same size of the labels using convolutional layers with stride 2. The discriminator network is trained to distinguish two kinds of labels obtained from different places. The loss function is calculated as:

$$L^D = \frac{1}{2}[L_{bce}(I, D(label_{GT}), 0) + L_{bce}(I, D(G(I)), 1)] \tag{2}$$

As usual, the binary cross entropy (bce) loss is calculated to differ two types of inputs. The batch size of the discriminator network is twice the size of the generator network. Therefore, the discriminator network could process both the synthetic labels and ground truth labels in a single batch.

Adversarial Loss. The discriminator network provides the adversarial loss by minimizing the probability that the adversarial predicts $D(label_{GT})$ are similar to the one of synthetic labels. The adversarial loss is calculated as:

$$L_{Ad}^G = L_{bce}(I, D(G(I)), 0) \tag{3}$$

The adversarial loss contains high order derivatives and are fed back to the generator network in (1) Gradients from the adversarial network encourage the generator network to correct the mistakes of the segmentation results with high-order terms. The discriminator network could assess the mutual information of many label varies and reinforce the spatial contiguity of the segmentation results with the global information. The adversarial loss is produced by the discriminator network after a long period of training and could not be assessed by the pixel-wise content loss.

The adversarial loss is produced along with the training process of the generator network and the discriminator network. However, the discriminator network with the poor discrimination ability may not provide the effective adjustment for the generator network. The effectiveness of pretrain of the model is evaluated in this study. During the pretrain procedure, the generator network is firstly trained for a while separately, and the discriminator is trained with settled generator network until the network is stable.

2.3   Pre-processing and Post-processing

Before entering the patches to the networks, some pre-processing procedures are taken to make the input data have similar distributions. The intensity of the patches are normalized to from 0 to 1 for each channel, separately. Then the mean values of the patches are subtracted and the variances of the patches are united, separately for each channel. In the post-processing stage, we want to reduce the false positive segmentation results. In particular, the tumor region is always gathered in a certain area. However, the network may mistake other regions as tumor because of the intensity inhomogeneity of MR images. Regions with similar gray intensity but in other brain areas could be likely to be mistaken. Therefore, the largest three-dimensional (3D) connection region of the segmentation results is firstly chosen as the tumor candidate. 3D bounding box slightly larger than the tumor candidate is built, and then recognized region inside the bounding box are finally identified as the tumor region.

3   Experimental Results

All the experiments were developed on the top of Matconvnet. Both the generator network and the discriminator network were trained using Adam optimizer with beta1 = 0.9, beta2 = 0.999 and epsilon = 1e-8. The primary learning rate was 1e-3 and

1e-4 for the generator network and discriminator network, separately. The learning rates were decreased exponentially. The two CNN networks were both initialized using Xavier method. The batch size of the generator network and the discriminator network is 128 and 256 respectively. About 280,000 patches are extracted from the training data. Patch samples inside and around tumor regions are more likely to be taken. Consequently, about 40% of the selected patches contain tumor regions.

3.1   Material

The presented tumor segmentation methods were evaluated on the Brats2017 training dataset [10–12]. The dataset consists of four MR images modalities (T1, T1c, T2 and Flair) of 285 patients. The tumor regions were manually segmented into three sub-regions including the enhancing tumor (label4), the peritumoral edema (label2) and the necrotic and non-enhancing tumor (label1). Whole regions (label1 + label2 + label4), core regions (label1 + label3) and enhancing regions (label4) of the segmentation results were evaluated, separately. The Dice similarity coefficient (DSC), positive predictive value (PPV) and sensitivity (Sen.) were calculated for segmentation results with the corresponding manual segmentation as the ground truth. Calculation details of those indices could be found in the previous study [1].

3.2   Evaluation on the BRATS2017 Training Dataset

The effectiveness of adversarial training. It is interesting for us to observe the effect of the addition of the discriminator network. Thus, two experiments were carried out with exactly the same condition except for the existence of the adversarial network. Qualitative results could be found in Fig. 3. With the help of adversarial loss, the amount of over segmentation is reduced. False positive segmentation results are also decreased. Moreover, the spatial contiguity of segmentation of all tumor sub-regions is enhanced. The segmentation results become smoother in the sub-regions and preserve good boundaries. It is hard to achieve by the post-processing of CRF with certain parameters.

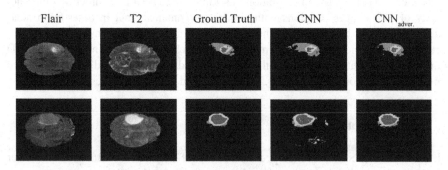

Fig. 3. Visual segmentation results of two examples using the direct outputs of CNN network.

To quantitative exhibit the effectiveness of the adversarial loss, the segmentation results of all 285 training data are summarized in Table 1. To better illustrate the effectiveness of the adversarial loss, the segmentation results were extracted directly from the generator network without any post-processing. We can see that the improvement by the adversarial loss is small but consistent in all sub-regions.

Table 1. Quantitative segmentation results of 285 training data using the direct outputs of a CNN network. $CNN_{adver.}$ corresponds to the network trained with the adversarial loss.

Method	Whole			Core			Enhancing		
	DSC	PPV	Sen.	DSC	PPV	Sen.	DSC	PPV	Sen.
CNN	86.1	82.2	90.0	86.3	85.5	87.2	77.1	74.2	80.1
$CNN_{adver.}$	**87.9**	**86.8**	89.0	**86.8**	**86.6**	87.0	**77.5**	**77.1**	77.9

To better illustrate the effectiveness of the loss from adversarial network, the losses are visualized in Fig. 4. The pixel-wise content loss, which is the most common loss for the neural network, is calculated simply by the derivatives between the feedforward network output and the given ground truth. The pixel-wise content losses directly represent the differences in the given cases but might not be the best for the overall dataset.

FLAIR	Ground Truth	Network Output	Pixel-wise Loss	Loss from the Discriminator Network

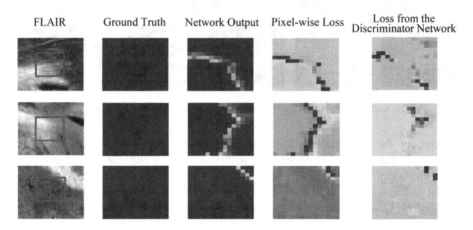

Fig. 4. Comparison between the pixel-wise content loss and the loss from the discriminator network. In the last two columns of image, the more obvious the color change, the greater the value of loss in the corresponding area.

On the other hand, loss from the discriminator network could be more perceptual. The discriminator network is trained by discriminating the synthetic labels from the ground truth labels with the use of plenty of MR image and corresponding label patches. The adversarial network can discover the mutual characteristics of the mistakes. As we can see from Fig. 4, the adversarial losses do not simply be obtained by the first-order derivative but generated in a high-order form. Actually, the adversarial loss could figure out the more important parts of the mistaken regions, which have the greater impact on the identification of the discriminator network. The adversarial loss would help the output of the generator network visually closer to the ground truth and more likely to fool the discriminator network. This would drive the generator network produce more realistic and space continuous results. The adversarial loss may be not the best option for the single given case but could lead the generator network to pursue the best solutions for the overall dataset. What is more, this kind of high-order loss has a stronger adaptability, contains more global information, and cannot be provided by per-pixel loss. Thus, this kind of loss is more meaningful.

Results of adding adversarial loss with pretrain. As mentioned in the method section, the pretrain of the model seems to be useful. Understandably, the better the discriminator is trained, the more effective the adversarial loss is. The experiment results illustrate this point. As demonstrated in Fig. 5, segmentation results of the pretrain model show more accurate recognition ability, especially in details.

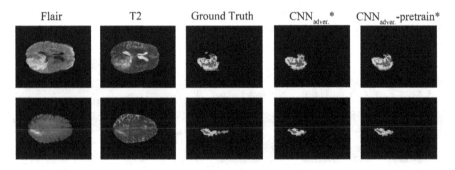

Fig. 5. Visual segmentation results of two examples using a CNN with the adversarial loss.

Similarly, the quantitative segmentation results of all 285 training data are summarized in Table 2. It could be seen that the post-processing procedure could improve the segmentation accuracy. Better segmentation results could be carried out with the pretrain of the model. Compared with the results of previous methods on the previous Brats dataset [1], segmentation results provided by the presented method is competitive.

Table 2. Quantitative segmentation results of 285 training data using a CNN with the adversarial loss. Results with post-processing is marked followed by *.

Method	Whole			Core			Enhancing		
	DSC	PPV	Sen.	DSC	PPV	Sen.	DSC	PPV	Sen.
CNN$_{adver.}$	87.9	86.8	89.0	86.8	86.6	87.0	77.5	77.1	77.9
CNN$_{adver.}$*	89.5	90.6	88.4	88.0	89.0	87.0	78.4	79.1	77.8
CNN$_{adver.}$-pretrain*	**89.7**	89.8	88.5	**88.4**	**89.7**	**87.2**	**79.1**	78.1	**80.0**

3.3   Cross Validation on the Brats2017 Training Dataset

The presented method was also evaluated on a separate dataset. The proposed model was trained once again using 250 cases randomly selected from the Brats2017 training dataset. The rest 35 cases were set as separate validation dataset. Quantitative results are summarized in Table 3. The experiment results also demonstrate the effectiveness of the adversarial network.

Table 3. Quantitative results of separate validation data from Brats2017 training dataset.

Method	Whole			Core			Enhancing		
	DSC	PPV	Sen.	DSC	PPV	Sen.	DSC	PPV	Sen.
CNN*	85.8	86.9	84.6	72.3	76.8	68.3	67.7	71.3	67.5
CNN$_{adver.}$*	**87.0**	86.7	**87.2**	72.0	71.4	**72.5**	**68.2**	68.3	**68.1**

4   Conclusion

In this study, a novel CNN-based tumor segmentation method with adversarial network is presented. A high-order adversarial loss provided simultaneously by the discriminator network is added to encourage the generator network to produce more precise results. Experiments on the Brats2017 training dataset demonstrate that the presented methods could enhance the spatial contiguity of the segmentation results in all tumor sub-regions and improve segmentation accuracy. Moreover, the effectiveness of pre-train of the model is demonstrated in this study. Compared with segmentation results of previous researches on the previous Brats dataset, our method could provide competitive segmentation results. It should be mentioned that the presented method is also efficient and energy-saving since the complexity is not added to the network at test time. In the future, we will extent the presented method into 3D to better make use of the 3D information of MR images. Further, we will exploit the best way to take advantage of the adversarial loss.

Acknowledgments.   This work was supported by the National Basic Research Program of China (2015CB755500), the National Natural Science Foundation of China (11474071).

References

1. Menze, B.H., Jakab, A., Bauer, S., Kalpathy-Cramer, J., Farahani, K., Kirby, J., et al.: The multimodal brain tumor image segmentation benchmark (BRATS). IEEE Trans. Med. Imaging **34**(10), 1993–2024 (2015)
2. Pereira, S., Pinto, A., Alves, V., Silva, C.A.: Brain tumor segmentation using convolutional neural networks in MR images. IEEE Trans. on Med. Imaging **35**(5), 1240–1251 (2016)
3. Zhao, X., Wu, Y., Song, G., Li, Z., Fan, Y., Zhang, Y.: Brain tumor segmentation using a fully convolutional neural network with conditional random fields. In: Crimi, A., Menze, B., Maier, O., Reyes, M., Winzeck, S., Handels, H. (eds.) BrainLes 2016. LNCS, vol. 10154, pp. 77–80. Springer, Cham (2016). https://doi.org/10.1007/978-3-319-55524-9_8

4. Havaei, M., Davy, A., Wardefarley, D., Biard, A., Courville, A., Bengio, Y., et al.: Brain tumor segmentation with deep neural networks. Med. Image Anal. **35**, 18–31 (2017)
5. Li, Z., Wang, Y., Yu, J., Shi, Z., Guo, Y., Chen, L., et al.: Low grade glioma segmentation based on CNN with fully connected CRF. J. Healthc. Eng. **2017** (2017). https://doi.org/10.1155/2017/9283480. Article No. 9283480
6. Kamnitsas, K., Ledig, C., Newcombe, V.F., Simpson, J.P., Kane, A.D., Menon, D.K., et al.: Efficient multi-scale 3D CNN with fully connected crf for accurate brain lesion segmentation. Med. Image Anal. **36**, 61–78 (2017)
7. Luc, P., Couprie, C., Chintala, S., Verbeek, J.: Semantic segmentation using adversarial networks. arXiv:1611.08408 (2016)
8. Goodfellow, I.J., Pouget-Abadie, J., Mirza, M., Xu, B., Warde-Farley, D., Ozair, S., et al.: Generative adversarial networks. In: NIPS, pp. 2672–2680 (2014)
9. Radford, A., Metz, L., Chintala, S.: Unsupervised representation learning with deep convolutional generative adversarial networks. arXiv:1511.06434 (2015)
10. Bakas, S., Akbari, H., Sotiras, A., Bilello, M., Rozycki, M., Kirby, J., et al.: Advancing The Cancer Genome Atlas glioma MRI collections with expert segmentation labels and radiomic features. Sci Data **4** (2017). https://doi.org/10.1038/sdata.2017.117. Article No.170117
11. Bakas, S., Akbari, H., Sotiras, A., Bilello, M., Rozycki, M., Kirby, J., at al.: Segmentation Labels and Radiomic Features for the Pre-operative Scans of the TCGA-GBM collection. The Cancer Imaging Archive (2017)
12. Bakas, S., Akbari, H., Sotiras, A., Bilello, M., Rozycki, M., Kirby, J., at al.: Segmentation Labels and Radiomic Features for the Pre-operative Scans of the TCGA-LGG collection. The Cancer Imaging Archive (2017)

Brain Cancer Imaging Phenomics Toolkit (brain-CaPTk): An Interactive Platform for Quantitative Analysis of Glioblastoma

Saima Rathore[✉], Spyridon Bakas, Sarthak Pati, Hamed Akbari,
Ratheesh Kalarot, Patmaa Sridharan, Martin Rozycki, Mark Bergman,
Birkan Tunc, Ragini Verma, Michel Bilello, and Christos Davatzikos

Department of Radiology, Perelman School of Medicine,
Center for Biomedical Image Computing and Analytics (CBICA),
University of Pennsylvania, Philadelphia, PA, USA
saima.rathore@uphs.upenn.edu

Abstract. Quantitative research, especially in the field of radio(geno)mics, has helped us understand fundamental mechanisms of neurologic diseases. Such research is integrally based on advanced algorithms to derive extensive radiomic features and integrate them into diagnostic and predictive models. To exploit the benefit of such complex algorithms, their swift translation into clinical practice is required, currently hindered by their complicated nature. brain-CaPTk is a modular platform, with components spanning across image processing, segmentation, feature extraction, and machine learning, that facilitates such translation, enabling quantitative analyses without requiring substantial computational background. Thus, brain-CaPTk can be seamlessly integrated into the typical quantification, analysis and reporting workflow of a radiologist, underscoring its clinical potential. This paper describes currently available components of brain-CaPTk and example results from their application in glioblastoma.

Keywords: Glioblastoma · Open-source software · Radiomics
Radiogenomics · Computational algorithms · Image analysis · Fiber tracking

1 Introduction

Quantitative computational research has helped us gain a comprehensive understanding of fundamental mechanisms of neurologic diseases, while providing substantive insight into the biological basis of disease susceptibility and treatment response, as well as potentially leading to the identification of new therapeutic targets. During the last decade there is mounting evidence that clinically acquired radiographic imaging can reveal visual (e.g., intensity, extent) and sub-visual (e.g., morphologic, textural, kinetic) features, which when integrated via advanced computational methods can identify *in vivo* imaging signatures of clinical outcomes, as well as of underlying tumor molecular characteristics (radiogenomic signatures) [1–10]. However, despite their widespread applicability in the scientific research community and the promising findings obtained with them, the increasingly complicated nature of advanced computational algorithms limits their accessibility in routine clinical practice. Thus, there is

© Springer International Publishing AG, part of Springer Nature 2018
A. Crimi et al. (Eds.): BrainLes 2017, LNCS 10670, pp. 133–145, 2018.
https://doi.org/10.1007/978-3-319-75238-9_12

a rising need for relatively easy-to-use software tools that can assist the translation of such algorithms in the clinical setting. Towards this end, we present brain-Cancer imaging Phenomics Toolkit (brain-CaPTk – www.med.upenn.edu/sbia/captk.html), which can provide a bridge for quick and efficient translation between academic image analysis research and clinical application, thereby enabling translation of cutting-edge academic research into clinically practical tools.

brain-CaPTk aims to derive extensively comprehensive sets of quantitative radiomic features and integrate them via advanced multivariate machine learning methods towards providing related neuroimaging biomarkers for integrative precision diagnosis and prediction of clinical outcome, while being seamlessly integrated into the typical quantification, analysis and reporting workflow of a radiologist, underscoring its clinical potential. Existing tools offering computational algorithms have not been designed to target specific diseases [11–14] and are neither modularized nor offer specialized analysis tools [12–14]. Although the rest of this paper focuses on example applications of brain-CaPTk in glioblastoma, its incorporated components can be applied in most neurological diseases, such as meningioma, multiple sclerosis, stroke, and trauma brain injuries, with the intention of linking quantitative imaging signatures with clinical outcome and molecular characteristics.

2   Platform and Components

The hereby presented platform, brain-CaPTk, leverages well-established open-source libraries, such as the Insight ToolKit (ITK), Visualization ToolKit (VTK) and OpenCV, to perform the data input/output, preprocessing tasks, rendering and machine learning. The advantage of using these well-established community- and industry-driven software libraries is their optimized algorithmic environment, allowing for further extension, interoperability and cross-platform usability. The overall design of brain-CaPTk is adaptable, allowing for packages developed using ITK and OpenCV to be incorporated within brain-CaPTk with minimal effort, thereby providing to imaging researchers a ready-to-use graphical front-end for their computational algorithms.

Although, brain-CaPTk is a dynamically growing software platform and can consider any anatomical site and image type, it currently focuses on analyzing multimodal Magnetic Resonance Imaging (MRI), such as native (T1) and contrast-enhanced T1-weighted (T1-Gd), T2-weighted (T2), T2 Fluid Attenuated Inversion Recovery (T2-FLAIR), Diffusion Tensor Imaging (DTI), Dynamic Susceptibility Contrast (DSC), and Dynamic Contrast-Enhanced (DCE). Furthermore, brain-CaPTk also supports visualization of DTI derivative measurements such as the tensor's apparent diffusion coefficient, axial diffusivity, radial diffusivity, and fractional anisotropy, as well as parametric maps extracted from DSC of relative cerebral blood volume, peak height and percentage signal recovery.

brain-CaPTk is based on a two-tier functionality: (1) Image processing and analysis algorithms enable the extraction of extensive radiomic features; (2) Machine learning methods integrate these features into diagnostic, prognostic and predictive biomarkers. Currently incorporated components for preprocessing, interaction, segmentation, feature extraction, and specialized diagnostic analysis, are described below.

2.1 Preprocessing

An essential component for such quantitative research is the appropriate image preprocessing. The related brain-CaPTk tools (Fig. 1) are fully-parameterizable and entail: (i) image denoising (i.e., intensity noise reduction in regions of uniform intensity profile) [15]; (ii) bias correction (i.e., correction for magnetic field inhomogeneity based on non-parametric non-uniform intensity normalization) [16]; (iii) co-registration of various modalities (i.e., for examining in tandem at the voxel level anatomically aligned signals); (iv) skull stripping; and (v) intensity normalization (scaling in a certain range, z-score, and histogram matching) [17].

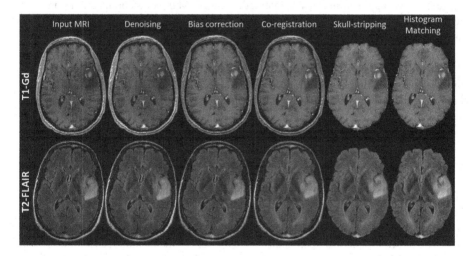

Fig. 1. Example application of the preprocessing tools available in brain-CaPTk.

2.2 Interaction

Part of brain-CaPTk's emphasis focuses in its lightweight and efficient operation without the burden of computationally expensive algorithms weighing in the interaction process. Its interaction tools include spherical approximation of abnormalities, coordinate definition, and region annotation that may be used as initialization of segmentation methods [18–20] and as region masks for further analysis (Fig. 2).

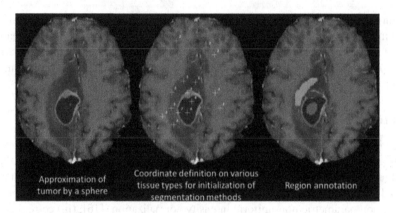

Fig. 2. Example of brain-CaPTk's interaction tools.

2.3   Image Segmentation

Representative applications of the interaction tools available in brain-CaPTk include two segmentation methods that require initialization, namely, GLISTRboost [18, 19] and geodesic distance transform (GDT) [20].

GLISTRboost is a hybrid generative-discriminative method developed for brain glioma segmentation and atlas registration in multimodal MRI, while incorporating tumor growth modeling via reaction-diffusion-advection [21]. The generative part creates the tumor and healthy-tissue segmentation labels based on expectation-maximization. The discriminative part refines tumor labels based on multiple patients, through a gradient boosting multi-class classification scheme [22]. A Bayesian strategy then finalizes the segmentation based on patient-specific intensity statistics from the multimodal MRI [23]. Specifically, brain-CaPTk enables the seamless initialization of GLISTRboost by (i) the definition of a sphere's center and radius that are used to initialize the growth model, and (ii) the coordinate definition on various tissue types that are used as prior knowledge to guide the segmentation process (Fig. 2). GLISTRboost, due to its complexity is not incorporated in brain-CaPTk yet, but is available for public use through the online Image Processing Portal (ipp.cbica.upenn.edu) of Center for Biomedical Image Computing and Analytics (CBICA), which allows users to perform their analyses without any software installation and whilst using CBICA's High Performance Computing resources.

The segmentation of brain structures based on the GDT [20], is a patient-based method fully incorporated in brain-CaPTk. In particular, a region is annotated to initialize the calculation of an "adaptive geodesic distance", which at a given voxel i is a joint quantification of intensity variation and spatial distance between i and the seed region. The calculation of this distance at every voxel in the image yields an "adaptive GDT image" on which a threshold is applied to generate the final segmentation label (Fig. 3). This method is appealing as it is computationally efficient and does not need high-performance computer hardware. Moreover, it does not require any preprocessing, is highly adaptable to any imaging modality, and remains insensitive to acquisition protocols. Thus, its "simplistic" nature supports its potential applicability in ample routine clinical settings for delineation of anatomical regions.

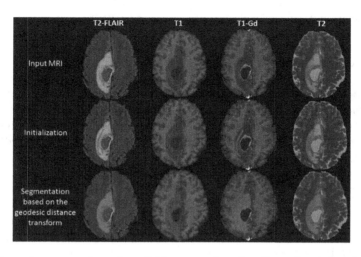

Fig. 3. Example segmentation of a glioblastoma sub-region (i.e., edema) based on GDT. "Initialization" denotes the region annotated manually for initiating the segmentation algorithm.

2.4 Feature Extraction

brain-CaPTk offers extraction of an extensively comprehensive panel of radiomic features both in 3D and 2D, depending on the operator's choice. The feature panel available in brain-CaPTk is continuously expanding, however, it currently comprises (i) intensity-based, (ii) textural, and (iii) volumetric/morphologic features (Table 1). The biological significance of the individual radiomic features remains unknown notwithstanding many related studies, and are provided to facilitate research on their association with molecular markers, clinical outcomes, treatment responses, and other endpoints. Via automated functionality provided by brain-CaPTk these features may enable clinicians and other researchers to extract feature measurements and conduct large-scale analyses in a repeatable manner.

Table 1. Radiomic features offered by brain-CaPTk for analysis of neurological diseases.

Feature type	Description
Intensity-Based	– 1st & 2nd order statistics (mean, standard deviation, skewness, kurtosis); – range and distributions of gray-level histograms [9]; – principal components of DSC image [24]
Textural	– gray-level co-occurrence matrix [25]; – gray-level run-length matrix [26]; – gray-level size zone matrix [26, 27]; – neighborhood gray-tone difference matrix [28]; – local binary patterns [29];
Volumetric/Morphologic	– shape descriptors (i.e., area/volume, eccentricity, sphericity, solidity, perimeter, elongation) [30, 31]

2.5   Specialized Analysis - Imaging Signature of EGFR Mutations

The radiogenomic marker currently integrated in brain-CaPTk allows the *in vivo* determination of mutations in the Epidermal Growth Factor Receptor (EGFR) in glioblastoma, through a quantitative within-patient/self-normalized peritumoral perfusion heterogeneity measure. The specific mutations that have been assessed so far comprise the splice variant III (EGFRvIII) [6, 10] and the amplification of the wild-type EGFR [7]. This marker requires the annotation of two regions; one near and another far from the enhancing tumor, but still within the peritumoral edema depicted by the abnormal T2-FLAIR signal. Principal components of the temporal perfusion dynamics of these regions are then estimated and the Bhattacharyya coefficient is used to represent the peritumoral heterogeneity index (PHI). The discovered non-invasive personalized *in vivo* imaging marker of EGFR mutations utilizes clinically-available imaging protocols, without the need to deliver radiolabeled probes, which renders it likely for immediate translation into the clinic as a first-line pre-operative detection of this molecular target.

2.6   Neuro-Oncological Planning Tools

Some of the major challenges faced by fiber tracking in the realm of neurosurgical planning is that the reconstruction of tracts is affected by mass effect, when the tracts are displaced and distorted, and edema and infiltration, when the tracts are broken, as a result of change of diffusion parameters due to pathology. This underlines the needs for methods that can track through edema and reconstruct even partial and displaced tracts. To this end, brain-CaPTk provides tools for tractography robust to edema [32, 33] and automated tract detection based on connectivity signatures [34, 35], to extract fiber tracts, even distorted or broken, in the presence of mass effect and edema (Fig. 4). The edema invariant tractography [32, 33] is based on the multi-compartment modeling of diffusion data (a free water component representative of the edema and another component representing the underlying tissue) that is fitted with a tensor or higher order diffusion model, based on the single/multishell acquisition. The automated tract detection framework defines a fiber bundle atlas that will emulate the expert, using white matter fibers of healthy individuals. The white matter tracts in any patient are then extracted based on the definitions encoded in the atlas, using connectivity signatures of the fibers [34, 35].

3   Results and Application

3.1   Image Segmentation

GLISTRboost is the top-performing method in the BraTS'15 challenge [18, 19, 36], thereby emphasizing the value of brain-CaPTk that allowed the initialization of numerous glioma scans in a short timeframe. The tumor regions evaluated during BraTS described the tumor part that enhances in the T1-Gd image (ET), the core of the tumor (TC) that is typically resected during surgery, and the whole tumor (WT) which comprised the TC and the peritumoral edema/invasion. Specifically, the median Dice score values with their corresponding Inter-Quartile Ranges (IQR) for the three evaluated regions, i.e. WT, TC, ET, were equal to 0.92 (IQR: 0.88–0.94), 0.88 (IQR: 0.81–0.93) and 0.88 (IQR: 0.81–0.91), respectively. Furthermore, such specialized algorithms as GLISTRboost enable the evaluation of tumor spatial distribution in standardized coordinate systems, which receive increasing attention as predictors of clinical outcome as well as markers of underlying tumor molecular characteristics [37].

The segmentation method incorporated in brain-CaPTk, based on GDT, was previously validated on T1-Gd images of 24 glioblastomas, 15 meningiomas, and 15 metastases, captured under diverse acquisition conditions, and reported Dice scores of 0.82, 0.83, and 0.69, respectively [20]. We have further evaluated GDT on 132 T2-FLAIR glioblastoma baseline images, from the BraTS'15 challenge training dataset. The optimal cut-off threshold was determined based on 10-fold cross-validation, yielding an average Dice score of 0.72 for the WT.

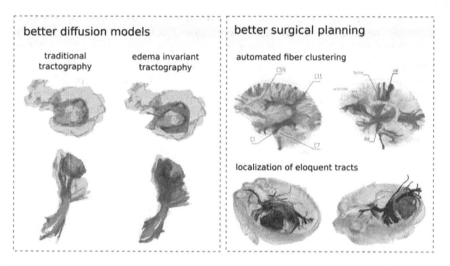

Fig. 4. Tools for edema invariant tractography and automated tract detection. (Left panel) Tracking through edema made possible with multi-compartment modeling of diffusion data; (Right panel) Atlas-based reconstruction of tracts, resilient to mass effect induced tract distortions, and the surgical plan with the tumor and surrounding eloquent tract.

3.2   Feature Extraction

Extensive literature over the past decade has shown that rich panels of quantitative imaging features can result in non-invasive imaging signatures with diagnostic, prognostic and predictive value for many types of cancer, such as lung [38, 39], neck [38] and brain [2, 6–10, 40–43]. Specifically, these features have shown evidence of imaging signatures relating to underlying molecular characteristics, treatment response, patient survival, with the potential of augmenting conventional prognostic and predictive assays.

Specifically about the intensity-based features offered in brain-CaPTk, the histogram distributions capture anatomical and functional changes caused by the tumor, and have demonstrated a connection to clinical endpoints, such as survival, and molecular subtypes [8, 9]. The principal component features of temporal perfusion dynamics have been related to recurrence and infiltration [24, 42], as well as molecular characteristics [6, 7, 10, 44]. Furthermore, the textural features available in brain-CaPTk capture characteristics of the local micro-architecture of tissue and have already demonstrated predictive and prognostic value [9, 38, 41, 44, 45].

3.3   Specialized Analysis - Imaging Signature of EGFR Mutations

The patient-based radiogenomic signature of EGFRvIII in glioblastoma integrated in brain-CaPTk was applied in independent discovery (γ) and replication (δ) cohorts, as well as their combination (ζ), and revealed highly significant distinctive results in all configurations ($p_\gamma = 1.57 \times 10^{-7}$, $p_\delta = 2.8 \times 10^{-4}$, $p_\zeta = 4 \times 10^{-10}$) (Fig. 5). Its accuracy (89.92%), specificity (92.53%), sensitivity (83.77%), as well as its independent sample repeatability (Intra-class Correlation Coefficient (ICC) = 0.825) and reproducibility (ICC = 0.775), supports its potential routine clinical use [6, 7, 10]. Such signatures contribute to personalized medicine, and can enable non-invasive patient selection for targeted therapy, stratification into clinical trials, and repeatable monitoring of mutations during the treatment course.

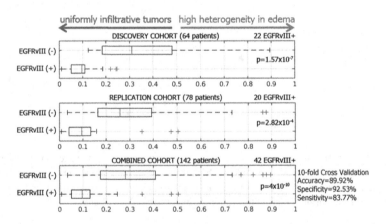

Fig. 5. Distributions of the PHI by EGFRvIII expression status.

3.4   Neuro-Oncological Planning Tools

The applicability, reliability and repeatability of the automated tract extraction tool integrated in brain-CaPTk, was validated in a dataset of healthy individuals acquired repeatedly [35]. Compared to the clustering of fibers for each scan independently, our framework provided better reproducibility (test-retest) results, with decreased (25%) mean intra-individual distance (i.e., disagreement of clusters between different time-points of the same individual), while preserving inter-individual differences.

Additionally, the framework was also tested in tumor patients [34] on six major fiber bundles: cingulum bundle; fornix, uncinate fasciculus (UF), arcuate fasciculus, inferior fronto-occipital fasciculus, and inferior longitudinal fasciculus (ILF). The agreement between clustering and experts as quantified by Cohen's kappa ranged between 0.6 and 0.76. Except two tracts, ILF and UF, the agreement between clustering and experts was higher than agreement between experts themselves, highlighting the reliability of the paradigm. When the tumor demonstrated significant mass effect or shift, the automated approach was useful to provide an initialization to guide the experts with the identification of the specific tract of interest.

4 Extendability

There are two mechanisms for integrating new applications into brain-CaPTk, each with its own advantages and disadvantages:

4.1 Source Level Integration

This is the tighest integration, providing memory-level access to all of brain-CaPTk interactive functionalities while allowing for maximum optimization. The external application should be written in C++ and compiled alongside brain-CaPTk.

4.2 Executable Level Integration

This level provides a graphical interface to an existing command-line application (not necessarily developed in C++), allowing users to leverage brain-CaPTk's functionality (e.g., interaction, feature extraction). Executable-level integration requires only minor additions to brain-CaPTk to create a menu option for the new application.

5 Conclusion and Future Work

Although, advanced computational algorithms have shown exciting clinically-significant findings in the research community, their complicated nature limits clinical applicability, revealing a need for software tools to help with translation of such complex algorithms into clinical practice, and hence to maximize their potential benefit.

brain-CaPTk describes a platform that can allow: (1) clinical use of computationally complex algorithms, (2) non-imaging experts (e.g., bioinformaticians, or clinicians who do not have sufficient computational background) to generate quantitative data useful for correlative clinical/genomic studies, and (3) imaging experts to integrate their advanced computational algorithms in an existing easy-to-use front-end, benchmark new algorithms and perform inter-institution comparisons.

Immediate future plans include the integration of various other specialized diagnostic analysis tools for glioblastoma, such as prediction of survival [9], potential recurrence [42], and characterization into distinct imaging subtypes [41], as well as application of existing brain-CaPTk components in other neurological diseases, i.e. meningioma and multiple sclerosis.

Acknowledgments. This work was supported by the NIH grants R01-NS042645 and U24-CA189523.

References

1. Aerts, H.J.: The potential of radiomic-based phenotyping in precision medicine: a review. JAMA Oncol. **2**, 1636–1642 (2016)
2. Zinn, P.O., Mahajan, B., Sathyan, P., Singh, S.K., Majumder, S., Jolesz, F.A., Colen, R.R.: Radiogenomic mapping of edema/cellular invasion MRI-phenotypes in glioblastoma multiforme. PLoS One **6**, e25451 (2011)
3. Gevaert, O., Mitchell, L.A., Achrol, A.S., Xu, J., Echegaray, S., Steinberg, G.K., Cheshier, S.H., Napel, S., Zaharchuk, G., Plevritis, S.K.: Glioblastoma multiforme: exploratory radiogenomic analysis by using quantitative image features. Radiology **273**, 168–174 (2014)
4. Jain, R., Poisson, L.M., Gutman, D., Scarpace, L., Hwang, S.N., Holder, C.A., Wintermark, M., Rao, A., Colen, R.R., Kirby, J., Freymann, J., Jaffe, C.C., Mikkelsen, T., Flanders, A.: Outcome prediction in patients with glioblastoma by using imaging, clinical, and genomic biomarkers: focus on the nonenhancing component of the tumor. Radiology **272**, 484–493 (2014)
5. Ellingson, B.M.: Radiogenomics and imaging phenotypes in glioblastoma: novel observations and correlation with molecular characteristics. Curr. Neurol. Neurosci. Rep. **15**, 506 (2015)
6. Bakas, S., Akbari, H., Pisapia, J., Martinez-Lage, M., Rozycki, M., Rathore, S., Dahmane, N., O'Rourke, D.M., Davatzikos, C.: In vivo detection of EGFRvIII in glioblastoma via perfusion magnetic resonance imaging signature consistent with deep peritumoral infiltration: the φ index. Clin. Cancer Res. **23**, 4724–4734 (2017)
7. Bakas, S., Binder, Z.A., Akbari, H., Martinez-Lage, M., Rozycki, M., Morrissette, J.J.D., Dahmane, N., O'Rourke, D.M., Davatzikos, C.: Highly-expressed wild-type EGFR and EGFRvIII mutant glioblastomas have similar MRI signature, consistent with deep peritumoral infiltration. Neuro-Oncol. **18**, vi125 (2016)
8. Akbari, H., Bakas, S., Rozycki, M., Da, X., Pisapia, J., Bilello, M., O'Rourke, D., Davatzikos, C.: Non-invasive determination of epidermal growth factor receptor variant III expression in glioblastoma through analysis of multi-parametric magnetic resonance imaging. In: Oral Presentation in 101st Scientific Assembly and Annual Meeting of the Radiological Society of North America (RSNA) (2015)
9. Macyszyn, L., Akbari, H., Pisapia, J.M., Da, X., Attiah, M., Pigrish, V., Bi, Y., Pal, S., Davuluri, R.V., Roccograndi, L., Dahmane, N., Biros, G., Wolf, R.L., Bilello, M., O'Rourke, D.M., Davatzikos, C.: Imaging patterns predict patient survival and molecular subtype in glioblastoma via machine learning techniques. Neuro-Oncol. **18**, 417–425 (2016)
10. Bakas, S., Akbari, H., Pisapia, J., Rozycki, M., O'Rourke, D., Davatzikos, C.: Identification of imaging signatures of the epidermal growth factor receptor variant III (EGFRvIII) in glioblastoma. Neuro-Oncol. **17**, 154 (2015)
11. Fedorov, A., Beichel, R., Kalpathy-Cramer, J., Finet, J., Fillion-Robin, J.C., Pujol, S., Bauer, C., Jennings, D., Fennessy, F., Sonka, M., Buatti, J., Aylward, S., Miller, J.V., Pieper, S., Kikinis, R.: 3D slicer as an image computing platform for the quantitative imaging network. Magn. Reson. Imaging **30**, 1323–1341 (2012)

12. Jenkinson, M., Beckmann, C.F., Behrens, T.E.J., Woolrich, M.W., Smith, S.M.: FSL. NeuroImage **62**, 782–790 (2012)
13. http://citeseerx.ist.psu.edu/viewdoc/summary?doi=10.1.1.180.3343
14. https://mipav.cit.nih.gov/
15. Smith, S.M., Brady, J.M.: SUSAN - a new approach to low level image processing. Int. J. Comput. Vis. **23**, 45–78 (1997)
16. Tustison, N.J., Avants, B.B., Cook, P.A., Zheng, Y., Egan, A., Yushkevich, P.A., Gee, J.C.: N4ITK: improved N3 bias correction. IEEE Trans. Med. Imaging **29**, 1310–1320 (2010)
17. Nyul, L.G., Udupa, J.K., Zhang, X.: New variants of a method of MRI scale standardization. IEEE Trans. Med. Imaging **19**, 143–150 (2000)
18. Bakas, S., Zeng, K., Sotiras, A., Rathore, S., Akbari, H., Gaonkar, B., Rozycki, M., Pati, S., Davatzikos, C.: GLISTRboost: combining multimodal MRI segmentation, registration, and biophysical tumor growth modeling with gradient boosting machines for glioma segmentation. In: Crimi, A., Menze, B., Maier, O., Reyes, M., Handels, H. (eds.) BrainLes 2015. LNCS, vol. 9556, pp. 144–155. Springer, Cham (2016). https://doi.org/10.1007/978-3-319-30858-6_13
19. Bakas, S., Zeng, K., Sotiras, A., Rathore, S., Akbari, H., Gaonkar, B., Rozycki, M., Pati, S., Davatzikos, C.: Segmentation of gliomas in multimodal magnetic resonance imaging volumes based on a hybrid generative-discriminative framework. In: Menze, B., Reyes, M., Farahani, K., Kalpathy-Cramer, J., Kwon, D. (eds.) Proceedings of the Multimodal Brain Tumor Image Segmentation Challenge Held in Conjunction with MICCAI 2015 (MICCAI-BRATS 2015), 5–9 October 2015, pp. 5–12. Technische Universität München (T.U.M.), Munich, Germany (2015)
20. Gaonkar, B., Macyszyn, L., Bilello, M., Sadaghiani, M.S., Akbari, H., Atthiah, M.A., Ali, Z. S., Da, X., Zhan, Y., Rourke, D.O., Grady, S.M., Davatzikos, C.: Automated tumor volumetry using computer-aided image segmentation. Acad. Radiol. **22**, 653–661 (2015)
21. Hogea, C., Davatzikos, C., Biros, G.: An image-driven parameter estimation problem for a reaction-diffusion glioma growth model with mass effects. J. Math. Biol. **56**, 793–825 (2008)
22. Friedman, J.H.: Stochastic gradient boosting. Comput. Statist. Data Anal. **38**, 367–378 (2002)
23. Bakas, S., Chatzimichail, K., Hunter, G., Labbe, B., Sidhu, P.S., Makris, D.: Fast semi-automatic segmentation of focal liver lesions in contrast-enhanced ultrasound, based on a probabilistic model. In: TCIV Computer Methods in Biomechanics and Biomedical Engineering: Imaging & Visualization (2015). ePub-ahead-of-print
24. Akbari, H., Macyszyn, L., Da, X., Wolf, R.L., Bilello, M., Verma, R., O'Rourke, D.M., Davatzikos, C.: Pattern analysis of dynamic susceptibility contrast MRI reveals peritumoral tissue heterogeneity. Radiology **273**, 502–510 (2014)
25. Haralick, R.M., Shanmugam, K., Dinstein, I.H.: Textural features for image classification. IEEE Trans. Syst. Man Cybern. **3**, 610–621 (1973)
26. Galloway, M.M.: Texture analysis using grey level run lengths. Comput. Graph. Image Process. **4**, 172–179 (1975)
27. Tang, X.: Texture information in run-length matrices. IEEE Trans. Image Process. **7**, 1602–1609 (1998)
28. Amadasun, M., King, R.: Textural features corresponding to textural properties. IEEE Trans. Syst. Man Cybern. **19**, 1264–1274 (1989)
29. Ojala, T., Pietikainen, M., Maenpaa, T.: Multiresolution gray-scale and rotation invariant texture classification with local binary patterns. IEEE Trans. Pattern Anal. Mach. Intell. **24**, 971–987 (2002)

30. Thibault, G., Fertil, B., Navarro, C., Pereira, S., Cau, P., Levy, N., Sequeira, J., Mari, J.-L.: Shape and texture indexes application to cell nuclei classification. Int. J. Pattern Recognit. Artif. Intell. **27**, 1357002 (2013)

31. Vallières, M., Freeman, C., Skamene, S., El Naqa, I.: A radiomics model from joint FDG-PET and MRI texture features for the prediction of lung metastases in soft-tissue sarcomas of the extremities. Phys. Med. Biol. **60**, 5471 (2015)

32. Lecoeur, J., Caruyer, E., Elliott, M., Brem, S., Macyszyn, L., Verma, R.: Addressing the challenge of edema in fiber tracking. In: Medical Image Computing and Computer-Assisted Intervention MICCAI 2014, DTI Tractography Challenge, Boston, MA (2014)

33. Lecoeur, J., Caruyer, E., Macyszyn, L., Verma, R.: Improving white matter tractography by resolving the challenges of edema. In: MICCAI Workshop: DTI Challenge 2013 (2013)

34. Tunc, B., Ingalhalikar, M., Parker, D., Lecoeur, J., Singh, N., Wolf, R.L., Macyszyn, L., Brem, S., Verma, R.: Individualized map of white matter pathways: connectivity-based paradigm for neurosurgical planning. Neurosurgery **79**, 568–577 (2016)

35. Tunc, B., Parker, W.A., Ingalhalikar, M., Verma, R.: Automated tract extraction via atlas based adaptive clustering. NeuroImage **102P2**, 596–607 (2014)

36. Menze, B.H., Jakab, A., Bauer, S., Kalpathy-Cramer, J., Farahani, K., Kirby, J., Burren, Y., Porz, N., Slotboom, J., Wiest, R., Lanczi, L., Gerstner, E., Weber, M.A., Arbel, T., Avants, B.B., Ayache, N., Buendia, P., Collins, D.L., Cordier, N., Corso, J.J., Criminisi, A., Das, T., Delingette, H., Ç, D., Durst, C.R., Dojat, M., Doyle, S., Festa, J., Forbes, F., Geremia, E., Glocker, B., Golland, P., Guo, X., Hamamci, A., Iftekharuddin, K.M., Jena, R., John, N.M., Konukoglu, E., Lashkari, D., Mariz, J.A., Meier, R., Pereira, S., Precup, D., Price, S.J., Raviv, T.R., Reza, S.M.S., Ryan, M., Sarikaya, D., Schwartz, L., Shin, H.C., Shotton, J., Silva, C.A., Sousa, N., Subbanna, N.K., Szekely, G., Taylor, T.J., Thomas, O.M., Tustison, N.J., Unal, G., Vasseur, F., Wintermark, M., Ye, D.H., Zhao, L., Zhao, B., Zikic, D., Prastawa, M., Reyes, M., Leemput, K.V.: The multimodal brain tumor image segmentation benchmark (BRATS). IEEE Trans. Med. Imaging **34**, 1993–2024 (2015)

37. Bilello, M., Akbari, H., Da, X., Pisapia, J.M., Mohan, S., Wolf, R.L., O'Rourke, D.M., Martinez-Lage, M., Davatzikos, C.: Population-based MRI atlases of spatial distribution are specific to patient and tumor characteristics in glioblastoma. Neuroimage Clin. **12**, 34–40 (2016)

38. Aerts, H.J., Velazquez, E.R., Leijenaar, R.T., Parmar, C., Grossmann, P., Carvalho, S., Bussink, J., Monshouwer, R., Haibe-Kains, B., Rietveld, D., Hoebers, F., Rietbergen, M.M., Leemans, C.R., Dekker, A., Quackenbush, J., Gillies, R.J., Lambin, P.: Decoding tumour phenotype by noninvasive imaging using a quantitative radiomics approach. Nat. Commun. **5**, 4006 (2014)

39. Gevaert, O., Xu, J., Hoang, C.D., Leung, A.N., Xu, Y., Quon, A., Rubin, D.L., Napel, S., Plevritis, S.K.: Non-small cell lung cancer: identifying prognostic imaging biomarkers by leveraging public gene expression microarray data–methods and preliminary results. Radiology **264**, 387–396 (2012)

40. Diehn, M., Nardini, C., Wang, D.S., McGovern, S., Jayaraman, M., Liang, Y., Aldape, K., Cha, S., Kuo, M.D.: Identification of noninvasive imaging surrogates for brain tumor gene-expression modules. Proc. Natl. Acad. Sci. USA **105**, 5213–5218 (2008)

41. Rathore, S., Akbari, H., Rozycki, M., Bakas, S., Davatzikos, C.: Imaging pattern analysis reveals three distinct phenotypic subtypes of GBM with different survival rates. Neuro-Oncol. **18**, vi128 (2016)

42. Akbari, H., Macyszyn, L., Da, X., Bilello, M., Wolf, R.L., Martinez-Lage, M., Biros, G., Alonso-Basanta, M., O'Rourke, D.M., Davatzikos, C.: Imaging surrogates of infiltration obtained via multiparametric imaging pattern analysis predict subsequent location of recurrence of glioblastoma. Neurosurgery **78**, 572–580 (2016)

43. Akbari, H., Macyszyn, L., Pisapia, J., Da, X., Attiah, M., Bi, Y., Pal, S., Davuluri, R., Roccograndi, L., Dahmane, N., Wolf, R., Bilello, M., O'Rourke, D., Davatzikos, C.: Survival Prediction in Glioblastoma Patients Using Multi-parametric MRI Biomarkers and Machine Learning Methods. ASNR, Chicago, IL (2015)

44. Binder, Z.A., Bakas, S., Wileyto, E.P., Akbari, H., Rathore, S., Rozycki, M., Morrissette, J.J. D., Martinez-Lage, M., Dahmane, N., Davatzikos, C., O'Rourke, D.M.: Extracellular EGFR289 activating mutations confer poorer survival and exhibit radiographic signature of enhanced motility in primary glioblastoma. Neuro-Oncol. **18**, vi105–vi106 (2016)

45. Assefa, D., Keller, H., Ménard, C., Laperriere, N., Ferrari, R.J., Yeung, I.: Robust texture features for response monitoring of glioblastoma multiforme on T1-weighted and T2-FLAIR MR images: a preliminary investigation in terms of identification and segmentation. Med. Phys. **37**, 1722–1736 (2010)

Brain Tumor Image Segmentation

Deep Learning Based Multimodal Brain Tumor Diagnosis

Yuexiang Li and Linlin Shen[(✉)]

College of Computer Science and Software Engineering,
Computer Vision Institute, Shenzhen University, Shenzhen, China
{yuexiang.li,llshen}@szu.edu.cn

Abstract. Brain tumor segmentation plays an important role in the disease diagnosis. In this paper, we proposed deep learning frameworks, i.e. MvNet and SPNet, to address the challenges of multimodal brain tumor segmentation. The proposed multi-view deep learning framework (MvNet) uses three multi-branch fully-convolutional residual networks (Mb-FCRN) to segment multimodal brain images from different view-point, i.e. slices along x, y, z axis. The three sub-networks produce independent segmentation results and vote for the final outcome. The SPNet is a CNN-based framework developed to predict the survival time of patients. The proposed deep learning frameworks was evaluated on BraTS 17 validation set and achieved competing results for tumor segmentation While Dice scores of 0.88, 0.75 0.71 were achieved for whole tumor, enhancing tumor and tumor core, respectively, an accuracy of 0.55 was obtained for survival prediction.

Keywords: Deep learning · Multi-view · Tumor segmentation
Survival prediction

1 Introduction

Brain tumor is a severe disease threating the health of human-being. An accurate automatic tumor segmentation framework can significantly improve the efficiency of disease diagnosis and help design appropriate treatment strategy. In recent years, we witnessed the development of deep learning algorithm and were impressed by its powerful performance. Increasing numbers of studies tried to employ deep learning algorithm to process medical images. In previous challenges, i.e. BraTS 15–16 [1–3], various 2D and 3D deep learning networks have been proposed for the segmentation of multimodal brain tumor. For example, Lun et al. evaluated three types of 2-D convolutional networks, i.e. Patch-Wise, FCN [4] and SegNet [5] for BraTS 15 dataset. Kamnitsas et al. extended a 3-D CNN architecture, i.e. DeepMedic [6], with residual connections for brain lesion segmentation. In more recent research, Havaei et al. split 3D brain MRI data into 2D slices and crop patches from 2D slices to train deep neural networks [7]. Fidon et al. proposed scalable multimodal convolutional networks for brain tumor segmentation, which can explicitly leverage deep features within or across modalities [8]. Tseng et al. proposed a Cross-Modality convolutional network for brain tumor segmentation [9]. The network utilizes convolutional LSTM to model a

© Springer International Publishing AG, part of Springer Nature 2018
A. Crimi et al. (Eds.): BrainLes 2017, LNCS 10670, pp. 149–158, 2018.
https://doi.org/10.1007/978-3-319-75238-9_13

sequence of 2D slices, and jointly learn the multi-modalities and convolutional LSTM in an end-to-end manner. The approach achieved an excellent result on BraTS 15 dataset. However, most of the proposed 2D networks only use the slices along z-axis, which do not fully explore the spatial information compared to the 3D approaches. As the 3D convolutional network is not computational-efficient, an efficient and accurate brain tumor automatic segmentation system is worthwhile to develop.

Using the brain tumor data to predict the survival days of patients is a new task announced in BraTS 17. Lots of related work has been proposed. For example, Zhou et al. developed a computational framework using tumor sub-regions and three classifiers, i.e. SVM, Naïve Bayes classifier and KNN classifier, to predict survival period of patients [10]. Lao et al. proposed a deep learning-based model for survival prediction of Glioblastoma Multiforme (GBM) patients in more recent research [11].

In this paper, we proposed deep learning frameworks to address the two tasks announced in BraTS 17, i.e. brain tumor segmentation and survival-days prediction. A 2.5D deep learning framework is proposed to address the task of brain tumor segmentation. The network has three sub-networks for different view-points, which takes the advantages of both 2D and 3D approaches. The sub-network adopts a novel architecture, namely multi-branch fully-convolutional ResNet (Mb-FCRN), for tumor segmentation. Henceforth, the proposed 2.5D framework is named as Multi-view net (MvNet). For the survival prediction, we proposed a CNN-based framework, namely SPNet, to address the challenge. The proposed deep learning frameworks have been evaluated on BraTS 17 validation set. The experimental results demonstrate the competing performances of our deep learning frameworks.

2   Multi-view Deep Learning Network (MvNet)

2.1   Image Pre-processing

BraTS 17 dataset is utilized in this work. The dataset contains multimodal MRI scans of glioblastoma (GBM/HGG) and lower grade glioma (LGG). We only adopt HGG data for network training. The HGG has 210 multimodal MRI scans with the resolution of $240 \times 240 \times 155$. We extract the 2D slices along different axis, i.e. x, y and z, to form the training sets for Mb-FCRNs. The approach proposed by Nyul [12] is applied to normalize the extracted MRI slices. No data augmentation is applied to the training sets.

2.2   Network Architecture

The proposed MvNet framework consisting of three sub-networks, which process multimodal brain images along different axis, is illustrated in Fig. 1. FLAIR voxel data is taken for example, though four brain image models, i.e. T1, T1Gd, T2 and FLAIR, are available. The slices from different modal were concatenated as input for each Mb-FCRN.

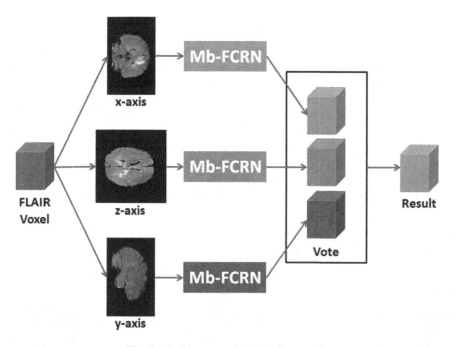

Fig. 1. Architecture of MvNet framework

2.3   Multi-branch Fully-Convolutional ResNet (Mb-FCRN)

MRI scans of different modalities enhance different tumor sub-regions for observation. For examples, the whole tumor is visible in T2-FLAIR (Fig. 2(d)), the tumor core is visible in T2 (Fig. 2(c)) and the enhancing tumor structures surrounding the cystic/necrotic components of the core are visible in T1Gd (Fig. 2(b)). Figure 2(a) is the native scan, i.e. T1. Hence, we proposed a multi-branch fully-convolutional residual network (Mb-FCRN), which has separate branch to independently extract features, to fully utilize the enhanced information in different modal MRI scans.

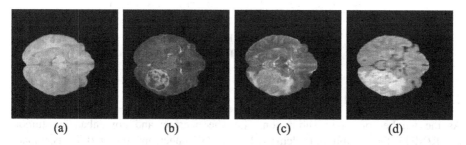

| (a) | (b) | (c) | (d) |

Fig. 2. Examples of different modal MRI scans. (a) native scan (T1). (b) post-contrast T1-weighted (T1Gd). (c) T2-weighted (T2). (d) T2 Fluid Attenuated Inversion Recovery (FLAIR) volumes.

Figure 3 presents the architecture of multi-branch fully-convolutional ResNet (Mb-FCRN). The green and blue rectangles represent the concatenation layer and convolutional layer, respectively. ReLU is used as the non-linear activation function. Batch Normalization layer [13] is placed between the convolutional layer and ReLU. The ResNet-101 [14] pre-trained on ImageNet [15] is converted to fully-convolutional network, i.e. FCRN-101, based on the U-net based architecture [16]. The MFE is modal feature extractor used to separately extract features from different modal MRI scans. The architecture of MFE is presented in Table 1. We use a Network in Network based architecture [17] to fuse the features extracted by MFEs and the original brain slices. The fused output is then fed to the fully-convolutional ResNet-101, i.e. FCRN-101, for tumor segmentation. The MRI scans are cropped to 224×224, 224×144 and 224×144 for z-axis, x-axis and y-axis Mb-FCRNs, respectively.

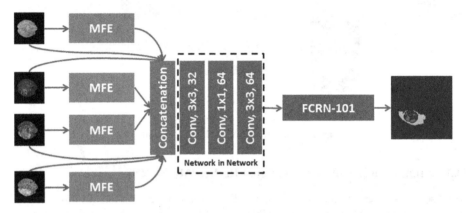

Fig. 3. Flowchart of Mb-FCRN. The MFE is modal feature extractor. ResNet-101 is converted to a U-net based fully-convolutional network, i.e. FCRN-101.

Table 1. Detailed information of MFE used in Mb-FCRN. The pipeline consists of Input layer (**I**), Convolutional layer (**C**), Batch Normalization layer (**BN**), ReLU layer (**R**).

Layer	Input size	Type	Kernel size & amount
1	224×224x1	I-C-BN-R	3×3, 4
2	224×224x4	C-BN-R	3×3, 4
3	224×224x4	C-BN-R	3×3, 4

2.4 Weighted Focal Loss

As the number of tumor sub-regions, i.e. the necrotic and non-enhancing tumor (NCR/NET), the peritumoral edema (ED) and GD-enhancing tumor (ET), is imbalanced, weighted Focal loss is applied for the supervision of Mb-FCRN to prevent the sub-regions with vast volume overwhelming the network during training. The original

Focal loss [18] is derived from softmax loss. Hence, we begin with the definition of softmax loss (L), as defined in Eq. (1).

$$L = \frac{1}{N}\sum_i L_i = \frac{1}{N}\sum_i -\log\left(\frac{e^{f_{y_i}}}{\sum_j e^{f_j}}\right) \tag{1}$$

where f_j denotes the j-th element ($j \in [1, K]$, K is the number of classes) of vector of class scores f, y_i is the label of i-th input feature and N is the number of training data. Let $p_i = \frac{e^{f_{y_i}}}{\sum_j e^{f_j}}$, the softmax loss (L) can be rewrote as $L = \frac{1}{N}\sum_i -\log(p_i)$. Therefore, the Focal loss (FL) can be defined as:

$$FL(p_i) = -(1 - p_i)^\gamma \log(p_i) \tag{2}$$

where $\gamma = 2$ in our experiments.

To further address the imbalance problem, according to the number of each sub-region, we assign different weights, i.e. 10, 5, 20, to NCR/NET, ED and ET, respectively.

2.5 Implementation

The proposed MvNet is established using PyTorch toolbox. The network is trained on two K80 with a mini-batch size of 30. Adam is used as the optimizer [19]. The start learning-rate is set to 0.0002. The BraTS 17 training dataset [20, 21] is separated to training and validation sets according to the ratio of 80:20. The three sub-networks are separately trained on training set and validated on validation set. Figure 4 presents the loss curves i.e. the blue lines are for training loss while green lines are for validation loss, for Mb-FCRN along different axis. From Fig. 4, the three sub-networks are found to produce the best performances on validation set after about 20 epochs of training.

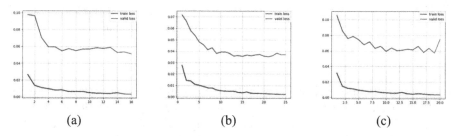

(a)   (b)   (c)

Fig. 4. Loss curves on validation set. (a) is for x-axis Mb-FCRN. (b) is for y-axis Mb-FCRN and (c) is for z-axis Mb-FCRN.

3   CNN for Survival Prediction (SPNet)

3.1   Network Architecture

Survival prediction is a new task introduced in BraTS 17. We developed a convolutional network, namely SPNet, to predict the survival days of patients. The convolutional network (CNN) takes the four brain image modals and the tumor segmentation result from MvNet as input and finally predicts the survival days. Figure 5 shows the flowchart of SPNet. The blue, red, orange and purple rectangles represent the convolutional layer, max pooling layer, average pooling layer and fully-connected layer, respectively. The framework concatenates the age information provided by challenge organizers and the features extracted by convolutions for final prediction of survival days. Batch Normalization layer and LeakyReLU are placed after each convolutional layer. The SPNet is optimized by the supervision of Mean Square Error Loss. The ground truths of survival days are normalized to [0, 1] by dividing the maximum value of days for SPNet training, which needs to be multiplied back to the prediction of SPNet during testing.

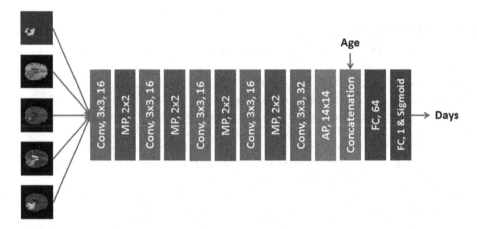

Fig. 5. Flowchart for survival prediction (Color figure online)

3.2   Implementation

The proposed SPNet is established using PyTorch toolbox. The network is trained on two K80 with a mini-batch size of 64. Adam is used as the optimizer [19]. While 80% of BraTS 17 dataset is used for network training, the remaining 20% is used for validation. The SPNet is observed to converge after 10 epochs of training.

4   Results

4.1   Dataset

Multimodal Brain Tumor Segmentation Challenge (BraTS) was continuously held since 2012. The datasets utilized in this year have been updated with more routine clinically-acquired 3T multimodal MRI scans and all the ground truth labels have been manually-labelled by expert board-certified neuroradiologists. As illustrated in Fig. 2, four modal brain MRI scans, i.e. native (**T1**), post-contrast T1-weighted (**T1Gd**), T2-weighted (**T2**), and T2 Fluid Attenuated Inversion Recovery (**FLAIR**) volumes, were acquired. The resolution of MRI scans is $240 \times 240 \times 155$.

The BraTS 17 training dataset contains 210 multimodal MRI scans of glioblastoma (GBM/HGG) and 75 scans of lower grade glioma (LGG). The BraTS 17 validation set contains 46 MRI scans. The competition participants need to test their algorithms on the validation set and send the segmentation results to the challenge organizers for evaluation. All the imaging datasets have been segmented manually, by one to four raters, following the same annotation protocol, and their annotations were approved by experienced neuro-radiologists. Annotations comprise the GD-enhancing tumor (ET — label 4), the peritumoral edema (ED — label 2), and the necrotic and non-enhancing tumor (NCR/NET — label 1), as described in [1]. The annotations of BraTS 17 training set is provided to the competition participants, while the annotations of BraTS 17 validation set is unpublished.

4.2   Evaluation Criterion

Brain Tumor Segmentation. The Dice score and the Hausdorff distance were used in BraTS 17 to evaluate the performance addressing tumor segmentation task, which is consistent with the previous BraTS challenges. Expanding upon this evaluation scheme, the metrics of Sensitivity and Specificity were also used in BraTS 17. In this paper, we mainly use 'Dice score' for the evaluation of segmentation performance.

Survival prediction. Two schemes based on classification and regression principles were involved for performance evaluation of survival prediction task in BraTS 17 challenge. For the evaluation based on the classification principle, the provided data is divided in three groups based on survival, i.e. long-survivors (e.g., >15 months), short-survivors (e.g., <10 months), and mid-survivors (e.g. between 10 and 15 months). The algorithms from participant teams are evaluated based on classification accuracy (i.e. the number of correctly classified survivors over all patients). For the evaluation based on the regression principle, the Mean Square Error is used to evaluate the predictions in a pairwise manner. In this paper, the classification accuracy is adopted to evaluate the performance of survival prediction.

4.3   Tumor Segmentation

Figure 6 presents the example of segmentation results produced by different Mb-FCRNs on BraTS 17 validation dataset. The labels in the results represent different regions of brain tumor. It can be observed from Fig. 6 that the final result (Fig. 6(d)) removes the segmentation errors by fusing results from different Mb-FCRNs (Fig. 6(a–c)).

To evaluate the performance of proposed MvNet, two well-known deep learning networks, i.e. U-net [16] and FCRN-101 [14], are selected for comparison. We calculate the Dice coefficient of z-axis only framework and our MvNet on the BraTS 17 validation set. In Table 2, ET represents enhancing tumor. WT represents whole tumor and TC represents tumor core. As the 2.5D MvNet adopts information along two more axes for tumor segmentation, the overall segmentation performances of MvNets with U-net/FRCN-101, are better than the z-axis only frameworks. Among the listed algorithms, the proposed MvNet with Mb-FCRN provides the best performance on BraTS 17 validation set, i.e. Dice coefficients of 0.75, 0.88 and 0.71 were achieved for ET, WT and TC, respectively.

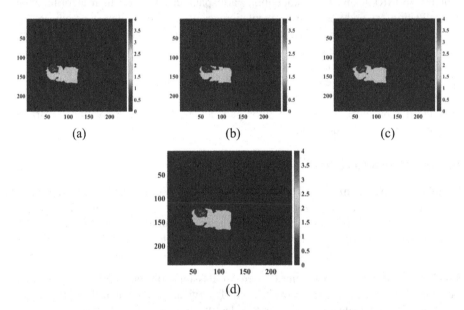

(a)   (b)   (c)

(d)

Fig. 6. Segmentation results (view from z-axis). (a) Result from x-axis Mb-FCRN. (b) Result from y-axis Mb-FCRN. (c) Result from z-axis Mb-FCRN. (d) Final result after voting.

Table 2. Dice coefficient of different frameworks on validation set

	Dice_ET	Dice_WT	Dice_TC
z-axis U-net	0.49	0.77	0.62
z-axis FCRN-101	0.65	0.86	0.68
MvNet (with U-net)	0.66	0.84	0.54
MvNet (with FCRN-101)	0.74	0.86	0.68
MvNet (with Mb-FCRN)	**0.75**	**0.88**	**0.71**

4.4 Survival Prediction

There are 18 submissions for the validation set of survival prediction in BraTS 17. The proposed SPNet achieved an accuracy of 0.55, which ranks the fifth place of the competition.

4.5 BraTS 17 Testing Set

BraTS 17 testing set contains 146 multimodal MRI scans. Participant teams ran their algorithms on the testing set and sent the results to the competition organizers for final ranking. The proposed MvNet achieved Dice coefficients of 0.69, 0.88 and 0.71 for ET, WT and TC, respectively, on BraTS 17 testing set. For the survival prediction, an accuracy of 0.45 was achieved by our SPNet.

5   Conclusion

In this paper, we proposed deep learning frameworks, so-called MvNet and SPNet, to address the tasks of multi-modal brain tumor segmentation and survival prediction of patients. The proposed MvNet employs three sub-networks to process the brain images along different axis. The results on BraTS 17 validation set show the competing performance of MvNet, i.e. Dice scores of 0.88, 0.75 and 0.71 were achieved for whole tumor, enhancing tumor and tumor core, respectively. The SPNet is a CNN-based network, which achieved an accuracy of 0.55 on BraTS 17 validation set.

Acknowledgement. The work was supported by Natural Science Foundation of China under grands no. 61672357 and 61702339, the Science Foundation of Shenzhen under Grant No. JCYJ20160422144110140, and the China Postdoctoral Science Foundation under Grant No. 2017M622779.

References

1. Menze, B.H., Jakab, A., Bauer, S., Kalpathycramer, J., Farahani, K., Kirby, J., Burren, Y., Porz, N., Slotboom, J., Wiest, R.: The multimodal brain tumor image segmentation benchmark (BRATS). IEEE Trans. Med. Imaging **34**, 1993–2024 (2015)
2. Previous BraTS Challenges. http://www.braintumorsegmentation.org/
3. Bakas, S., Akbari, H., Sotiras, A., Bilello, M., Rozycki, M., Kirby, J., Freymann, J., Farahani, K., Davatzikos, C.: Advancing the Cancer Genome Atlas glioma MRI collections with expert segmentation labels and radiomic features. Nature Scientific Data (2017, in press)
4. Shelhamer, E., Long, J., Darrell, T.: Fully convolutional networks for semantic segmentation. In: IEEE Conference on Computer Vision and Pattern Recognition, pp. 3431–3440 (2015)
5. Badrinarayanan, V., Kendall, A., Cipolla, R.: SegNet: a deep convolutional encoder-decoder architecture for scene segmentation. IEEE Trans. Pattern Anal. Mach. Intell. **39**(12), 2481–2495 (2017)

6. Kamnitsas, K., Ledig, C., Newcombe, V.F., Simpson, J.P., Kane, A.D., Menon, D.K., Rueckert, D., Glocker, B.: Efficient multi-scale 3D CNN with fully connected CRF for accurate brain lesion segmentation. Med. Image Anal. **36**, 61 (2016)
7. Havaei, M., Davy, A., Warde-Farley, D., Biard, A., Courville, A., Bengio, Y., Pal, C., Jodoin, P.M., Larochelle, H.: Brain tumor segmentation with Deep Neural Networks. Med. Image Anal. **35**, 18–31 (2017)
8. Fidon, L., Li, W., Garcia-Peraza-Herrera, L.C., Ekanayake, J., Kitchen, N., Ourselin, S., Vercauteren, T.: Scalable multimodal convolutional networks for brain tumour segmentation. In: International Conference on Medical Image Computing and Computer-Assisted Intervention, pp. 285–293 (2017)
9. Tseng, K.L., Lin, Y.L., Hsu, W., Huang, C.Y.: Joint sequence learning and cross-modality convolution for 3D biomedical segmentation. arXiv e-print arXiv:1704.07754 (2017)
10. Zhou, M., Chaudhury, B., Hall, L.O., Goldgof, D.B., Gillies, R.J., Gatenby, R.A.: Identifying spatial imaging biomarkers of glioblastoma multiforme for survival group prediction. J. Magn. Reson. Imaging **46**(1), 115–123 (2016)
11. Lao, J., Chen, Y., Li, Z.C., Li, Q., Zhang, J., Liu, J., Zhai, G.: A deep learning-based radiomics model for prediction of survival in glioblastoma multiforme. Sci. Rep. **7**, 10353 (2017)
12. Nyul, L.G., Udupa, J.K., Zhang, X.: New variants of a method of MRI scale standardization. IEEE Trans. Med. Imaging **19**, 143–150 (2000)
13. Ioffe, S., Szegedy, C.: Batch normalization: accelerating deep network training by reducing internal covariate shift. In: International Conference on Machine Learning, pp. 448–456 (2015)
14. He, K., Zhang, X., Ren, S., Sun, J.: Deep residual learning for image recognition. In: IEEE Conference on Computer Vision and Pattern Recognition, pp. 770–778 (2016)
15. Deng, J., Dong, W., Socher, R., Li, L.J., Li, K., Li, F.F.: ImageNet: a large-scale hierarchical image database. In: IEEE Conference on Computer Vision and Pattern Recognition, pp. 248–255 (2009)
16. Ronneberger, O., Fischer, P., Brox, T.: U-Net: convolutional networks for biomedical image segmentation. In: Navab, N., Hornegger, J., Wells, W.M., Frangi, A.F. (eds.) MICCAI 2015. LNCS, vol. 9351, pp. 234–241. Springer, Cham (2015). https://doi.org/10.1007/978-3-319-24574-4_28
17. Lin, M., Chen, Q., Yan, S.: Network in Network. arXiv e-print arXiv:1312.4400 (2013)
18. Lin, T.Y., Goyal, P., Girshick, R., He, K., Dollár, P.: Focal loss for dense object detection. In: IEEE International Conference on Computer Vision (2017)
19. Kingma, D.P., Ba, J.: Adam: a method for stochastic optimization. arXiv e-print arXiv:1412.6980 (2014)
20. Bakas, S., Akbari, H., Sotiras, A., Bilello, M., Rozycki, M., Kirby, J., Freymann, J., Farahani, K., Davatzikos, C.: Segmentation labels and radiomic features for the pre-operative scans of the TCGA-GBM collection. The Cancer Imaging Archive (2017). https://doi.org/10.7937/k9/tcia.2017.klxwjj1q
21. Bakas, S., Akbari, H., Sotiras, A., Bilello, M., Rozycki, M., Kirby, J., Freymann, J., Farahani, K., Davatzikos, C.: Segmentation labels and radiomic features for the pre-operative scans of the TCGA-LGG collection. The Cancer Imaging Archive (2017). https://doi.org/10.7937/k9/tcia.2017.gjq7r0ef

Multimodal Brain Tumor Segmentation Using Ensemble of Forest Method

Ashish Phophalia[1]([✉]) and Pradipta Maji[2]

[1] Indian Institute of Information Technology, Vadodara, Gandhinagar Campus,
Vadodara 382028, Gujarat, India
ashish_p@iiitvadodara.ac.in
[2] Machine Intelligence Unit, Indian Statistical Institute, Kolkata 700108, India
pmaji@isical.ac.in

Abstract. In this paper, we have proposed a cascaded ensemble method based on Random Forest, named as **Ensemble-of-Forest, (EoF)**. Instead of classifying huge amount of data with a single forest, we proposed two stage ensemble method for Multimodal Brain Tumor Segmentation problem. Identification of Tumor region and its sub-regions poses challenge in terms of variations in intensity, location etc. from patient to patient. We identify the initial region of interest (ROI) by linear combination of FLAIR and T2 modality. For each training scan/ROI, we define a Random Forest as first stage of ensemble method. For a test ROI, collect a set of similarly seen ROI and hence forest based on mutual information criteria and collect majority voting to classify voxels in it. We have reported results on BRATS 2017 dataset in this paper.

Keywords: Brain tumor segmentation · Ensemble method
Random Forest

1 Introduction

Gliomas is one of the well known form of brain tumor from glial cells. It is categorized as either Low Grade Gliomas (LGG) or High Grade Gliomas (HGG). HGG is found to be more aggressive in growth leading to death. The tumor region is also divided into sub-regions inside named as necrotic, enhancing and non-enhancing part. The automated methods must delineate tumor region and segment them from healthy brain. However, presence of tumor is highly varies in terms of intensity, texture, appearance etc. from patient to patient. Hence, one needs to take many parameters in to account for classification and segmentation task [1,2].

The Multimodal **B**rain **T**umor Image **S**egmentation (BraTS) challenge have seen various methods in past few years [3]. The Deep Learning/CNN, SVM, Random Forest and CRF based methods are most commonly used approaches [4–9].

Random Forest (RF) [10], being a supervised learning method has been explored in the brain tumor segmentation context led by work of Zikic et al. [11].

© Springer International Publishing AG, part of Springer Nature 2018
A. Crimi et al. (Eds.): BrainLes 2017, LNCS 10670, pp. 159–168, 2018.
https://doi.org/10.1007/978-3-319-75238-9_14

The authors have proposed Gaussian Mixture model based prior probability estimation for various tissues which are used to train Decision Forest in the later stage. Goetz et al. [12] have proposed their method based on Extremely Randomized Tree method [13] to leverage the selection of features in splitting in trees as in classical RF. Meier et al. [14] proposed RF method followed by Conditional Random Field (CRF) as spatial regularization. Malmi et al. [15] proposed two stage RF architecture where first stage classifies Tumor and Non-Tumor tissues. Second stage involve classification of tumorous tissues to various sub-parts. The method follows multiple post-processing steps using morphological operations and Markov Random Field (MRF) as spatial regularization. Folgoc et al. [16] proposed multilayer RF architecture where each layer sequentially refines predefined ROI in to sub parts of tumor region/classes. Ellwaa et al. [17] have proposed a new way to select sample from few patients only instead of selecting samples from whole database.

Inspired by previous methods with RF, we propose a novel method based on two stage architecture. The crux of method is to find the relevance of the tumor/patient seen in the past. In essence, we tries to capture the resemblance of the input patient/tumor from given database as a past examples. The proposed architecture is shown in Fig. 1. We model the characteristics each example via RF. Given an input test pattern, selected similar RF cast their votes and again ensemble in majority fashion as second stage predication. Since, brain tumor segmentation is a imbalanced class problem, the method give much scope to select samples from small classes. Also, the method can be extended easily with more data with respect to time for better predication.

The rest of the paper is organized as follows: Sect. 2 presents proposed method with all the steps involved in it. Section 3 presents results of proposed method in terms of qualitative and quantitative measures. The manuscript is concluded in Sect. 4.

2   Proposed Method

2.1   Pre-processing

The N4ITK bias correction method [18] was applied to all the images in dataset using 3DSlicer software. Afterward, all the images were rescaled in the range [0–255].

2.2   Initial Segmentation

We have considered linear combination of FLAIR and T2 imaging modalities as $I_{fused} = \alpha * I_{FLAIR} + (1 - \alpha) * I_{T2}$ (where α is adjusted experimentally) [9]. This helps to maintain the hyper-intensity of the tumor region and, at the same time, to suppress the intensity of other irrelevant areas [19]. An intensity at T^{th} percentile is defined as threshold in I_{fused}, τ, and volume intensity above τ is converted to 1, otherwise 0, thus converted to binary mask. Afterward, K largest

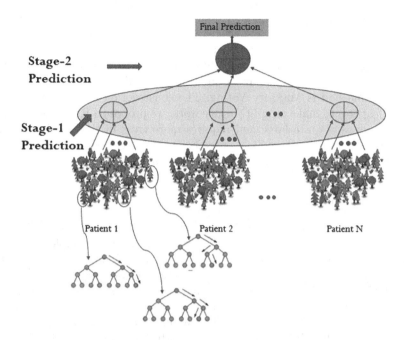

Fig. 1. The proposed architecture as Ensemble of Forest (EoF) method

connected components in 3D is extracted from the binary mask as initial region of interest (ROI). The selection of multiple components is done in order to capture presence of abnormal tissues at different locations. Here, we have considered $K = 3$ largest connected components in 3D. We have experimentally observed three largest components capture most of the tissue region and remove small disjoint regions. The image I_{fused} is also considered for feature generation along with those four modalities in the next step.

2.3 Feature Extraction

After extracting initial ROI for each patient, we have derived 280 features at each voxel locations. The features used are as follows:

1. Appearance - Intensity in each modality ($1 \times 5 = 5$ features)
2. Texture - (a) Image Gradient in three directions in each modality, (b) Min, Max, Mean, Median, Mode intensities after Gaussian smoothing at scale, $\in 0.5, 1.0, 1.5$, and window size $3 \times 3 \times 3$ and $5 \times 5 \times 5$ ($3 \times 5 = 15 + 5 \times 3 \times 2 \times 5 = 150$ features)
3. Statistical - Max, Min, Mean, Median, Mode, Standard deviation, kurtosis, skewness and three central order moments in each modality with window size $3 \times 3 \times 3$ and $5 \times 5 \times 5$ ($11 \times 5 \times 2 = 110$ features)

2.4   Forest Generation

Random Forest is ensemble method utilizing numerous of trained decision trees for decision making [10]. It pass test input to each tree and collect class information and aggregate them to make final decision. The most commonly used aggregation method is Majority Voting. The construction of RF takes limited subset of features to make an split. In this work, we propose a RF to each patient data. Since data is quite large and requires more trees in the training. Hence, we proposed two stage hierarchical ensemble method. For each training scan, a RF is constructed considering features at only initial ROI locations.

2.5   Ensemble of Forests

The idea is to find a resemblance with the patients in the database. Here, we tries to model given test example, with already seen past examples. Hence, a mutual information based criteria is used to find out M similar cases from the database. So, for each test case, class information is collected from each those *similar* forests and aggregated again in majority voting fashion as final class label with equal weights. Note that, mutual information with itself is considered to be zero and hence it is not considered in similar M cases for training database.

For each test ROI from fused modality, a Mutual Information is computed for each training ROI (from fused image only). The intensity values in both ROIs are considered as random variable here. Based on mutual information criteria, best M similar cases are selected (excluding itself). After that, only those M RFs are eligible to cast their vote of classification of each tissue in test ROI. Figure 2 outline the proposed pipeline processing.

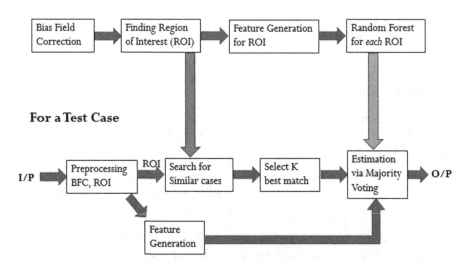

Fig. 2. The flowchart for proposed method

3   Results

3.1   Dataset

We have used MICCAI BRATS 2017 dataset in this work [3,20–22]. The dataset contains total 285 cases, 210 HGG and 75 LGG patients. Each patient has 4 modalities, namely, FLAIR, T1, T1-Contrast enhanced, T2 and ground truth label volume of size $240 \times 240 \times 155$. The database comprises of contribution from various organizations, this make challenging to cop-up with variety in data. The sub-regions considered for evaluation are: (1) the "Enhancing Tumor" (ET), (2) the "Tumor Core" (TC), and (3) the "Whole Tumor" (WT). The labels in the provided data are: 1 for Necrotic (NCR) and the Non-Enhancing Tumor (NET), 2 for Edema (ED), 4 for ET, and 0 for everything else. The TC entails the ET, as well as the necrotic (fluid-filled) and the non-enhancing (solid) parts of the tumor. The WT describes the complete extent of the disease, as it entails the TC and the peritumoral edema (ED). All the imaging data-sets have been segmented manually, by one to four raters, following the same annotation protocol. The provided data are distributed after their pre-processing, i.e. co-registered to the same anatomical template, interpolated to the same size ($1\,mm^3$) and skull-stripped.

3.2   Performance Analysis

The parameter values estimated experimentally as: $M = 11$, $\alpha = 0.7$ and $T = 98$ percentile. The value of M can be maximum up to number of patient in the database and hence make everyone eligible to vote for classification. This may cause over-fitting. However, $M = 1$ simply copy segmentation map from closet ROI. Hence, it fixed experimentally to $M = 11$. The value of $alpha$ governs the fusing ratio between Flair and T2 modality. The value of T, is used as extraction of ROI from each fused volume. It has been observed that, the value $T = 98$ percentile covers most of the tumor region under observation. The lower values of T fetches more region which are non-tumorous and undesirable.

Results on Training Database: The Fig. 3 shows the box-plots for Dice Coefficient and Robust Hausdorff Distance for all 285 patients. The mean value of Dice coefficient for whole tumor, tumor core and enhance part are 0.64, 0.49 and 0.47 respectively. Figure 4 shows comparison of slice 75 of $TCIA - 231$ patient ID with ground truth where Dice score of whole tumor is 0.9239. Figure 5 shows performance of proposed on various examples.

Results on Validation Data: Figure 6(a) shows performance of proposed method for each patient in dataset in terms of dice coefficient whereas Fig. 6(b) shows histogram of dice coefficient over all 46 patients. Figure 7 shows qualitative performance of few sample data TCIA-600 and UAB-3499 patient ID.

Results on Test Data: Table 1 shows performance of proposed method on unseen test data. The performance of proposed method is consistent in the Test data also.

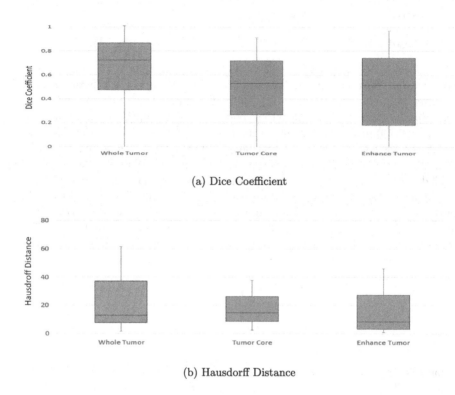

(a) Dice Coefficient

(b) Hausdorff Distance

Fig. 3. The performance of proposed method on BRATS 2017 training database. Parameters used are mentioned in the text.

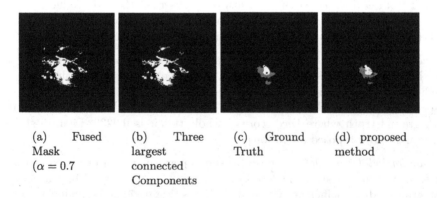

(a)   Fused
Mask
($\alpha = 0.7$

(b)   Three
largest
connected
Components

(c)   Ground
Truth

(d) proposed
method

Fig. 4. The result showing for case $TCIA - 231$ slice 75 with fused mask in (a), three largest connected component in (b), corresponding ground truth in (c) and proposed segmentation in (d) with dice score for whole tumor is 0.9239.

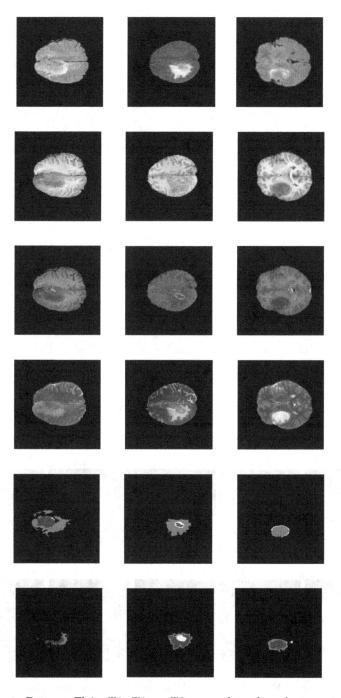

Fig. 5. Top-to-Bottom: Flair, T1, T1-ce, T2, ground truth and segmentation from proposed method. Left-to-Right: TCIA-282 patient ID, CBICA-ATD patient ID and 2013-24 patient ID.

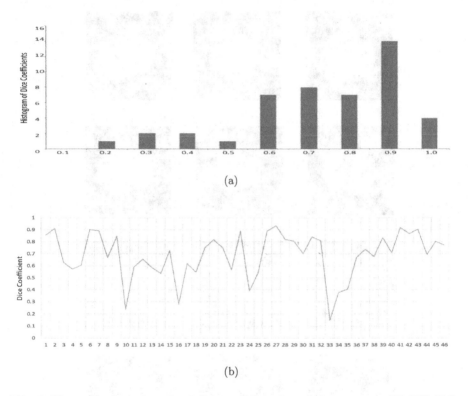

(a)

(b)

Fig. 6. The performance graph of dice coefficient for whole tumor on BRATS 2017 validation dataset

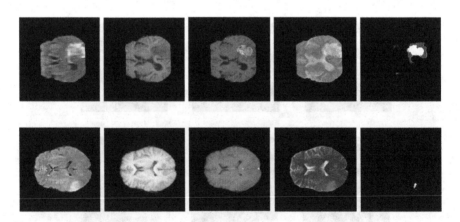

Fig. 7. Left-to-Right: Flair, T1, T1-ce, T2 and segmentation from proposed method. Top row - TCIA-600 patient ID and bottom row - UAB3499 patient ID. Both are example from Validation dataset, hence, ground truth is not provided.

Table 1. Performance of proposed method on Test Dataset

Label	Dice_ET	Dice_WT	Dice_TC	H95_ET	H95_WT	H95_TC
Mean	0.42	0.63	0.41	69.12	21.17	40.06
StdDev	0.32	0.23	0.27	130.21	23.07	83.07
Median	0.47	0.69	0.39	8.79	11.22	13.73
25quantile	0.06	0.49	0.17	3.74	6.16	8.14
75quantile	0.71	0.81	0.65	31.38	25.45	28.04

4   Conclusion

In this paper, a novel two stage based Random Forest method is proposed. A forest of small trained forests is build to classify test pattern aggregation voting from all such small forest. For each patient, a small forest is trained based on the features extracted from initial ROI. The proposed method is performing consistently on validation data and Test data. But still there is huge scope to improve the performance. A details analysis is sought for construction of those ensemble forests and trees inside in them.

Acknowledgement. This work was supported in part by the Dept. of Electronics and Information Technology, Govt. of India (PhD-MLA/4(90)/2015-16).

References

1. Despotović, I., Goossens, B., Philips, W.: MRI segmentation of the human brain: challenges, methods, and applications. Comput. Math. Methods Med. **2015**, 23 (2015)
2. Gordillo, N., Montseny, E., Sobrevilla, P.: State of the art survey on MRI brain tumor segmentation. Magn. Reson. Imaging **31**(8), 1426–1438 (2013)
3. Menze, B.H., Jakab, A., Bauer, S., Kalpathy-Cramer, J., Farahani, K., Kirby, J., Burren, Y., Porz, N., Slotboom, J., Wiest, R., et al.: The multimodal brain tumor image segmentation benchmark (BRATS). IEEE Trans. Med. Imaging **34**(10), 1993–2024 (2015)
4. Akkus, Z., Galimzianova, A., Hoogi, A., Rubin, D.L., Erickson, B.J.: Deep learning for brain MRI segmentation: state of the art and future directions. J. Digit. Imaging **30**, 1–11 (2017)
5. Işın, A., Direkoğlu, C., Şah, M.: Review of MRI-based brain tumor image segmentation using deep learning methods. Procedia Comput. Sci. **102**, 317–324 (2016)
6. Havaei, M., Davy, A., Warde-Farley, D., Biard, A., Courville, A., Bengio, Y., Pal, C., Jodoin, P.-M., Larochelle, H.: Brain tumor segmentation with deep neural networks. arXiv:1505.03540v3 [cs.CV] (2016)
7. Pereira, S., Pinto, A., Alves, V., Silva, C.A.: Brain tumor segmentation using convolutional neural networks in MRI images. IEEE Trans. Med. imaging **35**(5), 1240–1251 (2016)
8. Lefkovits, L., Lefkovits, S., Szilágyi, L.: Brain tumor segmentation with optimized random forest. In: Crimi, A., Menze, B., Maier, O., Reyes, M., Winzeck, S., Handels, H. (eds.) BrainLes 2016. LNCS, vol. 10154, pp. 88–99. Springer, Cham (2016). https://doi.org/10.1007/978-3-319-55524-9_9

9. Song, B., Chou, C.R., Chen, X., Huang, A., Liu, M.C.: Anatomy-guided brain tumor segmentation and classification. In: Crimi, A., Menze, B., Maier, O., Reyes, M., Winzeck, S., Handels, H. (eds.) BrainLes 2016. LNCS, vol. 10154, pp. 162–170. Springer, Cham (2016). https://doi.org/10.1007/978-3-319-55524-9_16

10. Breiman, L.: Random forests. Mach. Learn. **45**(1), 5–32 (2001)

11. Zikic, D., et al.: Decision forests for tissue-specific segmentation of high-grade Gliomas in multi-channel MR. In: Ayache, N., Delingette, H., Golland, P., Mori, K. (eds.) MICCAI 2012. LNCS, vol. 7512, pp. 369–376. Springer, Heidelberg (2012). https://doi.org/10.1007/978-3-642-33454-2_46

12. Goetz, M., Weber, C., Bloecher, J., Stieltjes, B., Meinzer, H.-P., Maier-Hein, K.: Extremely randomized trees based brain tumor segmentation. In: Proceeding of BRATS Challenge-MICCAI, pp. 006–011 (2014)

13. Geurts, P., Ernst, D., Wehenkel, L.: Extremely randomized trees. Mach. Learn. **63**(1), 3–42 (2006)

14. Meier, R., Bauer, S., Slotboom, J., Wiest, R., Reyes, M.: Appearance-and context-sensitive features for brain tumor segmentation. In: Proceedings of MICCAI BRATS Challenge, pp. 020–026 (2014)

15. Malmi, E., Parambath, S., Peyrat, J.-M., Abinahed, J., Chawla, S.: Cabs: a cascaded brain tumor segmentation approach. In: Proceedings of MICCAI BRATS Challenge, pp. 042–047 (2015)

16. Le Folgoc, L., Nori, A.V., Ancha, S., Criminisi, A.: Lifted auto-context forests for brain tumour segmentation. In: Crimi, A., Menze, B., Maier, O., Reyes, M., Winzeck, S., Handels, H. (eds.) BrainLes 2016. LNCS, vol. 10154, pp. 171–183. Springer, Cham (2016). https://doi.org/10.1007/978-3-319-55524-9_17

17. Ellwaa, A., Hussein, A., AlNaggar, E., Zidan, M., Zaki, M., Ismail, M.A., Ghanem, N.M.: Brain tumor segmantation using random forest trained on iteratively selected patients. In: International Workshop on Brainlesion: Glioma, Multiple Sclerosis, Stroke and Traumatic Brain Injuries, pp. 129–137. Springer (2016)

18. Tustison, N.J., Avants, B.B., Cook, P.A., Zheng, Y., Egan, A., Yushkevich, P.A., Gee, J.C.: N4ITK: improved N3 bias correction. IEEE Trans. Med. Imaging **29**(6), 1310–1320 (2010)

19. Saha, R., Phophalia, A., Mitra, S.K.: Brain tumor segmentation from multimodal MR images using rough sets. In: Mukherjee, S., Mukherjee, S., Mukherjee, D.P., Sivaswamy, J., Awate, S., Setlur, S., Namboodiri, A.M., Chaudhury, S. (eds.) ICVGIP 2016. LNCS, vol. 10481, pp. 133–144. Springer, Cham (2017). https://doi.org/10.1007/978-3-319-68124-5_12

20. Bakas, S., Akbari, H., Sotiras, A., Bilello, M., Rozycki, M., Kirby, J.S., Freymann, J.B., Farahani, K., Davatzikos, C.: Advancing the cancer genome atlas Glioma MRI collections with expert segmentation labels and radiomic features. Nat. Sci. Data **4**, 170117 (2017)

21. Bakas, S., Akbari, H., Sotiras, A., Bilello, M., Rozycki, M., Kirby, J.S., Freymann, J.B., Farahani, K., Davatzikos, C.: Segmentation labels and radiomic features for the pre-operative scans of the TCGA-GBM collection. The Cancer Imaging Archive (2017)

22. Bakas, S., Akbari, H., Sotiras, A., Bilello, M., Rozycki, M., Kirby, J.S., Freymann, J.B., Farahani, K., Davatzikos, C.: Segmentation labels and radiomic features for the pre-operative scans of the TCGA-LGG collection. The Cancer Imaging Archive (2017)

Pooling-Free Fully Convolutional Networks with Dense Skip Connections for Semantic Segmentation, with Application to Brain Tumor Segmentation

Richard McKinley[1(✉)], Alain Jungo[2], Roland Wiest[1], and Mauricio Reyes[2]

[1] Support Centre for Advanced Neuroimaging, Inselspital, University Hospital,
University of Bern, Bern, Switzerland
`RichardIain.McKinley@insel.ch`
[2] Institute for Surgical Technology and Biomechanics, University of Bern,
Bern, Switzerland

Abstract. Segmentation of medical images requires multi-scale information, combining local boundary detection with global context. State-of-the-art convolutional neural network (CNN) architectures for semantic segmentation are often composed of a downsampling path which computes features at multiple scales, followed by an upsampling path, required to recover those features at the same scale as the input image. Skip connections allow features discovered in the downward path to be integrated in the upward path. The downsampling mechanism is typically a pooling operation. However, pooling was introduced in CNNs to enable translation invariance, which is not desirable in segmentation tasks. For this reason, we propose an architecture, based on the recently proposed Densenet, for semantic segmentation, in which pooling has been replaced with dilated convolutions. We also present a variant approach, used in the 2017 BRATS challenge, in which a cascade of densely connected nets is used to first exclude non-brain tissue, and then segment tumor structures. We present results on the validation dataset of the Multimodal Brain Tumor Segmentation Challenge 2017.

1 Introduction

We present a network architecture for semantic segmentation, heavily inspired by the recent Densenet architecture for image classification [1], in which pooling layers are replaced by heavy use of dilated convolutions [2]. Densenet employs dense blocks, in which the output of each layer is concatenated with its input before passing to the next layer. A typical Densenet architecture consists of a number of dense blocks separated by transition layers: the transition layers contain a pooling operation, which allows some degree of translation invariance and downsamples the feature maps. A Densenet architecture adapted for semantic segmentation was presented in [3], which adopted the now standard approach of U-net [4]: a downsampling path, followed by an upsampling path, with skip

© Springer International Publishing AG, part of Springer Nature 2018
A. Crimi et al. (Eds.): BrainLes 2017, LNCS 10670, pp. 169–177, 2018.
https://doi.org/10.1007/978-3-319-75238-9_15

connections passing feature maps of the sample spatial dimension from the down-sampling path to the upsampling path.

In this paper, we describe an alternative architecture adapting Densenet for semantic segmentation: in this architecture, which we call DeepSCAN, there are no transition layers and no pooling operations. Instead, dilated convolutions are used to increase the receptive field of the classifier. The absence of transition layers means that the whole network can be seen as a single dense block, enabling gradients to pass easily to the deepest layers.

We describe the general architecture of DeepSCAN, plus the particular features of the network as applied to brain tumor segmentation, and report preliminary results on the validation portion of the BRATS 2017 dataset. We then discuss a major source of errors on the BRATS2017 dataset - namely, the imperfect stripping of non-brain tissue. We then introduce a cascade approach in which an initial network strips away remaining non-brain tissue, and a subsequent network to identify the tumor tissues.

2   The DeepSCAN Architecture

2.1   Densely Connected Layers and Densenet

Densenet [1] is a recently introduced architecture for image classification. The fundamental unit of a densenet architecture is the densely connected block, or dense block. In such a block, the output of each layer (where a layer here means some combination of convolutional filters, nonlinearities and perhaps batch normalization) is concatenated to its input before passing to the next layer. The goal behind Densenet is to build an architecture which supports the training of very deep networks: the skip connections implicit in the concatenation of filter maps between layers allows the flow of gradients directly to those layers, providing an implicit deep supervision of those layers.

In the original Densenet architecture, which has state-of-the-art performance on the CIFAR image recognition task, dense blocks are combined with transition blocks: non-densely connected convolutional layers, followed by a maxpooling layer. This helps to control parameter explosion (by limiting the size of the input to each dense block) and limit redundancy between features, but also means that the deep supervision is not direct, at the lowest layers of the network. This Dense-plus-transition architecture was also adopted by Jegou et al. [3], whose whimsically named Tiramisu network is a U-net-style variation of the Densenet architecture designed for semantic segmentation.

In contrast to the standard Densenet architecture, in our approach we dispense with the transition layers: this means, in effect that the whole network (except for the final one by one convolutions) is a single dense block. The layers in our dense blocks have the shape shown in Fig. 1. Depending on its position in the network, the convolution might have kernel size 3 by 3 or 5 by 5, and might or might not be dilated. At deeper levels of the network (where the feature depth is rather high) a "bottleneck" is used, meaning that before the 2D convolution a convolution with 1 by 1 kernels is performed to reduce the number of

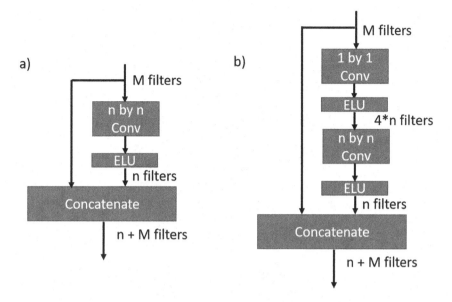

Fig. 1. Dense units, as used in the DeepSCAN architecture (a) a dense unit without bottleneck, and (b) a dense unit with bottleneck

parameters. As a nonlinearity, we use Exponential Linear Units (ELU) [5] rather than the combination of rectified linear unit and Batch Normalization [6] used in the original Densenet paper. There are two reasons for this: the first is that densenets are very memory intensive: removing batch norm layers reduces the overall memory footprint of network. Secondly eliminating batch normalization makes training less sensitive to high levels of variance in batches.

2.2 Dilated Convolutions

The role of pooling layers in CNNs is twofold: to efficiently increase the receptive field and to allow some translation invariance. Translation invariance is of course undesirable in semantic segmentation problems, where what is needed is instead translation equivariance: a translated input corresponding to a translated output. To that end, we use layers with dilated convolutions to aggregate features at multiple scales. Dilated convolutions, sometimes called atrous convolutions, can be best visualised as convolutional layers "with holes": a 3 by 3 convolutional layer with dilation 2 is a 5 by 5 convolution, in which only the centre and corner values of the filter are nonzero, as illustrated in Fig. 3. Dilated convolutions are a simple way to increase the receptive field of a classifier without losing spatial information.

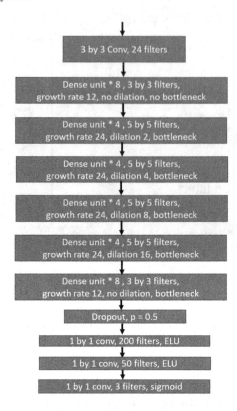

Fig. 2. The DeepSCAN architecture, as applied to brain tumor segmentation

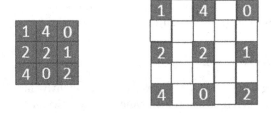

Fig. 3. Left, a 3 by 3 kernel. Right, a 3 by 3 kernel with dilation 2, visualised as a 5 by 5 kernel

2.3   Multi-task Learning and Data Imbalance

Data imbalance in classification in general, and in medical image analysis in particular, is an important theme: in a typical medical image, the background class (healthy appearing tissue) will typically outnumber pathological tissue by a factor of between 10 and 1000 to one. This can lead to the parameter updates arising from the target classes to be strongly diluted by updates from the background class, slowing learning, and can also lead to underidentification of the target class, if this leads to an overall increase in the accuracy of the classifier. Standard approaches to this imbalance problem include undersampling the background class, oversampling the target class(es), or weighting training examples according to their prevalence in the training set.

For training the DeepSCAN classifiers, we adopted a newer technique from the Bayesian theory of uncertainty in learning [7]. In this framework, one network is used to perform a number of different tasks, each with a loss $\mathcal{L}_i(W)$:, where W are the weights of the network. The *homoscedastic uncertainty* (the noise inherent in the model's output) σ_i of the network is a learned parameter for each task i, and the loss associated with each task is

$$\frac{1}{2\sigma_i^2}\mathcal{L}_i(W) + log(\sigma_i^2) \tag{1}$$

The factor $\frac{1}{2\sigma_i^2}$ provides an adaptive, rather than a fixed, weighting of the loss associated to task i, regularized by the term $log(\sigma_i^2)$. By recasting the segmentation problem in the language of multi-task learning, the appropriate weighting of the different components of the problem is therefore allowed to arise from the data, rather than being imposed.

3   Initial Application to Brain Tumor Segmentation

Brain Tumor segmentation has become a benchmark problem in medical image segmentation, due to the existence since 2012 of a long-running competition, BRATS, together with a large curated dataset [8–10] of annotated images. Both fully-automated and semi-automatic approaches to brain-tumor segmentation are accepted to the challenge, with supervised learning approaches dominating the fully-automated part of the challenge. A good survey of approaches which dominated BRATS up to 2013 can be found here [11]. More recently, CNN-based approaches have dominated the fully-automated approaches to the problem [12–14]

The network used is pictured in Fig. 2. The network was built using Keras [15] and Tensorflow [16], and trained using stochastic gradient descent with momentum for 100 epochs. Rather than using a softmax layer to classify the three labels (edema, enhancing, other tumor) we employ a multi-task approach to hierarchically segment the tumor into the three overlapping targets: whole tumor, tumor core and enhancing: thus the output of the network is three sigmoid units, one for each target. The multi-task uncertainty weighting approach as described above, was applied to each of these tasks.

3.1   Data Preparation and Homogenization

The raw values of MRI sequences cannot be compared across scanners and sequences, and therefore a homogenization is necessary across the training examples. In addition, learning in CNNs proceeds best when the inputs are standardized (i.e. mean zero, and unit variance). To this end, the nonzero intensities in the training, validation and testing sets were standardised, this being done across individual volumes rather than across the training set. This achieves both standardisation and homogenisation.

3.2   Training and Results

The network segments the volume slice-by slice: the input data is five consecutive slices from all four modalities, Ground truth for such a set of slices is the lesion mask of the central slice.

Slices from all three directions (sagittal, axial, coronal) were fed to the classifier for training, and in testing the results of these three directions were ensembled by averaging. When applied to the BRATS 2017 validation dataset, the mean Dice scores for Whole Tumor, Tumor core and enhancing tumor were 0.87, 0.68 and 0.71 respectively. After some mild postprocessing (removing small connected components), the Dice coefficient for whole tumor increased to 0.88, and for tumor core to 0.70.

4   Cascaded Network for Nonbrain-Tissue Removal

The BRATS dataset was assembled from a large number of datasources, and does not comprise raw imaging data: the volumes are resampled to 1 mm isovoxels, and in addition have been automatically skull-stripped (Fig. 4). Unfortunately, the results of this skull-stripping vary: see Fig. 5 for an example with large amounts of residual skull tissue. Other examples have remnants of the dura or optic nerves. This remaining tissue can confound classification in two ways: it can be misidentified by the classification algorithm (though this is increasingly less likely as classifiers improve) and it can affect the distribution of the

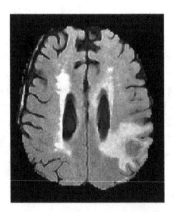

Fig. 4. An axial slice through the FLAIR acquisition for case TCIA_208_1, showing hyperintense nonbrain tissue which has not been removed by the skullstripping algorithm

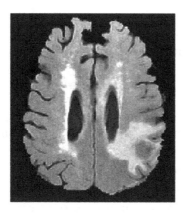

Fig. 5. The same axial slice, after masking with the output of our skullstripping network

intensities in a volume, adversely impacting the global standardisation of voxel values. To combat this effect, we used a cascade of networks to first segment the parenchymia from the poorly skull-stripped images, followed by a second network which identifies the tumor compartments as above. The ground truth for the first network in the cascade was obtained by applying FSL-FAST to the T1 post Gadolinium imaging, as this tended to have the best definition in all three planes. The brain tissue label was assembled by taking the union of tumor, white matter and grey matter labels, and then taking the largest connected component. This network was trained analogously to the tumor classification network above, and the four modalities of the training, validation and testing data were masked with its output. The masked modalities were then used to train a tumor

Label	Dice_ET	Dice_WT	Dice_TC
Mean	0.70985911	0.857922534	0.708739178
StdDev	0.26719754	0.142340453	0.275811784
Median	0.787695	0.90034	0.815625
25quantile	0.653735	0.84384	0.657485
75quantile	0.868275	0.9319575	0.88642

Label	Hausdorff95_ET	Hausdorff95_WT	Hausdorff95_TC
Mean	32.16084212	7.397078973	28.32401603
StdDev	98.1050951	11.26534053	83.88898478
Median	2.23607	4	6.40312
25quantile	1.73205	2.544225	3.4641
75quantile	5.3379075	6.40312	11.8573725

Fig. 6. Results of DeepSCAN on the BRATS 2017 test dataset

segmentation network, as above. For this cascade, the mean Dice scores for Whole Tumor, Tumor core and enhancing tumor were 0.88, 0.76 and 0.71, representing a substantial improvement in classification of the tumor core.

4.1 Challenge Results

The above cascaded network was used to compete the in the BRATS 2017 challenge: results on the testing data of that challenge are shown in Fig. 6.

5   Conclusions and Further Directions

Densely connected networks can provide a convincing tool for semantic segmentation of medical images. The problem of data imbalance in image segmentation can be helped by recasting the problem as a multi-task learning problem and using concepts from Bayesian learning to calibrate the weights on the various component problems. It would be interesting to compare the effects of homoscedastic uncertainty (which is calculated per task) and heteroscedastic uncertainty (which is calculated per datapoint) on quality of segmentation and speed of convergence.

This paper arose in the context of a challenge, where comparisons to other approaches are provided by the challenge leaderboard: while this is useful, it should not take the place of robust comparison against strong benchmarks, and as a result we are preparing further work in which the DeepSCAN architecture is rigorously compared to U-net, Tiramisu, and other existing architectures. We will also investigate the contribution of depth, nonlinearity used, and the contribution of the Bayesian loss function. In addition, we will apply the architecture to additional datasets, to confirm its broad applicability.

References

1. Huang, G., Liu, Z., van der Maaten, L., Weinberger, K.Q.: Densely connected convolutional networks. In: Proceedings of the IEEE Conference on Computer Vision and Pattern Recognition (2017)
2. Yu, F., Koltun, V.: Multi-scale context aggregation by dilated convolutions. In: Proceedings of International Conference on Learning Representations (ICLR 2017) (2017)
3. Jégou, S., Drozdzal, M., Vázquez, D., Romero, A., Bengio, Y.: The one hundred layers liramisu: fully convolutional denseNets for semantic segmentation. CoRR (2016)
4. Ronneberger, O., Fischer, P., Brox, T.: U-Net: convolutional networks for biomedical image segmentation. In: Navab, N., Hornegger, J., Wells, W.M., Frangi, A.F. (eds.) MICCAI 2015. LNCS, vol. 9351, pp. 234–241. Springer, Cham (2015). https://doi.org/10.1007/978-3-319-24574-4_28
5. Clevert, D., Unterthiner, T., Hochreiter, S.: Fast and accurate deep network learning by exponential linear units (eLUs). CoRR abs/1511.07289 (2015)

6. Ioffe, S., Szegedy, C.: Batch normalization: accelerating deep network training by reducing internal covariate shift. arXiv:1502.03167, pp. 1–11 (2015)
7. Kendall, A., Gal, Y., Cipolla, R.: Multi-task learning using uncertainty to weigh losses for scene geometry and semantics. arXiv:1705.07115 (2017)
8. Menze, B.H., Jakab, A., Bauer, S., Kalpathy-Cramer, J., Farahani, K., Kirby, J., Burren, Y., Porz, N., Slotboom, J., Wiest, R., Lanczi, L., Gerstner, E., Weber, M.A., Arbel, T., Avants, B.B., Ayache, N., Buendia, P., Collins, D.L., Cordier, N., Corso, J.J., Criminisi, A., Das, T., Delingette, H., Demiralp, Ç., Durst, C.R., Dojat, M., Doyle, S., Festa, J., Forbes, F., Geremia, E., Glocker, B., Golland, P., Guo, X., Hamamci, A., Iftekharuddin, K.M., Jena, R., John, N.M., Konukoglu, E., Lashkari, D., Mariz, J.A., Meier, R., Pereira, S., Precup, D., Price, S.J., Raviv, T.R., Reza, S.M.S., Ryan, M., Sarikaya, D., Schwartz, L., Shin, H.C., Shotton, J., Silva, C.A., Sousa, N., Subbanna, N.K., Szekely, G., Taylor, T.J., Thomas, O.M., Tustison, N.J., Unal, G., Vasseur, F., Wintermark, M., Ye, D.H., Zhao, L., Zhao, B., Zikic, D., Prastawa, M., Reyes, M., Leemput, K.V.: The multimodal brain tumor image segmentation benchmark (BRATS). IEEE Trans. Med. Imaging **34**, 1993–2024 (2015)
9. Bakas, S., Akbari, H., Sotiras, A., Bilello, M., Rozycki, M., Kirby, J.S., Freymann, J.B., Farahani, K., Davatzikos, C.: Advancing the cancer genome atlas glioma MRI collections with expert segmentation labels and radiomic features. Nat. Sci. Data (2017, in press)
10. Bakas, S., Akbari, H., Sotiras, A., Bilello, M., Rozycki, M., Kirby, J.S., Freymann, J.B., Farahani, K., Davatzikos, C.: Segmentation labels and radiomic features for the pre-operative scans of the TCGA-GBM collection. Cancer Imaging Archive (2017)
11. Bauer, S., Wiest, R., Nolte, L.-P., Reyes, M.: A survey of MRI-based medical image analysis for brain tumor studies. Phys. Med. Biol. **58**, R97–R129 (2013)
12. Havaei, M., Davy, A., Warde-Farley, D., Biard, A., Courville, A., Bengio, Y., Pal, C., Jodoin, P.M., Larochelle, H.: Brain tumor segmentation with deep neural networks. Med. Image Anal. **35**, 18–31 (2017)
13. Kamnitsas, K., Ledig, C., Newcombe, V.F., Simpson, J.P., Kane, A.D., Menon, D.K., Rueckert, D., Glocker, B.: Efficient multi-scale 3D CNN with fully connected CRF for accurate brain lesion segmentation. Med. Image Anal. **36**, 61–78 (2017)
14. Pereira, S., Pinto, A., Alves, V., Silva, C.A.: Brain tumor segmentation using convolutional neural networks in MRI images. IEEE Trans. Med. Imaging **35**, 1240–1251 (2016)
15. Chollet, F., et al.: Keras (2015)
16. Abadi, M., Agarwal, A., Barham, P., Brevdo, E., Chen, Z., Citro, C., Corrado, G.S., Davis, A., Dean, J., Devin, M., Ghemawat, S., Goodfellow, I., Harp, A., Irving, G., Isard, M., Jia, Y., Jozefowicz, R., Kaiser, L., Kudlur, M., Levenberg, J., Mané, D., Monga, R., Moore, S., Murray, D., Olah, C., Schuster, M., Shlens, J., Steiner, B., Sutskever, I., Talwar, K., Tucker, P., Vanhoucke, V., Vasudevan, V., Viégas, F., Vinyals, O., Warden, P., Wattenberg, M., Wicke, M., Yu, Y., Zheng, X.: TensorFlow: large-scale machine learning on heterogeneous systems (2015). http://tensorflow.org/

Automatic Brain Tumor Segmentation Using Cascaded Anisotropic Convolutional Neural Networks

Guotai Wang[1,2(✉)], Wenqi Li[1,2], Sébastien Ourselin[1,2], and Tom Vercauteren[1,2]

[1] Translational Imaging Group, CMIC, University College London, London, UK
guotai.wang.14@ucl.ac.uk
[2] Wellcome/EPSRC Centre for Interventional and Surgical Sciences, UCL, London, UK

Abstract. A cascade of fully convolutional neural networks is proposed to segment multi-modal Magnetic Resonance (MR) images with brain tumor into background and three hierarchical regions: whole tumor, tumor core and enhancing tumor core. The cascade is designed to decompose the multi-class segmentation problem into a sequence of three binary segmentation problems according to the subregion hierarchy. The whole tumor is segmented in the first step and the bounding box of the result is used for the tumor core segmentation in the second step. The enhancing tumor core is then segmented based on the bounding box of the tumor core segmentation result. Our networks consist of multiple layers of anisotropic and dilated convolution filters, and they are combined with multi-view fusion to reduce false positives. Residual connections and multi-scale predictions are employed in these networks to boost the segmentation performance. Experiments with BraTS 2017 validation set show that the proposed method achieved average Dice scores of 0.7859, 0.9050, 0.8378 for enhancing tumor core, whole tumor and tumor core, respectively. The corresponding values for BraTS 2017 testing set were 0.7831, 0.8739, and 0.7748, respectively.

Keywords: Brain tumor · Convolutional neural network
Segmentation

1 Introduction

Gliomas are the most common brain tumors that arise from glial cells. They can be categorized into two basic grades: low-grade gliomas (LGG) that tend to exhibit benign tendencies and indicate a better prognosis for the patient, and high-grade gliomas (HGG) that are malignant and more aggressive. With the development of medical imaging, brain tumors can be imaged by various Magnetic Resonance (MR) sequences, such as T1-weighted, contrast enhanced T1-weighted (T1c), T2-weighted and Fluid Attenuation Inversion Recovery (FLAIR) images. Different sequences can provide complementary information

© Springer International Publishing AG, part of Springer Nature 2018
A. Crimi et al. (Eds.): BrainLes 2017, LNCS 10670, pp. 178–190, 2018.
https://doi.org/10.1007/978-3-319-75238-9_16

to analyze different subregions of gliomas. For example, T2 and FLAIR highlight the tumor with peritumoral edema, designated "whole tumor" as per [22]. T1 and T1c highlight the tumor without peritumoral edema, designated "tumor core" as per [22]. An enhancing region of the tumor core with hyper-intensity can also be observed in T1c, designated "enhancing tumor core" as per [22].

Automatic segmentation of brain tumors and substructures has a potential to provide accurate and reproducible measurements of the tumors. It has a great potential for better diagnosis, surgical planning and treatment assessment of brain tumors [3,22]. However, this segmentation task is challenging because (1) the size, shape, and localization of brain tumors have considerable variations among patients. This limits the usability and usefulness of prior information about shape and location that are widely used for robust segmentation of many other anatomical structures [11,28]; (2) the boundaries between adjacent structures are often ambiguous due to the smooth intensity gradients, partial volume effects and bias field artifacts.

There have been many studies on automatic brain tumor segmentation over the past decades [30]. Most current methods use generative or discriminative approaches. Generative approaches explicitly model the probabilistic distributions of anatomy and appearance of the tumor or healthy tissues [17,23]. They often present good generalization to unseen images by incorporating domain-specific prior knowledge. However, accurate probabilistic distributions of brain tumors are hard to model. Discriminative approaches directly learn the relationship between image intensities and tissue classes, and they require a set of annotated training images for learning. Representative works include classification based on support vector machines [19] and decision trees [32].

In recent years, discriminative methods based on deep neural networks have achieved state-of-the-art performance for multi-modal brain tumor segmentation. In [12], a convolutional neural network (CNN) was proposed to exploit both local and more global features for robust brain tumor segmentation. However, their approach works on individual 2D slices without considering 3D contextual information. DeepMedic [16] uses a dual pathway 3D CNN with 11 layers for brain tumor segmentation. The network processes the input image at multiple scales and the result is post-processed by a fully connected Conditional Random Field (CRF) to remove false positives. However, DeepMedic works on local image patches and has a low inference efficiency. Recently, several ideas to improve the segmentation performance of CNNs have been explored in the literature. 3D U-Net [2] allows end-to-end training and testing for volumetric image segmentation. HighRes3DNet [20] proposes a compact end-to-end 3D CNN structure that maintains high-resolution multi-scale features with dilated convolution and residual connection [6,29]. Other works also propose using fully convolutional networks [8,13], incorporating large visual contexts by employing a mixture of convolution and downsampling operations [12,16], and handling imbalanced training data by designing new loss functions [9,27] and sampling strategies [27].

The contributions of this work are three-fold. First, we propose a cascade of CNNs to segment brain tumor subregions sequentially. The cascaded CNNs separate the complex problem of multiple class segmentation into three simpler binary segmentation problems, and take advantage of the hierarchical structure of tumor subregions to reduce false positives. Second, we propose a novel network structure with anisotropic convolution to deal with 3D images as a trade-off among receptive field, model complexity and memory consumption. It uses dilated convolution, residual connection and multi-scale prediction to improve segmentation performance. Third, we propose to fuse the output of CNNs in three orthogonal views for more robust segmentation of brain tumor.

2   Methods

2.1   Triple Cascaded Framework

The proposed cascaded framework is shown in Fig. 1. We use three networks to hierarchically and sequentially segment substructures of brain tumor, and each of these networks deals with a binary segmentation problem. The first network (WNet) segments the whole tumor from multi-modal 3D volumes of the same

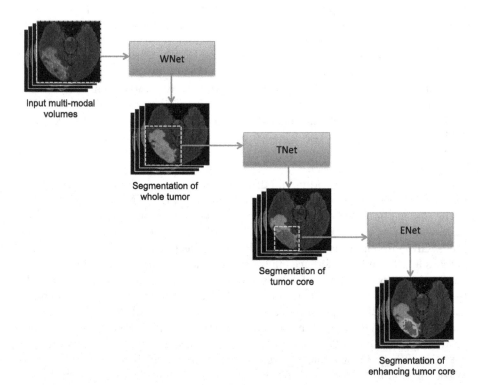

Fig. 1. The proposed triple cascaded framework for brain tumor segmentation. Three networks are proposed to hierarchically segment whole tumor (WNet), tumor core (TNet) and enhancing tumor core (ENet) sequentially.

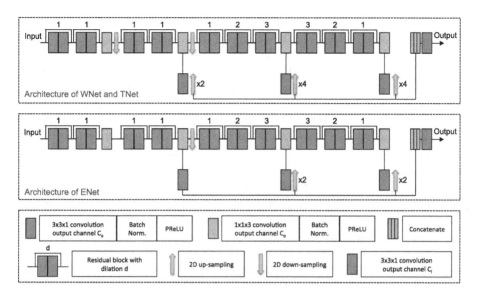

Fig. 2. Our anisotropic convolutional networks with dilated convolution, residual connection and multi-scale fusion. ENet uses only one downsampling layer considering its smaller input size. (Color figure online)

patient. Then a bounding box of the whole tumor is obtained. The cropped region of the input images based on the bounding box is used as the input of the second network (TNet) to segment the tumor core. Similarly, image region inside the bounding box of the tumor core is used as the input of the third network (ENet) to segment the enhancing tumor core. In the training stage, the bounding boxes are automatically generated based on the ground truth. In the testing stage, the bounding boxes are generated based on the binary segmentation results of the whole tumor and the tumor core, respectively. The segmentation result of WNet is used as a crisp binary mask for the output of TNet, and the segmentation result of TNet is used as a crisp binary mask for the output of ENet, which serves as anatomical constraints for the segmentation.

2.2   Anisotropic Convolutional Neural Networks

For 3D neural networks, the balance among receptive field, model complexity and memory consumption should be considered. A small receptive field leads the model to only use local features, and a larger receptive field allows the model to also learn more global features. Many 2D networks use a very large receptive field to capture features from the entire image context, such as FCN [21] and U-Net [26]. They require a large patch size for training and testing. Using a large 3D receptive field also helps to obtain more global features for 3D volumes. However, the resulting large 3D patches for training consume a lot of memory, and therefore restrict the resolution and number of features in the network, leading to limited model complexity and low representation ability. As a trade-off, we propose anisotropic networks that take a stack of slices as input with a large receptive field in 2D and a relatively small receptive field in the out-plane direction that is orthogonal to the 2D slices. The 2D receptive fields for WNet, TNet and ENet are 217×217, 217×217, and 113×113, respectively. During training and testing, the 2D sizes of the inputs are typically smaller than the corresponding 2D receptive fields. WNet, TNet and ENet have the same out-plane receptive field of 9. The architectures of these proposed networks are shown in Fig. 2. All of them are fully convolutional and use 10 residual connection blocks with anisotropic convolution, dilated convolution, and multi-scale prediction.

Anisotropic and Dilated Convolution. To deal with anisotropic receptive fields, we decompose a 3D kernel with a size of $3 \times 3 \times 3$ into an intra-slice kernel with a size of $3 \times 3 \times 1$ and an inter-slice kernel with a size of $1 \times 1 \times 3$. Convolution layers with either of these kernels have C_o output channels and each is followed by a batch normalization layer and an activation layer, as illustrated by blue and green blocks in Fig. 2. The activation layers use Parametric Rectified Linear Units (PReLU) that have been shown better performance than traditional rectified units [14]. WNet and TNet use 20 intra-slice convolution layers and four inter-slice convolution layers with two 2D downsampling layers. ENet uses the same set of convolution layers as WNet but only one downsampling layer considering its smaller input size. We only employ up to two layers of downsampling in order to avoid large image resolution reduction and loss of segmentation details. After the downsampling layers, we use dilated convolution for intra-slice kernels to enlarge the receptive field within a slice. The dilation parameter is set to 1 to 3 as shown in Fig. 2.

Residual Connection. For effective training of deep CNNs, residual connections [15] were introduced to create identity mapping connections to bypass the parameterized layers in a network. Our WNet, TNet and ENet have 10 residual blocks. Each of these blocks contains two intra-slice convolution layers, and the input of a residual block is directly added to the output, encouraging the block to learn residual functions with reference to the input. This can make information propagation smooth and speed the convergence of training [15,20].

Multi-scale Prediction. With the kernel sizes used in our networks, shallow layers learn to represent local and low-level features while deep layers learn to represent more global and high-level features. To combine features at different scales, we use three $3 \times 3 \times 1$ convolution layers at different depths of the network to get multiple intermediate predictions and upsample them to the resolution of the input. A concatenation of these predictions are fed into an additional $3 \times 3 \times 1$ convolution layer to obtain the final score map. These layers are illustrated by red blocks in Fig. 2. The outputs of these layers have C_l channels where C_l is the number of classes for segmentation in each network. C_l equals to 2 in our method. A combination of predictions from multiple scales has also been used in [9,31].

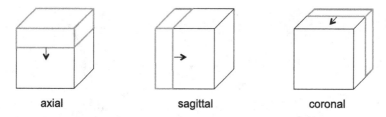

Fig. 3. Illustration of multi-view fusion at one level of the proposed cascade. Due to the anisotropic receptive field of our networks, we average the softmax outputs in axial, sagittal and coronal views. The orange boxes show examples of sliding windows for testing. Multi-view fusion is implemented for WNet, TNet, and ENet, respectively. (Color figure online)

Multi-view Fusion. Since the anisotropic convolution has a small receptive field in the out-plane direction, to take advantage of 3D contextual information, we fuse the segmentation results from three different orthogonal views. Each of WNet, TNet and ENet was trained in axial, sagittal and coronal views respectively. During the testing time, predictions in these three views are fused to get the final segmentation. For the fusion, we average the softmax outputs in these three views for each level of the cascade of WNet, TNet, and ENet, respectively. An illustration of multi-view fusion at one level is shown in Fig. 3.

3   Experiments and Results

Data and Implementation Details. We used the BraTS 2017[1] [3–5,22] dataset for experiments. The training set contains images from 285 patients (210 HGG and 75 LGG). The BraTS 2017 validation and testing set contain images from 46 and 146 patients with brain tumors of unknown grade, respectively. Each patient was scanned with four sequences: T1, T1c, T2 and FLAIR. All the images were skull-striped and re-sampled to an isotropic $1\,\text{mm}^3$ resolution, and the four sequences of the same patient had been co-registered. The ground truth were obtained by manual segmentation results given by experts. We uploaded the segmentation results obtained by the experimental algorithms to the BraTS 2017 server, and the server provided quantitative evaluations including Dice score and Hausdorff distance compared with the ground truth.

Our networks were implemented in Tensorflow[2] [1] using NiftyNet[3,4] [10]. We used Adaptive Moment Estimation (Adam) [18] for training, with initial learning rate 10^{-3}, weight decay 10^{-7}, batch size 5, and maximal iteration 30 k. Training was implemented on an NVIDIA TITAN X GPU. The training patch size was $144{\times}144{\times}19$, $96{\times}96{\times}19$, and $64{\times}64{\times}19$ for WNet, TNet and ENet, respectively.

---

[1] http://www.med.upenn.edu/sbia/brats2017.html.
[2] https://www.tensorflow.org.
[3] http://niftynet.io.
[4] https://cmiclab.cs.ucl.ac.uk/CMIC/NiftyNet/tree/dev/demos/BRATS17.

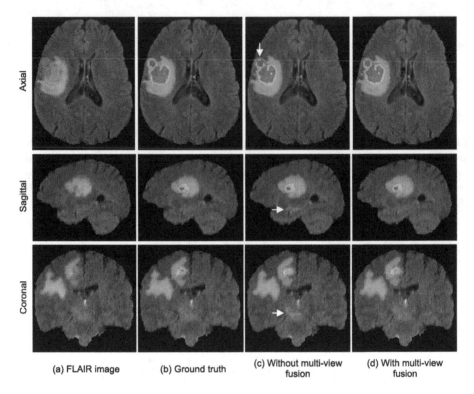

Fig. 4. Segmentation result of the brain tumor (HGG) from a training image. Green: edema; Red: non-enhancing tumor core; Yellow: enhancing tumor core. (c) shows the result when only networks in axial view are used, with mis-segmentations highlighted by white arrows. (d) shows the result with multi-view fusion. (Color figure online)

We set C_o to 32 and C_l to 2 for these three types of networks. For pre-processing, the images were normalized by the mean value and standard deviation of the training images for each sequence. We used the Dice loss function [9, 24] for training of each network.

Segmentation Results. Figures 4 and 5 show examples for HGG and LGG segmentation from training images, respectively. In both figures, for simplicity of visualization, only the FLAIR image is shown. The green, red and yellow colors show the edema, non-enhancing and enhancing tumor cores, respectively. We compared the proposed method with its variant that does not use multi-view fusion. For this variant, we trained and tested the networks only in axial view. In Fig. 4, segmentation without and with multi-view fusion are presented in the third and forth columns, respectively. It can be observed that the segmentation without multi-view fusion shown in Fig. 4(c) has some noises for edema and enhancing tumor core, which is highlighted by white arrows. In contrast, the segmentation with multi-view fusion shown in Fig. 4(d) is more accurate.

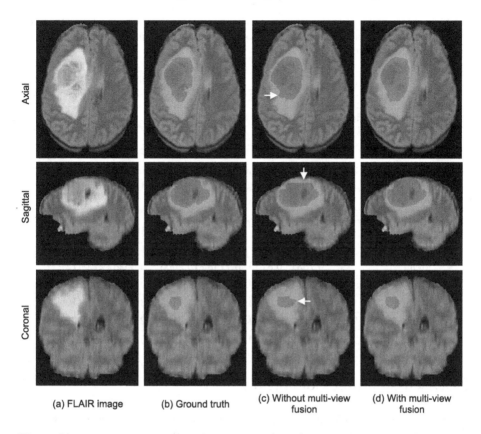

(a) FLAIR image	(b) Ground truth	(c) Without multi-view fusion	(d) With multi-view fusion

Fig. 5. Segmentation result of the brain tumor (LGG) from a training image. Green: edema; Red: non-enhancing tumor core; Yellow: enhancing tumor core. (c) shows the result when only networks in axial view are used, with mis-segmentations highlighted by white arrows. (d) shows the result with multi-view fusion. (Color figure online)

In Fig. 5, the LGG does not contain enhancing regions. The two counterparts achieve similar results for the whole tumor. However, it can be observed that the segmentation of tumor core is more accurate by using multi-view fusion.

Table 1 presents quantitative evaluations with the BraTS 2017 validation set. It shows that the proposed method achieves average Dice scores of 0.7859, 0.9050 and 0.8378 for enhancing tumor core, whole tumor and tumor core, respectively. For comparison, the variant without multi-view fusion obtains average Dice scores of 0.7411, 0.8896 and 0.8255 fore these three regions, respectively.

Table 2 presents quantitative evaluations with the BraTS 2017 testing set. It shows the mean values, standard deviations, medians, 25 and 75 quantiles of Dice and Hausdorff distance. Compared with the performance on the validation set, the performance on the testing set is lower, with average Dice scores of 0.7831, 0.8739, and 0.7748 for enhancing tumor core, whole tumor and tumor core, respectively. The higher median values show that good segmentation results are achieved for most images, and some outliers contributed to the lower average scores.

Table 1. Mean values of Dice and Hausdorff measurements of the proposed method on BraTS 2017 validation set. EN, WT, TC denote enhancing tumor core, whole tumor and tumor core, respectively.

	Dice			Hausdorff (mm)		
	ET	WT	TC	ET	WT	TC
Without multi-view fusion	0.7411	0.8896	0.8255	5.3178	12.4566	9.6616
With multi-view fusion	0.7859	0.9050	0.8378	3.2821	3.8901	6.4790

Table 2. Dice and Hausdorff measurements of the proposed method on BraTS 2017 testing set. EN, WT, TC denote enhancing tumor core, whole tumor and tumor core, respectively.

	Dice			Hausdorff (mm)		
	ET	WT	TC	ET	WT	TC
Mean	0.7831	0.8739	0.7748	15.9003	6.5528	27.0472
Standard deviation	0.2215	0.1319	0.2700	67.8552	10.6915	84.4297
Median	0.8442	0.9162	0.8869	1.7321	3.0811	3.7417
25 quantile	0.7287	0.8709	0.7712	1.4142	2.2361	2.0000
75 quantile	0.8882	0.9420	0.9342	3.1217	5.8310	8.4255

4   Discussion and Conclusion

There are several benefits of using a cascaded framework for segmentation of hierarchical structures [7]. First, compared with using a single network for all substructures of the brain tumor that requires complex network architectures, using three binary segmentation networks allows for a simpler network for each task. Therefore, they are easier to train and can reduce over-fitting. Second, the cascade helps to reduce false positives since TNet works on the region extracted by WNet, and ENet works on the region extracted by TNet. Third, the hierarchical pipeline follows anatomical structures of the brain tumor and uses them as spatial constraints. The binary crisp masks restrict the tumor core to be inside the whole tumor region and enhancing tumor core to be inside the tumor core region, respectively. In [9], the hierarchical structural information was leveraged to design a Generalised Wasserstein Dice loss function for imbalanced multi-class segmentation. However, that work did not use the hierarchical structural information as spatial constraints. One drawback of the cascade is that it is not end-to-end and requires longer time for training and testing compared with its multi-class counterparts using similar structures. However, we believe this is not an important issue for automatic brain tumor segmentation. Also, at inference time, our framework is more computationally efficient than most competitive approaches including ScaleNet [8] and DeepMedic [16].

The results show that our proposed method achieved competitive performance for automatic brain tumor segmentation. Figs. 4 and 5 demonstrate that the multi-view fusion helps to improve segmentation accuracy. This is mainly because our networks are designed with anisotropic receptive fields. The multi-view fusion is an ensemble of networks in three orthogonal views, which takes advantage of 3D contextual information to obtain higher accuracy. Considering the different imaging resolution in different views, it may be more reasonable to use a weighted average of axial, sagittal and coronal views rather than a simple average of them in the testing stage [25]. Our current results are not post-processed by CRFs that have been shown effective to get more spatially regularized segmentation [16]. Therefore, it is of interest to further improve our segmentation results by using CRFs.

In conclusion, we developed a cascaded system to segment glioma subregions from multi-modal brain MR images. We convert the multi-class segmentation problem to three cascaded binary segmentation problems, and use three networks to segment the whole tumor, tumor core and enhancing tumor core, respectively. Our networks use an anisotropic structure, which considers the balance among receptive field, model complexity and memory consumption. We also use multi-view fusion to reduce noises in the segmentation result. Experimental results on BraTS 2017 validation set show that the proposed method achieved average Dice scores of 0.7859, 0.9050, 0.8378 for enhancing tumor core, whole tumor and tumor core, respectively. The corresponding values for BraTS 2017 testing set were 0.7831, 0.8739, and 0.7748, respectively.

Acknowledgements. We would like to thank the NiftyNet team. This work was supported through an Innovative Engineering for Health award by the Wellcome Trust [WT101957], Engineering and Physical Sciences Research Council (EPSRC) [NS/A000027/1], the National Institute for Health Research University College London Hospitals Biomedical Research Centre (NIHR BRC UCLH/UCL High Impact Initiative), a UCL Overseas Research Scholarship, a UCL Graduate Research Scholarship, hardware donated by NVIDIA, and the Health Innovation Challenge Fund [HICF-T4-275, WT 97914], a parallel funding partnership between the Department of Health and Wellcome Trust.

References

1. Abadi, M., Barham, P., Chen, J., Chen, Z., Davis, A., Dean, J., Devin, M., Ghemawat, S., Irving, G., Isard, M., Kudlur, M., Levenberg, J., Monga, R., Moore, S., Murray, D.G., Steiner, B., Tucker, P., Vasudevan, V., Warden, P., Wicke, M., Yu, Y., Zheng, X., Brain, G.: TensorFlow: A system for large-scale machine learning. In: OSDI, pp. 265–284 (2016)
2. Abdulkadir, A., Lienkamp, S.S., Brox, T., Ronneberger, O.: 3D U-Net: Learning dense volumetric segmentation from sparse annotation. In: MICCAI, pp. 424–432 (2016)
3. Bakas, S., Akbari, H., Sotiras, A., Bilello, M., Rozycki, M., Kirby, J., Freymann, J., Farahani, K., Davatzikos, C.: Advancing the cancer genome atlas glioma MRI collections with expert segmentation labels and radiomic features. Nature Sci. Data 170117 (2017)

4. Bakas, S., Akbari, H., Sotiras, A., Bilello, M., Rozycki, M., Kirby, J., Freymann, J., Farahani, K., Davatzikos, C.: Segmentation labels and radiomic features for the pre-operative scans of the TCGA-LGG collection. The Cancer Imaging Archive (2017)
5. Bakas, S., Akbari, H., Sotiras, A., Bilello, M., Rozycki, M., Kirby, J., Freymann, J., Farahani, K., Davatzikos, C.: Segmentation labels for the pre-operative scans of the TCGA-GBM collection. The Cancer Imaging Archive (2017)
6. Chen, H., Dou, Q., Yu, L., Heng, P.A.: Voxresnet: Deep voxelwise residual networks for volumetric brain segmentation. NeuroImage (2017). https://doi.org/10.1016/j.neuroimage.2017.04.041. ISSN 1053-8119
7. Christ, P.F., Elshaer, M.E.A., Ettlinger, F., Tatavarty, S., Bickel, M., Bilic, P., Rempfler, M., Armbruster, M., Hofmann, F., Anastasi, M.D., Sommer, W.H., Ahmadi, S.A., Menze, B.H.: Automatic liver and lesion segmentation in CT using cascaded fully convolutional neural networks and 3D conditional random fields. In: MICCAI, pp. 415–423 (2016)
8. Fidon, L., Li, W., Garcia-Peraza-Herrera, L.C., Ekanayake, J., Kitchen, N., Ourselin, S., Vercauteren, T.: Scalable multimodal convolutional networks for brain tumour segmentation. In: MICCAI, pp. 285–293 (2017)
9. Fidon, L., Li, W., Garcia-Peraza-Herrera, L.C.: Generalised Wasserstein Dice score for imbalanced multi-class segmentation using holistic convolutional networks (2017). arXiv preprint arXiv:1707.00478
10. Gibson, E., Li, W., Sudre, C., Fidon, L., Shakir, D., Wang, G., Eaton-Rosen, Z., Gray, R., Doel, T., Hu, Y., Whyntie, T., Nachev, P., Barratt, D.C., Ourselin, S., Cardoso, M.J., Vercauteren, T.: NiftyNet: A deep-learning platform for medical imaging (2017). arXiv preprint arXiv:1709.03485
11. Grosgeorge, D., Petitjean, C., Dacher, J.N., Ruan, S.: Graph cut segmentation with a statistical shape model in cardiac MRI. Comput. Vis. Image Underst. 117(9), 1027–1035 (2013)
12. Havaei, M., Davy, A., Warde-Farley, D., Biard, A., Courville, A., Bengio, Y., Pal, C., Jodoin, P.M., Larochelle, H.: Brain tumor segmentation with deep neural networks. Med. Image Anal. 35, 18–31 (2016)
13. Havaei, M., Guizard, N., Chapados, N., Bengio, Y.: HeMIS: Hetero-modal image segmentation. In: MICCAI, pp. 469–477 (2016)
14. He, K., Zhang, X., Ren, S., Sun, J.: Delving deep into rectifiers: surpassing human-level performance on ImageNet classification. In: ICCV, pp. 1026–1034 (2015)
15. He, K., Zhang, X., Ren, S., Sun, J.: Deep residual learning for image recognition. In: CVPR, pp. 770–778 (2016)
16. Kamnitsas, K., Ledig, C., Newcombe, V.F.J., Simpson, J.P., Kane, A.D., Menon, D.K., Rueckert, D., Glocker, B.: Efficient multi-scale 3D CNN with fully connected CRF for accurate brain lesion segmentation. Med. Image Anal. 36, 61–78 (2017)
17. Kaus, M.R., Warfield, S.K., Nabavi, A., Black, P.M., Jolesz, F.A., Kikinis, R.: Automated segmentation of MR images of brain tumors. Radiology 218(2), 586–591 (2001)
18. Kingma, D.P., Ba, J.L.: Adam: A method for stochastic optimization. In: ICLR (2015)
19. Lee, C.-H., Schmidt, M., Murtha, A., Bistritz, A., Sander, J., Greiner, R.: Segmenting brain tumors with conditional random fields and support vector machines. In: Liu, Y., Jiang, T., Zhang, C. (eds.) CVBIA 2005. LNCS, vol. 3765, pp. 469–478. Springer, Heidelberg (2005). https://doi.org/10.1007/11569541_47

20. Li, W., Wang, G., Fidon, L., Ourselin, S., Cardoso, M.J., Vercauteren, T.: On the compactness, efficiency, and representation of 3D convolutional networks: brain parcellation as a pretext task. In: Niethammer, M., Styner, M., Aylward, S., Zhu, H., Oguz, I., Yap, P.-T., Shen, D. (eds.) IPMI 2017. LNCS, vol. 10265, pp. 348–360. Springer, Cham (2017). https://doi.org/10.1007/978-3-319-59050-9_28

21. Long, J., Shelhamer, E., Darrell, T.: Fully convolutional networks for semantic segmentation. In: CVPR, pp. 3431–3440 (2015)

22. Menze, B.H., Jakab, A., Bauer, S., Kalpathy-Cramer, J., Farahani, K., Kirby, J., Burren, Y., Porz, N., Slotboom, J., Wiest, R., Lanczi, L., Gerstner, E., Weber, M.A., Arbel, T., Avants, B.B., Ayache, N., Buendia, P., Collins, D.L., Cordier, N., Corso, J.J., Criminisi, A., Das, T., Delingette, H., Demiralp, Ç., Durst, C.R., Dojat, M., Doyle, S., Festa, J., Forbes, F., Geremia, E., Glocker, B., Golland, P., Guo, X., Hamamci, A., Iftekharuddin, K.M., Jena, R., John, N.M., Konukoglu, E., Lashkari, D., Mariz, J.A., Meier, R., Pereira, S., Precup, D., Price, S.J., Raviv, T.R., Reza, S.M., Ryan, M., Sarikaya, D., Schwartz, L., Shin, H.C., Shotton, J., Silva, C.A., Sousa, N., Subbanna, N.K., Szekely, G., Taylor, T.J., Thomas, O.M., Tustison, N.J., Unal, G., Vasseur, F., Wintermark, M., Ye, D.H., Zhao, L., Zhao, B., Zikic, D., Prastawa, M., Reyes, M., Van Leemput, K.: The multimodal brain tumor image segmentation benchmark (BRATS). TMI **34**(10), 1993–2024 (2015)

23. Menze, B.H., van Leemput, K., Lashkari, D., Weber, M.-A., Ayache, N., Golland, P.: A generative model for brain tumor segmentation in multi-modal images. In: Jiang, T., Navab, N., Pluim, J.P.W., Viergever, M.A. (eds.) MICCAI 2010. LNCS, vol. 6362, pp. 151–159. Springer, Heidelberg (2010). https://doi.org/10.1007/978-3-642-15745-5_19

24. Milletari, F., Navab, N., Ahmadi, S.A.: V-Net: Fully convolutional neural networks for volumetric medical image segmentation. In: IC3DV, pp. 565–571 (2016)

25. Mortazi, A., Karim, R., Rhode, K., Burt, J., Bagci, U.: CardiacNET: Segmentation of left atrium and proximal pulmonary veins from MRI using multi-view CNN. In: MICCAI, pp. 377–385 (2017)

26. Ronneberger, O., Fischer, P., Brox, T.: U-Net: Convolutional networks for biomedical image segmentation. In: MICCAI, pp. 234–241 (2015)

27. Sudre, C.H., Li, W., Vercauteren, T., Ourselin, S., Jorge Cardoso, M.: Generalised dice overlap as a deep learning loss function for highly unbalanced segmentations. In: Cardoso, M.J., Arbel, T., Carneiro, G., Syeda-Mahmood, T., Tavares, J.M.R.S., Moradi, M., Bradley, A., Greenspan, H., Papa, J.P., Madabhushi, A., Nascimento, J.C., Cardoso, J.S., Belagiannis, V., Lu, Z. (eds.) DLMIA/ML-CDS -2017. LNCS, vol. 10553, pp. 240–248. Springer, Cham (2017). https://doi.org/10.1007/978-3-319-67558-9_28

28. Wang, G., Zhang, S., Xie, H., Metaxas, D.N., Gu, L.: A homotopy-based sparse representation for fast and accurate shape prior modeling in liver surgical planning. Med. Image Anal. **19**(1), 176–186 (2015)

29. Wang, G., Zuluaga, M.A., Li, W., Pratt, R., Patel, P.A., Aertsen, M., Doel, T., Klusmann, M., David, A.L., Deprest, J., Ourselin, S., Vercauteren, T.: DeepIGeoS: A deep interactive geodesic framework for medical image segmentation (2017). arXiv preprint arXiv:1707.00652

30. Wang, J., Liu, T.: A survey of MRI-based brain tumor segmentation methods. Tsinghua Sci. Technol. **19**(6), 578–595 (2014)

31. Xie, S., Diego, S., Jolla, L., Tu, Z., Diego, S., Jolla, L.: Holistically-nested edge detection. In: ICCV, pp. 1395–1403 (2015)
32. Zikic, D., Glocker, B., Konukoglu, E., Criminisi, A., Demiralp, C., Shotton, J., Thomas, O.M., Das, T., Jena, R., Price, S.J.: Decision forests for tissue-specific segmentation of high-grade gliomas in multi-channel MR. In: Ayache, N., Delingette, H., Golland, P., Mori, K. (eds.) MICCAI 2012. LNCS, vol. 7512, pp. 369–376. Springer, Heidelberg (2012). https://doi.org/10.1007/978-3-642-33454-2_46

3D Brain Tumor Segmentation Through Integrating Multiple 2D FCNNs

Xiaomei Zhao[1,2(✉)], Yihong Wu[1(✉)], Guidong Song[3], Zhenye Li[4],
Yazhuo Zhang[3,4,5,6], and Yong Fan[7]

[1] National Laboratory of Pattern Recognition, Institute of Automation,
Chinese Academy of Sciences, Beijing, China
yhwu@nlpr.ia.ac.cn
[2] University of Chinese Academy of Sciences, Beijing, China
zhaoxiaomei14@mails.ucas.ac.cn
[3] Beijing Neurosurgical Institute, Capital Medical University, Beijing, China
[4] Department of Neurosurgery, Beijing Tiantan Hospital,
Capital Medical University, Beijing, China
[5] Beijing Institute for Brain Disorders Brain Tumor Center, Beijing, China
[6] China National Clinical Research Center for Neurological Diseases, Beijing, China
[7] Department of Radiology, Perelman School of Medicine,
University of Pennsylvania, Philadelphia, PA, USA

Abstract. The Magnetic Resonance Images (MRI) which can be used
to segment brain tumors are 3D images. To make use of 3D information,
a method that integrates the segmentation results of 3 2D Fully Convolutional Neural Networks (FCNNs), each of which is trained to segment
brain tumor images from axial, coronal, and sagittal views respectively,
is applied in this paper. Integrating multiple FCNN models by fusing
their segmentation results rather than by fusing into one deep network
makes sure that each FCNN model can still be tested by 2D slices, guaranteeing the testing efficiency. An averaging strategy is applied to do
the fusing job. This method can be easily extended to integrate more
FCNN models which are trained to segment brain tumor images from
more views, without retraining the FCNN models that we already have.
In addition, 3D Conditional Random Fields (CRFs) are applied to optimize our fused segmentation results. Experimental results show that,
integrating the segmentation results of multiple 2D FCNNs obviously
improves the segmentation accuracy, and 3D CRF greatly reduces false
positives and improves the accuracy of tumor boundaries.

Keywords: Brain tumor segmentation
Fully Convolutional Neural Networks · 3D Conditional Random Fields
Multi-views

1 Introduction

Brain tumor segmentation results provide the volume, shape, and localization
of brain tumors, which are crucial for brain tumor diagnosis and monitoring.

© Springer International Publishing AG, part of Springer Nature 2018
A. Crimi et al. (Eds.): BrainLes 2017, LNCS 10670, pp. 191–203, 2018.
https://doi.org/10.1007/978-3-319-75238-9_17

Automatic brain tumor segmentation methods can emancipate doctors from the manual segmentation work, which is tedious and time-consuming [1]. Brain tumor segmentation technologies develop fast in recent years [2], especially those methods based on deep learning.

Up to now, many types of deep learning models have been successfully used in medical image analysis areas. According to statistics, segmentation is the most common subject among the literatures that apply deep learning to analyze medical images, and Convolutional Neural Networks (CNNs) are the most successful type of deep learning models for image analysis [3]. CNNs based methods have won many medical image segmentation challenges, such as Multimodal Brain Tumor Segmentation Challenge (BRATS) [4] and International Symposium on Biomedical Imaging (ISBI) cell tracking challenge [5].

Many kinds of medical images, such as the Magnetic Resonance Images (MRI), which can be used to segment brain tumors, are 3D images. To take full use of 3D information for medical image analysis, it is better to use 3D CNNs. However, 3D CNNs have large memory and training time requirements [6]. Therefore, many researchers have tried to integrate multi-view 2D CNNs for 3D medical images analysis, such as [6,7]. These methods integrated their multi-view 2D CNNs into one deep network, and sent the 2D patches in multi-views centered at the same voxel into their deep networks at the same time, predicting the label of these 2D patches' common center voxel. Under this situation, 3D images could only be segmented patch by patch, which is a very slow testing strategy, even if we change their CNNs into FCNNs. To improve the segmentation efficiency, multiple FCNN models, each of which is trained to segment slices in different views, can be combined by fusing their segmentation results, such as [8,9], rather than by fusing into one deep network. In this way, each FCNN model can still be tested by 2D slices, guaranteeing the testing efficiency. In this paper, we integrate multiple 2D FCNNs by integrating their segmentation results.

This paper is developed from our previous work [10]. In [10], 3 integrated networks of FCNNs and CRF-RNN [11] were used to segment brain images slice by slice from axial, coronal, and sagittal views respectively, and then their segmentation results were fused by voting. While in this paper, the segmentation results of multiple FCNNs are fused by averaging and then 3D CRF [12] is used to optimize the fused results. 3D CRF costs much more time than CRF-RNN, but it has a much better performance. The details of our method are given in the following sections.

2   Materials and Methods

2.1   Materials

We use the dataset provided by Multimodal Brain Tumor Segmentation Challenge (BraTS) 2017 [13–15] to train and test our segmentation method. The multimodal Magnetic Resonance Imaging (MRI) scans for each patient include native (T1), post-contrast T1-weighted (T1Gd), T2-weighted, and T2-weighted fluid attenuated inversion recovery (Flair) volumes. Different from the datasets provided during BraTS 2014-2016, which include both pre- and post-operative scans, the dataset provided in this year only includes pre-operative MRI scans. BraTS 2017 has separated its dataset into 3 subsets: training subset, validation subset and testing subset. The training subset contains 210 High Grade Gliomas (HGG) cases and 75 Low Grade Gliomas (LGG) cases. The validation and the testing subsets contain 46 and 146 cases respectively, with unknown grades. All the ground truths of these subsets are produced by manual segmentation. Annotations include: enhancing tumor (label = 4), edema (label = 2), necrosis and non-enhancing tumor (label = 1), and others (label = 0). There is no tissue labeled as 3.

2.2 Methods

The proposed segmentation method consists of 5 main steps: pre-processing, segmenting brain images slice by slice from 3 different views using 3 2D FCNN models respectively, fusing segmentation results obtained in 3 different views, optimizing the fused segmentation results by 3D CRF, and post-processing. In the following we will introduce each of our segmentation steps in detail.

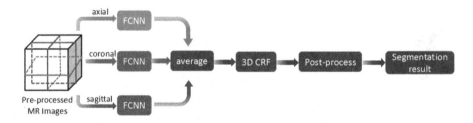

Fig. 1. Flowchart of our brain tumor segmentation method

Pre-process. To make similar intensities in MRI scans of the same modality have similar tissue meanings, pre-processing steps are utilized. Our pre-processing steps include N4ITK [16] and intensity normalization. The applied intensity normalization method normalize each image' intensity by normalizing its gray value of the highest histogram bin $\hat{I}$ and robust deviation $\tilde{\sigma} = \sqrt{\sum_{k=1}^{N}(I_k - \hat{I})^2/N}$ [10], where N denotes the total number of voxels in an image, I_k denotes the intensity value of the kth voxel in the image. We also change intensity range of each image to 0-255 linearly. For more details of our pre-processing steps, please refer to [10].

Segment Brain Images by FCNNs. Our FCNNs brain tumor segmentation method is a patch-based segmentation method. A patch is a local region extracted from an image. It can be 2D or 3D. In this paper, we use 2D square patches. A patch-based segmentation method transforms a segmentation task to a classification task. Patches are the objects to be classified. The label of a patch is same as the label of its center pixel. During testing, the traditional patch-based CNNs segmentation methods segment images by classifying patches one by one [17]. To accelerate the testing speed, Fully Convolutional Neural Networks (FCNNs), whose stride of each layer is set to 1, can be used. These FCNN networks can be trained by patches and tested by slices, improving the testing efficiency greatly [10,18].

In this paper, we use the same FCNN structure proposed in [19] as shown in Fig. 2, which has two different sizes of inputs. The large inputs pass through several convolutional and pooling layers and turn into small feature maps. These feature maps together with small inputs are used to predict their center pixel's label. Different from [19], we train 3 FCNN models in this paper, using 2D patches extracted from axial, coronal, and sagittal slices respectively. During testing, we use these 3 segmentation models to segment brain images slice by slice from 3 different views and obtain 3 segmentation probability maps.

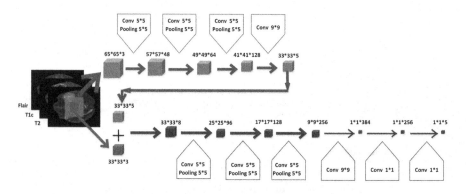

Fig. 2. The structure of the FCNN model used in this paper [19]

Fuse Segmentation Results Obtained in 3 Different Views. As described in the last subsection, 3 FCNN models are trained to segment brain images from 3 different views. During testing, their segmentation probability maps are fused by averaging to make better use of the 3D information provided by the 3D MRI scans.

Let P_a, P_c, and P_s denote the outputs of 3 the FCNN segmentation models respectively, $P_a = \{P_a^u | u = 0, 1, 2, 4\}$, $P_c = \{P_c^u | u = 0, 1, 2, 4\}$, $P_s = \{P_s^u | u = 0, 1, 2, 4\}$, where u denotes one of the four labels (enhancing tumor: label $= 4$; edema: label $= 2$; necrosis and non-enhancing tumor: label $= 1$; others: label $= 0$). P_a^u, P_c^u, and P_s^u are 3D probability images which have the same size as the 3D MRI scans to be segmented. The intensity value of each voxel in P_a^u, P_c^u, and P_s^u denotes the predicted probability of assigning label u to this voxel. We fuse these 3 segmentation results by averaging, that is $P = (P_a + P_c + P_s)/3$. P consists of

4 components $\{P^u | u = 0, 1, 2, 4\}$. Each $P^u = \{p_i^u\}$, where i is the index of voxel v_i in the 3D MRI scans and p_i^u is the fused predicted probability of assigning label u to voxel v_i.

We fuse the segmentation results as a post-processing step rather than fuse the 3 FCNN networks into one deep network, aiming to make sure that each FCNN model still has the ability to segment brain images slice by slice for efficiency. In this way, this method improves the efficiency of integrating multi-view 2D CNNs while achieves better accuracy than using a single 2D CNN network.

Optimize the Fused Segmentation Results by 3D CRF. To make sure the appearance and spatial consistency of segmentation results, we use fully connected 3D CRF [12] to optimize our segmentation results. CRF optimize the segmentation results by minimizing an energy function, which contains a unary term and a pairwise term. The energy function is shown as following:

$$E(a) = \sum_i \Phi(a_i^u) + \sum_{\forall i,j, i<j} \Psi(a_i^u, a_j^o) \tag{1}$$

where, i and j are indexes of two voxels v_i and v_j; a_i^u denotes assigning label u to voxel v_i, so does a_j^o; $\Phi(a_i^u)$ is the unary term, denoting the cost of assigning label u to voxel v_i; $\Psi(a_i^u, a_j^o)$ is the pairwise term, denoting the cost of assigning label u and o to voxels v_i and v_j respectively.

The unary term is calculated by $\Phi(a_i^u) = -\log p_i^u$, where, p_i^u denotes the fused probability of assigning label u to voxel v_i, which has been described in the last subsection. The pairwise term is formulated as a linear combination of Gaussian kernels [12]:

$$\Psi(a_i^u, a_j^o) = \mu(u, o)[\omega^{(1)} k^{(1)}(f_i, f_j) + \omega^{(2)} k^{(2)}(f_i, f_j)] \tag{2}$$

$$k^{(1)}(f_i, f_j) = exp(-\sum_d \frac{|s_{i,d} - s_{j,d}|^2}{2\sigma_{\alpha,d}^2}) \tag{3}$$

$$k^{(2)}(f_i, f_j) = exp(-\sum_d \frac{|s_{i,d} - s_{j,d}|^2}{2\sigma_{\beta,d}^2} - \sum_c \frac{|I_{i,c} - I_{j,c}|^2}{2\sigma_{\gamma,c}^2}) \tag{4}$$

$\mu(u, o)$ indicates the compatibility of labels u and o, $\mu(u, o) = [u \neq o]$; f_i and f_j denote feature vectors of v_i and v_j respectively, including their intensity $I_{i,c}$, $I_{j,c}$, and coordinates $s_{i,d}$, $s_{j,d}$; $c = flair, t1Gd,$ or $t2$ indicates different MRI modalities; $d = x, y,$ or z denotes different axles; $(s_{i,x}, s_{i,y}, s_{i,z})$ indicates the coordinate of voxel v_i, so does $(s_{j,x}, s_{j,y}, s_{j,z})$. Other parameters, such as $\omega^{(1)}$, $\omega^{(2)}$, $\sigma_{\alpha,d}$, $\sigma_{\beta,d}$, and $\sigma_{\gamma,c}$, are optimized by grid searching. The values of these parameters used in our experiments will be shown in Table 2 in Subsect. 3.1.

Post-process. We remove small isolated areas and correct some voxels' labels to post-process our segmentation results automatically by a simple thresholding method [10]. The thresholding parameters used in this paper have the same values as the parameters used in our previous paper [10].

3   Experiment

Our FCNN models are built upon caffe [20], and we use a computing server with multiple Tesla K80 GPUs and Intel E5-2620 CPUs. The dataset provided by BraTS 2017 are used to train and test our segmentation method. The details of this dataset have been described in Subsect. 2.1.

We use 80% of BraTS 2017 HGG training cases, including 168 HGG cases (hereinafter called 168 HGGs), to train our segmentation models, and use the rest of HGG training cases, including 42 HGG cases (hereinafter called 42 HGGs), as a validation dataset. Our FCNN networks are trained by patches and tested by slices. During training, we train 3 FCNN models, using 2D patches extracted from axial, coronal, and sagittal slices respectively. The numbers of extracted patches for different classes are equal. In our experiments, for the training of each view network, we extract 1000 * 4 patches from each training case. Our FCNN networks need two different sizes of input patches, as shown in Fig. 2. The size of the larger patch is 65 * 65 * 3, and the size of the smaller patch is 33 * 33 * 3. Images in these 3 channels are extracted from pre-processed Flair, T1Gd, and T2 respectively. T1 scans are not used, because experiments in [10] showed that T1 scans couldn't improve segmentation performance. In our experiments, the training batch size is set to 300, and the initial learning rate is set to 10^{-4}. The learning rate is divided by 10 after each 20 epochs. During testing, slices are padded with 0 intensities before segmentation to make sure that the outputs of FCNN models have the same size as the original slices. For example, if the size of an original slice is 240 * 240, we pad it with 0 intensities before segmentation to make two larger slices with sizes of $(240 + 64) * (240 + 64)$ and $(240 + 32) * (240 + 32)$ respectively. These two larger slices are used as the inputs of FCNN network, and then FCNN network outputs its prediction result with the size of 240 * 240. The stride of each layer in our FCNN networks has been set to 1. That is why the outputs of our FCNN networks can have the same resolution as the original slices just by padding the original slices with 0 intensities before segmentation.

In our primary experiments that are tested on the 42 HGGs, we use Dice, Positive Predictive Value (PPV), and Sensitivity to measure the performance of our segmentation models. These 3 metrics are commonly used in BraTS evaluation websites: BraTS 2012[1], BraTS 2013[2], and BraTS 2015[3]. These metrics are calculated as following: $Dice(P_*, T_*) = \frac{|P_* \cap T_*|}{(|P_*| + |T_*|)/2}$, $PPV(P_*, T_*) = \frac{|P_* \cap T_*|}{|P_*|}$, $Sensitivity(P_*, T_*) = \frac{|P_* \cap T_*|}{|T_*|}$, where $*$ indicates complete, core, or enhancing regions. T_* denotes the true region of $*$. P_* denotes the segmented $*$ region. $|P_* \cap T_*|$ denotes the overlap area between P_* and T_*. $|P_*|$ and $|T_*|$ denotes the areas of P_* and T_* respectively. Particularly, the complete region includes enhancing core, edema, no-enhancing core and necrosis; the core region includes enhancing core, non-enhancing core and necrosis; the enhancing region only

---

[1]   https://www.virtualskeleton.ch/BRATS/Start2012.

[2]   https://www.virtualskeleton.ch/BRATS/Start2013.

[3]   https://www.virtualskeleton.ch/BRATS/Start2015.

includes enhancing core. The 42 HGGs come from BraTS 2017 training dataset, and their ground truths are available. Therefore, we calculate the evaluation scores of the 42 HGGs by ourselves.

We also report our models' Dice scores on BraTS 2017 Validation dataset and Testing dataset. BraTS 2017 doesn't provide the ground truths of these two datasets. In this paper, the evaluation scores of Validation dataset are calculated on its evaluation website[4], and the evaluation scores of Testing dataset are provided by BraTS 2017 organizer. Even though there exist a number of LGG cases in BraTS 2017 Validation and Testing datasets, we still use our segmentation models trained only by the 168 HGGs to segment all the cases in these two datasets. Segmentation results of validation and testing datasets show that our models also work well for segmenting LGG cases. Therefor we only use HGG cases to train our segmentation models.

3.1   Primary Experiments Tested on the 42 HGGs

The evaluation scores of our models on the 42 HGGs are shown in Table 1, where the method called Fusing(FCNNs)+3D CRF fuses the segmentation results of 3 FCNN models by averaging, and then uses 3D CRF to optimize the fused results, as shown in Fig. 1; the method called Fusing(FCNNs+3D CRF) uses 3D CRF to optimize the segmentation results of each FCNN model, and then fuses the optimized results by voting.

Table 1. The average evaluation scores of 42 HGG cases

Methods	Dice			PPV			Sensitivity		
	Comp.	Core	Enh.	Comp.	Core	Enh.	Comp.	Core	Enh.
FCNNs(axial)	0.623	0.701	0.633	0.480	0.602	0.530	0.971	**0.916**	0.877
FCNNs(coronal)	0.666	0.738	0.675	0.578	0.664	0.594	0.963	0.896	0.865
FCNNs(sagittal)	0.662	0.703	0.653	0.526	0.607	0.574	0.957	0.912	0.846
Fusing(FCNNs)	0.713	0.805	0.733	0.585	0.753	0.663	**0.972**	0.912	0.887
Fusing(FCNNs)+3D CRF	0.865	0.867	0.821	0.912	**0.906**	0.800	0.841	0.856	0.884
Fusing(FCNNs)+3D CRF +post-process	**0.873**	**0.868**	**0.830**	**0.925**	0.904	**0.819**	0.843	0.860	0.877
FCNNs(axial)+3D CRF	0.857	0.843	0.787	0.873	0.840	0.731	0.857	0.875	**0.895**
FCNNs(coronal)+3D CRF	0.862	0.843	0.800	0.898	0.869	0.765	0.845	0.850	0.880
FCNNs(sagittal)+3D CRF	0.845	0.848	0.797	0.887	0.853	0.762	0.827	0.869	0.874
Fusing(FCNNs+3D CRF)	0.865	0.864	0.816	0.906	0.894	0.784	0.845	0.861	0.887
Fusing(FCNNs+3D CRF) +post-process	**0.873**	**0.868**	0.828	0.920	0.895	0.813	0.846	0.865	0.879

The scores in Table 1 indicate that fusing the segmentation results obtained from different views obviously improves the segmentation accuracy, no matter the fusing operation is performed before or after 3D CRF. But from the

---

[4] https://ipp.cbica.upenn.edu/.

view of Dice scores, Fusing(FCNNs)+3D CRF performs slightly better than Fusing(FCNNs+3D CRF). Note that, the performance of Fusing(FCNNs)+3D CRF reported in this paper is slightly different from the performance that we have reported in our pre-conference short paper of BraTS 2017 [21]. It is because that, at the beginning of our experiments, the same values of parameters in 3D CRF, which were optimized based on the experiments of Fusing(FCNNs+3D CRF), were applied in all of our experiments. But now, the parameters of 3D CRF are optimized separately in our experiments of Fusing(FCNNs)+3D CRF and Fusing(FCNNs+3D CRF). The values of parameters in 3D CRF used in our experiments are shown in Table 2. In addition, in [21], Fusing(FCNNs) fused segmentation results of FCNNs by voting, while in this paper, Fusing(FCNNs) fuses segmentation results of FCNNs by averaging.

Table 2. The values of parameters in 3D CRF used in our experiments (in this table, $d = x$, y,or z, and $c = flair$, $t1Gd$,or $t2$)

Experiments	$\omega^{(1)}$	$\omega^{(2)}$	$\sigma_{\alpha,d}$	$\sigma_{\beta,x}$	$\sigma_{\beta,y}$	$\sigma_{\beta,z}$	$\sigma_{\gamma,c}$
Fusing(FCNNs)+3D CRF	2.5	4.0	24	17	12	10	8
Fusing(FCNNs+3D CRF)	3.0	4.0	24	17	12	10	8

To show the effectiveness of integrating multiple FCNNs and multiple FCNNs+3D CRF, we show some segmentation examples in Fig. 3. Images in the first and second columns are used to show the effectiveness of fusing multiple FCNNs. Images in the third and fourth columns are used to show the effectiveness of fusing multiple FCNNs+3D CRF. Figure 3 shows that, fusing the 3 segmentation results of multi-view models can remove some obvious false positives, which just appear in one of the three results and do not appear in the other two results.

To show the effectiveness of 3D CRF and post-processing steps, we show some segmentation results in Fig. 4. Images in the first and second rows show that 3D CRF makes the segmentation labels have appearance and spatial consistency, and post-processing steps can remove false positives by removing small isolated areas. Images in the third and fourth rows show that 3D CRF also has the ability to remove many false positives caused by bias field. In this case, even though the segmentation result which has been optimized by 3D CRF still has much difference from the ground truth, it is already much better than the segmentation result without 3D CRF.

3.2 Segmentation Performance on BraTS 2017 Validation Dataset

We test our segmentation results of BRATS 2017 Validation dataset on its evaluation website. The Dice scores are shown in Table 3. Table 3 shows that, on BraTS 2017 Validation dataset, Fusing(FCNNs)+3D CRF+post-process has a better performance on enhancing region and core region, while Fusing(FCNNs+3D CRF)+post-process has a slightly better performance on complete tumor region.

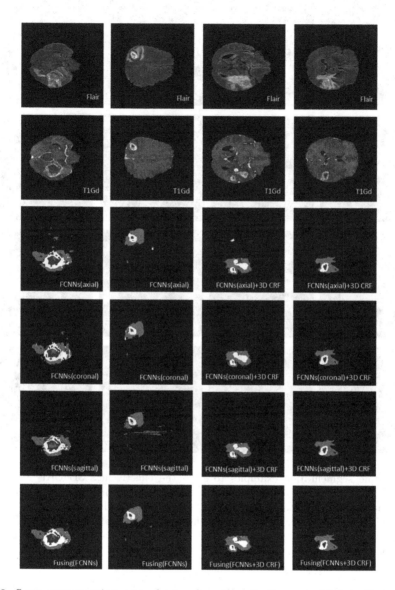

Fig. 3. Some segmentation examples to show the effectiveness of integrating multiple FCNNs and FCNNs+3D CRF. The type of each image has been labeled on the image. Images in the first and second columns are used to show the effectiveness of fusing multiple FCNNs. Images in the third and fourth columns are used to show the effectiveness of fusing multiple FCNNs+3D CRF. From left to right, the subjects ID are: Brats17_CBICA_ABE_1, Brats17_CBICA_AOZ_1, Brats17_CBICA_AME_1, Brats17_CBICA_AQD_1. In the segmentation results, each gray level represents a tumor class, from high to low: enhancing core, edema, necrosis and non-enhancing core.

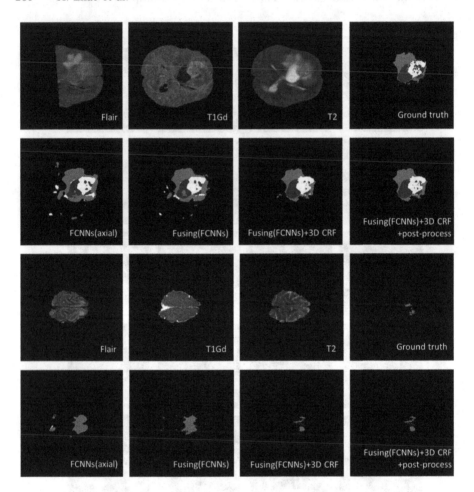

Fig. 4. Some segmentation examples to show the effectiveness 3D CRF and post-processing step. The type of each image has been labeled on the image. Images in the first and second rows come from the subject of Brats17_2013_20_1, and the images in the third and fourth rows come from the subject of Brats17_CBICA_ARZ_1. In the segmentation results, each gray level represents a tumor class, from high to low: enhancing core, edema, necrosis and non-enhancing core.

3.3   Segmentation Performance on BraTS 2017 Testing Dataset

The ground truths of BraTS 2017 Testing dataset are not available. The evaluation scores of our method on BraTS 2017 Testing dataset are provided by its organizer. We show the Dice scores of our method in Table 4.

During BraTS 2017, we used the segmentation model of Fusing(FCNNs)+3D CRF, not only because Fusing(FCNNs)+3D CRF has a slightly better performance, but also because Fusing(FCNNs)+3D CRF has a higher segmentation efficiency than Fusing(FCNNs+3D CRF). Fusing(FCNNs)+3D CRF only

Table 3. The average Dice scores of BRATS 2017 validation dataset (46 cases)

Methods	Dice		
	Comp.	Core	Enh.
FCNNs(axial)	0.648	0.601	0.543
FCNNs(coronal)	0.669	0.605	0.544
FCNNs(sagittal)	0.650	0.606	0.553
Fusing(FCNNs)	0.717	0.665	0.613
Fusing(FCNNs)+3D CRF	0.882	0.694	0.702
Fusing(FCNNs)+3D CRF+post-process	0.887	**0.794**	**0.754**
FCNNs(axial)+3D CRF	0.878	0.683	0.657
FCNNs(coronal)+3D CRF	0.871	0.677	0.647
FCNNs(sagittal) +3D CRF	0.870	0.694	0.668
Fusing(FCNNs+3D CRF)	0.881	0.694	0.696
Fusing(FCNNs+3D CRF)+post-process	**0.888**	0.792	0.749

Table 4. The average Dice scores of BRATS 2017 testing dataset (146 cases)

Methods	Dice		
	Comp.	Core	Enh.
Fusing(FCNNs)+3D CRF+post-process	0.876	0.752	0.764

performs 3D CRF once, while Fusing(FCNNs+3D CRF) performs 3D CRF three times. The 3D CRF is performed on CPU. Performing 3D CRF once costs about 3 min per case.

4   Conclusion

In this paper, 3D brain images are segmented by integrating the segmentation results of multiple 2D FCNNs, which are trained to segment brain images from axial, coronal, and sagittal views respectively. Each of the 2D FCNN networks is tested slice by slice, guaranteeing the segmentation efficiency. In addition, 3D CRF is used to optimize our fused segmentation results. Experimental results show that 3D CRF and the integrating strategy help a lot to improve segmentation accuracy. Moreover, this integrating method is not limited to fuse the 3 segmentation results from 3 different views. It can be extended to fuse the more from more views.

Acknowledgements. This work was supported by the National High Technology Research and Development Program of China (2015AA020504) and the National Natural Science Foundation of China under Grant No. 61572499, 61421004.

References

1. Bauer, S., Wiest, R., Nolte, L.-P., Reyes, M.: A survey of MRI-based medical image analysis for brain tumor studies. Phys. Med. Biol. **58**, 97–129 (2013)
2. Menze, B.H., Jakab, A., Bauer, S., Kalpathy-Cramer, J., Farahani, K., Kirby, J., Burren, Y., Porz, N., Slotboom, J., Wiest, R., et al.: The multimodal brain tumor image segmentation benchmark (BRATS). IEEE Trans. Med. Imaging **34**, 1993–2024 (2015)
3. Litjens, G., Kooi, T., Bejnordi, B.E., Setio, A.A.A., Ciompi, F., Ghafoorian, M., van der Laak, J.A., van Ginneken, B., Snchez, C.I.: A survey on deep learning in medical image analysis (2017). arXiv preprint arXiv:1702.05747
4. Chang, P.D.: Fully convolutional deep residual neural networks for brain tumor segmentation. In: Crimi, A., Menze, B., Maier, O., Reyes, M., Winzeck, S., Handels, H. (eds.) BrainLes 2016. LNCS, vol. 10154, pp. 108–118. Springer, Cham (2016). https://doi.org/10.1007/978-3-319-55524-9_11
5. Ronneberger, O., Fischer, P., Brox, T.: U-Net: Convolutional networks for biomedical image segmentation. In: Navab, N., Hornegger, J., Wells, W.M., Frangi, A.F. (eds.) MICCAI 2015. LNCS, vol. 9351, pp. 234–241. Springer, Cham (2015). https://doi.org/10.1007/978-3-319-24574-4_28
6. Prasoon, A., Petersen, K., Igel, C., Lauze, F., Dam, E., Nielsen, M.: Deep feature learning for knee cartilage segmentation using a triplanar convolutional neural network. In: Mori, K., Sakuma, I., Sato, Y., Barillot, C., Navab, N. (eds.) MICCAI 2013. LNCS, vol. 8150, pp. 246–253. Springer, Heidelberg (2013). https://doi.org/10.1007/978-3-642-40763-5_31
7. Fritscher, K., Raudaschl, P., Zaffino, P., Spadea, M.F., Sharp, G.C., Schubert, R.: Deep neural networks for fast segmentation of 3D medical images. In: Ourselin, S., Joskowicz, L., Sabuncu, M.R., Unal, G., Wells, W. (eds.) MICCAI 2016. LNCS, vol. 9901, pp. 158–165. Springer, Cham (2016). https://doi.org/10.1007/978-3-319-46723-8_19
8. Mortazi, A., Karim, R., Rhode, K., Burt, J., Bagci, U.: *CardiacNET*: Segmentation of left atrium and proximal pulmonary veins from MRI using multi-view CNN. In: Descoteaux, M., Maier-Hein, L., Franz, A., Jannin, P., Collins, D.L., Duchesne, S. (eds.) MICCAI 2017. LNCS, vol. 10434, pp. 377–385. Springer, Cham (2017). https://doi.org/10.1007/978-3-319-66185-8_43
9. Wang, G., Li, W., Ourselin, S., Vercauteren, T.: Automatic brain tumor segmentation using cascaded anisotropic convolutional neural networks (2017). arXiv preprint arXiv: 1709.00382
10. Zhao, X., Wu, Y., Song, G., Li, Z., Zhang, Y., Fan, Y.: A deep learning model integrating FCNNs and CRFs for brain tumor segmentation. Med. Image Anal. **43**, 98–111 (2018)
11. Zheng, S., Jayasumana, S., Romera-Paredes, B., Vineet, V., Su, Z., Du, D., Huang, C., Torr, P.H.: Conditional random fields as recurrent neural networks. In: Proceedings of the IEEE International Conference on Computer Vision, pp. 1529–1537 (2015)
12. Kamnitsas, K., Ledig, C., Newcombe, V.F., Simpson, J.P., Kane, A.D., Menon, D.K., Rueckert, D., Glocker, B.: Efficient multi-scale 3D CNN with fully connected CRF for accurate brain lesion segmentation. Med. Image Anal. **36**, 61–78 (2017)
13. Bakas, S., Akbari, H., Sotiras, A., Bilello, M., Rozycki, M., Kirby, J., Freymann, J., Farahani, K., Davatzikos, C.: Segmentation Labels and Radiomic Features for the Pre-operative Scans of the TCGA-GBM collection. The Cancer Imaging Archive (2017). https://doi.org/10.7937/K9/TCIA.2017.KLXWJJ1Q

14. Bakas, S., Akbari, H., Sotiras, A., Bilello, M., Rozycki, M., Kirby, J., Freymann, J., Farahani, K., Davatzikos, C.: Segmentation Labels and Radiomic Features for the Pre-operative Scans of the TCGA-LGG collection. The Cancer Imaging Archive (2017). https://doi.org/10.7937/K9/TCIA.2017.GJQ7R0EF
15. Bakas, S., Akbari, H., Sotiras, A., Bilello, M., Rozycki, M., Kirby, J.S., Freymann, J.B., Farahani, K., Davatzikos, C.: Advancing the cancer genome atlas glioma MRI collections with expert segmentation labels and radiomic features. Sci. Data **4** (2017)
16. Tustison, N.J., Avants, B.B., Cook, P.A., Zheng, Y., Egan, A., Yushkevich, P.A., Gee, J.C.: N4ITK: improved N3 bias correction. IEEE Trans. Med. Imaging **29**, 1310–1320 (2010)
17. Pereira, S., Pinto, A., Alves, V., Silva, C.A.: Brain tumor segmentation using convolutional neural networks in MRI images. IEEE Trans. Med. Imaging **35**, 1240–1251 (2016)
18. Havaei, M., Davy, A., Warde-Farley, D., Biard, A., Courville, A., Bengio, Y., Pal, C., Jodoin, P.-M., Larochelle, H.: Brain tumor segmentation with deep neural networks. Med. Image Anal. **35**, 18–31 (2017)
19. Zhao, X., Wu, Y., Song, G., Li, Z., Fan, Y., Zhang, Y.: Brain tumor segmentation using a fully convolutional neural network with conditional random fields. In: Crimi, A., et al. (eds.) Brainlesion Glioma Multiple Sclerosis Stroke and Traumatic Brain Injuries 2016. LNCS, vol. 10154, pp. 75–87. Springer, Cham (2016). https://doi.org/10.1007/978-3-319-55524-9_8
20. Jia, Y., Shelhamer, E., Donahue, J., Karayev, S., Long, J., Girshick, R., Guadarrama, S., Darrell, T.: Caffe: Convolutional architecture for fast feature embedding. In: Proceedings of the 22nd ACM International Conference on Multimedia, pp. 675–678. ACM (2014)
21. Zhao, X., Wu, Y., Song, G., Li, Z., Zhang, Y., and Fan, Y.: 3D brain tumor segmentation through integrating multiple 2D FCNNs. In: Pre-conference Proceedings of MICCAI-BraTS (Brain Tumor Segmentation Challenge), pp. 321–327 (2017)

MRI Brain Tumor Segmentation and Patient Survival Prediction Using Random Forests and Fully Convolutional Networks

Mohammadreza Soltaninejad[1](✉), Lei Zhang[1], Tryphon Lambrou[1],
Guang Yang[2], Nigel Allinson[1], and Xujiong Ye[1]

[1] Laboratory of Vision Engineering, School of Computer Science,
University of Lincoln, Lincoln, UK
{msoltaninejad,lzhang,tlambrou,nallinson,xye}@lincoln.ac.uk
[2] National Heart and Lung Institute, Imperial College London, London, UK
g.yang@imperial.ac.uk

Abstract. In this paper, we propose a learning based method for automated segmentation of brain tumor in multimodal MRI images, which incorporates two sets of machine-learned and hand-crafted features. Fully convolutional networks (FCN) forms the machine-learned features and texton based histograms are considered as hand-crafted features. Random forest (RF) is used to classify the MRI image voxels into normal brain tissues and different parts of tumors. The volumetric features from the segmented tumor tissues and patient age applying to an RF is used to predict the survival time. The method was evaluated on MICCAI-BRATS 2017 challenge dataset. The mean Dice overlap measures for segmentation of validation dataset are 0.86, 0.78 and 0.66 for whole tumor, core and enhancing tumor, respectively. The validation Hausdorff values are 7.61, 8.70 and 3.76. For the survival prediction task, the classification accuracy, pairwise mean square error and Spearman rank are 0.485, 198749 and 0.334, respectively.

Keywords: Fully convolutional networks · Random forest
Deep learning · Texton · MRI · Brain tumor segmentation

1 Introduction

Delineation of the tumor boundary and assessment of tumor size are needed for patient management in terms of treatment planning [1] and monitoring treatment response [2], and current guidelines incorporate the use of Magnetic Resonance Images (MRI) [3,4]. Tumor assessment requires accurate full 3D volume measurement of the tumor. However, automated segmentation of brain tumors is a very challenging task due to their high variation in size, shape and appearance (e.g. image uniformity and texture) [5].

Most of the classification-based brain tumor segmentation techniques used hand-crafted features which are fed into a classifier such as random forests

© Springer International Publishing AG, part of Springer Nature 2018
A. Crimi et al. (Eds.): BrainLes 2017, LNCS 10670, pp. 204–215, 2018.
https://doi.org/10.1007/978-3-319-75238-9_18

(RF), support vector machines, etc. [6,7]. Among the conventional classifiers, RF presents the best segmentation results [7,8]. However, one limitation of these types of methods is that a large number of features are required in order to provide better description of the different types of classes (tissues) in the images. Therefore, they result in a high dimensional problem which makes the process more complicated and time consuming.

Due to the recent advances in deep convolutional neural networks (CNNs) they have been widely used for recognition of the patterns in the images. Several CNN-based methods have been developed for medical image analysis, especially for segmentation of brain tumors in MRI [9–11].

Recently, fully convolutional networks (FCN) have been suggested for dense (i.e. per-pixel) classification with the advantage of end-to-end learning [12]. Despite the advantage of dense pixel classification, FCN-based methods still have limitations of considering the local dependencies in higher resolution (pixel) level. The loss of spatial information, which occurs in the pooling layers, results in coarse segmentation. This limitation will be addressed in this paper by incorporating high resolution hand-crafted textural features which consider local dependencies of the pixel. Texton feature maps [13] provides significant information on multi-resolution image patterns in both spatial and frequency domains. This is an inspiration to combine texton features to a partially end-to-end learning process in order to improve the segmentation.

In this paper, a novel fully automatic learning based segmentation method is proposed, by applying hand-crafted and machine-learned features to an RF classifier. The machine-learned FCN based features detect the coarse region of the tumor while the hand-crafted texton descriptors consider the spatial features and local dependencies to improve the accuracy for segmentation of tumor tissue subtypes. Also, the survival time of the patients is predicted using the volumetric features extracted from the segmented images and the patient information (in this paper, age).

2   Methods

The proposed segmentation method is comprised of four major steps (preprocessing, CNN design, Texton map extraction, RF classifier) that are depicted in Fig. 1.

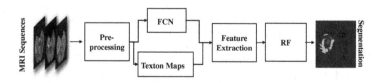

Fig. 1. The overall flowchart of the proposed method which uses hand-designed and machine-learned features for automatic brain tumor segmentation in MRI images.

2.1   Preprocessing

Firstly, the 1% highest and lowest intensity values for each image are eliminated. The 1% highest values correspond to the hyper intensities of the remaining voxels related to the skull, and the 1% lowest values correspond to the elimination of the background noise. The intensities were normalized for each protocol by subtracting the average of intensities of the image and dividing by their standard deviation. Then, the histogram of each image was normalized and matched to the one of the patient images which is selected as the reference. The normalization procedure for each individual protocol is illustrated in Fig. 2. To eliminate the bias of the matched histogram to the reference case, another block ("Histogram Matching 2" in Fig. 2.) is added to the process according to [14]. In this procedure, the average of all the new histograms including the initial reference case is calculated for each protocol and the histograms are again matched to the new reference, i.e. the average histogram for each protocol. In the second stage, for each case, the intensities of new images of all the protocols obtained from the first step are linearly normalized to the range [0, 255]. The protocols that are used in this study are Fluid Attenuated Inversion Recovery (FLAIR), post-contrast T1-weighted (T1-contrast), and T2-weighted.

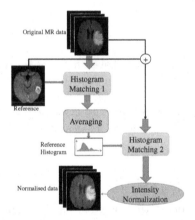

Fig. 2. Flowchart of the multimodal normalization and histogram matching of the MR dataset for one protocol.

2.2   Feature Extraction Form the FCN Layers

The FCN network is modified by eliminating the final classifier layer and converting all the fully connected (FC) layers to convolution layers (CONVs). This is realized by adding a CONV of size 1×1 with channel dimension 4 (i.e. number of output classes). A deconvolution layer is added to upsample the coarse output bilinearly to predict the scores for each pixels of multimodal MRI images that provides the pixel-wise fine segmentation.

The output stride is divided in half by predicting from a 16-pixel stride layer. A 1×1 convolution is added to the *POOL4* to further predict the classes. The corresponding output is combined with the output of *CONV7* at stride 32 by adding a 2x upsampling layer. The upsampling layer is initially a bilinear interpolation and its parameters can be learned later. The stride 16 predictions are then upsampled back to the image. This structure is called FCN-16.

The same procedure is applied on the *POOL3*, the predictions at 8 stride is then combined with the 2x upsampling of the combinations of the predictions derived from stride 16 and 32 that results in FCN-8s architecture. The FCN-8s provides relatively finer segmentation compared with the FCN-16s. In the same way, to produce finer predictions, we could decrease the strides of the pooling layers. However, it makes network training inefficient, since such implementation will increase the computational cost and increase the network convergence time.

The architecture of FCN based on VGG16 [15] for brain tumor segmentation is presented in Fig. 3. The predictions at shallow layers are produced using a skip layer that combines coarse predictions at deep layers to improve segmentation details.

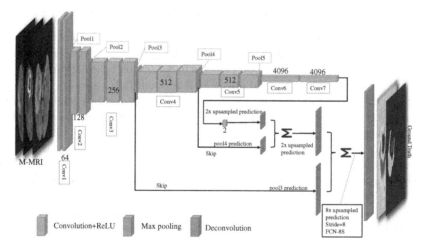

Fig. 3. The detailed architecture of the FCN used for segmentation of brain tumor in multimodal MRI.

The VGG model is designed based on natural image with intensities with bit depth $= 8$ (i.e. the intensity range is $[0, 255]$). The VGG model has also the capability of being further trained by adding more datasets to the existing pre-trained model. The initialization using a pre-trained model decreases the training time. Furthermore, the shallower layer of any CNNs learn more common features of images which are more likely domain-independent, thus such features could be used among different kinds of images. In this case, a pre-trained model could improve the model accuracy for new images. In order to use the pre-trained

VGG16 model for the case of medical MR images, some modifications should be taken into account. The intensities of the images are normalized into the range of a natural image which is [0, 255]. The pre-trained VGG model is trained on RGB images which has three channels. Therefore, three protocols were selected to build the input data, i.e. FLAIR, T1-contrast and T2-weighted according to the annotation protocol described in [8]. T2-weighted was selected since it was used mainly to segment the "edema". FLAIR was used to discriminate the edema from ventricles and fluid-filled structures. T1-contrast was utilized to distin-guish other tumor subtypes. The "enhancing tumor" appears as hyper-intensities and the "necrosis" appears as low intensities within the enhancing borders in T1-contrast.

The feature vector is generated for each voxel based on the score map from the FCN. For each class label, a score map is generated. Overall, 4 maps are generated using the standard MICCAI-BRATS17 labelling system, i.e. background plus normal brain, necrosis plus non-enhancing, edema, and enhancing tumor. The values of each map layer corresponding to each voxel are considered as machine-learned features of that voxel.

2.3   Spatial Feature Extraction Using Textons

The coarse results of the FCN-based segmentation are due to the down-sampling that occurs in the pooling layers. Given that the local dependency is not sufficiently considered in the FCN, a new pipeline using texton based feature descriptor derived from the convolutional operator is proposed. Textons are used since they are powerful feature descriptors that represent the local dependencies and neighborhood system information in all phases, i.e. convolution, k-means clustering and histogram calculation. Textons are obtained by convolving the image with a Gabor filter bank. To cover all orientations six different filter directions were used: $[0°, 30°, 45°, 60°, 90°, 120°]$. Filter sizes were $[0.3, 0.6, 0.9, 1.2, 1.5]$ and the wavelength of sinusoid coefficients of the Gabor filters were $[0.8, 1.0, 1.2, 1.5]$.

The MR images are convolved with the Gabor filters, then the filter responses are merged together and clustered using k-means clustering. The number of clusters 16 was selected as the optimum value for the number of clusters in texton map. The texton map is created by assigning the cluster number to each voxel of the image.

Each pixel in the image is described by its intensity and neighborhood pixels. For each pixel, its neighborhood with size $n \times n$ pixel is represented by the histogram of texton while the center pixel is represented by its normalized intensity. This descriptor of each pixel implicitly encodes the information that the center pixel conditionally depends on its neighborhood, thus incorporates the local dependencies into feature representation. The texton histogram is a vector with the size of k-means clusters (i.e. 16 in this paper). The procedure of mapping the connectivity based on the texton IDs (in the neighborhood window) to the histogram is illustrated in Fig. 4. The texton feature for each voxel is the histogram of textons in a neighborhood window of 5×5 around that voxel.

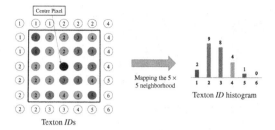

Fig. 4. The connectivity of the adjacent pixels from the histogram of the texton *ID*s in a 5 × 5 neighborhood of the center pixel. The texton clusters are integers in the range [1, 16]. This is a simplified example and the texton histogram values are zero for *ID*s from 6 to 16.

Figure 5 shows the FCN based score maps for each class layer and the protocols used to generate the corresponding score maps. Figure 5 also shows the corresponding texton maps.

It should be noted that the histogram of texton is considered for the adjacent pixels in the neighborhood and the target pixel (in the center) is not counted. Therefore, the normalized intensity value of the voxels in each protocol which is obtained from the preprocessing stage is also included in the feature vector. In total, 55 features were collected (4 FCN score maps, 3 protocol intensities and 48 texton histograms from three protocols) for usage in the classification stage. Figure 6 shows a graphic presentation of feature vector generation and presents how machine-learned and hand-designed features are integrated together.

2.4   Random Forest Classification

The potential tumor area detected by the FCN output was considered as the initial region of interest (ROI). This ROI was selected as a confidence margin of 10 voxels in 3D space around the detected initial tumor area which was calculated by morphological dilation. The feature vectors for voxels in this ROI were fed to an RF [16]. The main parameters in designing RF are tree depth and the number of trees. RF parameters were tuned by examining different tree depths and number of trees on training datasets and evaluating the classification accuracy using 5-fold cross validation. The number of 50 trees with depth 15 provided an optimum generalization and accuracy. Based on the classes assigned for each voxel in the validation dataset, the final segmentation mask was created by mapping back the voxel estimated class to the segmentation mask volume. Finally, the bright regions in the healthy part of the brain near to the skull were eliminated using a connected component analysis.

2.5   Patient Overall Survival Prediction

A new task is introduced in MICCAI-BRATS 2017 challenge which is prediction of patients' overall survival (OS) from the pre-operative scans. The features

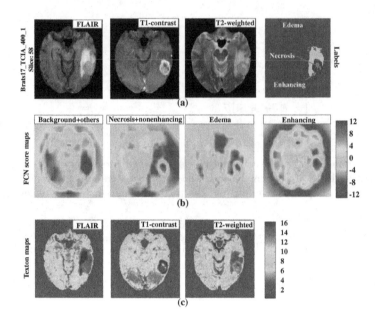

Fig. 5. The FCN-based score maps and texton maps generated from the multimodal MRI protocols: FLAIR, T1-contrast and T2-weighted. (a) The original images and the corresponding brain tissue labels, (b) FCN score maps generated from all three protocols together for each individual class, (c) texton maps generated from each individual protocol.

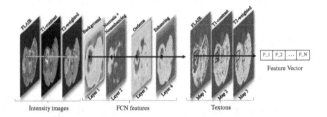

Fig. 6. The details of feature vector generation for the hybrid method. Machine based features from FCN are extracted based on pixel and the hand-designed texton features extracted from the neighborhood around the pixel and considers the local dependencies.

which are used for this task are the relative volume size of each tumor subtype after segmentation. The number of voxels within each segmented volume related to each tumor is divided by the total number of voxels within the brain. The age of patients is considered as another feature. Since RF can handle the categorical data and features with different ranges and they present promising classification and regression tasks, they are used for the prediction of survival time. An RF with the number of 1000 trees and with depth 15 is used as a regression model.

3   Results

The experiments were implemented on a PC with CPU Intel Core i7 and RAM 16 GB with the operating system windows 8.1. GPU GeForce gtx980i was used for reducing the training time of the FCN. The FCN was implemented using MatCovNet toolbox [17]. The VGG16 network was implemented using the Caffe model [18]. The network weights were initialized using pre-trained VGG16 model. The mini-batch stochastic gradient descent (SGD) with momentum was employed to train the FCN. The learning rate and momentum were set to 0.0001 and 0.9, respectively. The batch size was set to 20 and the total number of 150 epochs were used. The dropper layers with the rate of 0.5 were used to reduce overfitting. Other sections of the proposed method were performed using MAT-LAB 2016b. RF open source code provided in [19], which is a specialized toolbox for RF classification based on MATLAB, was utilized for the classification.

3.1   Segmentation Task

Both FCN and RF were trained on BRATS 2017 [8, 20–22] training dataset which include 220 high grade glioma (HGG) and 75 low grade glioma (LGG) patient cases. The method was evaluated on BRTAS 2017 validation (46 patient cases) and testing (146 patient cases) datasets.

The evaluation measures which are provided by the CBICA's Image Processing Portal (IPP) [23], i.e. Dice score, sensitivity, specificity, Hausdorff distance, were used to compare the segmentation results with the gold standard (blind testing). Figure 7 shows segmentation results of the proposed method on some cases of BRATS 2017 validation and testing datasets. The segmentation results of using only FCN are also shown in Fig. 7(c) to provide a comparison between both methods. As can be seen in Fig. 7(d), the proposed method provides finer segmentations compared to FCN only segmentation (Fig. 7(c)).

Table 1 provides the evaluation results obtained by applying the proposed method on BRATS 2017 validation dataset. The results of this paper appear as the team name "LoVE" on the CBICA portal leaderboard [24]. Table 2 provides the evaluation results for the testing dataset. It should be noted that only Dice and Hausdorff measures were provided by the challenge organizers at the time of submission of this paper. The mean Dice overlap measures for segmentation of validation dataset against ground truth are 0.86, 0.78 and 0.66 for the whole tumor, core and enhancing tumor, respectively. The corresponding Dice score results for the testing dataset are 0.85, 0.69 and 0.67, respectively. The average Hausdorff distance for segmentation of validation dataset against ground truth is for 7.61, 8.70 and 3.76 for the whole tumor, core and enhancing tumor, respectively. The corresponding Hausdorff distances for the testing dataset are 6.12, 28.72 and 23.55, respectively.

3.2   Survival Prediction Task

The training dataset includes 163 patients provided with overall survival time and the age of patients. The validation and test datasets include 33 and 95

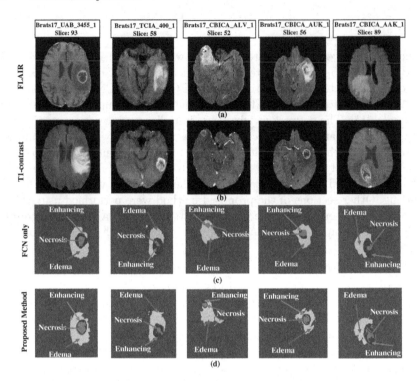

Fig. 7. Segmentation masks for some validation and test datasets, using the proposed method. The case names and the slice number are mentioned on the top of the images. (a) FLAIR images, (b) T1-contrast images, (c) segmentation masks and labels using FCN only, (d) segmentation masks and labels using the proposed method.

Table 1. Segmentation results for validation dataset which was provided by CBICA portal. ET: enhancing tumor, WT: whole tumor, TC: tumor core.

	Dice			Sensitivity			Specificity			Hausdorff (95%)		
	ET	WT	TC	ET	WT	TC	ET	WT	TC	ET	WT	TC
Mean	0.66	0.86	0.78	0.57	0.83	0.72	1.00	1.00	1.00	3.76	7.61	8.70
STD	0.28	0.09	0.19	0.28	0.13	0.21	0.00	0.01	0.00	4.38	12.99	13.52
Median	0.73	0.90	0.88	0.61	0.88	0.82	1.00	1.00	1.00	3.00	3.00	3.19
25 quantile	0.60	0.86	0.83	0.43	0.81	0.75	1.00	0.99	1.00	1.93	2.18	2.24
75 quantile	0.84	0.93	0.90	0.74	0.92	0.87	1.00	1.00	1.00	3.81	5.17	6.10

patients, respectively. For the evaluation on the training dataset, a 5-fold cross-validation was used. Then the RF was trained using all the training dataset and evaluated on the validation and testing datasets. The results were uploaded and the evaluation reports were provided by the CBICA system. Two evaluation procedures were considered based on classification and regression. In the

Table 2. Segmentation results for the test dataset (provided by CBICA portal).

	Dice			Hausdorff (95%)		
	ET	WT	TC	ET	WT	TC
Mean	0.67	0.85	0.69	23.55	6.12	28.72
STD	0.29	0.13	0.26	79.41	7.75	83.75
Median	0.76	0.89	0.80	2.83	4.12	6.63
25 quantile	0.57	0.81	0.60	1.41	3.00	4.12
75 quantile	0.86	0.92	0.87	6.85	5.87	12.20

Table 3. Survival prediction results for training, validation and test dataset.

Dataset	Accuracy	MSE	Median SE	STD SE	Spearman rank
Training	0.638	54063.061	17689	131754.325	0.809
Validation	0.485	198749.091	25921	480095.255	0.334
Testing	0.411	235546.432	45796	745532.757	0.389

classification scheme, the data were provided in three groups, i.e. long (more than 15 months), short (less than 10 months) and mid-survival (between, 10 and 15 months). Then the results were evaluated using accuracy of classification. In the regression scheme, the pairwise mean square error (MSE), median SE, standard deviation of SE, and Spearman rank were used. The corresponding results for all dataset types are provided in Table 3. The classification accuracy values are 0.638, 0.485, and 0.411 for training, validation, and testing datasets, respectively. The corresponding Spearman rank values are 0.809, 0.334, and 0.389, respectively.

4   Conclusion

In this paper, a novel method was proposed in which the machine-learned features extracted using FCN were combined with hand-crafted texton features to encode global information and local dependencies into feature representation. The score map with pixel-wise predictions was used as a feature map which was learned from multimodal MICCAI-BRATS 2017 training dataset using the FCN. The machine-learned features, along with hand-crafted texton features were then applied to random forests to classify each MRI image voxel.

The proposed method was tested on two independent MICCAI-BRATS 2017 challenge datasets, i.e. validation and testing, by uploading the results on the CBICA IPP portal and getting the evaluation results from the provided system (blind test). The results of the FCN based method showed that the application of the RF classifier to multimodal MRI images using machine-learned features based on FCN and hand-crafted features based on textons provides promising segmentations. The Dice overlap measure for the whole tumor was obtained 0.86

and 0.85 for validation and testing dataset, with the Hausdorff distances of 7.61 and 6.21, respectively.

The patient overall survival prediction task was performed with a regression based RF. The classification accuracy and regression evaluation were reported. The classification accuracy values of 0.638, 0.485, and 0.411 were obtained for training, validation, and testing datasets, respectively.

References

1. Gordillo, N., Montseny, E., Sobrevilla, P.: State of the art survey on MRI brain tumor segmentation. Magn. Reson. Imaging **31**, 1426–1438 (2013)
2. Eisele, S.C., Wen, P.Y., Lee, E.Q.: Assessment of brain tumor response: RANO and its offspring. Curr. Treat. Options Oncol. **17**, 35 (2016)
3. Wen, P.Y., Macdonald, D.R., Reardon, D.A., Cloughesy, T.F., Sorensen, A.G., Galanis, E., DeGroot, J., Wick, W., Gilbert, M.R., Lassman, A.B., Tsien, C., Mikkelsen, T., Wong, E.T., Chamberlain, M.C., Stupp, R., Lamborn, K.R., Vogelbaum, M.A., van den Bent, M.J., Chang, S.M.: Updated response assessment criteria for high-grade gliomas: response assessment in neuro-oncology working group. JCO **28**, 1963–1972 (2010)
4. Niyazi, M., Brada, M., Chalmers, A.J., Combs, S.E., Erridge, S.C., Fiorentino, A., Grosu, A.L., Lagerwaard, F.J., Minniti, G., Mirimanoff, R.O., Ricardi, U., Short, S.C., Weber, D.C., Belka, C.: ESTRO-ACROP guideline "target delineation of glioblastomas". Radiother Oncol. **118**, 35–42 (2016)
5. Patel, M.R., Tse, V.: Diagnosis and staging of brain tumors. Semin. Roentgenol. **39**, 347–360 (2004)
6. Pinto, A., Pereira, S., Correia, H., Oliveira, J., Rasteiro, D.M.L.D., Silva, C.A.: Brain tumour segmentation based on extremely randomized forest with high-level features. In: 2015 37th Annual International Conference of the IEEE Engineering in Medicine and Biology Society (EMBC), pp. 3037–3040 (2015)
7. Gotz, M., Weber, C., Blocher, J., Stieltjes, B., Meinzer, H., Maier-Hein, K.: Extremely randomized trees based brain tumor segmentation. In: Proceeding of BRATS Challenge-MICCAI, pp. 006–011 (2014)
8. Menze, B.H., Jakab, A., Bauer, S., Kalpathy-Cramer, J., Farahani, K., Kirby, J., Burren, Y., Porz, N., Slotboom, J., Wiest, R., Lanczi, L., Gerstner, E., Weber, M.A., Arbel, T., Avants, B.B., Ayache, N., Buendia, P., Collins, D.L., Cordier, N., Corso, J.J., Criminisi, A., Das, T., Delingette, H., Demiralp, Ç., Durst, C.R., Dojat, M., Doyle, S., Festa, J., Forbes, F., Geremia, E., Glocker, B., Golland, P., Guo, X., Hamamci, A., Iftekharuddin, K.M., Jena, R., John, N.M., Konukoglu, E., Lashkari, D., Mariz, J.A., Meier, R., Pereira, S., Precup, D., Price, S.J., Raviv, T.R., Reza, S.M.S., Ryan, M., Sarikaya, D., Schwartz, L., Shin, H.C., Shotton, J., Silva, C.A., Sousa, N., Subbanna, N.K., Szekely, G., Taylor, T.J., Thomas, O.M., Tustison, N.J., Unal, G., Vasseur, F., Wintermark, M., Ye, D.H., Zhao, L., Zhao, B., Zikic, D., Prastawa, M., Reyes, M., Leemput, K.V.: The multimodal brain tumor image segmentation benchmark (BRATS). IEEE Trans. Med. Imaging **34**, 1993–2024 (2015)
9. Pereira, S., Pinto, A., Alves, V., Silva, C.A.: Brain tumor segmentation using convolutional neural networks in MRI images. IEEE Trans. Med. Imaging **35**, 1240–1251 (2016)

10. Havaei, M., Davy, A., Warde-Farley, D., Biard, A., Courville, A., Bengio, Y., Pal, C., Jodoin, P.M., Larochelle, H.: Brain tumor segmentation with deep neural networks. Med. Image Anal. **35**, 18–31 (2017)
11. Kamnitsas, K., Ledig, C., Newcombe, V.F.J., Simpson, J.P., Kane, A.D., Menon, D.K., Rueckert, D., Glocker, B.: Efficient multi-scale 3D CNN with fully connected CRF for accurate brain lesion segmentation. Med. Image Anal. **36**, 61–78 (2017)
12. Long, J., Shelhamer, E., Darrell, T.: Fully convolutional networks for semantic segmentation. Presented at the Proceedings of the IEEE Conference on Computer Vision and Pattern Recognition (2015)
13. Arbelaez, P., Maire, M., Fowlkes, C., Malik, J.: Contour detection and hierarchical image segmentation. IEEE Trans. Pattern Anal. Mach. Intell. **33**, 898–916 (2011)
14. Nyúl, L.G., Udupa, J.K., Zhang, X.: New variants of a method of MRI scale standardization. IEEE Trans. Med. Imaging **19**, 143–150 (2000)
15. Simonyan, K., Zisserman, A.: Very deep convolutional networks for large-scale image recognition. arXiv:1409.1556 [cs] (2014)
16. Liaw, A., Wiener, M.: Classification and regression by randomForest. R News **2**, 18–22 (2002)
17. Vedaldi, A., Lenc, K.: MatConvNet: convolutional neural networks for MATLAB. In: Proceedings of the 23rd ACM International Conference on Multimedia, pp. 689–692. ACM, New York (2015)
18. Jia, Y., Shelhamer, E., Donahue, J., Karayev, S., Long, J., Girshick, R., Guadarrama, S., Darrell, T.: Caffe: convolutional architecture for fast feature embedding. In: Proceedings of the 22nd ACM International Conference on Multimedia, pp. 675–678. ACM, New York (2014)
19. Taormina, R.: MATLAB_ExtraTrees - File Exchange - MATLAB Central. http://uk.mathworks.com/matlabcentral/fileexchange/47372-rtaormina-matlab-extratrees
20. Bakas, S., Akbari, H., Sotiras, A., Bilello, M., Rozycki, M., Rozycki, M., Freymann, J., Farahani, K., Davatzikos, C.: Advancing the cancer genome atlas glioma MRI collections with expert segmentation labels and radiomic features. Nature Sci. Data (2017, in Press)
21. Bakas, S., Akbari, H., Sotiras, A., Bilello, M., Rozycki, M., Kirby, J., Freymann, J., Farahani, K., Davatzikos, C.: Segmentation labels and radiomic features for the pre-operative scans of the TCGA-GBM collection. The Cancer Imaging Archive (2017). https://doi.org/10.7937/K9/TCIA.2017.KLXWJJ1Q
22. Bakas, S., Akbari, H., Sotiras, A., Bilello, M., Rozycki, M., Kirby, J., Freymann, J., Farahani, K., Davatzikos, C.: Segmentation labels and radiomic features for the pre-operative scans of the TCGA-LGG collection. The Cancer Imaging Archive (2017). https://doi.org/10.7937/K9/TCIA.2017.GJQ7R0EF
23. Penn Imaging - Home. https://ipp.cbica.upenn.edu/
24. MICCAI-BraTS 2017 Leaderboard. https://www.cbica.upenn.edu/BraTS17/

Automatic Segmentation and Overall Survival Prediction in Gliomas Using Fully Convolutional Neural Network and Texture Analysis

Varghese Alex⬤, Mohammed Safwan⬤, and Ganapathy Krishnamurthi$^{(\boxtimes)}$

Indian Institute of Technology Madras, Chennai, India
gankrish@iitm.ac.in

Abstract. In this paper, we use a Fully Convolutional Neural Network (FCNN) for the segmentation of gliomas from Magnetic Resonance Images (MRI). A fully automatic, voxel based classification was achieved by training a 23 layer deep FCNN on 2-D slices extracted from patient volumes. The network was trained on slices extracted from 130 patients and validated on 50 patients. For the task of survival prediction, texture and shape based features were extracted from T1 post contrast volume to train an Extremely Gradient Boosting (XGBoost) regressor. On the BraTS 2017 validation set, the proposed scheme achieved a mean whole tumor, tumor core and active dice score of 0.83, 0.69 and 0.69 respectively, while for the task of overall survival prediction, the proposed scheme achieved an accuracy of 52%.

Keywords: Deep learning · Gliomas · MRI · FCNN
Survival prediction · XGBoost

1 Introduction

In this work, we utilize a 23 layer deep FCNN for the task of segmentation of gliomas from MR scans. In the field of medical image analysis, U-net [1] is one of the oft used architecture. The network used in this work has a similar architecture as that of the aforementioned network. The network was trained on 2-D axial slices (240×240) extracted from FLAIR, T2, T1, and T1 post contrast sequences. The architecture of the network enables semantic segmentation, i.e., classification of all voxels in a slice in a single forward pass. Therefore, the inference time associated with FCNN based networks are lower when compared to traditional patch based CNNs.

Convolutional neural network and its variants being deterministic techniques often tend to mis-classify voxels as lesion in regions like brain stem, cerebellum where occurrence of gliomas is anatomically impossible. We utilize 3-D connected component analysis to discard components below a certain threshold for false positive reduction.

All authors have contributed equally.

Unlike previous BraTS competitions, apart from segmentation of gliomas from MR volumes, BraTS 2017 comprised of an additional challenge for predicting the prognosis associated with subjects with glioma using pre-operative scans. For the prognosis challenge, the overall survival rate was categorized into three groups namely short survivors (prognosis, $p < 10$ months), mid survivors (10 months $< p < 15$ months) and long survivors ($p > 15$ months). The segmentations produced by the FCNN were used as masks to extract first order texture and shape based features such as entropy, skewness, circularity of lesion constituent, etc. from the T1 post contrast sequence. The extracted features along with 5 additional features including the age of the subject were fed to an Extreme Gradient Boosting (XGBoost) regressor to predict the survival of the subject.

2   Materials and Methods

The proposed technique comprises of the following stages:

1. Pre-processing of data.
2. Segmentation of gliomas using FCNN.
3. Post-processing using 3-D connected components.
4. Feature extraction for survival rate prediction.
5. Prediction of survival rate using XGBoost regressor.

The flowchart of the proposed technique is given in Fig. 1.

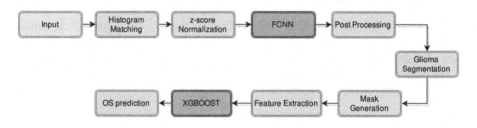

Fig. 1. Flow chart of the proposed technique

2.1   Data

The network was trained and validated on the BraTS 2017 training data [2–5]. The training data comprises of 210 HGG volumes and 75 LGG volumes collected from multiple centers. Each patient comprises of FLAIR, T2, T1, T1 post contrast and the associated ground truth labeled by experts. Each sequence was skull stripped and was re-sampled to 1 mm × 1 mm × 1 mm (isotropic resolution).

For the overall survival challenge, age and prognosis of the patient post treatment were supplied by the organizers. The training set for the challenge comprised of 163 High Grade Glioma patients of which 43 patients had survival rate between 10 and 15 months (mid survivors), while 65 patients had prognosis less than 10 months (short survivors) and 56 patients had prognosis greater than 15 months (long survivors).

2.2   Fully Convolutional Neural Network

A typical FCNN comprises of convolution operations, max pooling layers and transpose convolution layers. The absence of fully connected layers in FCNNs reduces the number of parameters in the network and in-turn accepts inputs of arbitrary sizes. The max pooling layer helps in reducing the spatial dimension of the feature maps in the deeper layers and also aids in capturing translational invariant features in the data.

The dimensionality of the feature maps are brought back to size of the input by either using up-sampling modules such as bilinear interpolation of feature maps or by utilizing transposed convolution. The use of transposed convolution in the networks makes the scaling procedure of feature maps a parameter to be learned during the training process. Concatenation of feature maps between different layers of the network enables the classifier in the network to make use of both low and complex level features for better classification results.

FCNNs have an inherent advantage of classifying all pixels in the image by using single forward pass of the image and thus makes FCNNs an ideal choice for semantic segmentation related tasks. Similar to traditional CNNs, the parameters of the network are learned by minimizing the cross entropy.

3   Preprocessing of Data

3.1   Histogram Matching

Multi center data and magnetic field inhomogeneities contribute to the non-uniform intensity variation in MR images. The voxel intensities of all volumes were standardized by matching histograms to an arbitrary chosen reference image from the training database (Fig. 2).

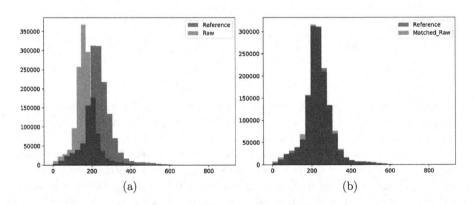

Fig. 2. Histogram Matching. (a) Raw histograms of reference volume and test volume. (b) Histograms of reference and test volume post histogram matching.

3.2 Z-score Normalization

The histogram matched volumes were normalized to have zero mean and unit variance using Eq. 1, where X is the MR volume, μ and σ are the mean and standard deviation of the volume and X_{norm} is the normalized volume.

$$X_{norm} = \frac{X - \mu}{\sigma} \tag{1}$$

4 Segmentation of Gliomas Using Proposed Network

4.1 Network Architecture

The architecture of the network is given in Fig. 3(a). Each **Conv** block in the network comprises of 2 sets of convolution by 3×3 kernels, batch normalization and a non linearity (ReLU) (Fig. 3(b)). The number of filters in each layer is given inside parenthesis in the **Conv** and **UpConv** block. The concatenation of feature maps is presented in the architecture as blue arrows.

The stride, kernel size and padding of the transposed convolution were chosen so as to produce feature maps of similar dimensions as that of the feature maps of the adjoining **Conv** block. This enables concatenation of feature maps without the need of cropping feature maps from the **Conv** block. The network makes use of convolution with 1×1 filters in the hindmost convolution block and results in generating the segmentation map.

4.2 Training

The network was trained and validated using slices extracted from 130 and 50 HGG patients respectively. The weights and biases in each layer was initialized using the Xavier initialization [6]. The network was trained for 30 epochs and the weights and biases were learned by minimizing the cross entropy loss function with ADAM [7] as the optimizer.

The imbalance amongst classes in the dataset were addressed by:

1. Training and validating the network using slices that comprises of atleast one pixel of lesion.
2. Performing data augmentation on the extracted slices which include horizontal flipping of the data.
3. Using a weighted cross entropy as the loss function for training the network. The weight assigned to the pixels corresponding to normal, necrotic, edema and enhancing were 1, 5, 2 and 3 respectively.

4.3 Testing

During the testing phase, axial slices from all 4 sequences were fed to the trained network to generate the segmentation mask/volumes.

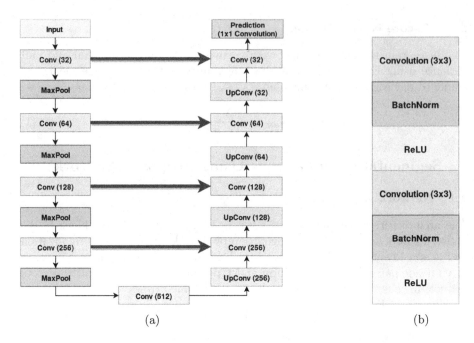

Fig. 3. Architecture of the proposed network. (a) Proposed FCNN. (b) Composition of the **Conv** block. (Color figure online)

4.4   Post Processing

CNN's being deterministic techniques tend to predict presence of lesion by learning various intensity based features. Henceforth, CNN based techniques tend to mis-classify voxels as lesions at certain locations such as cerebellum, brain stem etc. were occurrence of gliomas is physiologically impossible. The false positives in predictions made by the trained network were reduced by using 3-D connected component analysis. All components below a certain threshold (T = 2000) were discarded while the rest were retained.

4.5   Survival Prediction

The segmentation mask generated by the network was binarized to form 4 different volumes namely the whole lesion mask, edema mask, necrosis mask and enhancing mask (Fig. 4). A total of 19 first order texture based features (Table 1) and 16 shape based features of the lesion (Table 2), were extracted from T1 post contrast sequences using each of the aforementioned masks. The texture and shape based features were extracted from MR volume using a python package called Pyradiomics [8]. Apart from the extracted 76 texture based features and 64 shape based features, the age of subject, number of whole lesion voxels, number of voxels corresponding to edema, necrosis and enhancing tumor were used as additional features by the regressor to train and predict the prognosis.

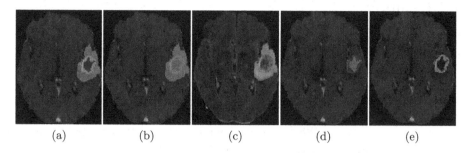

| (a) | (b) | (c) | (d) | (e) |

Fig. 4. Mask generated from segmentation maps. (a) Prediction made by the segmentation network. (b) whole lesion mask. (c) edema mask. (d) necrosis mask. (e) enhancing mask. In figure (a), green, red and yellow indicate edema, necrotic core and enhancing tumor in the lesion respectively. (Color figure online)

Table 1. First order texture features extracted from T1 post contrast sequence to predict overall survival of a subject.

First order texture based feature	
1. Volume	11. Range
2. Total Energy	12. Mean Absolute Deviation
3. Entropy	13. Robust Mean Absolute Deviation
4. Minimum	14. Root Mean Squared
5. 10th percentile	15. Standard Deviation
6. 90th percentile	16. Skewness
7. Maximum	17. Kurtosis
8. Mean	18. Variance
9. Median	19. Uniformity
10. Interquartile Range	

Table 2. Shape based features used to predict prognosis of a subject

Shape based feature	
1. Volume	9. Maximum 2D diameter (coronal)
2. Surface area	10. Maximum 2D diameter (sagital)
3. Surface area to Volume Ratio	11. Major Axis
4. Sphericity	12. Minor Axis
5. Spherical Disproportion	13. Least Axis
6. Compactness 1	14. Elongation
7. Maximum 3D diameter	15. Flatness
8. Maximum 2D diameter (axial)	16. Compactness 2

5   Results

The performance of network on the local test set (n = 40) [HGG-25, LGG-15] is given in Table 3. Figure 5 shows the performance of the network on 2 different patients from the local test data.

Table 3. Performance of the network on local test data (HGG = 25 and LGG = 15)

	Whole tumor	Tumor core	Active tumor
Mean	0.84	0.84	0.77
Std. Dev.	0.19	0.20	0.19
Median	0.90	0.90	0.83

The post processing technique helps in reducing false positives in the prediction and thereby improves the performance of the network. On the local test data, the improvement in performance was in the order of 2.44% for whole tumor dice score, 2.44% for tumor core and 1.31% for active tumor. Figure 6 shows an example were the proposed post processing technique aids in eliminating false positives.

For the task of overall survival rate prediction, it was observed that texture based and shape based features extracted from T1 post contrast sequence performed better than extracting features from other MR sequences. We observed that using features extracted all four sequences had negative impact on performance of the regressor. From a total of 145 features used to train the regressor, Fig. 7 illustrates the top 10 features along with their respective importance to accurately predict the survival of a subject. It was observed that the volume of the cuboid encompassing the lesion, lesion load, compactness of the lesion, maximum diameter (3-D) of the lesion and the minimum intensity of enhancing tumor in the lesion formed the top 5 features required by the regressor.

The performance of the network on the BraTS 2017 validation set is given in Table 4. It was observed that the network maintains similar whole tumor scores on the local test data and on the validation data. However, a dip in performance was observed in the tumor core and active tumor compartments. The performance of the proposed technique for survival prediction on the validation data is given in Table 5.

The trained network was tested on BraTS 2017 challenge data (n = 146). The performance of the proposed algorithm for the task of segmentation of gliomas from multi modal MR images is given in Table 6. For the overall survival prediction, the proposed technique achieved an accuracy of 47% and a Spearman coefficient of 0.41 (Table 7).

On comparing the performance of the network on the BraTS 2017 validation and test data, we observed a 4, 4 and 9% difference in whole tumor, tumor core and active tumor dice score. This deviation in performance is an indicator of the possibility of the network over-fitting on the training data due to presence of large number (approximately 65,00,000) parameters.

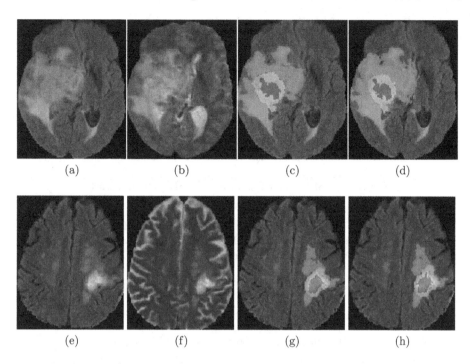

(a)   (b)   (c)   (d)

(e)   (f)   (g)   (h)

Fig. 5. Performance of the network on local test data. (a) FLAIR. (b) T2. (c) Prediction. (d) Ground Truth. In figures c, d, g and h, Green, Yellow and Red represent the Edema, Enhancing Tumor and Necrosis found in the lesion. (Color figure online)

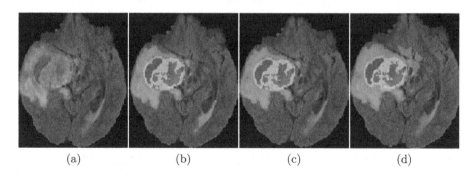

(a)   (b)   (c)   (d)

Fig. 6. Reduction of False positive using connected components. (a) FLAIR. (b) Raw Prediction. (c) Post Processed image. (d) Ground Truth. In figures b, c, d, Green, Yellow and Red represent the Edema, Enhancing Tumor and the Necrosis in the lesion. (Color figure online)

Table 4. Performance of FCNN on BraTS 2017 validation data for the task of segmentation of gliomas.

	Whole tumor	Tumor core	Active tumor
Mean	0.83	0.69	0.72
Std. Dev.	0.16	0.30	0.32
Median	0.90	0.83	0.85

Table 5. Survival prediction on BraTS 2017 validation data

Accuracy	MSE	Median SE	Std. SE	SpearmanR
0.52	221203.54	59035.10	505184.81	0.27

Table 6. Performance of the network on BraTS 2017 testing data (n = 146) for the task of segmentation of gliomas from MR images

	Whole tumor	Tumor core	Active tumor
Mean	0.79	0.65	0.63
Std. Dev.	0.20	0.33	0.33
Median	0.87	0.82	0.77

Table 7. Survival prediction on BraTS 2017 testing data (n = 95)

Accuracy	MSE	Median SE	Std. SE	SpearmanR
0.47	217755.772	39264.206	668015.465	0.411

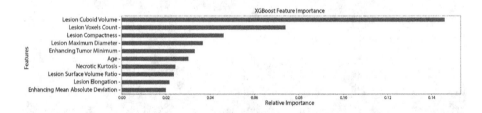

Fig. 7. Feature importance based on f-score for the task of overall survival prediction.

6   Conclusion

In this paper, we propose a fully automatic technique for segmentation of gliomas from MR volume and predict the prognosis of the patient using first order texture and shape based features. A fully convolutional neural network was utilized for task segmentation of gliomas into its various constituents namely edema, necrotic core and enhancing tumor. A 3-D connected component analysis was used to remove false positives in the predictions made by the network. The network produces good segmentation on the BraTS test data and achieved a whole tumor, tumor core and active tumor dice score of 0.79, 0.65 and 0.63 respectively. The segmentation produced by the network was used to generate 4 different masks namely whole tumor mask, edema mask, necrotic mask, enhancing mask. Using each mask 19 different first order texture features and 16 shaped based features were extracted from T1 post contrast sequence to train a XGBOOST regressor to predict the prognosis of a subject. On the BraTS 2017 validation data and test data, the regressor achieved an accuracy of 52% and 47% respectively.

References

1. Ronneberger, O., Fischer, P., Brox, T.: U-Net: convolutional networks for biomedical image segmentation. In: Navab, N., Hornegger, J., Wells, W.M., Frangi, A.F. (eds.) MICCAI 2015, Part III. LNCS, vol. 9351, pp. 234–241. Springer, Cham (2015). https://doi.org/10.1007/978-3-319-24574-4_28
2. Menze, B.H., Jakab, A., Bauer, S., Kalpathy-Cramer, J., Farahani, K., Kirby, J., Burren, Y., Porz, N., Slotboom, J., Wiest, R., Lanczi, L., Gerstner, E., Weber, M.A., Arbel, T., Avants, B.B., Ayache, N., Buendia, P., Collins, D.L., Cordier, N., Corso, J.J., Criminisi, A., Das, T., Delingette, H., Demiralp, Ç., Durst, C.R., Dojat, M., Doyle, S., Festa, J., Forbes, F., Geremia, E., Glocker, B., Golland, P., Guo, X., Hamamci, A., Iftekharuddin, K.M., Jena, R., John, N.M., Konukoglu, E., Lashkari, D., Mariz, J.A., Meier, R., Pereira, S., Precup, D., Price, S.J., Raviv, T.R., Reza, S.M., Ryan, M., Sarikaya, D., Schwartz, L., Shin, H.C., Shotton, J., Silva, C.A., Sousa, N., Subbanna, N.K., Szekely, G., Taylor, T.J., Thomas, O.M., Tustison, N.J., Unal, G., Vasseur, F., Wintermark, M., Ye, D.H., Zhao, L., Zhao, B., Zikic, D., Prastawa, M., Reyes, M., Van Leemput, K.: The multimodal brain tumor image segmentation benchmark (BRATS). IEEE Trans. Med. Imaging 34(10), 1993–2024 (2015)
3. Bakas, S., et al.: Advancing the Cancer Genome Atlas glioma MRI collections with expert segmentation labels and radiomic features, Nature Scientific Data (2017, in press)
4. Bakas, S., Akbari, H., Sotiras, A., Bilello, M., Rozycki, M., Kirby, J., Freymann, J., Farahani, K., Davatzikos, C.: Segmentation Labels and Radiomic Features for the Pre-operative Scans of the TCGA-GBM collection, The Cancer Imaging Archive (2017). https://doi.org/10.7937/K9/TCIA.2017.KLXWJJ1Q
5. Bakas, S., Akbari, H., Sotiras, A., Bilello, M., Rozycki, M., Kirby, J., Freymann, J., Farahani, K., Davatzikos, C.: Segmentation Labels and Radiomic Features for the Pre-operative Scans of the TCGA-LGG collection, The Cancer Imaging Archive (2017). https://doi.org/10.7937/K9/TCIA.2017.GJQ7R0EF
6. Glorot, X., et al.: Understanding the difficulty of training deep feedforward neural networks. In: International Conference on Artificial Intelligence and Statistics, pp. 249–256 (2010)
7. Kingma, D., Ba, J.: Adam: A method for stochastic optimization, 22 December 2014. arXiv preprint: arXiv:1412.6980
8. van Griethuysen, J.J.M., et al.: Computational Radiomics System to Decode the Radiographic Phenotype; Accepted Cancer Research (2017)

Multimodal Brain Tumor Segmentation Using 3D Convolutional Networks

R. G. Rodríguez Colmeiro[1,2,3](✉) 🆔, C. A. Verrastro[1,2], and T. Grosges[3] 🆔

[1] Universidad Tecnológica Nacional, Buenos Aires, Argentina
rrodriguezcolmeiro@frba.utn.edu.ar
[2] Comisión Nacional de Energía Atómica, Buenos Aires, Argentina
rodriguezcolmeiro@cae.cnea.gov.ar
[3] GAMMA3 (UTT-INRIA), ICD-UMR CNRS 6281,
University of Technology of Troyes, Troyes, France
ramiro_german.rodriguez_colmeiro@utt.fr

Abstract. Volume segmentation is one of the most time consuming and therefore error prone tasks in the field of medicine. The construction of a good segmentation requires cross-validation from highly trained professionals. In order to address this problem we propose the use of 3D deep convolutional networks (DCN). Using a 2 step procedure we first segment whole the tumor from a low resolution volume and then feed a second step which makes the fine tissue segmentation. The advantages of using 3D-DCN is that it extracts 3D features form all neighbouring voxels. In this method all parameters are self-learned during a single training procedure and its accuracy can improve by feeding new examples to the trained network. The training dice-loss value reach 0.85 and 0.9 for the coarse and fine segmentation networks respectively. The obtained validation and testing mean dice for the *Whole Tumor* class are 0.86 and 0.82 respectively.

Keywords: 3D convolutional network · Deep learning
Medical image segmentation · Volumetric semantic segmentation

1 Introduction

The manual segmentation of medical images is an exhausting and error prone procedure which is known to have a low inter-professional agreement [1]. The development of a fully automated and reliable segmentation procedure presents a great advance and is one of the most challenging tasks in the field of medical imaging.

In the last years the deep convolutional networks (DCN) have been applied to image recognition tasks pushing the state-of-the-art [2]. More recently DCN have been applied to semantic segmentation and classification in 2-D images and 3D volumes, achieving once more state-of-the-art performances in biomedical domains such as, cancer metastases cell segmentation [3], lung pattern and

© Springer International Publishing AG, part of Springer Nature 2018
A. Crimi et al. (Eds.): BrainLes 2017, LNCS 10670, pp. 226–240, 2018.
https://doi.org/10.1007/978-3-319-75238-9_20

nodule classification [4,5], alzheimer disease detection [6] and also anatomy classification [7]. Among the applied topologies, the U-Net [8], is one of the most successful topologies in the semantic segmentation of biomedical images. More recently novel DCN topologies that take into account the volumetric nature of biological data have been proposed, among those is the 3D U-Net [9] derived from the original U-Net which replaces all 2-D convolutional layers with 3D convolutional ones and was tested in the volumetric segmentation of Xenopus kidney. Other really close topology to the U-Net is the V-Net [10], which also uses 3D convolutional layers and was applied on prostate segmentation task. The success of this previous studies show the fitness of 3D DCN for segmentation in volumetric data.

The use of 3D convolutional operations allow them to generate volumetric filters that are able to capture features with a high correlation in volume. The tomographic images like PET, CT and MRI present such correlation between neighbouring voxels, since they are representations of physical volumes. It is then promising to apply a 3D DCN to the segmentation task on this type of images, where the objective segmentation is a volume rather than an accumulation of 2D images or textures.

The DCN were also applied in the task of brain tumor segmentation. In previous editions of the BRATS challenge DCM have been proposed as an end to end classification scheme. In BRATS 2013 a 2D DCN topology achieved state-of-the-art results [11] and a patch driven 2D DCN won the competition [12]. In BRATS 2013 and BRATS 2014 a 3D patch driven DCN was applied to the task [13] showing promising results in the use of 3D convolutions. In the previous edition, BRATS 2016, a fully convolutional residual neural network (FCR-NN) achieved state-of-the-art performance using an slice driven approach [14].

The BRATS challenge offers a unique opportunity to test this technique against other state-of-the-art automatic segmentation methods. The challenge dataset offers 285 training samples with FLAIR, T1, T1ce and T2 MRI studies. The data comes from several sources and is annotated by experts providing labels for three different tissues, enhancing tumor (ET), whole tumor (WT) and tumor core (TC) [15–17].

In the following sections we describe the implementation of a topology, similar to the 3D U-Net, for this particular task. Section two summarizes the proposed method, starting with the overall view of the segmentation process, then explains the data preprocessing, then the topology of the networks that compose the segmentation procedure (coarse and fine segmentation) followed by the training methods and data enhancement techniques applied. In section three the training and validation accuracy is presented along with other metrics. In section four the results are discussed and several segmented volumes are shown. Finally a conclusion is drawn and future work is proposed.

2 Methods

This section describes the operations of the automated segmentation process, starting with the description of the full segmentation process, followed by the input data and objective data treatment and construction of the coarse and fine segmentation networks and finally the training procedure.

2.1   Segmentation Process

The proposed segmentation procedure consists of a two-step process. Each step presents a 3D U-Net which realizes a different task. The complete process is described in Fig. 1. The process starts with the input preprocessing which normalizes the input volumes for the *Coarse Segmentation Network (CSN)*. Then the CSN is applied, its task is to detect the whole tumor within the brain volume. Using CSNs output, the input volume is masked and cropped. The resulting volume, presumably, consist of only tumorous tissue. The masked input is finally feed to the *Fine Segmentation Network (FSN)* which is responsible of generating the desired output labels; *enhancing tumor, tumor core* and *whole tumor*.

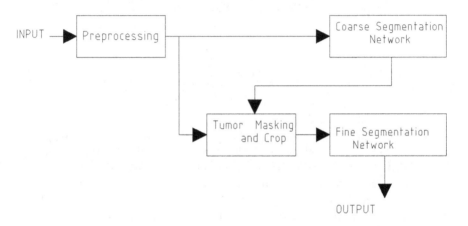

Fig. 1. Block diagram of the full segmentation process.

2.2   Data Preprocessing

The input data consist of a set of volumes acquired from four different MRI modalities; *FLAIR, T1, T1ce and T2*. This set of volumes are treated as different channels of a unique volume. Each volume of $240 \times 240 \times 155$ voxels is processed as a single volume with 4 channels, just as the RGB channels of a photograph. Voxels values are also normalized between 0 and 1 and coded with a 32 bit floating point number.

The objective data, which consists of a single volume with labels from 1 to 4, is decomposed into several objective volumes. For the CSN all labels are fussed in a single label, which represented the whole tumor, in the case of the FSN all labels with different values are converted to different objective volumes, creating

4 binary objective volumes. In each case two new objective classes are added, one is non-tumorous tissue and an other class is *background*, their function is to help the convergence of the CNN.

A problem-specific normalization is also applied to the dataset. BRATS17 training, testing and validation sets are composed from data of 6 different institutions, and therefore data distribution in the studies is not uniform. In Fig. 2 we see two histograms corresponding to the *FLAIR* modality of two studies from different institutions, there is a noticeable disalignment of gray and white matter distributions. To lower the impact of using data from several institutions, all volumes dynamic ranges of the same study type are rescaled and shifted before being normalized. The rescaling procedure is done by normalizing in height each histogram and matching it to a reference shape (in this work the reference was a hand-picked sample) using the correlation measure. The result of the normalization of histograms showed in Fig. 2 can be seen in Fig. 3.

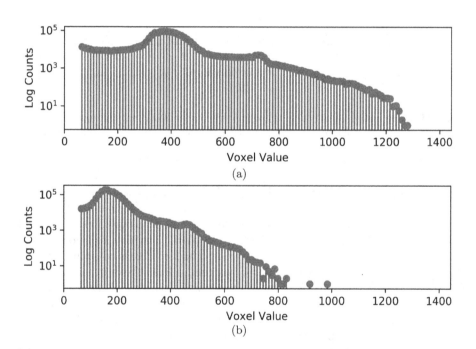

Fig. 2. FLAIR image voxel value histogram. Histogram (a) corresponds to sample volume *Brats17_2013_10_1*, histogram (b) corresponds to sample volume *Brats17_CBICA_ALN_1*.

2.3 Deep Convolutional Network

The topology selected for the segmentation task is a 3D version of the U-Net. Since all volumes are co-registered the proposed input is a 4 channel volume instead of 4 different intensity volumes, this allows the net to be more compact.

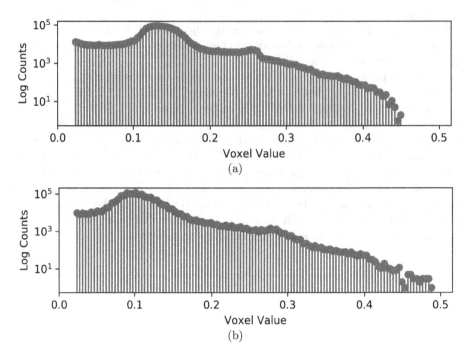

Fig. 3. FLAIR image voxel value histogram after normalization. Histogram (a) corresponds to sample volume *Brats17_2013_10_1*, histogram (b) corresponds to sample volume *Brats17_CBICA_ALN_1*.

The same structures are more or less visible in the different volume channels, therefore the same filters are applied to every volume channel, reducing the final amount of filters used by the convolutional layers. This topology can be explained following Fig. 4. The topology consists of two parts. The first one, follows the shape of a typical image recognition network, which performs convolutions over the input image then applies a non linear function (a ReLU layer in this case) and finally performs a pooling operation. Its function is to extract features from the input volume. In this implementation the common *max-pooling* operation was replaced by a 2-voxel stride convolution operation as suggested in [10]. This first part decomposes the input volume in lower resolution volumes, dividing by two its dimensions in each step but duplicating the number of channels. The second part starts at the lowest level (referred as base level) and is where the semantic segmentation starts. In the base level instead of a 2-voxel stride convolution the network applies a 2-voxel stride up-convolution, which duplicates the image size and infers the values of the new voxels. The following levels of this part not only receive information of the lower levels but also high-detailed information which is broadcast from the levels of first part of the network which operate at their own precision (volume size) making possible detail rich segmentation of the input volume (see Fig. 4). The broadcast detail rich volume is concatenated at channel level with the volume coming from the lower level, i.e. if the volume at the current level has a size of $64 \times 64 \times 16$ voxels and 16 channels, then the concatenated volume will have a size of $64 \times 64 \times 16$ voxels and 32 channels. The final segmentation is done by a convolutional layer followed by a *softmax* operation among the objective classes.

Both networks are constructed with the same number of levels, 4 levels in the downward path, 4 levels in the upward path and a base level. Each level consists of a convolution part, for feature extraction and a down or up sampling procedure. The feature extraction part consists of two layers with a 3D convolution followed by a ReLU layer. The network input has four channels (one per input volume type) which is decomposed into 8 channels in the first level, and ends in 64 channels at the base level. The convolutional filters had a size of $3 \times 3 \times 3$ voxels and the final segmentation filters had a size of $2 \times 2 \times 2$ voxels.

In the following sub-sections some particularities of each net are explained.

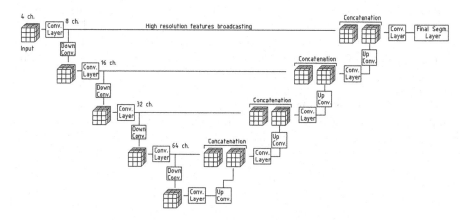

Fig. 4. 3D U-Net topology.

Coarse Segmentation Network. This network takes as input a volume of size $128 \times 128 \times 64$ voxels with 4 channels, this volume is generated by down-sampling the input. Since coarse segmentation does not produce the final segmentation we are able to reduce its resolution in order to reduce the memory requirements of the network and allow a faster processing. The output of the network is a binary mask volume of size $128 \times 128 \times 64$ voxels.

Fine Segmentation Network. This network receives a 4 channel $96 \times 96 \times 96$ voxel volume at original resolution. When the network is in production, its input is built using the output of the CSN and the original input. The output of the CSN is up-sampled to the original volume resolution ($240 \times 240 \times 155$ voxels) and then used as a binary mask for the original input. Once the input volume is masked it is cropped to a $96 \times 96 \times 96$ voxel volume aligned to the tumor center of mass. If the tumor is larger than the *field of view (FOV)* of the FSM, it is divided into as many $96 \times 96 \times 96$ cubes are needed to describe it. These cubes are partially overlapped. After the FSN is applied, the output on the overlapped areas is averaged and rounded to the most probable class.

When the network is being trained, instead of the CSN output, the ground truth is used to mask the volume.

2.4   Training

As objective function the dice loss running over all outputs was chosen. The objective function can be seen in Eq. 1, where N_c is the number of objective classes, N_v the number of voxels in the volume, $g_{i,c}$ are the voxels of the ground truth and $p_{i,c}$ the values of the softmaxed output of the network. The dice loss metric based on the dice coefficient. This metric was adapted from [10] in order to be used in multi-class segmentation problems. The dice loss ranges from 0 to 1. It produces it maximum value when all voxels of the ground truth $(g_{i,c})$ have the same value as the softmaxed output voxels $(p_{i,c})$. Since the output is softmaxed the denominator of Eq. 1 is always larger than its numerator except when $g_{i,c}$ and $p_{i,c}$ are identical. In the case of a multi-class problem $(N_c > 1)$ the final value is divided by the number of classes.

The training of both networks are trained separately using the ADAM optimizer [18] and with learning rate decay following $\alpha = \alpha_{ini}/\sqrt{n_{step}}$, where n_{step} is the step number. Batch normalization [19] is applied at each convolutional layer.

$$D = \frac{1}{N_c} \sum_{c=0}^{N_c} \frac{2 \sum_i^{N_v} p_{i,c} g_{i,c}}{\sum_i^{N_v} p_{i,c}^2 + \sum_i^{N_v} g_{i,c}^2} \tag{1}$$

2.5   Data Enhancement

Since the training of the 3D DCN requires thousands of samples to converge, new input samples are generated from the original data. This new samples are created by applying two transformations: rotation and elastic deformation.

Both transformations are performed by operating on a uniform mesh which extends over the whole input volume. The first operation applied to it is a random rotation in an interval of $-\pi/4$ to $\pi/4$ in the direction of a random versor. Then the deformation procedure is applied to the rotated mesh. The deformation consists of a sinusoidal distortion in every axis, this sinusoidal distortion has a random period between 10 and 25 voxel size and a peak between 2 and 4 voxel size.

After the fully transformed mesh is created, it is used to remap the coordinates of all voxels in the input volumes and segmentation labels to their new position in the transformed sample. The transformed sample mapping is created using a trilinear interpolation.

3 Results

This section summarises the results of the train and validation accuracy. Train accuracy is given in terms of Eq. 1. Validation and Test values are given according to BRATS17 challenge metrics.

The CSN was trained with 13000 examples achieving a dice loss of $D_c = 0.85$ while the FSN was trained with 16000 examples and achieved a dice loss over $D_f = 0.95$. The number of examples represent the amount of transformed volumes that each network required to converge.

The Tables 1 and 2 show the results of the segmentation performed using the BRATS17 metrics. Figure 5 shows the box plots of validation and test dice metrics.

Table 1. BRATS17 validation results

	Dice			Sensitivity			Specificity			Hausdorff95		
	ET	WT	TC	ET	WT	TC	ET	WT	TC	ET	WT	TC
Mean	0.66	0.86	0.69	0.76	0.87	0.73	0.997	0.993	0.996	11.1	9.28	14.0
Median	0.80	0.89	0.76	0.86	0.91	0.85	0.998	0.994	0.997	3.74	3.87	8.6

Table 2. BRATS17 test results

	Dice			Hausdorff95		
	ET	WT	TC	ET	WT	TC
Mean	0.60	0.82	0.67	56.4	11.34	30.66
Median	0.72	0.88	0.80	3.53	4.12	7.17

The time to process a single volume depends on the tumor size. A whole volume can be processed in 20 s if the tumor fit in the FOV of the FSN. If the tumor is larger than the FOV of the FSN, then the process takes between 35 and 70 s due to the multiple calls to the FSN.

4 Discussion

The results show a good generalization of the network and avoiding overfitting. It can be seen that the train, validation and test results, shown in Tables 1 and 2, agree overall. The final training dice value of the CSN largely agrees with the *Whole Tummor* dice coefficient for the validation and testing datasets, showing that the network is not overfitting on the training samples. This also shows that the data enhancement procedure was able to enlarge the initial dataset to thousands examples despite the basic transformations applied to the original dataset.

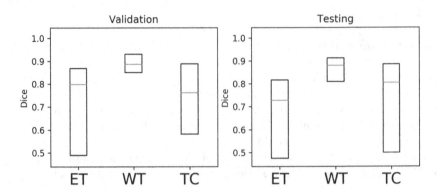

Fig. 5. Validation and test dataset boxplots of dice metric for the three target classes, constructed using Median, 25-quantile and 75-quantile.

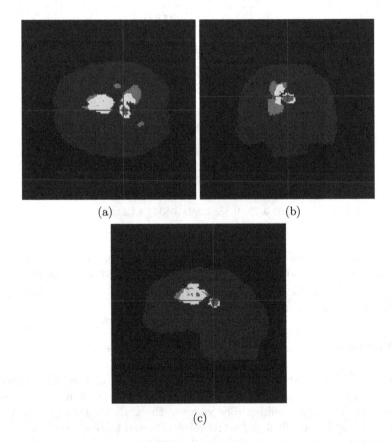

Fig. 6. Transverse (a), Coronal (b), Sagital (c) views of sample BRATS_2013_12_1 segmentation, Training set. Edema is represented in teal color, enhancing core regions in yellow and tumor core in red. (Color figure online)

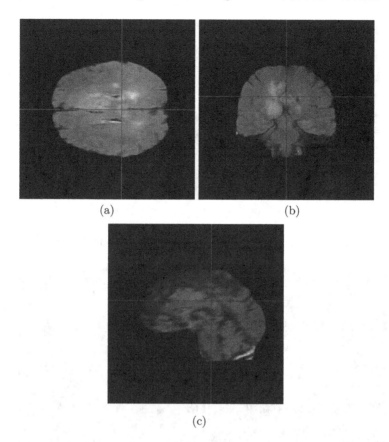

(a)   (b)

(c)

Fig. 7. Transverse (a), Coronal (b), Sagital (c) views of sample BRATS_2013_12_1 FLAIR.

The time needed process a single sample is little more than a minute in tumors that greatly surpass the FOV of the FSN and below 20 s for most examples in the datasets. After being trained, the network needs only 2.2 GB of GPU memory to be used in production, which is conventionally found in consume gaming GPUs.

An example of the segmentation is shown in Fig. 6. It can be seen that all classes are separated. The teal coloured areas represents the edema, yellow areas are the enhancing core regions and finally tumor core is shown in red. The FLAIR modality slices corresponding to the segmentation can be seen in Fig. 7.

In Fig. 8 the resulting segmentation is compared to the ground truth data, it can be seen that the sharp edges of the objective volume are met and also some small and isolated areas are also segmented showing that the process is able to create volumes with complex borders.

This behaviour is also observed on Fig. 9 which shows the segmentation on a sample of the validation set. The segmented structures are complex and match the structures seen in the MRI slices showed in Fig. 10, showing that

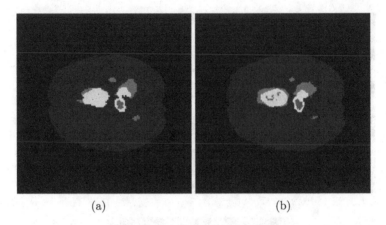

(a)   (b)

Fig. 8. Generated segmentation (a) and ground truth (b) of sample BRATS_2013_12_1.

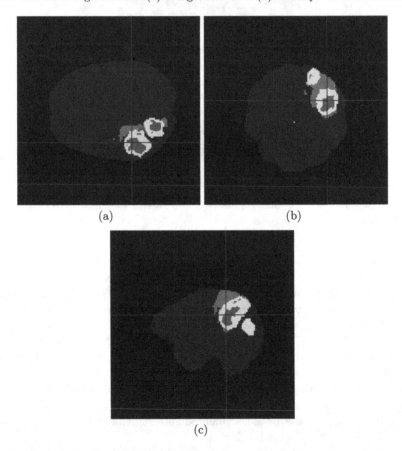

(a)   (b)

(c)

Fig. 9. Transverse (a), Coronal (b), Sagital (c) views of sample CBICA_APM_1 segmentation. Edema is represented in teal color, enhancing core regions in yellow and tumor core in red. (Color figure online)

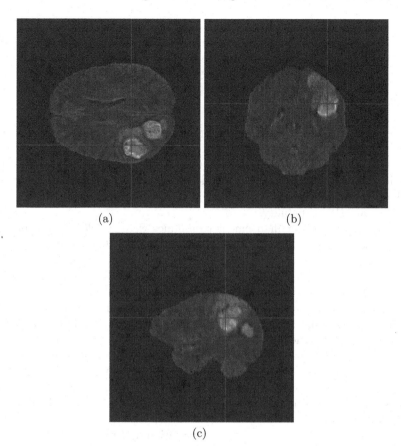

Fig. 10. Transverse (a), Coronal (b), Sagital (c) views of sample CBICA_APM_1 FLAIR.

no overfitting was done during training. The method was also able to separate multiple regions, it can be seen that there are two separated tumor core regions correctly detected by the network as distinct structures. The ground truth for this sample is not available at the time of writing this report.

As an explanation to the lower precision during the fine segmentation tasks in the validation phase against the training error, we presume that it can be cause by the lower precision of the CSN (due to the lower volumes) to the FSN during production phase. Since the FSN expects a tumor that is more or less centred in its FOV, a bad coarse segmentation can lead to a wrong calculation of the tumor center of mass and hence generate a non centred input to the FSN. This misalignement and tumor tissue occlusions form an imperfect coarse tumor masking may result in lower dice values in the validation phase of the FSN.

The Fig. 5 shows that the distribution of the segmentation accuracy is far from normal, this may be due to the normalization process which may be failing in some of the samples. Nevertheless the median values are rather high.

5 Conclusions

The proposed automatic segmentation procedure based on a 3D U-Net topology has shown to be effective when applied to the BRATS17 dataset. The networks were able to perform segmentation without any other information than the given examples and no specific knowledge of the problem was used to create the topology. The trained network is simple and fast, it can be run in desktop PC with relatively low GPU capability.

Even when the data enhancement techniques were simple and not problem specific they were capable of produce new valid data. Generating a problem specific data enhancement technique which focuses on the transformation of the tumor areas might speed up the process and reduce the final training error.

The data normalization probed to be one of the critical points in the network training. One of the major difficulties in medical imaging is the relatively low number of images annotated by experts, being able to combine information from different scanners is crucial if deep learning techniques are to be used.

Probably one of the most promising paths to improve the segmentation accuracy resides in the field of data enhancement and representation. This work has shown that with a more or less standard topology, the network achieved good results when it was trained using a few hundred original samples and only simple transformations were applied.

Better and problem specific data representation techniques are expected to be applied. By using a re-meshing technique on the data it is expected to obtain representations which focus on the tumor structures and thus enhance the expressive power of the data for the tumor segmentation task. The description of MRI volumes with meshing techniques was already proposed in [20] but such method required user-defined initial seeds. Using a modified version of the re-meshing technique presented in [21] it is expected to obtain such meshes in an unsupervised manner. This additional information generated by the mesh representation can be used by the network by means of a node density map or by a filtered tumor map in the case of the coarse segmentation task and to achieve sub-pixel accuracy on the fine segmentation task by remapping the input.

Further refinement of the network topology is also expected to be done, in order to further lower its complexity and explore the effects of including the masking and fine segmentation process as additional layers.

References

1. Foster, B., Bagci, U., Mansoor, A., Xu, Z., Mollura, D.J.: A review on segmentation of positron emission tomography images. Comput. Biol. Med. **50**, 76–96 (2014)
2. Schmidhuber, J.: Deep learning in neural networks: an overview. Neural Netw. **61**, 85–117 (2015)
3. Liu, Y., Gadepalli, K., Norouzi, M., Dahl, G.E., Kohlberger, T., Boyko, A., Venu-gopalan, S., Timofeev, A., Nelson, P.Q., Corrado, G.S., et al.: Detecting cancer metastases on gigapixel pathology images (2017). arXiv preprint: arXiv:1703.02442
4. Anthimopoulos, M., Christodoulidis, S., Ebner, L., Christe, A., Mougiakakou, S.: Lung pattern classification for interstitial lung diseases using a deep convolutional neural network. IEEE Trans. Med. Imaging **35**(5), 1207–1216 (2016)
5. Kim, B.-C., Sung, Y.S., Suk, H.-I.: Deep feature learning for pulmonary nodule classification in a lung CT. In: 2016 4th International Winter Conference on Brain-Computer Interface (BCI), pp. 1–3. IEEE (2016)
6. Gao, X.W., Hui, R.: A deep learning based approach to classification of CT brain images (2016)
7. Roth, H.R., Lee, C.T., Shin, H.-C., Seff, A., Kim, L., Yao, J., Lu, L., Summers, R.M.: Anatomy-specific classification of medical images using deep convolutional nets. In: 2015 IEEE 12th International Symposium on Biomedical Imaging (ISBI), pp. 101–104. IEEE (2015)
8. Ronneberger, O., Fischer, P., Brox, T.: U-Net: convolutional networks for biomed-ical image segmentation. In: Navab, N., Hornegger, J., Wells, W.M., Frangi, A.F. (eds.) MICCAI 2015, Part III. LNCS, vol. 9351, pp. 234–241. Springer, Cham (2015). https://doi.org/10.1007/978-3-319-24574-4_28
9. Çiçek, Ö., Abdulkadir, A., Lienkamp, S.S., Brox, T., Ronneberger, O.: 3D U-Net: learning dense volumetric segmentation from sparse annotation. In: Ourselin, S., Joskowicz, L., Sabuncu, M.R., Unal, G., Wells, W. (eds.) MICCAI 2016, Part II. LNCS, vol. 9901, pp. 424–432. Springer, Cham (2016). https://doi.org/10.1007/978-3-319-46723-8_49
10. Milletari, F., Navab, N., Ahmadi, S.-A.: V-net: fully convolutional neural networks for volumetric medical image segmentation. In: 2016 Fourth International Confer-ence on 3D Vision (3DV), pp. 565–571. IEEE (2016)
11. Havaei, M., Davy, A., Warde-Farley, D., Biard, A., Courville, A., Bengio, Y., Pal, C., Jodoin, P.-M., Larochelle, H.: Brain tumor segmentation with deep neural networks. Med. Image Anal. **35**, 18–31 (2017)
12. Pereira, S., Pinto, A., Alves, V., Silva, C.A.: Brain tumor segmentation using convolutional neural networks in MRI images. IEEE Trans. Med. Imaging **35**(5), 1240–1251 (2016)
13. Zikic, D., Ioannou, Y., Brown, M., Criminisi, A.: Segmentation of brain tumor tissues with convolutional neural networks. In: Proceedings MICCAI-BRATS, pp. 36–39 (2014)
14. Chang, P.D.: Fully convolutional deep residual neural networks for brain tumor segmentation. In: Crimi, A., Menze, B., Maier, O., Reyes, M., Winzeck, S., Han-dels, H. (eds.) Brainlesion: Glioma, Multiple Sclerosis, Stroke and Traumatic Brain Injuries. LNCS, vol. 10154, pp. 108–118. Springer, Cham (2016). https://doi.org/10.1007/978-3-319-55524-9_11
15. Bakas, S., Akbari, H., Sotiras, A., Bilello, M., Rozycki, M., Kirby, J.S., Freymann, J.B., Farahani, K., Davatzikos, C.: Advancing the cancer genome atlas glioma MRI collections with expert segmentation labels and radiomic features. Nat. Sci. Data **4**, 170117 (2017)

16. Bakas, S., Sotiras, A., Bilello, M., Rozycki, M., Kirby, J.S., Freymann, J.B., Farahani, K., Davatzikos, C.: Segmentation labels and radiomic features for the preoperative scans of the TCGA-GBM collection. Nat. Sci. Data (2017). https://doi.org/10.7937/K9/TCIA.2017.KLXWJJ1Q

17. Bakas, S., Akbari, H., Sotiras, A., Bilello, M., Rozycki, M., Kirby, J.S., Freymann, J.B., Farahani, K., Davatzikos, C.: Segmentation labels and radiomic features for the pre-operative scans of the TCGA-LGG collection. Nat. Sci. Data (2017). https://doi.org/10.7937/K9/TCIA.2017.GJQ7R0EF

18. Kingma, D., Ba, J.: Adam: A method for stochastic optimization (2014). arXiv preprint: arXiv:1412.6980

19. Ioffe, S., Szegedy, C.: Batch normalization: Accelerating deep network training by reducing internal covariate shift (2015). arXiv preprint: arXiv:1502.03167

20. del Fresno, M., Vénere, M., Clausse, A.: A combined region growing and deformable model method for extraction of closed surfaces in 3D CT and MRI scans. Comput. Med. Imaging Graph. 33(5), 369–376 (2009)

21. Grosges, T., Borouchaki, H., Barchiési, D.: New adaptive mesh development for accurate near-field enhancement computation. J. Microsc. 229(2), 293–301 (2008)

A Conditional Adversarial Network for Semantic Segmentation of Brain Tumor

Mina Rezaei$^{(\boxtimes)}$ ⓘ, Konstantin Harmuth, Willi Gierke, Thomas Kellermeier, Martin Fischer, Haojin Yang, and Christoph Meinel

Hasso-Plattner Institute for Digital Engineering,
Prof.-Dr.-Helmert-Strae 2-3, 14482 Potsdam, Germany
{mina.rezaei,haojin.yang,christoph.meinel}@hpi.de,
{konstantin.harmuth,willi.gierke,thomas.kellermeier,
martin.fischer}@student.hpi.uni-potsdam.de

Abstract. Automated brain lesion detection is an important and very challenging clinical diagnostic task, due to the lesions'different sizes, shapes, contrasts, and locations. Recently deep learning has shown promising progresses in many application fields, thereby motivating us to apply this technique for such an important problem. In this paper, we propose an automatic end-to-end trainable architecture for heterogeneous brain tumor segmentation through adversarial training for the BraTS-2017 challenge. Inspired by classical generative adversarial network, the proposed network has two components: the "Discriminator" and the "Generator". We use a patient-wise fully convolutional neural networks (FCNs) as the segmentor network to generate segmentation label maps. The discriminator network is patient-wise fully convolutional neural networks (FCNs) with L1 loss that discriminates segmentation maps coming from the ground truth or from the segmentor network. We propose an end-to-end trainable CNNs for survival day prediction based on deep learning techniques. The experimental results demonstrate the ability of the propose approaches for both tasks of BraTS-2017 challenge. Our patient-wise cGAN achieved competitive results in the BraTS-2017 challenges.

Keywords: Conditional generative adversarial network
Brain tumor semantic segmentation · Survival day prediction

1 Introduction

Medical imaging plays an important role in disease diagnosis, treatment planning and clinical monitoring. The diverse magnetic resonance imaging (MRI) acquisition method regarding their settings (e.g. echo time, repetition time) and geometry (2D vs. 3D), as well as the difference in hardware (e.g. field strength, gradient performance) can yield variation in the appearance of the tumor, making automated segmentation challenging [1].

An accurate brain lesion segmentation algorithm based on multi-modal MR images might be able to improve the prediction accuracy and efficiency for better treatment planning and monitoring of the disease progress. As mentioned

© Springer International Publishing AG, part of Springer Nature 2018
A. Crimi et al. (Eds.): BrainLes 2017, LNCS 10670, pp. 241–252, 2018.
https://doi.org/10.1007/978-3-319-75238-9_21

by Menze et al. [2], in the last few decades the number of clinical studies for automatic brain lesion detection has grown significantly.

Over the last three years, Generative Adversarial Networks (GANs) [3] have received increased attention in different computer vision applications such as classification [4,5], object detection [6,7], video prediction [8–10], image segmentation [11], and medical image segmentation [12]. In this paper, we address the two tasks from the BraTS-2017 [2,13–15] challenge. Semantic segmentation is the task of classifying parts of images together that belong to the same object class. Inspired by the power of GANs [11,12], we designed an end-to-end trainable adversarial network to perform brain High and Low Grade Glioma (HGG/LGG) tumor segmentation.

Our proposed model for segmentation takes multi-modal images as input in arbitrary sizes and the output semantic segmented mask. To this end, we consider patient-wise FCNs with skip connection in layers like "U-Net" [16] as a segmentor network. The patient-wise discriminator comprises FCNs with L2 loss like "Markovian GAN" [17].

For the second task of BraTS-2017 [2,13–15], we design an end-to-end trainable FCNs architecture on heterogeneous data (clinical data and multi-modal images) that enables predicting the survival day. The architecture has a parallel fully convolutional layer, which is responsible for learn multi-modal patient images with the segmented mask, while simultaneously the second pathway learns clinical data representation. Both paths are concatenated, and the extracted features pass to the fully convolutional network to learn the survival rate. A detailed evaluation of the parameters' variations and network architecture is provided. The contribution of this work can be summarized as follows:

- We propose a robust solution for brain tumor segmentation by patient-wise conditional GANs. We achieved promising results on two kinds of brain tumor segmentation. The achieved accuracy in terms of Dice is 0.80 and it is 8.7 for the Hausdorff-95 in the whole tumor region at test data reported by the BraTS-2017 organizer.
- We propose an automatic and trainable heterogeneous deep learning architecture for survival day prediction based on clinical data and multi-modal MR images.

The rest of the paper is organized as follows: Sect. 2 describes the proposed method for semantic segmentation and survival day prediction, Sect. 3 presents the details of experiments and results. Section 4 concludes the paper and gives an outlook on future work.

2   Methodology

In this chapter, we describe the patient-wise cGAN approach to the semantic segmentation of brain tumor and our solution for the survival day prediction. The core techniques applied in our approach are depicted as well.

Machine learning approaches can be divided into two categories of generative and discriminative modal. The basic idea of GAN [3] is to train the discriminator model (D) and the generator model (G) simultaneously in a single network via adversarial loss. According to GAN theory, the discriminator network tries to identify whether a certain input is sourced from the reference distribution, or has been generated by the generator network. In the conditional version of GANs, both G and D are conditioned on specific data y. The training procedure in the generator (G) uses the pixel's label of certain multi-modal images, while D tries to distinguish if this certain boundary regions comes from reference distribution or generative network.

In order to incorporate more classes in this output while maintaining the GAN spirit of distinguishing distribution class instead of one example class, we could add additional input sources. As suggested by Goodfellow et al. [3], one can consider the cGAN models with multi-class labels as:

1. GAN model with class-conditional models which makes the input label rather than the output. We ask GAN to generate specific classes [18].
2. GAN model with N different output classes which the network trains by N different "real" and no "fake" classes [19].
3. GAN models with N + 1 different output classes which the network trains by N different "real" and an additional "fake" class. This type works well for semi-supervised learning when combined with feature matching GANs, e.g. [20].

Therefore, our proposed approach lies in the second category as we consider for each multi-modality image three segmentation class conditions. Figure 1 describes the proposed approach to the brain tumor segmentation. In continue we describe in detail the techniques of pixel label classes for prediction in Sect. 2.2 and for survival day prediction in Sect. 2.3.

2.1 Patient Wise Batch Normalization

The main purpose of batch normalization [21,22] is to improve the optimization of the model. Batch normalization 3 involves re-parametrizing the model with the mean Eq. (1) and variance Eq. (2) of each feature.

We introduce patient-wise batch normalization where the mean and variance are computed on specific patient from the same acquisition plane (Saggital, Cronal, Axial) and from all available image modalities (t1,t1ce,Flair,t2). For example, for the mini-batch with the size of 128, all images selected from the same patient and the same acquisition plane on four available modalities. In other words, we restricted the mini-batch normalization [21] by setting conditions on the patient and acquisition planes for the normalization process. Patient-wise batch normalization Eq. (3) helps in re-parametrizing the model for faster learning and higher overall accuracy.

$$Mean : \mu_x \leftarrow \frac{1}{m}\sum_{i=1}^{n} x_i \tag{1}$$

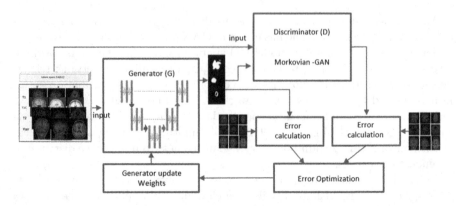

Fig. 1. The propose architecture for brain tumor semantic segmentation with two components of segmentor and discriminator

$$Variance : \sigma_x^2 \leftarrow \frac{1}{m} \sum_{i=1}^{n} (x_i - \mu_x)^2 \qquad (2)$$

$$Normalize : \hat{x}_i \leftarrow \frac{x_i - \mu_x}{\sqrt[2]{\sigma_x^2 + \varepsilon}} \qquad (3)$$

2.2   Brain Tumor Semantic Segmentation Architecture

As illustrated in Fig. 1, the proposed approach has two components a generator network and a discriminator network.

The generator is a fully convolutional encoder-decoder network with skip connection in the layer that generates a probability label map from input multi-modal images. The discriminator network takes original mask annotated by expert (ground truth) and predicted mask from segmentor network. Our discriminator is a binary classifier. The both network simultaneously train via adversarial loss Eq. (4) with the well know strategy, min-max two-player game.

$$L_{GAN}(G, D) = E_y \, pdata(y)[logD(y)] + E_x \, pdata(x), z \, p_z(z)[log1 - D(x, z)] \quad (4)$$

We choose the auto-encoder with skip connection like "U-Net" architecture [16] as generator because most of the deep learning approaches are patchwise learning models, that ignore the contextual information within the whole image region. Like the winner of BraTS-2016 [23], we come over this problem by leveraging global-based CNN methods (e.g. Seg-Net, Encoder-Decoder, and FCN) and incorporating multi-modal of MRI data. The discriminative network extracted hierarchical features from multi-layers of FCNs and used to compute the l1 loss.

We confirmed the suggested solution by "Markovian GAN" [24] that l1 loss can capture long and short range spatial relations between pixels. Then two models are trained simultaneously through back propagation. The training of the generator and the discriminator is like playing a min-max game: while G's is goal to minimize the loss, D tries to maximize it. This training process makes both networks more and more powerful. The generator will be able to produce predicted label maps very close to the ground truth as labeled by medical expert.

2.3   Survival Day Prediction Architecture

Figure 2 describes our solution for survival day prediction. This task is more challenging since the learning procedure is based on heterogeneous data. To this end, we propose a two-path-way architecture that takes multi-modal images, while another processes the clinical data from same patient.

The first pathway has nine convolutional layers with dropout and l2-norm pooling layers in between with the fully connected layer before the concatenation. At the same time, the clinical data (text data) enter the process on two convolutional and one dropout layers. The extracted features from each path-way, are concatenated in the next step to share the extracted features. As Fig. 2 shows, the shared features passed to the two fully connected layers to learn the survival day. We do mini-batch normalization patient-wise in each epoch to accelerate the training process and improve accuracy. To prevent over-fitting, we generate augmented images through horizontal and vertical flipping and re-scaling, and also use the dropout layer. Our loss function is a mean squared error. We map the clinical data (ages and survival days) into float[0,1].

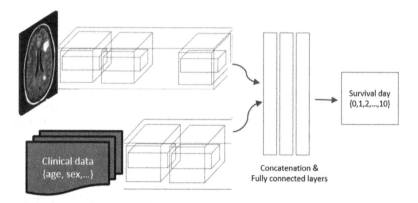

Fig. 2. The propose architecture for the task of survival day prediction. We designed an end-to-end trainable two pathway network to process parallel a clinical data and related images. The extracted features from each way concatenated later to flatten layer and mean squared error is the final loss function.

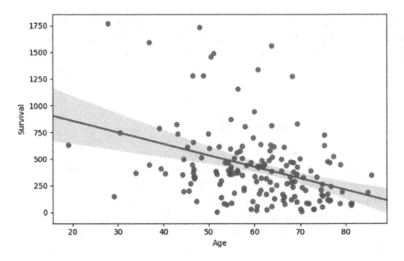

Fig. 3. Clinical data distribution from training set of BraTS-2017, second task of challenge which shows survival day versus age.

3   Experiment and Results

In the experiment, we applied real patient data with two types of brain tumors provided by the BraTS-2017 challenge [2,13–15]. The challenge is organized in two sections heterogeneous brain tumor segmentation, and overall survival day prediction.

3.1   Dataset

The BraTS-2017 benchmark [2,13–15] prepared the data in High and Low Grade Glioma (HGG/LGG) tumors collected from multiple centers. All images were aligned to the same anatomical template and interpolated to 1-mm, 3-voxel resolution. The training dataset for the task of segmentation, consisted of 220 HGG and 108 LGG MRI images, for which each patient's T1, T1contrast, T2, FLAIR, and ground truth labeled by medical experts were provided. For the task of survival day prediction, the training set for the challenge comprised of 163 HGG patients. As Fig. 3 shows, 41 of these patients had prognosis less than 180 days, 84 had a survival rate between 180 and 540 days, and 38 patients had prognosis more than 540 days.

3.2   Preprocessing

In the first of pre-processing, we prepared 2D slices in sagittal, axial, and coronal views. We applied a bias field correction on the MR images to correct the intensity non-uniformity in MR images by using N4ITK [25]. In the next step of pre-processing we applied histogram matching normalization [26].

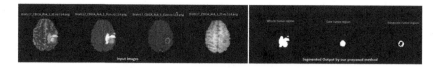

Fig. 4. Examples of segmentation results from BraTS-2017 Validation Data [2, 13–15] which our propose method takes four image modalities from same plane and the output is three predicted binary masks.

3.3 Training, Validation, and Test

The proposed approach is trained on all training data [2, 13–15] released by the BraTS-2017 benchmark which is 328 MR images. We used all provided image-modalities from the axes of x, y, and z for training, validation, and testing respectively. In the segmentation task in the training phase, we provided the three sub-region masks of tumor core, active tumor (enhanced tumor), and whole tumor for each 2D input image. Both the proposed generator and discriminator have four input channels and map the output in three channels (4-3), which each channel output represented as the segmented mask from the core of the tumor, active tumor, and whole tumor Fig. 4. In the generator network, the sign function aides in noise reduction. The generator for all layers used ReLU acti-vation function except the output layer, which used Tanh. Qualitative results are shown in Fig. 4. The training took five days for 100 epochs on parallel Pas-cal Titan X GPUs for the segmentation task. For the validation and test time respectively 47 and 114 MR images without ground truth file were provided by BraTS-2017 challenge. The predicted binary mask for each region of validation and test were provided on the basis of the trained model. The proposed network provided three predicted masks for each 2D images less than 3 ms. In the second task, the training took 12 h on a single Pascal Titan X GPU.

3.4 Evaluation and Results

Tables 1 and 2 describe the results of the models evaluated in the BraTS 2017 online judge system. Owing to practical clinical applications, the tumor struc-tures are grouped in three different sub-regions. As described by BraTS-2017, the tumor regions are defined as:

1. WT: the whole tumor region represents the area with labels 1, 2, 3, 4, where 0 for normal tissue, 1 for edema, 2 for non-enhancing core, 3 for necrotic core, and 4 for the enhancing core.
2. CT: The core tumor region represents only tumor core region, and measures labels 1, 3, 4.
3. ET: The enhancing tumor region or active area of tumor (label 4).

There are four kinds of evaluation criteria for the segmentation task, namely F1 score or Dice coefficient Eq. (5), Hausdorff distance Eq. (8), sensitivity Eq. (6)

and specificity Eq. (7) which have been provided by the BraTS-2017 challenge organizer as an online judgment system for training, validation, and test (Fig. 5).

$$Dice : \frac{\mid P_1 \mid \wedge \mid T_1 \mid}{\frac{\mid P_1 \mid + \mid T_1 \mid}{2}} \tag{5}$$

$$Sensitivity : \frac{\mid P_1 \mid \wedge \mid T_1 \mid}{\mid T_1 \mid} \tag{6}$$

$$Specificity : \frac{\mid P_0 \mid \vee \mid T_0 \mid}{\mid T_0 \mid} \tag{7}$$

$$Haus(P,T) \leftarrow max\{sup - inf - d(p,t), sup - inf - d(t,p)\} \tag{8}$$

Table 1. The achieved accuracy for the task of semantic segmentation in the term of Dice, Sensitivity, Specificity and Hausdorff distance on unseen data of validation set and test set [2, 13–15] reported by BraTS-2017 organizer

Evaluation	Validation			Test		
	WT	ET	CT	WT	ET	CT
Dice	0.80	0.61	0.61	0.80	0.54	0.59
Sens	0.75	0.61	0.55	-	-	-
Spec	0.99	0.99	0.99	-	-	-
Hdfd	7.22	9.30	12.04	8.73	59.2	25.9

Table 2. The achieved accuracy for the task of semantic segmentation in the term of Dice and Hausdorff95 distance on Test data [2, 13–15] reported by BraTS-2017 organizer

Label	Dice-ET	Dice-WT	Dice-CT	Hausdorff95-ET	Hausdorff95-WT	Hausdorff95-CT
Mean	0.54	0.80	0.59	59.2	8.7	25.9
StdDev	0.30	0.17	0.31	129.6	12.8	73.0
Median	0.68	0.86	0.72	4.12	4.8	8.4
25quantile	0.36	0.77	0.34	2.23	3.3	5.4
75quantile	0.76	0.90	0.84	13.33	8.9	14.1

Table 3 describes the survival day prediction results. The first path way of CNN has seven input channels which four from multi-modal images and three from segmented regions. We translated ages from interval [0, 100] into float [0, 1] and also for survival day did from [0–1750] days into float of [0, 1] (Fig. 6).

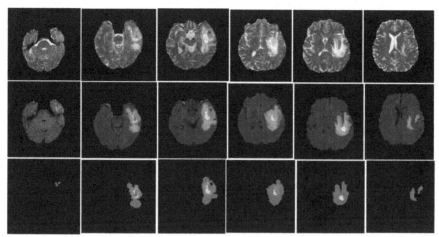

Brats17.TCIA.288.nz.53 Brats17.TCIA.288.nz.65 Brats17.TCIA.288.nz.75 Brats17.TCIA.288.nz.87 Brats17.TCIA.288.nz.95 Brats17.TCIA.288.nz.104

(a)

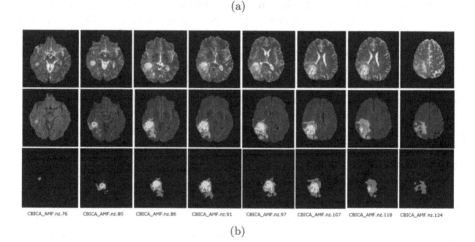

CBICA_AMF.nz.76 CBICA_AMF.nz.80 CBICA_AMF.nz.86 CBICA_AMF.nz.91 CBICA_AMF.nz.97 CBICA_AMF.nz.107 CBICA_AMF.nz.118 CBICA_AMF.nz.124

(b)

Fig. 5. Examples of segmentation results from BraTS-2017 Validation Data [2, 13–15]. Segmentation images are overlaid on unprocessed Flair images. Each image is an axial slice taken from two patients. The yellow label is core of tumor. Pink color shows the active region of tumor (enhanced tumor) and the red part is whole tumor. (Color figure online)

Table 3. The survival day prediction results on unseen data of validation set and test set reported by BraTS-2017 organizer

	casesEvaluated	Accuracy	MSE	medianSE	stdSE	SpearmanR
Validation	33	0.33	325285.78	94249.0	719523.522	0.075
Test	95	0.38	332052.116	68644.0	974571.141	0.228

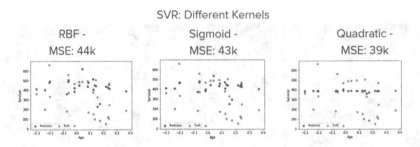

Fig. 6. Different regression techniques (e.g. Support Vector Regression, Polynomial Regression, ...) for survival day prediction.

4 Conclusion

In this paper, we introduced and evaluated two trainable and end-to-end approaches to two important clinical tasks heterogeneous brain tumor segmentation and the prediction of survival day after tumor diagnosis. Our proposed approach to tumor segmentation is fully automatic based on the newly proposed conditional generative adversarial network. We propose an automatic trainable parallel convolution neural network to predict the survival day(s) as the second task in the BraTS-2017 challenge. These networks learn a loss adapted to the task and data at hand, which makes it applicable to unseen data. In future work, we plan to improve both generative and discriminative network by incorporating recurrent neural networks (RNNs) inside of the Encoder-Decoder. This framework can be extended as voxel-GANs for end-to-end 3D medical image segmentation.

References

1. Inda, Maria-del-Mar, R.B., Seoane, J.: Glioblastoma multiforme: a look inside its heterogeneous nature. In: Cancer Archive, pp. 226–239 (2014)
2. Menze, B., Jakab, A., Bauer, S., Kalpathy-Cramer, J., Farahani, K., Kirby, J., Burren, Y., Porz, N., Slotboom, J., Wiest, R., Lanczi, L., Gerstner, E., Weber, M., Arbel, T., Avants, B., Ayache, N., Buendia, P., Collins, D., Cordier, N., Corso, J., Criminisi, A., Das, T., Delingette, H., Demiralp, Ç., Durst, C., Dojat, M., Doyle, S., Festa, J., Forbes, F., Geremia, E., Glocker, B., Golland, P., Guo, D., Hamamci, A., Iftekharuddin, K., Jena, R., John, N., Konukoglu, E., Lashkari, D., Mariz, J., Meier, R., Pereira, S., Precup, D., Price, S., Raviv, T., Reza, S., Ryan, S., Sarikaya, D., Schwartz, L., Shin, H., Shotton, J., Silva, C., Sousa, N., Subbanna, N., Szekely, G., Taylor, T., Thomas, O., Tustison, N., Unal, G., Vasseur, F., Wintermark, M., Ye, D., Zhao, L., Zhao, B., Zikic, D., Prastawa, M., Reyes, M., Van Leemput, K.: The multimodal brain tumor image segmentation benchmark (BRATS). IEEE Trans. Med. Imaging **34**(10), 1993–2024 (2015)
3. Goodfellow, I.J., Pouget-Abadie, J., Mirza, M., Xu, B., Warde-Farley, D., Ozair, S., Courville, A., Bengio, Y.: Generative Adversarial Networks. ArXiv e-prints (2014)

4. Reed, S.E., Akata, Z., Mohan, S., Tenka, S., Schiele, B., Lee, H.: Learning what and where to draw. In: Lee, D.D., Sugiyama, M., Luxburg, U.V., Guyon, I., Garnett, R. (eds.) Advances in Neural Information Processing Systems, vol. 29, pp. 217–225. Curran Associates, Inc. (2016). http://papers.nips.cc/paper/6111-learning-what-and-where-to-draw.pdf

5. Makhzani, A., Shlens, J., Jaitly, N., Goodfellow, I.J.: Adversarial autoencoders. CoRR abs/1511.05644 (2015). http://arxiv.org/abs/1511.05644

6. Li, J., Liang, X., Wei, Y., Xu, T., Feng, J., Yan, S.: Perceptual Generative Adversarial Networks for Small Object Detection. ArXiv e-prints, June 2017

7. Wang, X., Shrivastava, A., Gupta, A.: A-Fast-RCNN: hard positive generation via adversary for object detection. arXiv preprint arXiv:1704.03414 (2017)

8. Mathieu, M., Couprie, C., LeCun, Y.: Deep multi-scale video prediction beyond mean square error. CoRR abs/1511.05440 (2015). http://arxiv.org/abs/1511.05440

9. Finn, C., Goodfellow, I.J., Levine, S.: Unsupervised learning for physical interaction through video prediction. CoRR abs/1605.07157 (2016). http://arxiv.org/abs/1605.07157

10. Vondrick, C., Pirsiavash, H., Torralba, A.: Generating videos with scene dynamics. CoRR abs/1609.02612 (2016). http://arxiv.org/abs/1609.02612

11. Isola, P., Zhu, J., Zhou, T., Efros, A.A.: Image-to-image translation with conditional adversarial networks. CoRR abs/1611.07004 (2016). http://arxiv.org/abs/1611.07004

12. Zhu, W., Xie, X.: Adversarial deep structural networks for mammographic mass segmentation. CoRR abs/1612.05970 (2016). http://arxiv.org/abs/1612.05970

13. Bakas, S., Akbari, H., Sotiras, A., Bilello, M., Rozycki, M., Kirby, J.S., Freymann, J.B., Farahani, K., Davatzikos, C.: Advancing the Cancer Genome Atlas glioma MRI collections with expert segmentation labels and radiomic features. Sci. Data **4**, 170117 (2017)

14. Bakas, S., Akbari, H., Sotiras, A., Bilello, M., Rozycki, M., Kirby, J., Freymann, J., Farahani, K., Davatzikos, C.: Segmentation labels and radiomic features for the pre-operative scans of the TCGA-GBM collection. The Cancer Imaging Archive (2017)

15. Bakas, S., Akbari, H., Sotiras, A., Bilello, M., Rozycki, M., Kirby, J., Freymann, J., Farahani, K., Davatzikos, C.: Segmentation labels and radiomic features for the pre-operative scans of the TCGA-LGG collection. The Cancer Imaging Archive (2017)

16. Ronneberger, O., Fischer, P., Brox, T.: U-Net: convolutional networks for biomedical image segmentation. In: Navab, N., Hornegger, J., Wells, W.M., Frangi, A.F. (eds.) MICCAI 2015. LNCS, vol. 9351, pp. 234–241. Springer, Cham (2015). https://doi.org/10.1007/978-3-319-24574-4_28

17. Li, C., Wand, M.: Precomputed real-time texture synthesis with Markovian generative adversarial networks. CoRR abs/1604.04382 (2016). http://arxiv.org/abs/1604.04382

18. Mirza, M., Osindero, S.: Conditional generative adversarial nets. CoRR abs/1411.1784 (2014). http://arxiv.org/abs/1411.1784

19. Springenberg, J.T.: Unsupervised and Semi-supervised Learning with Categorical Generative Adversarial Networks. ArXiv e-prints, November 2015

20. Salimans, T., Goodfellow, I.J., Zaremba, W., Cheung, V., Radford, A., Chen, X.: Improved techniques for training gans. CoRR abs/1606.03498 (2016). http://arxiv.org/abs/1606.03498

21. Ioffe, S., Szegedy, C.: Batch normalization: Accelerating deep network training by reducing internal covariate shift. In: International Conference on Machine Learning, pp. 448–456 (2015)
22. Goodfellow, I.J.: NIPS 2016 tutorial: Generative adversarial networks. CoRR abs/1701.00160 (2017)
23. https://www.cbica.upenn.edu/sbia/Spyridon.Bakas/MICCAI_BraTS/MICCAI_BraTS_2016_proceedings.pdf
24. Radford, A., Metz, L., Chintala, S.: Unsupervised representation learning with deep convolutional generative adversarial networks. CoRR abs/1511.06434 (2015). http://arxiv.org/abs/1511.06434
25. Tustison, N.J., Avants, B.B., Cook, P.A., Zheng, Y., Egan, A., Yushkevich, P.A., Gee, J.C.: N4ITK: improved N3 bias correction. IEEE Trans. Med. Imaging **29**(6), 1310–1320 (2010)
26. Nyúl, L.G., Udupa, J.K., Zhang, X.: New variants of a method of MRI scale standardization. IEEE Trans. Med. Imaging **19**(2), 143–150 (2000)

Dilated Convolutions for Brain Tumor Segmentation in MRI Scans

Marc Moreno Lopez(ID) and Jonathan Ventura(✉)(ID)

Department of Computer Science,
University of Colorado, Colorado Springs, USA
{mmorenol,jventura}@uccs.edu

Abstract. We present a novel method to detect and segment brain tumors in Magnetic Resonance Imaging scans using a novel network based on the Dilated Residual Network. Dilated convolutions provide efficient multi-scale analysis for dense prediction tasks without losing resolution by downsampling the input. To the best of our knowledge, our work is the first to evaluate a dilated residual network for brain tumor segmentation in magnetic resonance imaging scans. We train and evaluate our method on the Brain Tumor Segmentation (BraTS) 2017 challenge dataset. To address the severe label imbalance in the data, we adopt a balanced, patch-based sampling approach for training. An ablation study establishes the importance of residual connections in the performance of our network.

Keywords: Deep learning · Brain tumor segmentation
Dilated convolutions · Residual network

1 Introduction

Brain tumor segmentation in magnetic resonance imaging (MRI) scans is a significant challenge problem for medical image analysis with many benchmark datasets available [16,19–21]. Dense prediction problems such as image segmentation depend on multi-scale analysis in order to identify both large-scale and small-scale effects. This issue is particularly relevant to brain tumor segmentation, where the objects to be identified vary widely in shape and size.

When applying convolutional neural networks, there are three dominant approaches to achieve multi-scale analysis. The first is to use a sequence of fixed-size filters and pooling layers [22], so that the network proceeds from local to global analysis in the forward pass. Pereira et al. [17] applied this concept to brain tumor segmentation in MRI scans using 3×3 convolutional filters. Using small filters is a form of regularization to prevent overfitting, by minimizing the number of parameters in the network [22]. Using the BraTS validation tool, Pereira et al. achieved Dice scores of 88% for whole tumor, 83% for tumor core, and 77% for active tumor.

© Springer International Publishing AG, part of Springer Nature 2018
A. Crimi et al. (Eds.): BrainLes 2017, LNCS 10670, pp. 253–262, 2018.
https://doi.org/10.1007/978-3-319-75238-9_22

A second option for multi-scale analysis is to use separate "columns" of differently-sized filters to analyze the image at different scales [2]. One of the most successful examples of this approach in the context of MRI brain tumor segmentation is the work of Havaei et al. [6]. They propose a cascaded two-pathway CNN architecture that extracts smaller and larger sized patches at the same time. The cascaded CNN processes local and global details of the brain MRI. While being centered at the same point, the local and global patches are extracted. A CNN processes the global patches first, and then the out is concatenated with the local patches and fed into a two-pathway CNN, with 7×7 filters in one of the paths and 13×13 in the other. To avoid class imbalance, they propose a two phase training. It consists on training the CNN first with a balanced distribution of classes and then training it with a representative distribution of the original images. The reported dice scores using the BRATS validation tool are 88% for whole tumor region, 79% for core tumor region and 73% for active tumor. Kamnitsas et al. [12,13] also use a multi-path network but use 3D filters.

When using these networks in a fully convolutional manner [15], the pooling layers cause a loss of resolution in the output. Because of this loss of resolution, it is common to add an upsampling path with skip connections to aid in recovering high-resolution detail [15]. The popular U-Net architecture uses a symmetric network with downsampling followed by upsampling with skip connections in between [10,18].

An interesting but relatively unexplored alternative to downsampling and upsampling is the use of dilated convolutions [23,24]. Dilated convolutions allow the network to look at larger receptive fields without an exponential increase in parameters. They have been shown to achieve excellent results on general image segmentation datasets. However, the application of dilated convolutional neural networks to medical image analysis has not been well-studied so far.

In this work, we introduce a modification of the Dilated Residual Network by Yu et al. [24] and apply it to brain tumor segmentation in MRI scans. We evaluate our network by training and testing on the BraTS 2017 challenge dataset [16]. To address the severe label imbalance in the dataset, we adopt a balanced patch-based sampling approach for training. We also perform an ablation study which confirms the importance of residual connections in the network design. We believe our work points to an interesting new research direction for the development of deep learning approaches to brain tumor segmentation in MRI scans and medical image segmentation in general.

2   Method

We apply a fully convolutional network [14] approach in order to produce a per-pixel segmentation output. Our network uses 2D convolutions and is applied to each slice in a scan separately. For every scan, we use all four modalities together as the input to the network; i.e., the four channels of the input image are the four MRI imaging modalities.

2.1 Dilation

An issue with traditional convolutional neural network architectures that use max pooling is that they downsample the image and thus produce a segmentation with resolution smaller than the input size. While down-sampling is useful for multi-scale analysis, it also leads to a loss of resolution in the output.

Without down-sampling, the receptive field of the network grows linearly as layers are added. For example, if only 3×3 filters are used, each added convolutional layer will increase the receptive field of the network by one pixel on each side. Larger filters would grow the receptive field more quickly, but would also greatly increase the number of parameters in the network, possibly leading to over-fitting. In this way, small filters act as a form of regularization and introduce more non-linearity in the network through the increased number of activation functions [22].

Yu et al. [23] point out that dilated convolutional filters allow for exponential increase in the receptive field of the network with a linear increase in number of parameters. Thus, dilated convolutional neural networks can have a large receptive field, small number of parameters and high amount of non-linearity, all without the loss of resolution caused by down-sampling. Dilated convolutional neural networks have been shown to produce competitive performance on general image segmentation tasks [23,24].

A dilated filter is a generalization of the convolutional filter that introduces a stride between input pixels. Formally, a $k \times k$ convolutional filter[1] with dilation d is defined as follows:

$$F_{k,d}(r,c) = \sum_{i=-k}^{k} \sum_{j=-k}^{k} W(i,j)I(r+di, c+dj) \tag{1}$$

where I is the input image and W are the filter weights.

Figure 1 illustrates the effect of dilation on a 3×3 filter. A 3×3 filter with dilation of 2 results in a receptive field of 5×5. Dilating by 4 results in a receptive field of 9×9. However, the number of parameters in each filter is identical. Yu et al. [23] propose using a sequence of $k \times k$ filters with exponentially growing dilation $(1, 2, 4, \ldots)$, so that the receptive field grows exponentially while the number of parameters grows linearly.

2.2 Dilated Residual Network

In [24], Yu et al. present a Dilated Residual Network (DRN) architecture which is based on the ResNet architecture [8] but uses dilated convolutions. They also noted that dilated convolutions can cause gridding artifacts. Figure 2 illustrates why dilated filters cause gridding artifacts. The artifacts are essentially the result of an aliasing problem which happens when a filters with large dilation are not followed by filters with smaller dilation. Applying a sequence of filters with progressively lower dilation will eliminate such artifacts.

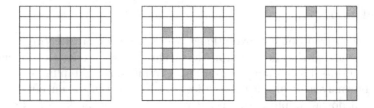

Fig. 1. Filter dilation example. *Left:* 3 × 3 filter with no dilation (dilation = 1). *Center:* 3 × 3 filter with dilation of size 2. *Right:* 3 × 3 filter with a dilation of size 4.

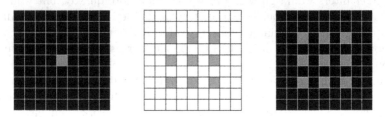

Fig. 2. Gridding artifacts. *Left:* Input: black indicates zeros and blue is non-zero. *Center:* 3 × 3 filter with dilation of 2. *Right:* Result of convolving the input with the filter, showing the gridding artifact caused by the dilated filter. (Color figure online)

The original DRN architecture uses max pooling to downsample the image, and upsamples the prediction by interpolation. To avoid upsampling and the resulting loss of segmentation resolution, we modified the DRN architecture by removing the max pooling layers. We also shortened the network by removing eight layers in the middle levels. Our modified DRN architecture has a receptive field of 59 × 59.

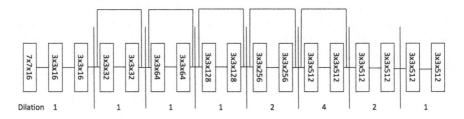

Fig. 3. Our adapted Dilated Residual Network. The layers are separated in level using vertical lines. The dilation is indicated underneath every level. The connecting lines above the network indicate residual connections.

Figure 3 illustrates the network design. Each rectangle is a Convolution - Batch Normalization [9] - ReLU group. The numbers in each rectangle specify

---

[1] This is actually a cross-correlation but we call it a convolution as is common in the literature today.

the filter size and the number of channels in that layer. The networks are divided into levels, such that all layers within a given level have the same dilation and number of filters.

2.3 Patch-Based Training

The dataset exhibits severe class imbalance, because the tumor pixels are vastly outnumbered by the non-tumor pixels. This poses a problem when training the network, because the non-tumor pixels influence the total loss function much more strongly than the tumor pixels.

To address this issue, we adopt a patch-based training approach. During training, we randomly sample patches from the images to form a batch. Each patch is exactly the size of receptive field of the network. We sample patches using a uniform distribution over the classes. In other words, we ensure that each batch has the same number of examples of each class. This effectively remedies the class imbalance that would be caused by simply randomly sampling the patches. Moreover, we don't sample patches from pixels with zero intensity.

Because the network is fully convolutional, we can use the same network trained on patches to test on images. At test time, we use whole images as input to the network to produce the full-resolution output.

2.4 Preprocessing

For preprocessing, we subtract from each slice the per-channel mean.

3 Results

3.1 Implementation Details

To develop the experiment, we used Keras for Python 2.7. All training was done in one machine with Ubuntu and Nvidia Titan X card with 12 GB of memory.

To train the network, we used a batch size of 120 patches, and trained for 1,000,000 iterations. We used an Adagrad optimizer [5] with a learning rate of 0.01. Each training iteration takes about 150 ms.

3.2 Evaluation on Validation Dataset

To evaluate our algorithm, we used the BraTS evaluation tool. To measure the performance of the algorithms, we computed recall (or sensitivity), specificity, the Dice score (also called F1-measure) and the Hausdorff95 distance [4]. Recall is the fraction of relevant instances that are retrieved, therefore it measures the proportion of positives that are correctly identified as such. Specificity measures the proportion of negatives that are correctly identified as such. The Dice score or F1-measure, is a statistic used for comparing the similarity of two samples.

It is calculated using the precision and recall parameters. Precision is the fraction of relevant instances among the retrieved instances. The Hausdorff distance measures how far two subsets of a metric space are from each other.

We performed an ablation study on the validation data to test the importance of residual connections. Table 1 compares the results of our method on the validation dataset with and without residual connections. The network achieves a better score in almost all tests when residual connections are used. This indicates that residual connections are critical for the performance of the network.

Table 1. Mean validation results. The bold number indicates the better result for each measure and class. Note that for the Hausdorff95 metric, smaller is better.

		Dice	Sensitivity	Specificity	Hausdorff95
With residual connections	Enhanced tumor	**0.56669**	**0.65688**	**0.99664**	**23.82812**
	Tumor core	**0.68537**	**0.91858**	0.97277	38.07678
	Whole tumor	**0.78331**	0.73782	**0.99267**	**30.3156**
No residual connections	Enhanced tumor	0.49685	0.64413	0.99576	28.08775
	Tumor core	0.59215	0.68962	**0.98891**	**33.87923**
	Whole tumor	0.73112	**0.87517**	0.96864	34.45454

Table 2. Mean test results - DRN. Sensitivity and specificity were not provided in the test results.

	Dice	Hausdorff95
Enhanced tumor	0.51881	87.91993
Tumor core	0.61747	53.10582
Whole tumor	0.69089	42.79233

Table 2 gives the results of our method (with residual connections) on the test dataset. Note that scores for the sensitivity and specificity measures were not provided for the test set.

4   Discussion

Figure 4 shows example MRI slices from the validation set and the segmentation predicted by our method. Because these slices are from the validation dataset, we do not have access to the gold standard segmentation and are unable to show it here. Figures 4b and d show how our network can predict complicated tumor shapes.

Figure 4f shows a failure case where the network likely over-predicted the edema class. The edema regions are similar in appearance to adjacent brain pixels as shown in Fig. 4f. However, this effect of over-prediction may also be caused

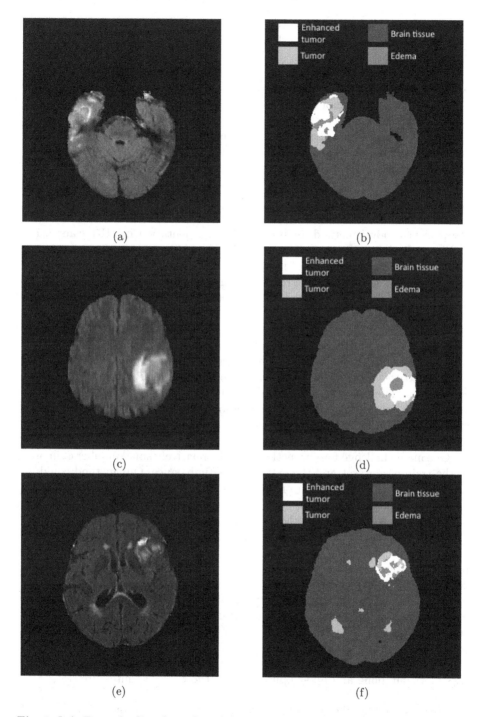

Fig. 4. *Left:* Example slices from the validation dataset. *Right:* Segmentation predicted by our method.

by the balanced sampling employed during training, which over-represents the minority classes during training. This problem could be addressed by score calibration [3] or fine-tuning [7].

The boundaries between regions are also often not well-segmented by our technique. Many tumor pixels are labeled as edema, and many enhanced tumor pixels are labeled as tumor core. This problem could be addressed using a structured prediction approach [1].

Our performance on enhanced tumor pixels is low. This is likely because there are very few examples of enhanced tumor pixels in the dataset. This problem could be addressed through data augmentation [18].

5   Conclusions and Future Work

We present a novel method for brain tumor segmentation in MRI scans using a Dilated Residual Network. The network uses a dilated convolution operator to increase the receptive field of the network without an exponential increase in the number of parameters. The residual connections allow us to effectively train a deeper network. We use balanced, patch-based training to cope with the class imbalance in the dataset.

Our method achieved a Dice score of 0.69 for whole tumor, 0.61 for tumor core and 0.51 for enhanced tumor on the test set.

To the best of our knowledge, we are the first to apply a Dilated Residual Network to the problem of brain tumor segmentation in MRI scans. Dilated convolutions offer several benefits for multi-scale analysis which make them a good choice for medical image segmentation problems. Future work includes evaluating our network on other image segmentation problems in the medical and scientific domain.

One main challenge for our method was the relatively small number of images in the training dataset and the extreme class imbalance. Our method could be improved with data augmentation strategies to increase the number of examples of the tumor pixels.

Our balanced sampling method allowed us to effectively learn a classifier on imbalanced data, but led to over-prediction of the minority classes. To avoid detecting small clusters as edema-tumor tissue, we could apply some postprocessing steps to remove spurious clusters based on their size or inter-slice consistency [11]. We also could use fine-tuning or per-class weights.

Our work shows that dilated convolutional neural networks are interesting alternative for multi-scale analysis in medical image segmentation. Because brain tumor segmentation is an inherently three-dimensional problem, future work could include using 3D convolutional filters instead of 2D filters. In addition, there might be benefits to combining dilated convolutions with a network which uses down-sampling and up-sampling such as the U-Net architecture [18].

Acknowledgments. We gratefully acknowledge the support of the UCCS Center of the BioFrontiers Institute, the Balsells Foundation, and National Science Foundation Grant No. 1659788.

References

1. Chen, L.C., Papandreou, G., Kokkinos, I., Murphy, K., Yuille, A.L.: DeepLab: semantic image segmentation with deep convolutional nets, atrous convolution, and fully connected CRFs. In: arXiv preprint arXiv:1606.00915 (2016)
2. Ciregan, D., Meier, U., Schmidhuber, J.: Multi-column deep neural networks for image classification. In: 2012 IEEE Conference on Computer Vision and Pattern Recognition (CVPR), pp. 3642–3649. IEEE (2012)
3. Ciresan, D., Giusti, A., Gambardella, L.M., Schmidhuber, J.: Deep neural networks segment neuronal membranes in electron microscopy images. In: Advances in Neural Information Processing Systems, pp. 2843–2851 (2012)
4. Davis, J., Goadrich, M.: The relationship between precision-recall and ROC curves. In: Proceedings of the 23rd International Conference on Machine Learning, ICML 2006, pp. 233–240. ACM, Pittsburgh, Pennsylvania, USA (2006). http://doi.acm.org/10.1145/1143844.1143874, https://doi.org/10.1145/1143844.1143874, ISBN 1-59593-383-2
5. Duchi, J.: Adaptive subgradient methods for online learning and stochastic optimization. J. Mach. Learn. Res. **12**, 2121–2159 (2011)
6. Havaei, M., Davy, A., Warde-Farley, D., Biard, A., Courville, A., Bengio, Y., Pal, C., Jodoin, P.M., Larochelle, H.: Brain tumor segmentation with deep neural networks. In: CoRR abs/1505.03540 (2015). http://arxiv.org/abs/1505.03540
7. Havaei, M., Davy, A., Warde-Farley, D., Biard, A., Courville, A., Bengio, Y., Pal, C., Jodoin, P.M., Larochelle, H.: Brain tumor segmentation with deep neural networks. Med. Image Anal. **35**, 18–31 (2017). arXiv: 1505.03540
8. He, K., Zhang, X., Ren, S., Sun, J.: Deep residual learning for image recognition. In: Proceedings of the IEEE Conference on Computer Vision and Pattern Recognition, pp. 770–778 (2016)
9. Ioffe, S., Szegedy, C.: Batch normalization: accelerating deep network training by reducing internal covariate shift. In: International Conference on Machine Learning, pp. 448–456 (2015)
10. Isensee, F., Kickingereder, P., Bonekamp, D., Bendszus, M., Wick, W., Schlemmer, H.-P., Maier-Hein, K.: Brain tumor segmentation using large receptive field deep convolutional neural networks. Bildverarbeitung für die Medizin 2017. Informatik aktuell, pp. 86–91. Springer, Heidelberg (2017). https://doi.org/10.1007/978-3-662-54345-0_24
11. Işin, A., Direkoğlu, C., Şah, M.: Review of MRI-based brain tumor image segmentation using deep learning methods. In: 12th International Conference on Application of Fuzzy Systems and Soft Computing, ICAFS 2016, Procedia Computer Science, 29–30 August 2016, Vienna, Austria, vol. 102, no. Supplement C, pp. 317–324 (2016). http://www.sciencedirect.com/science/article/pii/S187705091632587X, https://doi.org/10.1016/j.procs.2016.09.407, ISSN 1877-0509
12. Kamnitsas, K., Chen, L., Ledig, C., Rueckert, D., Glocker, B.: Multi-scale 3D convolutional neural networks for lesion segmentation in brain MRI. Ischemic Stroke Lesion Segmentation **13**, 46 (2015)
13. Kamnitsas, K., Ledig, C., Newcombe, V.F., Simpson, J.P., Kane, A.D., Menon, D.K., Rueckert, D., Glocker, B.: Efficient multi-scale 3D CNN with fully connected CRF for accurate brain lesion segmentation. Med. Image Anal. **36**, 61–78 (2017)
14. Long, J., Shelhamer, E., Darrell, T.: Fully convolutional networks for semantic segmentation. In: IEEE Transactions on Pattern Analysis and Machine Intelligence (TPAMI) (2015). arXiv: 1605.06211

15. Long, J., Shelhamer, E., Darrell, T.: Fully convolutional networks for semantic segmentation. In: Proceedings of the IEEE Conference on Computer Vision and Pattern Recognition, pp. 3431–3440 (2015)
16. Bjoern, M., Jakab, A., Bauer, S., Kalpathy-Cramer, J., Farahani, K., Kirby, J., Burren, Y., Porz, N., Slotboom, J., Wiest, R., Lanczi, L., Gerstner, E., Weber, M.-A., Arbel, T., Avants, B., Ayache, N., Buendia, P., Collins, L., Cordier, N., Corso, J., Criminisi, A., Das, T., Delingette, H., Demiralp, C., Christopher, D., Michel, D., Doyle, S., Festa, J., Forbes, F., Geremia, E., Glocker, B., Golland, P., Guo, X., Hamamci, A., Iftekharuddin, K., Jena, R., John, N., Konukoglu, E., Lashkari, D., Mariz, J.A., Meier, R., Pereira, S., Precup, D., Price, S.J., Riklin-Raviv, T., Reza, S., Ryan, M., Schwartz, L., Shin, H.-C., Shotton, J., Silva, C., Sousa, N., Subbanna, N., Szekely, G., Taylor, T., Thomas, O., Tustison, N., Unal, G., Vasseur, F., Wintermark, M., Ye, D.H., Zhao, L., Zhao, B., Zikic, D., Prastawa, M., Reyes, M., Van Leemput, K.: The multi-modal brain tumor image segmentation benchmark (BRATS). IEEE Trans. Med. Imaging **34**(10), 1993–2024 (2015)
17. Pereira, S., Pinto, A., Alves, V., Silva, C.A.: Brain tumor segmentation using convolutional neural networks in MRI images. IEEE Trans. Med. Imaging **35**(5), 1240–1251 (2016)
18. Ronneberger, O., Fischer, P., Brox, T.: U-Net: convolutional networks for biomedical image segmentation. In: Navab, N., Hornegger, J., Wells, W.M., Frangi, A.F. (eds.) MICCAI 2015. LNCS, vol. 9351, pp. 234–241. Springer, Cham (2015). https://doi.org/10.1007/978-3-319-24574-4_28
19. Bakas, S., Akbari, H., Sotiras, A., Bilello, M., Rozycki, M., Kirby, J.S., Freymann, J.B., Farahani, K., Davatzikos, C.: Advancing the cancer genome atlas glioma MRI collections with expert segmentation labels and radiomic features. Nat. Sci. Data **4**, 170117 (2017)
20. Bakas, S., Akbari, H., Sotiras, A., Bilello, M., Rozycki, M., Kirby, J., Freymann, J., Farahani, K., Davatzikos, C.: Segmentation labels and radiomic features for the pre-operative scans of the TCGA-GBM collection. In: The Cancer Imaging Archive (2017). https://doi.org/10.7937/K9/TCIA.2017.KLXWJJ1Q
21. Bakas, S., Akbari, H., Sotiras, A., Bilello, M., Rozycki, M., Kirby, J., Freymann, J., Farahani, K., Davatzikos, C.: Segmentation labels and radiomic features for the pre-operative scans of the TCGA-LGG collection. In: The Cancer Imaging Archive (2017). https://doi.org/10.7937/K9/TCIA.2017.GJQ7R0EF
22. Simonyan, K., Zisserman, A.: Very deep convolutional networks for large-scale image recognition. In: arXiv preprint arXiv: 1409.1556 (2014)
23. Yu, F., Koltun, V.: Multi-scale context aggregation by dilated convolutions. In: International Conference on Learning Representations (ICLR) (2016). arXiv: 1511.07122v3
24. Yu, F., Koltun, V., Funkhouser, T.: Dilated residual networks. In: Computer Vision and Pattern Recognition (CVPR) (2017). arXiv: 1705.09914

Residual Encoder and Convolutional Decoder Neural Network for Glioma Segmentation

Kamlesh Pawar[1,2(✉)] , Zhaolin Chen[1,3], N. Jon Shah[1,4], and Gary Egan[1,2]

[1] Monash Biomedical Imaging, Monash University, Melbourne, Australia
kamlesh.pawar@monash.edu
[2] School of Psychological Sciences, Monash University, Melbourne, Australia
[3] Electrical and Computer System Engineering, Monash University,
Melbourne, Australia
[4] Research Centre Juelich, Institute of Medicine, Juelich, Germany

Abstract. A deep learning approach to glioma segmentation is presented. An encoder and decoder pair deep learning network is designed which takes T1, T2, T1-CE (contrast enhanced) and T2-Flair (fluid attenuation inversion recovery) images as input and outputs the segmented labels. The encoder is a 49 layer deep residual learning architecture that encodes the $240 \times 240 \times 4$ input images into $8 \times 8 \times 2048$ feature maps. The decoder network takes these feature maps and extract the segmented labels. The decoder network is fully convolutional network consisting of convolutional and upsampling layers. Additionally, the input images are downsampled using bilinear interpolation and are inserted into the decoder network through concatenation. This concatenation step provides spatial information of the tumor to the decoder, which was lost due to pooling/downlsampling during encoding. The network is trained on the BRATS-17 training dataset and validated on the validation dataset. The dice score, sensitivity and specificity of the segmented whole tumor, core tumor and enhancing tumor is computed on validation dataset. The mean dice score for whole tumor, core tumor and enhancing tumor for validation dataset were 0.824, 0.627 and 0.575, respectively.

Keywords: Deep learning · Image segmentation · Computer vision
CNN

1 Introduction

Gliomas are the tumors of the central nervous system which arises from glial cells. The gliomas are classified into two types depending on the aggressiveness of the tumor: high grade (HGG) and low grade (LGG) gliomas, both

---

Caffe model and code available at: https://github.com/kamleshpawar17/BratsNet-2017.

A. Crimi et al. (Eds.): BrainLes 2017, LNCS 10670, pp. 263–273, 2018.
https://doi.org/10.1007/978-3-319-75238-9_23

types of tumors are malignant and need treatment [1]. The accurate segmentation of gliomas is important in grading, treating and monitoring tumor progression. Multiple magnetic resonance (MR) image contrasts are used to evaluate the type and extent of tumors. The different contrasts T1, T2, T1-CE and T2-Flair are analysed by a radiologist and tumor regions are manually segmented. Segmenting brain tumor is a comprehensive task, and large intra-rater variability is often reported, e.g. 20% [2]. Thus it is imperative to have a reliable automatic segmentation algorithm that standardizes the process of segmentation, resulting in more precise planning, treatment and monitoring.

Manual segmentation by an expert is a time consuming and expensive process, thus computer assisted tumor segmentation is imperative to the problem of brain tumor segmentation. Computer assisted methods [3–8] can be broadly classified into two categories: semiautomatic brain tumor segmentation and automatic brain tumor segmentation. Semiautomatic approach involves seeding some initial information by an expert such as a location of the tumor and the fine delineation and computational task is offloaded to a computer. This approach minimises the time spent by human experts. However large number of MR images are generated routinely in clinics, demanding fully automatic segmentation methods. The automatic segmentation methods require no human intervention and can segment the brain tumor into different classes such as necrotic tumor, enhancing tumor, tumor core and edema.

In this work, we present a deep learning based approach to brain tumor segmentation on the BRATS-17 dataset [9–12]. Deep learning methods [13,14] based on convolutional neural networks (CNN) [15,16] have demonstrated highly accurate results in image classification [17,18] and segmentation [19,20]. However, selection of the number of CNN layers is a complex task. On one hand, increasing the number of layers improves complexity of the network and leads to more accurate results. On the other hand, designing deeper CNN may result in performance degradation due to exploding/vanishing gradients. This problem is partially solved by the batch normalization layers [21] that minimize the chances of exploding/vanishing gradients. Another limitation of designing deep neural network is that the training process becomes difficult and, after a certain depth the network ceases to converge. However recently introduced residual networks [22], consisting of short cut connections, can be trained to the larger depths. In this paper we present an encoder-decoder based CNN architecture to solve the tumor segmentation problem.

2   Deep Residual Learning Networks

Deep learning CNN uses the layers of convolution as a feature extractor. The initial layers extract the basic features such as horizontal, vertical and slanted edges, the later layers extract more complicated features by combining the basic features. Thus increasing the depth results in more complicated features being extracted, hence better performance in classification/segmentation. However, it is found that increasing the network depth does not always increase the accuracy. The training error reduces with the depth of the network to a certain

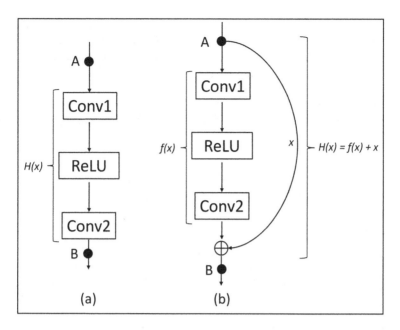

Fig. 1. If there exist a nonlinear function $H(x)$ between point A and B. **(a):** a network with no shortcut connection, here the layers Conv1 and Conv2 approximate the non linear function $H(x)$; **(b):** a network with shortcut connection, here the layers Conv1 and Conv2 approximate the nonlinear residual function $f(x) = H(x) - x$. Both (a) and (b) approximate the same non-linear function $H(x)$ between A and B, however individual layers learn different nonlinear functions.

level but the error increasing as further layers are added to the network [23,24]. This behaviour is counter intuitive, one may expect the error to decrease or stay constant after certain depth. The network may just learn identity mapping after certain depth and keep the error constant with even further increasing the depth of the network. Deep learning residual networks overcome this problem, by inserting the bottleneck units to increase the depth of the network. The bottleneck units learn the residual function that minimises the error.

Residual functions are realised with shortcut connection (Fig. 1(b)), a shortcut connection is a direct connection between two layers in a network skipping one or few layers. Consider that there exists a nonlinear relationship between the two points A and B in the network given by $H(x)$ as shown in Fig. 1. The conventional CNN without the shortcut connection (Fig. 1(a)), would train the layers (Conv1 and Conv2) such that the combined effect of the learning represents $H(x)$. However in case of the network with shortcut connection (Fig. 1(b)), the same layers (Conv1 and Conv2) would learn a residual function given by:

$$F(x) = H(x) - x \qquad (1)$$

In both the cases the relationship between the point A and B remains the same, however the convolution layers have learned different functions. The advantage of using a residual network is that it may approximate an identity relationship between the point A and B, if the convolution layers Conv1 and Conv2 are deemed to be unnecessary. Thus the residual learning in effect avoids the performance degradation on going to arbitrarily large depths.

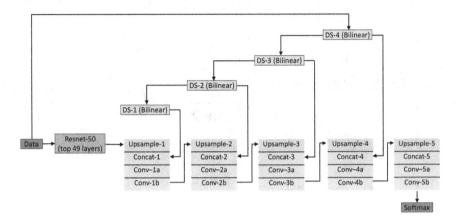

Fig. 2. Residual encoder and convolutional decoder network; the encoder is a 49 layer deep residual network and the decoder is a 10 layer deep fully convolutional network with bilinear upsampling layers. The input data is also downsampled using bilinear interpolation and is inserted back into the decoder through concatenation.

3   Proposed Segmentation Method

The method presented here is based on residual learning convolutional neural network [22] and the design is similar to the Unet encoder-decoder architecture [25]. The network is a 2D CNN, which performs segmentation on individual slices taken one by one from the full 3D dataset. The network is designed as an encoder-decoder pair, the four input images of size 240 × 240 are given as input to the encoder that encodes them into 8 × 8 × 2048 data. This encoded data are provided to a fully convolutional decoder network that predict the labels for the glioma segmentation. The Resent-50 [22] which was the winner of ILSRVC 2015 image classification challenge is used as an encoder network followed by fully convolutional layers of decoder network.

3.1   Deep Learning Network Architecture

Fig. 2, shows the network architecture; it consists of the first 49 layers of Resnet-50 as the encoder. Each convolutional layer in the encoder is followed by a batch normalization and scaling layers [21], which avoids vanishing/exploding gradients. The first layer of the encoder consists of a larger kernel size 7 × 7 with a stride of 2, and this reduces the input 240 × 240 image to 120 × 120. The first layer is followed by a max-pooling layer that further reduces the size of the data to 60 × 60. The use of larger kernel increases the field of view, at the same time the stride of 2 and max pooling reduces the size of the data, which results in reduction on memory requirement and reduces the training time. The layer parameters for encoder network, which is derived from first 49 layers of Resnet-50 are presented in [22].

The decoder network consists of upsampling layers that enlarges the dimension of image by a factor of 2. The weights of upsampling layer are fixed to bilinear upsampling and were not learned. During the encoding process the spatial information is lost due to pooling/downsampling, therefore the spatial information is reintroduced into the decoding network by concating the original images scaled by bilinear interpolation after each upsampling layer. After each convolutional layer, the batch normalization and scaling is performed followed by an ReLU non linear activation function. The last layer in the network is a multinomial logistic layer that predicts the probability of a given pixel being either normal (label 0), necrotic/non-enhancing tumor (NCR/NET, label 1), edema (label 2) or enhancing tumor (label 4). The decoder networks' input and output dimensions of the feature maps and convolutional kernel sizes are shown in the Table 1. The input to the decoder network is 2048 features of size 8 × 8, which are

Table 1. Decoder network input and output dimensions for each layer, the blob dimensions are *width × height × features*

Layer	Input dimension	Output dimension	Kernel size, Stride
Upsample-1	8 × 8 × 2048	15 × 15 × 2048	3x3, 2 (weights fixed to bilinear)
Concat-1	15 × 15 × 2048	15 × 15 × 2052	
Conv-1a	15 × 15 × 2052	15 × 15 × 1024	3x3, 1
Conv-1b	15 × 15 × 1024	15 × 15 × 1024	3x3, 1
Upsample-2	15 × 15 × 1024	30 × 30 × 1024	3x3, 2 (weights fixed to bilinear)
Concat-2	30 × 30 × 1024	30 × 30 × 1028	
Conv-2a	30 × 30 × 1028	30 × 30 × 512	3x3, 1
Conv-2b	30 × 30 × 512	30 × 30 × 512	3x3, 1
Upsample-3	30 × 30 × 512	60 × 60 × 512	3x3, 2 (weights fixed to bilinear)
Concat-3	60 × 60 × 512	60 × 60 × 516	
Conv-3a	60 × 60 × 516	60 × 60 × 256	3x3, 1
Conv-3b	60 × 60 × 256	60 × 60 × 256	3x3, 1
Upsample-4	60 × 60 × 256	120 × 120 × 256	3x3, 2 (weights fixed to bilinear)
Concat-4	120 × 120 × 256	120 × 120 × 260	
Conv-4a	120 × 120 × 260	120 × 120 × 128	3x3, 1
Conv-4b	120 × 120 × 128	120 × 120 × 128	3x3, 1
Upsample-5	120 × 120 × 128	240 × 240 × 128	3x3, 2 (weights fixed to bilinear)
Concat-5	240 × 240 × 128	240 × 240 × 132	
Conv-5a	240 × 240 × 132	240 × 240 × 64	3x3, 1
Conv-5b	240 × 240 × 64	240 × 240 × 64	3x3, 1
SotmaxwithLoss	240 × 240 × 64	240 × 240 × 4	

then passed successively through a series of convolution and upsampling layers, eventually generating a probability maps for the segmentation labels.

3.2 Dataset

The training dataset [9–12] used to train the network was provided by organisers of BRATS-17 challenge. The data consisted of 3D brain images from 285 subjects with four different contrast: T1, T1-CE, T2 and T2-Flair. There were 210 HGG subjects and 75 LGG subjects. The manually segmented labels were also provided for each subject. We divided the dataset into two groups:

– Train dataset: 259 subjects consisting of 192 HGG and 67 HGG subjects, used to train the network
– Test dataset: 26 subjects consisting of 18 HGG and 8 LGG subjects, used to evaluate the generalisation of the network.

Another two datasets for which the ground truth was not known were provided: one for validation consisting of 46 subjects and other for testing consisting of 147 subjects.

3.3 Pre-processing

The Caffe [26] deep learning library was used to train the network. The images provided by the organisers were in the NIFTI format, which were first converted to HDF5 file format, so that it can be read by Caffe. All the 3D volumes were normalised using histogram matching [27], the reference histogram for matching was obtained by averaging histograms of all the training dataset. Only the voxels with signal were used for computing the reference histogram and matching the histogram.

3.4 Training

The training was performed on the train dataset using stochastic gradient descent with momentum in Caffe. The training parameters were: base learning rate $(lr_{base}) = 0.01$, momentum $= 0.9$. The weights were decayed using the formula:

$$lr_{iter} = lr_{base} * (1 + \gamma * iter)^{(-power)} \qquad (2)$$

where, lr_{iter} is learning rate during $iter^{th}$ iteration, $\gamma = 0.0001$, and $power = 0.75$. The network was trained for 45 K iterations with the batch size of 8. The weights were regularized with l_2 regularization of 0.0005 during the training. Different base learning rate were experimented and the one that provided minimum loss was used for the final training.

3.5   Evaluation Method

The results of segmentation were evaluated using the dice score, sensitivity (true positive rate) and specificity (true negative rate). All the evaluation matrices were computed locally to test the local dataset of 26 subjects. The evaluation on the validation and test dataset was calculated on an online web-portal provided by the BRATS-17 organisers.

4   Results

The trained network was tested on the validation data and the results of segmentation were uploaded on the computing portal provided by the organisers. The dice score, sensitivity, specificity and Hausdorff distance were computed on the segmented labels. The Tables 2 and 3 show the result of segmentation of 46 subjects on the validation dataset and 147 subjects on the test dataset, respectively. The results of the segmentation from 2 different subjects on the local testing dataset are shown in Fig. 3. The whole tumor is defined as union of label 1, 2, and 4; the tumor core is defined as the union of label 1 and 4; and enhancing tumor is defined as label 4.

Table 2. Dice score, sensitivity, specificity and Hausdorfffor distance the segmentation on online validation dataset of 46 subjects

Metric	Whole tumor	Core tumor	Enhancing tumor
Dice Score (mean)	0.824	0.627	0.575
Dice Score (median)	0.865	0.728	0.724
Sensitivity (mean)	0.831	0.669	0.595
Sensitivity (median)	0.885	0.746	0.690
Specificity (mean)	0.993	0.994	0.999
Specificity (median)	0.994	0.997	0.999
Hausdorff (median)	35.38	39.45	25.11

Table 3. Dice scores and Hausdorfffor distance for the segmentation on online test dataset of 147 subjects

	Whole tumor	Core tumor	Enhancing tumor
Dice Score (mean)	0.784	0.577	0.502
Dice Score (Std. Dev)	0.152	0.280	0.315
Dice Score (median)	0.835	0.667	0.627
Dice Score (25 quantile)	0.731	0.359	0.200
Dice Score (75 quantile)	0.888	0.803	0.760
Hausdorff (median)	38.37	55.57	75.07

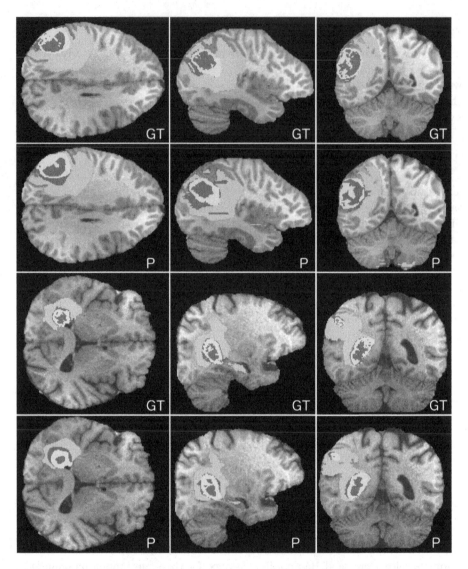

Fig. 3. Segmentation results on the test dataset for 2 different subjects; **GT**: represents the ground truth segmentation; **P**: represents the segmentation predicted by the proposed residual encoder-decoder network. Colour coding scheme: magenta (label 0, NCR/NET), yellow (label 4, enhancing tumor) and cyan (label 2, edema). (Color figure online)

5   Discussion

The median of dice score, sensitivity and specificity are all greater than the mean, which indicates that the proposed method performed well for most of the dataset but did not performed well for a few, that reduces the overall mean.

The boundaries of the labels segmented by the proposed algorithm are smooth compared to the ground truth (Fig. 3), and this may be due to the fact that some of the ground truth were created using automated algorithms rather than a human rater.

The network was trained only on the 2D axial slices of the 3D volume, thus it considered each slice as a separate instance and does not learn any correlation across the slices. This is evident from the predicted labels in the sagittal and coronal slices (Fig. 3), where there are few isolated false positive prediction. These false positive predictions can be suppressed by incorporating 3D information during training. One way to achieve this is to design a 3D residual network which takes a 3D volume and predicts a 3D label. This approach however would require large internal memory to store the network and 3D data/feature maps, which may not be feasible for a large depth. A moderate approach would be to use more than one slices at a time instead of full 3D volume for training. This approach would not increase the memory requirement and at the same time provide 3D information to the network. The number of slices to be used for this moderate approach would be determined by the available memory of the computing hardware. Ideally, all the slices should be used for the 3D architecture, but given the limitation of GPU internal memory a trade of would be required between accuracy and memory.

6   Conclusion

In this paper, we developed a 59-layer deep residual encoder-decoder convolutional neural network that takes 2D slices of 3D MRI images as input and outputs the segmented labels. The bottleneck residual units make it feasible to train a 49-layer deep encoder. The bilinear scaling of input images serves as a guidance for the decoder network to spatially locate the tumor within a image.

Supporting information
The trained caffe model and all the scrips to train/finetune the network presented in this work are available at: https://github.com/kamleshpawar17/BratsNet-2017

References

1. Louis, D.N., Ohgaki, H., Wiestler, O.D., Cavenee, W.K., Burger, P.C., Jouvet, A., Scheithauer, B.W., Kleihues, P.: The 2007 who classification of tumours of the central nervous system. Acta Neuropathol. **114**(2), 97–109 (2007)
2. Mazzara, G.P., Velthuizen, R.P., Pearlman, J.L., Greenberg, H.M., Wagner, H.: Brain tumor target volume determination for radiation treatment planning through automated MRI segmentation. Int. J. Radiat. Oncol. Biol. Phys. **59**(1), 300–312 (2004)
3. Liu, J., Li, M., Wang, J., Wu, F., Liu, T., Pan, Y.: A survey of MRI-based brain tumor segmentation methods. Tsinghua Sci. Technol. **19**(6), 578–595 (2014)

4. Angelini, E.D., Clatz, O., Mandonnet, E., Konukoglu, E., Capelle, L., Duffau, H.: Glioma dynamics and computational models: a review of segmentation, registration, and in silico growth algorithms and their clinical applications. Current Med. Imaging Rev. **3**(4), 262–276 (2007)
5. Gupta, M.P., Shringirishi, M.M., et al.: Implementation of brain tumor segmentation in brain MR images using K-means clustering and fuzzy C-means algorithm. Int. J. Comput. Technol. **5**(1), 54–59 (2013)
6. Corso, J.J., Sharon, E., Dube, S., El-Saden, S., Sinha, U., Yuille, A.: Efficient multilevel brain tumor segmentation with integrated Bayesian model classification. IEEE Trans. Med. Imaging **27**(5), 629–640 (2008)
7. Sharma, N., Aggarwal, L.M.: Automated medical image segmentation techniques. J. Med. Phys./Assoc. Med. Physicists India **35**(1), 3 (2010)
8. Pham, D.L., Xu, C., Prince, J.L.: Current methods in medical image segmentation. Annu. Rev. Biomed. Eng. **2**(1), 315–337 (2000)
9. Menze, B.H., Jakab, A., Bauer, S., Kalpathy-Cramer, J., Farahani, K., Kirby, J., Burren, Y., Porz, N., Slotboom, J., Wiest, R., Lanczi, L., Gerstner, E., Weber, M.-A., Arbel, T., Avants, B.B., Ayache, N., Buendia, P., Collins, D.L., Cordier, N., Corso, J.J., Criminisi, A., Das, T., Delingette, H., Demiralp, C., Durst, C.R., Dojat, M., Doyle, S., Festa, J., Forbes, F., Geremia, E., Glocker, B., Golland, P., Guo, X., Hamamci, A., Iftekharuddin, K.M., Jena, R., John, N.M., Konukoglu, E., Lashkari, D., Mariz, J.A., Meier, R., Pereira, S., Precup, D., Price, S.J., Raviv, T.R., Reza, S.M.S., Ryan, M., Sarikaya, D., Schwartz, L., Shin, H.-C., Shotton, J., Silva, C.A., Sousa, N., Subbanna, N.K., Szekely, G., Taylor, T.J., Thomas, O.M., Tustison, N.J., Unal, G., Vasseur, F., Wintermark, M., Ye, D.H., Zhao, L., Zhao, B., Zikic, D., Prastawa, M., Reyes, M., Leemput, K.V.: The multimodal brain tumor image segmentation benchmark (brats). IEEE Trans. Med. Imaging **34**(10), 1993–2024 (2015)
10. Bakas, S., Akbari, H., Sotiras, A., Bilello, M., Rozycki, M., Kirby, J., Freymann, J., Farahani, K., Davatzikos, C.: Advancing the cancer genome atlas glioma MRI collections with expert segmentation labels and radiomic features. Nat. Sci. Data **4** (2017)
11. Bakas, S., Sotiras, H., Bilello, M., Kirby, J., Freymann, J., Farahani, K., Davatzikos, C.: Segmentation labels and radiomic features for the pre-operative scans of the TCGA-GBM collection. The Cancer Imaging Archive (2017). https://doi.org/10.7937/K9/TCIA.2017.KLXWJJ1Q
12. Bakas, S., Sotiras, H., Bilello, M., Kirby, J., Freymann, J., Farahani, K., Davatzikos, C.: Segmentation labels and radiomic features for the pre-operative scans of the TCGA-LGG collection. The Cancer Imaging Archive (2017). https://doi.org/10.7937/K9/TCIA.2017.GJQ7R0EF
13. LeCun, Y., Bengio, Y., Hinton, G.: Deep learning. Nature **521**(7553), 436–444 (2015)
14. Schmidhuber, J.: Deep learning in neural networks: an overview. Neural Networks **61**, 85–117 (2015)
15. LeCun, Y., Boser, B.E., Denker, J.S., Henderson, D., Howard, R.E., Hubbard, W.E., Jackel, L.D.: Handwritten digit recognition with a back-propagation network. In: Advances in Neural Information Processing Systems, pp. 396–404 (1990)
16. LeCun, Y., Bottou, L., Bengio, Y., Haffner, P.: Gradient-based learning applied to document recognition. Proc. IEEE **86**(11), 2278–2324 (1998)
17. Krizhevsky, A., Sutskever, I., Hinton, G.E.: ImageNet classification with deep convolutional neural networks. In: Advances in Neural Information Processing Systems, pp. 1097–1105 (2012)

18. Ciregan, D., Meier, U., Schmidhuber, J.: Multi-column deep neural networks for image classification. In: 2012 IEEE Conference on Computer Vision and Pattern Recognition (CVPR), pp. 3642–3649. IEEE (2012)
19. Long, J., Shelhamer, E., Darrell, T.: Fully convolutional networks for semantic segmentation. In: Proceedings of the IEEE Conference on Computer Vision and Pattern Recognition, pp. 3431–3440 (2015)
20. Tajbakhsh, N., Shin, J.Y., Gurudu, S.R., Hurst, R.T., Kendall, C.B., Gotway, M.B., Liang, J.: Convolutional neural networks for medical image analysis: full training or fine tuning? IEEE Trans. Med. Imaging $35(5)$, 1299–1312 (2016)
21. Ioffe, S., Szegedy, C.: Batch normalization: accelerating deep network training by reducing internal covariate shift. In International Conference on Machine Learning, pp. 448–456 (2015)
22. He, K., Zhang, X., Ren, S., Sun, J.: Deep residual learning for image recognition. In: Proceedings of the IEEE Conference on Computer Vision and Pattern Recognition, pp. 770–778 (2016)
23. He, K., Sun, J.: Convolutional neural networks at constrained time cost. In: Proceedings of the IEEE Conference on Computer Vision and Pattern Recognition, pp. 5353–5360 (2015)
24. Srivastava, R.K., Greff, K., Schmidhuber, J.: Training very deep networks. In: Advances in Neural Information Processing Systems, pp. 2377–2385 (2015)
25. Ronneberger, O., Fischer, P., Brox, T.: U-Net: convolutional networks for biomedical image segmentation. In: Navab, N., Hornegger, J., Wells, W.M., Frangi, A.F. (eds.) MICCAI 2015. LNCS, vol. 9351, pp. 234–241. Springer, Cham (2015). https://doi.org/10.1007/978-3-319-24574-4_28
26. Jia, Y., Shelhamer, E., Donahue, J., Karayev, S., Long, J., Girshick, R., Guadarrama, S., Darrell, T.: Caffe: convolutional architecture for fast feature embedding, arXiv preprint arXiv:1408.5093 (2014)
27. Shapira, D., Avidan, S., Hel-Or, Y.: Multiple histogram matching. In: 2013 20th IEEE International Conference on Image Processing (ICIP), pp. 2269–2273. IEEE (2013)

TPCNN: Two-Phase Patch-Based Convolutional Neural Network for Automatic Brain Tumor Segmentation and Survival Prediction

Fan Zhou[2] , Tengfei Li[1], Heng Li[1], and Hongtu Zhu[1,2](✉)

[1] Department of Biostatistics, University of Texas, MD Anderson Cancer Center,
Houston, USA
hzhu5@mdanderson.org
[2] Department of Biostatistics, University of North Carolina at Chapel Hill,
Chapel Hill, USA

Abstract. The aim of this paper is to integrate some advanced statistical methods with modern deep learning methods for tumor segmentation and survival time prediction in the BraTS 2017 challenge. The goals of the BraTS 2017 challenge are to utilize multi-institutional pre-operative MRI scans to segment out different tumor subregions and then to use tumor information to predict patient's overall survival. We build a two-phase patch-based convolutional neural network (TPCNN) model to classify all the pixels in the brain and further refine the segmentation results by using XGBoost and a post-processing procedure. The segmentation results are then used to extract various informative radiomic features for prediction of the survival time by using the XGBoost method.

Keywords: Convolutional neural network · Patch-based · XGBoost

1 Introduction

Brain region segmentation plays an important role in accurate diagnosis and efficient treatment of brain related diseases, such as stroke, Alzheimer, and glioblastoma multiforme, which has received a lot of attention in the field of computer vision, medical image analysis, and cancer imaging. Certain kinds of brain tumors such as gliomas and glioblastomas are often difficult to localize, since they are often diffused, poorly contrasted, and variously shaped without a fixed size or appearing location. Moreover, manual segmentation can be very time consuming and laborious, and therefore there is a great interest in the development of various reliable automatic brain tumor segmentation methods.

The BraTS 2017 challenge is one of such platforms, in which different segmentation methods could be extensively tested and evaluated [6,9,10]. Besides the brain tumor sub-region segmentation competition in previous years' challenges, BraTS 2017 includes an additional task of predicting patient's overall survival time by integrating radiomic features extracted from different imaging

© Springer International Publishing AG, part of Springer Nature 2018
A. Crimi et al. (Eds.): BrainLes 2017, LNCS 10670, pp. 274–286, 2018.
https://doi.org/10.1007/978-3-319-75238-9_24

modalities, locations of different tumor regions, and other demographic information, such as age. A number of segmentation methods have been proposed to integrate information from different imaging modalities for automatic tumor segmentation [13]. For instance, the winner of BraTS 2013 challenge introduced a supervised segmentation framework by using multiple modality intensity, geometry, and asymmetry features, which generate the probability maps of each class by a random-forest algorithm.

With the development of deep learning methods, convolutional neural network has became more and more popular in dealing with the image segmentation problems. [7] divided the whole image of each modality into 33×33 small patches each labeled as the center annotation of the corresponding patch, and generates a single-branch CNN network with six convolutional layers, which achieves good performance on BraTS 2013 data. [3] extended the network to two-branch structure by adding another kind of patches with the same center, but larger patch size as the input, where the two branches were merged together at a certain layer before the final softmax layer. The two branch structure improves the segmentation results compared to the one-branch setting by simultaneously providing a global view and catching the location information of the corresponding pixels. [15] also adopted this two-branch framework, but they added more layers and used conditional random field, which achieve the best performance in the BraTS 2015 challenge.

Different from strategies above which predict a single pixel with a corresponding patch, fully convolutional neural network (FCNN) is proved to be a good deep learning structure in neural image segmentation since it is more efficient by dealing with a small region each time instead of the center only and thus provides a more smooth segmentation results [4]. Moreover, 2D patches are replaced by 3D patches in order to fully exploit dense-inference. However, 3D models have many more parameters compared to 2D models, which may require much longer time to train. Therefore, these kind of 'deep' 3D CNN models are not always acceptable with the limitation in computation power and time. The aim of this paper is to build a two-step strategy, in which the first step is to use a 2D model to mask out the tumor regions, and the second step is to use XGBoost to integrate the results of several simple 2D or 3D models for further refinement [1].

Although there are a lot of efforts in predicting patient's survival by using all kinds of informative radiomic features [5,14], most existing studies only use traditional quantitative features directly calculated from raw images. Little has been done on the use of abstract imaging features learned by deep learning methods for survival prediction. We integrate both quantitative radiomic features and highly abstract imaging features extracted by training a CNN model for predicting the overall survival time. Our final prediction model is built under the framework of XGBoost algorithm, which selects the most significant features, while reducing the potential risk of overfitting caused by the small sample size.

2 Data Description

The BraTS 2017 challenge data set includes subjects from three different resources, which are labeled as '2013', 'CBICA', and 'TCIA'. Specially, in the training data set, there are 20 high-grade gliomas subjects (HGGs) from group '2013', 88 HGGs from group 'CBICA', and 102 HGGs from 'TCIA', whereas 75 other subjects from group '2013' and 'TCIA' are with low-grade gliomas (LGG), which are less aggressive and infiltrative. Each patient has T2-weighted fluid attenuated inversion recovery (Flair), T1-weighted (T1), post-contrast T1-weighted (T1Gd), and T2-weighted (T2) images.

Same as the previous BraTS challenges, a validation data set is provided to test all segmentation methods and tune their associated parameters, while the final prediction on an independent test data set will be used to evaluate the finite sample performance of each participating team. Any information about the HGG/LGG status is unknown about the 46 subjects in the validation data set and the other 146 subject in the test data set.

All the four kinds of MRI scans are roughly registered to a common $240 \times 240 \times 155$ template and resampled at 1 mm resolution level. In the training data set, the annotation of three tumor regions, namely, the GD-enhancing tumor (ET, labeled 4), the peritumoral edema (ED, labeled 2), and the necrotic and non-enhancing tumor (NCR/NET, labeled 1), are provided along with the MRI scans. For the survival time prediction part, age information of 165 selected patients are also provided, which can be combined with the imaging modalities and segmented tumor regions to build and train a survival prediction model. The final predictive model is evaluated using the test data set.

3 Two-Phase Convolutional Neural Network

In this section, we discuss the details of our framework for brain tumor segmentation and how the two-phase procedures work in steps. Specifically, we use a two-branch convolutional neural network with two kinds of input patches in different sizes to briefly mask out the tumor regions, and four other 2D and 3D CNN (FCNN) models to jointly refine the segmentation within the mask determined at the first phase. Furthermore, we also discuss how we do the pre-processing to prepare the data for the deep learning models and post-processing to smooth and optimize the segmentation results.

3.1 Data Preprocessing

We find that due to the multi-institutional data origin, the raw MRI scans from different subjects suffer from varied intensity ranges. To achieve consistency in dynamic range and to ensure comparability across subjects, we use the robust intensity normalization method proposed by [15] to preprocess the images. The details of the procedures are described in the following steps:

1. Linearly transfer the original intensities of each individual MRI scans ($I_1(v)$) to the range between 0 and 255 ($I_2(v)$).
2. Calculate the intensity histogram with 256 bins. Then find the gray-value of highest histogram bin $x \in [0, 255]$ of $I_2(v)$.
3. Calculate the robust deviation which is formulated as $\sigma^2 = [\sum(v_i - x)^2]^{-1}$, $v_i \in I_2(v)$
4. Update the image value by $v_i^* = (v_i - x)/\sigma * c_1 + c_2$
5. Update the image value by $v_i^* = \min(\max(v_i^*, 0), 255)$

Figure 1 demonstrates comparison between before and after preprocessment for T1, FLAIR and T2 (left to right) images of a randomly selected subject.

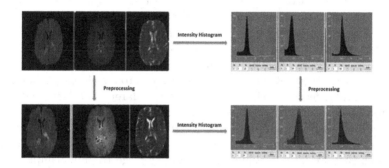

Fig. 1. Visualization of intensities before and after pre-processing

3.2   Method and Framework

After the preprocessing of the raw MRI images, we propose a patch-based two-phase convolutional neural network (TPCNN) to label all the pixels within the brain regions as non-tumor or the three tumor classes: ecrosis core, edema, enhancing core. Specifically, the second-phase could be seen as a conditional optimization procedure, which is to refine the segmentation results within the tumor mask built by the first-phase CNN model.

The input for first-phase CNN model will be the squared patches extracted from the axial slices of the MR images, where the corresponding label for each individual patch will be the label of its center pixel. In the second phase, we only need to pay attention to the regions masked by phase one. Both 3d and 2d models with different architectures and input dimensions are used, so the input patches can not only be the squares like phase one but also be cubics.

Since the four modalities T1, T2, T1Gd and Flair are co-registered to a common template, for pixels at the same location of T1Gd, T2 and Flair, we generate three patches from each of them as the three channels of the input X for the CNN models, where T1 is dropped since the performance of our method with and without T1 do not show much difference and the model with fewer image channels have fewer parameters, which may drastically reduce computational time in training and testing.

In the first phase of our CNN models, we extract patches in two different sizes, where the smaller one is $(18 + 3n) \times (18 + 3n)$ and the larger one is $(35 + 6n) \times (35 + 6n)$, where n here is a kernel parameter, which determines the sizes of the two patches. The reason of this architecture choice is that we want the class prediction of a pixel to be decided by both the local features within a small region around the pixel and the larger 'context': the comparative location of the pixel inside the brain. We adopt the structure of the CNN model described in [15] in the first phase, where the larger input is merged with the small input at a certain layer after passing through several convolutional and pooling layers. The layer settings are shown in Fig. 2. By comparing the mean dice-ratios achieved by different n from experiment, we eventually choose $n = 5$ to be optimal kernel size, with which we are able to roughly mask out the whole tumor regions as the starting point for the second-phase procedure.

One major issue we find with only one-phase CNN model is that we could only briefly mask out the whole tumor region but many non-tumor pixels are misclassified as tumors. Also, the boundaries between different classes are difficult to classify, since pixels belonging to different groups along the boundaries may share similar features when the patch size is large. The high sensitivities of the first-phase results motivate us to add the second phase to refine the segmentation by resampling within the mask built by phase 1 and reduce the patch size to cover more local variations. Another advantage of using the two-phase approach is that we do not require an extremely large training sample at each individual phase which may help reduce the computation cost and save a considerable amount of running time.

We adopt four convolutional neural networks at phase two with different input sizes and try to combine the prediction results by each of them. The first model still uses the same setting as the model in phase 1, but all the sampled points are within six-pixel distance from the tumor mask built by step 1. The second model has a single-size patch input, which is 13 by 13, and we combine classes 1 and 4 into a bigger class which helps us to better determine the regions of tumor core.

The third and fourth models jump from 2D models to 3D ones, and adopts the FCNN setting instead of labeling only the center of the corresponding input patch. For the third model, we choose the patch size to be $25 \times 25 \times 25$, with 8 convolutional layers of kernel size being $3 \times 3 \times 3$, and 3 convolutional layers with $1 \times 1 \times 1$ kernel size after that before the final softmax layer which produces the probability map in a $9 \times 9 \times 9$ region. This model enables us to get the labeling of the $9 \times 9 \times 9$ pixels around the center of the input $25 \times 25 \times 25$ cubic other than predicting only the center of input patch as the normal CNN model. The numbers of filters for the first 8 convolutional layers are 30, 30, 40, 40, 40, 50, 50, 50 and for the latter 3 convolutional layers are 400, 200, 150. We pick $3 \times 3 \times 3$ because replacing one convolutional layer with $5 \times 5 \times 5$ kernel by two layers with $3 \times 3 \times 3$ kernel can do the same dimension reduction but having much fewer parameters to estimate during the training process to the model with $5 \times 5 \times 5$ ones, which meets our aim of using simple but efficient model design.

The fourth model still uses the FCNN architecture but the size of input patch becomes $13 \times 13 \times 13$ and the output size is reduced to $3 \times 3 \times 3$, with five convolutional layers of $5 \times 5 \times 5$ kernel. The smaller input and output sizes may help catch more local features compared to the third model.

To combine the results of the four models used in phase2, we extract the probability of the four classes non-tumor, necrosis core, edema, enhancing core at each pixel predicted by each individual method as the candidate 'voters' and then use XGBoost to train a classification model and decide the important probabilities by cross-validation to refine the pixel-level classification. Specifically, all the sample points used by XGBoost here are selected from those pixels which have different prediction labels by the four CNN (FCNN) models in phase 2. Our empirical results shows that XGBoost could do a better job in combing the prediction results of the four models than the majority voting or averaging their probabilities. The framework diagram of our method is depicted in Fig. 2 and illustrated in Fig. 3 by one example, which shows how the initial segmentation is improved after each segmentation step.

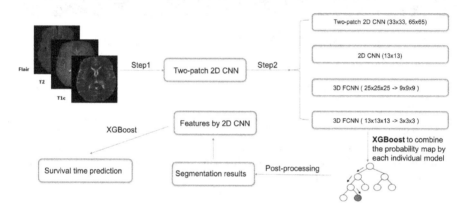

Fig. 2. Framework of TPCNN procedure

3.3 Post-processing

After using XGBoost to refine the results by combing several models in phase 2, we further improve the segmentation results by employing the following post-processing techniques. The idea is to fill in the holes and delete the small isolated clusters which are proved useful by [15]:

1. Segment the tumor mask into all connected components/clusters. Voxels in clusters whose volume is less than 0.2 times the largest connected cluster volume will be reclassified as non-tumor.
2. Segment the enhancing core mask into all connected components/clusters. Voxels in clusters whose volume is less than 0.01 times the largest connected cluster volume will be reclassified as the necrosis.

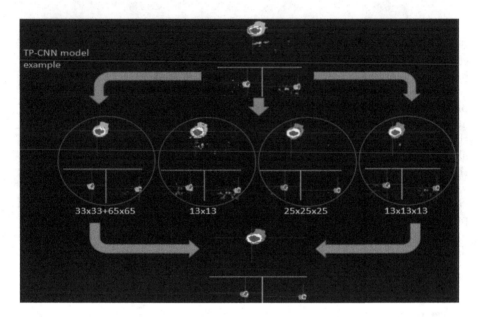

Fig. 3. Example segmentation through TPCNN procedure

3. Fill in the holes within the tumor mask and assign voxels within the holes to necrosis area.

By comparing the dice-ratios of the defined tumor sub-regions by our TPCNN model with and without the three-step post-processing, we find that the performance could be improved by applying the post-processing on the existing TPCNN results after the two-phase prediction.

4   CNN-Based Survival Time Prediction

The basic idea of our procedure to do the overall survival prediction with the brain scans is to extract the important features by training a CNN model whose input is a selected axial slice with biggest tumor regions for each subject. Continuous survival time of training subjects is divided into three categories ($<15, 10-15$ and >15) for the CNN model training. After the training is done, the last fully-connected layer before the softmax layer is considered as important features, which will be incorporated with age and some other quantitive features to predict the survival time by XGBoost regression model.

XGBoost is short for Extreme 'Gradient Boosting', where the term 'Gradient Boosting' is proposed in the paper Greedy Function Approximation: A Gradient Boosting Machine, by Friedman [2]. In brief, XGBoost is a tree-based boosting algorithm, which performs well in supervised learning problems and previous challenges. The advantage of using XGBoost here to predict the survival time for each patient is that we could throw out the unimportant features by based on AUC value and avoid over-fitting.

We extract various quantitative imaging features directly from the tumor regions of the brain scans by simply measuring the shape, volume or other potentially important parameters as predictors to add in the survival time prediction model. Among these features, nine are describing the shape of the tumor regions, including the volume of the whole tumor, superficial area of the whole tumor, roundness and ratio between different subregions. In the training data set, all these features are computed based on the provided true annotations, but only using the segmentation results by our TPCNN model discussed in last section for the subjects in validation set. We also consider other 10 intensity statistics features (such as maximum, minimum, median, kurtosis), 57 texture features(13 gray-level co-occurrence matrix features, 8 statistics of local binary patterns and 36 threshold adjacency statistics) and 72 wavelet transform features, all of which are computed according to the tumor subregions from the corresponding modality.

Besides the global feature mentioned above, we also train a 2D convolutional neural network and extract the last dense layer as supplementary features. We take five successive 2-D slices in X-Y space with the largest number pixels belonging to class 1 and 4 for each of T1Gd, T2 and Flair scan as the three input channels. Considering the small sample size we have for the survival time prediction task (163 subjects in the training set with survival time information), we augment the sample by flipping, rotating and doing pixel shifting to the original five slides for each subject. According to the evaluation scheme based on classification principle, the continuous survival time will be divided into three groups, i.e. long-survivors (e.g., ≥ 15 months), short-survivors (e.g., ≤ 10 months), and mid-survivors (e.g. between 10 and 15 months). So we do the same way to divide the survival time for all the subjects into three classes, which are used as output to train a 2D-CNN model by borrowing the VGG-16 setting [11] and extract the dense layer before the softmax layer as the hidden image features, which will be combined with the global features and age for each subject as predictors to build the final prediction model (Fig. 4).

We also try to move to 3D CNN model instead of the current 2D to extract the feature within the tumor regions roughly masked out by segmentation results because the way we use to select 2-D slices depend more on the accuracy of segmentation predictions on validation data. However, according to the results of empirical study, the features by 3D model does not work better than those by 2D model, so we keep the 2D setting which may also help reduce a lot of computational complexity.

Before building the XGBoost prediction model, we first use Pearson chi-square test to analyze the marginal correlation between all the candidate predictors with the survival time, and sort them by p-value from small to large, where the covariate with smaller p-value may show more significant association with the survival time, and we then use the XGBoost to gradually add in covariates until the mean squared error value will not decrease after a certain

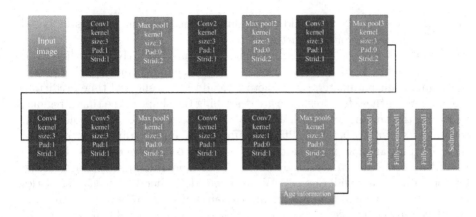

Fig. 4. 2D CNN architecture to extract important image features for survival time prediction

number of steps. To test the performance of our model, we still randomly split the training data into two parts, one of which is used to train the model and the other used to evaluate the prediction accuracy. We do 10-fold cross-validation to test the performance of our method and use the classification evaluation by dividing the survival time into three classes using threshold 10 and 15 to compute the prediction accuracy. According to the results of cross-validation, the whole tumor volume, the tumor core (necrosis core plus enhancing core) volume, the enhancing tumor volume, the longest diameter along the X-Y and X-Z space, supplementary 120 latent features achieved by CNN model are considered important and selected out, which are used to train the final model with all the training subjects to predict the survival time of subjects in validation and testing data set.

5   Empirical Study

We use the BraTS 2017 data set to test the performance of our method. We include all the 285 released subjects in the training data set to generate the training sample for phase 1 and phase 2. In particular, we split the whole training set into a sub-training set which is used to train the two-patch CNN model in the first phase and the four 2D or 3D CNN (FCNN) models in phase 2, and a sub-testing set used to validate the performance of the trained model. Specifically, the sub-training set contains 200 subjects while the other 85 subjects make up the sub-testing set. To guarantee the validation of the sub-testing data, we include 50 LGG subjects in the sub-training set and the other 25 in the sub-testing set to make sure that the proportions of LGG and HGG subjects are roughly the same in both sides.

In phase 1, we pick out 100 subjects from all the five groups, and within each of the four classes randomly sample 500 pixels from each of the four classes as the centers to generate the 33×33 and 65×65 patches around them for each of the three modalities T2, T1Gd and Flair, where the two sizes are determined by our experiment when comparing with other sizes. The total sample size will be around $2 \times 100 \times 4 \times 1000$ where non-tumor and background pixels are combined into one class. There are many more pixels belonging to the non-tumor class in brain regions, but we sample equal number for the four classes to avoid the unbalanced bias. We do not use T1 here since the prediction result is not significantly improved when it was added in, which may occupy more computation resources and increase the running time. Besides the two kinds of input patches with different sizes as the three-channel input, we also record the label of the center voxel for each patch as the output to train the model.

At each training epoch, a small sample consists of 200 randomly selected patches (100 for each size) is used to update the model parameters. The learning rate is set to be 10^{-3} at first and then reduced to 10^{-4} after several epochs. The training process is terminated until the overall prediction accuracy of the sub-testing set when applied the updated model does not change within 20 successive training epochs.

In phase 2, within the mask built by the two-branch CNN model in phase 1, we sample the same number of patches as phase one for the first two models, while for the third and fourth 3D FCNN model, we only sample 100 patches for each class and each subject because of the memory limitation of the machines since the 3D patches takes much more space than a 2D patch. As comparison with the performance achieved by phase-one model only, we still use the same sub-training and sub-testing sets divided before the first stage. For all these four CNN (FCNN) models with different settings, we still initialize the learning rate as 10^{-3}, which will be reduced to 10^{-4} after several epochs and choose the batch size as 100. Early stopping is also applied when the performance on the sub-testing set does not improve within 20 epochs.

After training and validating the model by using the 285 training subjects, we apply the saved optimal model on the validation data which is separated from the whole training set to test the transferring ability of our model. Different from the training subjects, all the 46 subjects in the validation set do not provide the information that whether they are classified as LGG or HGG. More HGG or LGG proportions of the validation set compared to the training set may result in the lower prediction accuracy since the important features may be changed. The performance by phase-one CNN only, phase-two CNN only and our TPCNN method is shown in Table 1 in terms of the dice-ratio of each tumor regions, corresponding sensitivities and 'Hausdorff distance' statistic.

All the training and predictions are done by using a GPU sever with Nvidia K80 cards, 2496 CUDA cores, and 12 GB RAMs. The training of Phase 1 takes around 6–7 h when taking around 500 epochs until the loss value does not change within 20 successive steps. The four models in phase 2 will only take 2–3 h before we terminate the training, which costs much less time compared with the models with more complicated structures.

Table 1. Results comparison among step1, step2 and final combined two-phase results

Method	Dice_ET	Dice_WT	Dice_TC	Sensitivity_ET	Sensitivity_WT	Sensitivity_TC
Phase1	0.472	0.630	0.526	0.722	0.921	0.668
Phase2 Model1	0.594	0.832	0.670	0.674	0.911	0.759
Phase2 Model2	0.632	0.843	0.654	0.669	0.813	0.716
Phase2 Model3	0.670	0.856	0.670	0.767	0.856	0.719
Phase2 Model4	0.620	0.818	0.658	0.787	0.915	0.743
TP-CNN XGBoost	0.730	0.880	0.722	0.783	0.916	0.789

For the task of survival time prediction. We do 10-fold cross validation with the training data to test the performance of our approach and the highest prediction among the 10-times could reach 85% and the mean accuracy is around 74% (while the lowest accuracy could be around 60%). The average MSE (mean square error) of the 10-times experiments is around 89572.0. Then we use all the 160 subjects from the training sample to train the model and make predictions for the 33 validation subjects based on our segmentation results and the results are shown in Table 2.

Table 2. Evaluation of the survival prediction model by cross-validation

Survival Prediction	Accuracy	MSE	MedianSE	stdSE	SpearmanR
	0.636	216572.0	44742.6	475483.1	0.38

6 Conclusion and Discussion

Our two-phase convolutional neural network together with the XGBoost and postprocessing refinement is an automatic brain tumor segmentation method using deep learning. According to the performance of our method on the validation data set, our method could make an acceptable segmentation prediction for the non-tumor and three tumor regions in terms of dice-ratio and Hausdorff distance. One advantage is that we could achieve a high sensitivity, which means that we do not have much tumor regions to be considered as non-tumor part. Another important characteristic of our method is that we adopt some models with complicated structures, which may require a lot of computation power, but to combine the results from several simple models by using XGBoost, which is much cheaper in time consuming and machine cost. For the survival time prediction task, we use CNN model to extract the features from each of the four modalities and then use XGBoost to build the regression model, which could provide a relatively good prediction accuracy considering the small sample size we have.

We have to admit that there are several obvious weaknesses of our method. First, the pixel-based prediction procedure may result in some singular points with a misclassified label within a regions having correct predictions, which may cause a huge reduction in the tumor core dice-ratio. Second, compared with U-Net [8] or other slice-based method, our TPCNN model could not acquire a smooth segmentation results, even though it can be improved by doing post-processing. Third, we only use simple post-processing procedures to refine the segmentation acquired by the two-phase CNN model, while some other more complicated techniques such as Conditional Random Filed (CRF) [12] are proved to greatly improve the results. Fourth, with the limitation in the machine memory, we do not sample enough patches for each individual subject compared to the total number of pixels from a corresponding modality, which may affect the power of the trained model in predicting the validation and testing data set. Despite these potential disadvantages, the simple structure and the combining idea of our method will still be valuable when there are limited computing power and time, to build a reasonable results in segmenting tumor regions and predicting survival time of patients.

References

1. Chen, T., Guestrin, C.: XGBoost: a scalable tree boosting system. In: Proceedings of the 22nd ACM SIGKDD International Conference on Knowledge Discovery and Data Mining, pp. 785–794. ACM (2016)
2. Friedman, J.H.: Greedy function approximation: a gradient boosting machine. Ann. Stat. **29**, 1189–1232 (2001)
3. Havaei, M., Davy, A., Warde-Farley, D., Biard, A., Courville, A., Bengio, Y., Pal, C., Jodoin, P.-M., Larochelle, H.: Brain tumor segmentation with deep neural networks. Med. Image Anal. **35**, 18–31 (2017)
4. Kamnitsas, K., Ledig, C., Newcombe, V.F.J., Simpson, J.P., Kane, A.D., Menon, D.K., Rueckert, D., Glocker, B.: Efficient multi-scale 3D CNN with fully connected CRF for accurate brain lesion segmentation. Med. Image Anal. **36**, 61–78 (2017)
5. Liu, Y., Xu, X., Yin, L., Zhang, X., Li, L., Lu, H.: Relationship between Glioblastoma Heterogeneity and survival time: an MR imaging texture analysis. Am. J. Neuroradiol. **38**, 1695–1701 (2017)
6. Menze, B.H., Jakab, A., Bauer, S., Kalpathy-Cramer, J., Farahani, K., Kirby, J., Burren, Y., Porz, N., Slotboom, J., Wiest, R., et al.: The multimodal brain tumor image segmentation benchmark (BRATS). IEEE Trans. Med. Imaging **34**(10), 1993–2024 (2015)
7. Pereira, S., Pinto, A., Alves, V., Silva, C.A.: Brain tumor segmentation using convolutional neural networks in MRI images. IEEE Trans. Med. Imaging **35**(5), 1240–1251 (2016)
8. Ronneberger, O., Fischer, P., Brox, T.: U-Net: convolutional networks for biomedical image segmentation. In: Navab, N., Hornegger, J., Wells, W.M., Frangi, A.F. (eds.) MICCAI 2015. LNCS, vol. 9351, pp. 234–241. Springer, Cham (2015). https://doi.org/10.1007/978-3-319-24574-4_28
9. Bakas, S., Sotiras, A., Akbari, H., Rozycki, M., Bilello, M., Kirby, J., Freymann, J., Farahani, K., Davatzikos, C.: Segmentation labels and radiomic features for the pre-operative scans of the TCGA-GBM collection. The Cancer Imaging Archive (2017)

10. Bakas, S., Akbari, H., Bilello, M., Sotiras, A., Rozycki, M., Freymann, J.B., Kirby, J.S., Farahani, K., Davatzikos, C.: Advancing the Cancer Genome Atlas glioma MRI collections with expert segmentation labels and radiomic features. Nature Scientific Data (2017)
11. Simonyan, K., Zisserman, A.: Very deep convolutional networks for large-scale image recognition. arXiv preprint arXiv:1409.1556 (2014)
12. Sutton, C., McCallum, A., et al.: An introduction to conditional random fields. Found. Trends®in Mach. Learn. 4(4), 267–373 (2012)
13. Tustison, N.J., Shrinidhi, K.L., Wintermark, M., Durst, C.R., Kandel, B.M., Gee, J.C., Grossman, M.C., Avants, B.B.: Optimal symmetric multimodal templates and concatenated random forests for supervised brain tumor segmentation (simplified) with ANTsR. Neuroinformatics 13(2), 209–225 (2015)
14. Wangaryattawanich, P., Wang, J., Thomas, G.A., Chaddad, A., Zinn, P.O., Colen, R.R.: Survival analysis of pre-operative GBM patients by using quantitative image features. In: 2014 International Conference on Control, Decision and Information Technologies (CoDIT), pp. 625–627. IEEE (2014)
15. Zhao, X., Wu, Y., Song, G., Li, Z., Zhang, Y., Fan, Y.: A deep learning model integrating FCNNs and CRFs for brain tumor segmentation. arXiv preprint arXiv:1702.04528 (2017)

Brain Tumor Segmentation and Radiomics Survival Prediction: Contribution to the BRATS 2017 Challenge

Fabian Isensee[1](✉), Philipp Kickingereder[2], Wolfgang Wick[3],
Martin Bendszus[2], and Klaus H. Maier-Hein[1]

[1] Division of Medical Image Computing, German Cancer Research Center (DKFZ),
Heidelberg, Germany
f.isensee@dkfz-heidelberg.de
[2] Department of Neuroradiology, Heidelberg University Hospital,
Heidelberg, Germany
[3] Neurology Clinic, Heidelberg University Hospital, Heidelberg, Germany

Abstract. Quantitative analysis of brain tumors is critical for clinical decision making. While manual segmentation is tedious, time consuming and subjective, this task is at the same time very challenging to solve for automatic segmentation methods. In this paper we present our most recent effort on developing a robust segmentation algorithm in the form of a convolutional neural network. Our network architecture was inspired by the popular U-Net and has been carefully modified to maximize brain tumor segmentation performance. We use a dice loss function to cope with class imbalances and use extensive data augmentation to successfully prevent overfitting. Our method beats the current state of the art on BraTS 2015, is one of the leading methods on the BraTS 2017 validation set (dice scores of 0.896, 0.797 and 0.732 for whole tumor, tumor core and enhancing tumor, respectively) and achieves very good Dice scores on the test set (0.858 for whole, 0.775 for core and 0.647 for enhancing tumor). We furthermore take part in the survival prediction subchallenge by training an ensemble of a random forest regressor and multilayer perceptrons on shape features describing the tumor subregions. Our approach achieves 52.6% accuracy, a Spearman correlation coefficient of 0.496 and a mean square error of 209607 on the test set.

Keywords: CNN · Brain tumor · Glioblastoma · Deep learning

1 Introduction

Quantitative assessment of brain tumors provides valuable information and therefore constitutes an essential part of diagnostic procedures. Automatic segmentation is attractive in this context, as it allows for faster, more objective and potentially more accurate description of relevant tumor parameters, such as the volume of its subregions. Due to the irregular nature of tumors, however, the development of algorithms capable of automatic segmentation remains challenging.

© Springer International Publishing AG, part of Springer Nature 2018
A. Crimi et al. (Eds.): BrainLes 2017, LNCS 10670, pp. 287–297, 2018.
https://doi.org/10.1007/978-3-319-75238-9_25

The brain tumor segmentation challenge (BraTS) [1] aims at encouraging the development of state of the art methods for tumor segmentation by providing a large dataset of annotated low grade gliomas (LGG) and high grade glioblastomas (HGG). Unlike the previous years, the BraTS 2017 training dataset, which consists of 210 HGG and 75 LGG cases, was annotated manually by one to four raters and all segmentations were approved by expert raters [2–4]. For each patient a T1 weighted, a post-contrast T1-weighted, a T2-weighted and a FLAIR MRI was provided. The MRI originate from 19 institutions and were acquired with different protocols, magnetic field strengths and MRI scanners. Each tumor was segmented into edema (label 2), necrosis and non-enhancing tumor (label 1) and active/enhancing tumor (label 4). The segmentation performance of participating algorithms is measured based on the DICE coefficient, sensitivity, specificity and Hausdorff distance. Additional to the segmentation challenge, BraTS 2017 also required participants to develop an algorithm for survival prediction. For this purpose the survival (in days) of 163 training cases was provided as well.

Inspired by the recent success of convolutional neural networks, an increasing number of deep learning based automatic segmentation algorithms have been proposed. Havaei et al. [5] use a multi-scale architecture by combining features from pathways with different filter sizes. They furthermore improve their results by cascading their models. Pereira et al. [6] stack more convolutional layers with smaller (3×3) filter sizes. They develop separate networks for segmenting low grade and high grade glioblastomas (LGG and HGG, respectively). Their LGG network consists of 4 convolutional layers, followed by two dense and a classification network. The HGG network is composed of 7 convolutional layers. Both [5,6] use 2D convolutions. Kamnitsas et al. [7] proposed a fully connected multiscale CNN that was among the first to employ 3D convolutions. It comprises a high resolution and a low resolution pathway that are recombined to form the final segmentation output. For their submission to the brain tumor segmentation challenge in 2016 [8], they enhanced their architecture through the addition of residual connections, yielding minor improvements. They addressed the class imbalance problem through a sophisticated training data sampling strategy. Kayalibay et al. [9] developed very successful adaptation of the popular U-Net architecture [10] and achieved state of the art results for the BraTS 2015 dataset. Notably, they employed a Jaccard loss function that intrinsically handles class imbalances. They make use of the large receptive field of their architecture to process entire patients at once, at the cost of being able to train with only one patient per batch.

Here we propose our contribution to the BraTS 2017 challenge that is also based on the popular U-Net architecture [10]. Being both based on the U-Net, our network architecture shares some similarities with [9]. However, there are a multitude of different design choices that me made regarding the exact architecture of the context pathway, normalization schemes, number of feature maps throughout the network, nonlinearity and the structure of the upsampling pathway. Particularly through optimizing the number of feature maps in the localization pathway, our network uses twice as many filters than [9] while being trained with only a slightly smaller input patch size and a larger batch size. We furthermore employ a multiclass adaptation of the dice loss [11] and make extensive use of data augmentation.

Image based tumor phenotyping and derived clinically relevant parameters such as predicted survival is typically done by means of radiomics. Intensity, shape and texture features are thereby computed from segmentation masks of the tumor subregions and subsequently used to train a machine learning algorithm. These features may also be complemented by other measures handcrafted to the problem at hand, such as the distance of the tumor to the ventricles and critical structures in the brain [12]. Although our main focus was put on the segmentation part of the challenge, we developed a simple radiomics based approach combined with a random forest regressor and a multilayer perceptron ensemble for survival prediction.

2   Methods

2.1   Segmentation

Data Preprocessing. With MRI intensity values being non standardized, normalization is critical to allow for data from different institutes, scanners and acquired with varying protocols to be processed by one single algorithm. This is particularly true for neural networks where imaging modalities are typically treated as color channels. Here we need to ensure that the value ranges match not only between patients but between the modalities as well in order to avoid initial biases of the network. We found the following simple workflow to work surprisingly well. First, we normalize each modality of each patient independently by subtracting the mean and dividing by the standard deviation of the brain region. We then clip the resulting images at $[-5, 5]$ to remove outliers and subsequently rescale to $[0, 1]$, with the non-brain region being set to 0.

Network Architecture. Our network is inspired by the U-Net architecture [10]. We designed the network to process large 3D input blocks of $128 \times 128 \times 128$ voxels. In contrast to many previous approaches who manually combined different input resolutions or pathways with varying filter sizes, the U-Net based approach allows the network to intrinsically recombine different scales throughout the entire network.

Just like the U-Net, our architecture comprises a context aggregation pathway that encodes increasingly abstract representations of the input as we progress deeper into the network, followed by a localization pathway that recombines these representations with shallower features to precisely localize the structures of interest. We refer to the vertical depth (the depth in the U shape) as level, with higher levels being lower spatial resolution, but higher dimensional feature representations.

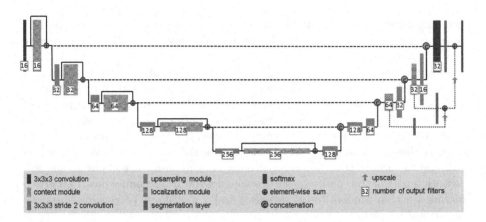

Fig. 1. Network architecture. Our architecture is derived from the U-Net [10]. The context pathway (left) aggregates high level information that is subsequently localized precisely in the localization pathway (right). Inspired by [9] we inject gradient signals deep into the network through deep supervision.

The activations in the context pathway are computed by context modules. Each context module is in fact a pre-activation residual block [13] with two $3 \times 3 \times 3$ convolutional layers and a dropout layer ($p_{\text{drop}} = 0.3$) in between. Context modules are connected by $3 \times 3 \times 3$ convolutions with input stride 2 to reduce the resolution of the feature maps and allow for more features while descending down the aggregation pathway.

As stated previously, the localization pathway is designed to take features from lower levels of the network that encode contextual information at low spatial resolution and transfer that information to a higher spatial resolution. This is achieved by first upsampling the low resolution feature maps, which is done by means of a simple upscale that repeats the feature voxels twice in each spatial dimension, followed by a $3 \times 3 \times 3$ convolution that halves the number of feature maps. Compared to the more frequently employed transposed convolution we found this approach to deliver similar performance while preventing checkerboard artifacts in the network output. We then recombine the upsampled features with the features from the corresponding level of the context aggregation pathway via concatenation. Following the concatenation, a localization module recombines these features together. It also further reduces the number of feature maps which is critical for reducing memory consumption. A localization module consists of a $3 \times 3 \times 3$ convolution followed by a $1 \times 1 \times 1$ convolution that halves the number of feature maps.

Inspired by [9] we employ deep supervision in the localization pathway by integrating segmentation layers at different levels of the network and combining them via elementwise summation to form the final network output. Throughout the network we use leaky ReLU nonlinearities with a negative slope of 10^{-2} for all feature map computing convolutions. We furthermore replace the traditional batch with instance normalization [14] since we found that the stochasticity induced by our small batch sizes may destabilize batch normalization.

Training Procedure. Our network architecture is trained with randomly sampled patches of size $128 \times 128 \times 128$ voxels and batch size 2. We refer to an epoch as an iteration over 100 batches and train for a total of 300 epochs. Training is done using the adam optimizer [15] with an initial learning rate $lr_{init} = 5 \cdot 10^{-4}$, the following learning rate schedule: $lr_{init} \cdot 0.985^{epoch}$ and a l2 weight decay of 10^{-5}.

One challenge in medical image segmentation is the class imbalance in the data that hampers the training when using the conventional categorical crossentropy loss. In the BraTS 2017 training data for example, there is 166 times as much background (label 0) as there is enhancing tumor (label 4). We approach this issue by formulating a multiclass Dice loss function, similar to the one employed in [11], that is differentiable and can be easily integrated into deep learning frameworks:

$$\mathcal{L}_{dc} = -\frac{2}{|K|} \sum_{k \in K} \frac{\sum_i u_{i,k} v_{i,k}}{\sum_i u_{i,k} + \sum_i v_{i,k}} \tag{1}$$

where u is the softmax output of the network and v is a one hot encoding of the ground truth segmentation map. Both u and v have shape I by K with $i \in I$ being the voxels in the training patch and $k \in K$ being the classes. $u_{i,k}$ and $v_{i,k}$ denote the softmax output and ground truth for class k at voxel i, respectively.

When training large neural networks from limited training data, special care has to be taken to prevent overfitting. We address this problem by utilizing a large variety of data augmentation techniques. Whenever possible, we initialize these techniques using aggressive parameters that we subsequently attenuate over the course of the training. The following augmentation techniques were applied on the fly during training: random rotations, random scaling, random elastic deformations, gamma correction augmentation and mirroring.

The fully convolutional nature of our network allows to process arbitrarily sized inputs. At test time we therefore segment an entire patient at once, alleviating problems that may arise when computing the segmentation in tiles with a network that has padded convolutions. We furthermore use test time data augmentation by mirroring the images and averaging the softmax outputs over several dropout samples.

2.2 Survival Prediction

The task of survival prediction underpins the clinical relevance of the BraTS challenge, but at the same time is very challenging, particularly due to the absence of treatment information and the small size of the available dataset. For this subchallenge, only the image information and the age of the patients was provided.

Our approach to survival prediction is based on radiomics. We characterize the tumors using image based features that are computed on the segmentation masks. We compute shape features (13 features), first order statistics (19 features) and gray level co-occurence matrix features (28 features) with the pyradiomics package [16]. The tumor regions for which we computed the features were the edema (ede), enhancing tumor (enh), necrosis (nec), tumor core (core) and whole tumor (whole). We computed only shape features for edema and the whole tumor, shape and first order features for tumor core and the entire feature set for non-enhancing and necrosis and enhancing tumor. With the image features being computed for all modalities, we extracted a total of 517 features.

These features are then used for training a regression ensemble for survival prediction. Random forests are well established in the radiomics community for performing well, especially when many features but only few training data are available. These properties make random forest regressors the prime choice for the scenario at hand (518 features, 163 training cases). We train a random forest regressor (RFR) with 1000 trees and the mean squared error as split criterion. Additionally, we designed an ensemble of small multilayer perceptrons (MLP) to complement the output of the regression forest. The ensemble consists of 15 MLPs, each with 3 hidden layers, 64 units per layer and trained with a mean squared error loss function. We use batch normalization, dropout ($p_{drop} = 0.5$) and add gaussian noise ($\mu = 0, \sigma = 0.1$) in each hidden layer. The outputs of the RFR and the MLP ensemble are averaged to obtain our final prediction.

3 Results

3.1 Segmentation

We trained and evaluated our architecture on the BraTS 2017 and 2015 training datasets via five fold cross-validation. No external data was used and the networks were trained from scratch. Furthermore, we used the five networks obtained by the corresponding cross-validation as an ensemble to predict the respective validation (BraTS 2017) and test (BraTS 2015 and 2017) set. Both the training set and validation/test set results were evaluated using the online evaluation platforms to ensure comparability with other participants.

Table 1 compares the performance of our algorithm to other state of the art methods on the BraTS 2015 test set. Our method compares favorably to other state of the art neural networks and is currently ranked first in the BraTS 2015 test set online leaderboard. In Table 2 we show an overview over the segmentation performance of our model on the BraTS 2017 dataset.

Table 1. BraTS 2015 test set results. We used the five models obtained by training a five fold cross-validation on the BraTS 2015 training data as an ensemble.

	Dice			Sensitivity			PPV		
	whole	core	enh.	whole	core	enh.	whole	core	enh.
Kamnitsas et al. [7]	**0.85**	0.67	0.63	0.88	0.60	0.67	**0.85**	**0.86**	**0.63**
Kayalibay et al. [9]	**0.85**	0.72	0.61	**0.91**	**0.73**	0.67	0.82	0.77	0.61
Ours	**0.85**	**0.74**	**0.64**	**0.91**	**0.73**	**0.72**	0.83	0.80	**0.63**

Table 2. Results for the BraTS 2017 dataset. Train: 5 fold cross-validation on the training data (285 cases). Val: Result on the validation dataset using the five models from the training cross-validation as an ensemble (46 cases).

Dataset	Dice			Sensitivity			Specificity			Hausdorff Dist.		
	whole	core	enh.	whole	core	enh.	whole	core	enh.	whole	core	enh.
BraTS 2017 Train	0.895	0.828	0.707	0.890	0.831	0.800	0.995	0.997	0.998	6.04	6.95	6.24
BraTS 2017 Val	0.896	0.797	0.732	0.896	0.781	0.790	0.996	0.999	0.998	6.97	9.48	4.55

Qualitative segmentation results are presented in Figs. 2 and 3. Our network is capable of accurately segmenting large tumor regions (such as the necrotic cores in Fig. 2) as well as fine grained details (scattered necrotic regions in the tumor core). Note how the thin wall of the enhancing region in the uppermost part of the tumor in Fig. 2 was segmented with voxel-level accuracy whereas the manual ground truth label spilled into the bordering edema region. Furthermore, the small spot of enhancing tumor that is surrounded by edema in the ground truth segmentation can, upon closer inspection of the raw data (see patient Brats17_TCIA_469_1), be identified as a blood vessel that has been erroneously included in the enhancing tumor region by the annotator. Figure 3 demonstrates the main mode of error of our model. The former non-enhancing tumor label, which was integrated into the necrosis label for the BraTS 2017 challenge, is often not well defined in the training data. As a result, our algorithm learns where to predict this label from the context rather than based on image evidence and seems to sometimes guess where to place it.

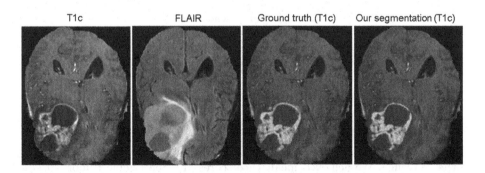

Fig. 2. Qualitative segmentation result. Our approach is capable of segmenting the large necrotic cores while also detecting the small structures within the tumor core. Edema is shown in blue, enhancing tumor in green and non-enhancing and necrotic tumor in red. (Color figure online)

T1c   FLAIR   Ground truth (T1c)   Our segmentation (T1c)

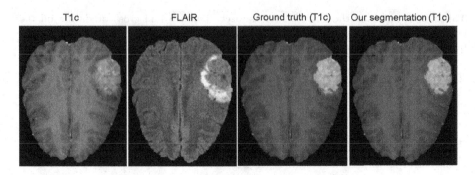

Fig. 3. The most prominent mode of error for the tumor core is the non enhancing tumor region. Edema is shown in blue, enhancing tumor in green and non-enhancing and necrotic tumor in red. (Color figure online)

Quantitatively, we achieve Dice scores of 0.896, 0.797 and 0.732 for whole, core and enhancing, respectively, on the BraTS 2017 validation set. This result places us among the best performing methods according to the online validation leaderboard. When comparing these values to the Dice scores achieved on the training set (0.895, 0.828, 0.707) we conclude that our model, together with the extensive data augmentation used during training, does not overfit to the training dataset. We purposefully did not submit more than once to the validation set in order to ensure that we do not overfit by adapting our hyper parameters to the validation data.

Table 3. BraTS 2017 test set results. The scores were computed by the organizers of the challenge based on our submitted segmentations.

	Dice		
	enh.	whole	core
Mean	0.647	0.858	0.775
StdDev.	0.326	0.161	0.269
Median	0.795	0.910	0.886
25 quantile	0.619	0.856	0.764
75 quantile	0.863	0.940	0.932

Table 3 shows the test set results as reported back to us by the organizers of the challenge. We achieved mean Dice scores of 0.858 (whole tumor), 0.775 (tumor core) and 0.647 (enhancing tumor). These scores are lower than the ones obtained on either training or validation set, which is surprising provided that we did not observe overfitting during training and on the validation set. Based on the high median Dice scores we hypothesize that the test set contained a significant number of very difficult cases. Also, we are uncertain how cases with no enhancing tumor in the ground truth segmentation are aggregated into the mean since their Dice score is always zero by definition.

3.2   Survival Prediction

We extensively evaluated the components of our regression ensemble as well as different feature sets with the aim of minimizing the mean squared error by running 5-fold cross-validations on the 163 provided training cases. A summary of our findings for both the ground truth and our segmentations is shown in Table 4. We observed that the random forest regressor performs very well across all feature sets while the MLP ensemble is much less stable with an increasing number of features. The overall best results were obtained by averaging the MLP ensemble output with the one from the random forest regressor (column *combined*) and using only shape features and the age of a patient. Interestingly, while the random forest performance is almost identical between ground truth and our segmentations, the MLP ensemble performs better on our segmentations for all feature sets, which is also reflected by the *combined* results. The best root mean squared error we achieved was 335.08 (mean absolute error 232.76) in a five-fold cross-validation on the training set. On the test set we obtained 457.83 RMSE (MSE 209607), an accuracy of 52.6% and a Spearman correlation coefficient of 0.496.

Table 4. Survival prediction experiments. We trained a random forest regressor (RFR) and a MLP ensemble (MLP ens). Averaging the regression outputs of the RFR and MLP ensemble yields the *combined* result. The best root mean squared error is achieved when using RFR and MLP ensemble together with only shape features and the patients age.

Features	Ground truth segmentation			Our segmentation		
	RFR	MLP ens	combined	RFR	MLP ens	combined
shape, age (66)	344.89	**352.00**	**339.61**	353.12	**343.19**	**335.08**
glcm, age (225)	348.14	462.16	381.25	350.78	388.99	357.41
first order, age (229)	358.69	388.44	362.20	354.66	381.42	355.89
shape, glcm, age (290)	**344.86**	431.96	367.14	**346.40**	378.73	349.13
shape, first order, age (294)	352.64	372.59	350.62	351.56	360.24	342.46
glcm, first order, age (453)	353.18	443.64	378.83	354.30	383.82	356.25
all (518)	350.40	385.66	354.86	352.95	372.04	348.55

4   Discussion

In this paper we presented contribution to the BraTS 2017 challenge. For the segmentation part of the challenge we developed a U-Net inspired deep convolutional neural network architecture which was trained from scratch using only the provided training data, extensive data augmentation and a dice loss formulation. We achieve state of the art results on BraTS 2015 and presented promising scores on the BraTS 2017 validation set. On the test set we obtained mean dice scores of 0.858 for whole tumor, 0.775 for tumor core and 0.647 for the contrast enhancing tumor. Training time was about five days per network. Due to time restrictions we were limited in the number of architectural variants and data augmentation methods we could explore. Careful architecture optimizations already allowed us to train with large $128 \times 128 \times 128$ patches and a batch size of 2 with 16 filters at full resolution, which is significantly more than in [9]. Training with larger batch sizes and more convolutional filters in a multi-GPU setup should yield further improvements, especially provided that we did not observe significant overfitting in our experiments. While most of our effort was concentrated on the segmentation part of the challenge, we also proposed an ensemble of a random forest regressor and a multilayer perceptron ensemble for the survival prediction subchallenge. By using only shape based features, we achieved a root mean squared error of 335.08 and a mean absolute error of 232.76 in a five fold cross-validation on the training data and using our segmentations. On the test set, our survival prediction approach obtained 457.83 rmse (209607 mse), an accuracy of 52.6% and a Spearman correlation coefficient of 0.496. The survival prediction task could be improved further by considering the position in the tumor relative to other structures in the brain such as the ventricles, optical nerve fibers or other important fibre tracts. Furthermore, our group based manual feature selection should be replaced by a proper feature selection algorithm such as forward/backward selection [17] or a feature filter based approach [18].

References

1. Menze, B.H., Jakab, A., Bauer, S., Kalpathy-Cramer, J., Farahani, K., Kirby, J., Burren, Y., Porz, N., Slotboom, J., Wiest, R., et al.: The multimodal brain tumor image segmentation benchmark (BRATS). IEEE Trans. Med. Imaging **34**(10), 1993–2024 (2015)
2. Bakas, S., Akbari, H., Sotiras, A., Bilello, M., Rozycki, M., Kirby, J., Freymann, J., Farahani, K., Davatzikos, C.: Advancing the cancer genome Atlas Glioma MRI collections with expert segmentation labels and radiomic features. Nature Scientific Data (2017, in Press)
3. Bakas, S., Akbari, H., Sotiras, A., Bilello, M., Rozycki, M., Kirby, J., Freymann, J., Farahani, K., Davatzikos, C.: Segmentation labels and radiomic features for the pre-operative scans of the TCGA-GBM collection. In: TCIA (2017)
4. Bakas, S., Akbari, H., Sotiras, A., Bilello, M., Rozycki, M., Kirby, J., Freymann, J., Farahani, K., Davatzikos, C.: Segmentation labels and radiomic features for the pre-operative scans of the TCGA-LGG collection. In: TCIA (2017)
5. Havaei, M., Davy, A., Warde-Farley, D., Biard, A., Courville, A., Bengio, Y., Pal, C., Jodoin, P.-M., Larochelle, H.: Brain tumor segmentation with deep neural networks. Med. Image Anal. **35**, 18–31 (2017)
6. Pereira, S., Pinto, A., Alves, V., Silva, C.A.: Brain tumor segmentation using convolutional neural networks in MRI images. IEEE Trans. Med. Imaging **35**(5), 1240–1251 (2016)
7. Kamnitsas, K., Ledig, C., Newcombe, V.F., Simpson, J.P., Kane, A.D., Menon, D.K., Rueckert, D., Glocker, B.: Efficient multi-scale 3D CNN with fully connected CRF for accurate brain lesion segmentation. Med. Image Anal. **36**, 61–78 (2017)

8. Kamnitsas, K., Ferrante, E., Parisot, S., Ledig, C., Nori, A.V., Criminisi, A., Rueckert, D., Glocker, B.: DeepMedic for brain tumor segmentation. In: Crimi, A., Menze, B., Maier, O., Reyes, M., Handels, H. (eds.) BrainLes 2015. LNCS, vol. 9556. Springer, Cham (2016). https://doi.org/10.1007/978-3-319-30858-6

9. Kayalibay, B., Jensen, G., van der Smagt, P.: CNN-based segmentation of medical imaging data. arXiv preprint arXiv:1701.03056 (2017)

10. Ronneberger, O., Fischer, P., Brox, T.: U-Net: convolutional networks for biomedical image segmentation. In: Navab, N., Hornegger, J., Wells, W.M., Frangi, A.F. (eds.) MICCAI 2015. LNCS, vol. 9351, pp. 234–241. Springer, Cham (2015). https://doi.org/10.1007/978-3-319-24574-4_28

11. Milletari, F., Navab, N., Ahmadi, S.-A.: V-Net: fully convolutional neural networks for volumetric medical image segmentation. In: International Conference on 3D Vision, pp. 565–571. IEEE (2016)

12. Macyszyn, L., Akbari, H., Pisapia, J.M., Da, X., Attiah, M., Pigrish, V., Bi, Y., Pal, S., Davuluri, R.V., Roccograndi, L., et al.: Imaging patterns predict patient survival and molecular subtype in glioblastoma via machine learning techniques. Neuro-oncology 18(3), 417–425 (2015)

13. He, K., Zhang, X., Ren, S., Sun, J.: Identity mappings in deep residual networks. In: Leibe, B., Matas, J., Sebe, N., Welling, M. (eds.) ECCV 2016. LNCS, vol. 9908, pp. 630–645. Springer, Cham (2016). https://doi.org/10.1007/978-3-319-46493-0_38

14. Ulyanov, D., Vedaldi, A., Lempitsky, V.: Instance normalization: the missing ingredient for fast stylization. arXiv preprint arXiv:1607.08022 (2016)

15. Kingma, D., Ba, J.: Adam: a method for stochastic optimization. arXiv preprint arXiv:1412.6980 (2014)

16. van Griethuysen, J.J.M., Fedorov, A., Parmar, C., Hosny, A., Aucoin, N., Narayan, V., Beets-Tan, R.G.H., Fillion-Robin, J.-C., Pieper, S., Aerts, H.J.W.L.: Computational radiomics system to decode the radiographic phenotype. Cancer Research (2017, accepted)

17. Kohavi, R., John, G.H.: Wrappers for feature subset selection. Artif. Intell. 97(1–2), 273–324 (1997)

18. Brown, G.: A new perspective for information theoretic feature selection. In: Artificial Intelligence and Statistics, pp. 49–56 (2009)

Multi-modal PixelNet for Brain Tumor Segmentation

Mobarakol Islam[1]([⊠]) [iD] and Hongliang Ren[2]

[1] Department of NUS Graduate School for Integrative Sciences and Engineering (NGS), National University of Singapore, Singapore, Singapore
mobarakol@u.nus.edu
[2] Department of Biomedical Engineering, National University of Singapore, Singapore, Singapore
ren@nus.edu.sg

Abstract. Brain tumor segmentation using multi-modal MRI data sets is important for diagnosis, surgery and follow up evaluation. In this paper, a convolutional neural network (CNN) with hypercolumns features (e.g. PixelNet) utilizes for automatic brain tumor segmentation containing low and high-grade glioblastomas. Though pixel level convolutional predictors like CNNs, are computationally efficient, such approaches are not statistically efficient during learning precisely because spatial redundancy limits the information learned from neighboring pixels. PixelNet extracts features from multiple layers that correspond to the same pixel and samples a modest number of pixels across a small number of images for each SGD (Stochastic gradient descent) batch update. PixelNet has achieved whole tumor dice accuracy 87.6% and 85.8% for validation and testing data respectively in BraTS 2017 challenge.

Keywords: Brain tumor segmentation · Gliomas · BraTS · Deep learning
Convolutional neural network · Pixel level segmentation · Hypercolumn

1 Introduction

It is very important to segment the gliomas and its intra-tumoral structures as well as estimate relative volume to monitor the progression, assessment, treatment planning and follow-up studies. Generally, the segmentation of gliomas observes in various regions such as active tumorous tissue, necrotic tissue, and the peritumoral edematous which defined through intensity changes relative to the surrounding normal tissue. However, gliomas or glioblastomas are usually spread out, poorly contrasted and intensity information being disseminated across various modalities that make them difficult to segment [1]. The tumor intensity also differs across the patients like HGG patients the tumor consists of enhancing, non-enhancing and necrotic parts, while in the LGG patients it is not necessarily to include an enhancing part [2]. Due to inconsistency and diversity of MRI acquisition parameters [3] and hardware variations, there are large difference in appearance, shape and intensity ranges among the same sequences and acquisition scanners [5], which make the segmentation more challenging. Thus, physicians conventionally use rough evaluation or manual segmentation; however, manual segmentation is time-consuming and laborious task that is inclined to misinterpretation and observer bias [4].

In recent years, Deep Learning (DL) have drawn increasing attention medical applications such as in object detection [6, 7], semantic segmentation [8] and classification [9]. DL models like convolutional neural networks (CNN) and Fully convolutional network (FCN) are capable of learning high level and task adaptive hierarchical features from training data and take part as an effective approach. Specially in segmentation task, FCN models achieve state of art results for natural image [22, 23] as well as biomedical images [33–35]. Havae et al. [10] build a CNN based two-pathway cascade network which performs a two-phase training using both local and global contextual features and tackle difficulties related to the imbalance of tumor labels in data. Another similar approach DeepMedic [11] uses two convolutional parallel pathways and 3D CNN architecture with 11-layers for brain lesion segmentation. Later, modified version of DeepMedic with residual connection utilize for brain tumor segmentation [12]. On the other hand, Pandian et al. [13] and Casamitjana et al. [14] use 3D volumetric CNN to train sub- volume of multi-modal MRIs and show that 3D CNN performs well for segmentation as MRI acquires 3D information. The benefit of these architectures is that they performed well with a comparatively smaller dataset. However, they are computationally expensive as it needs 3D kernels and a large number of trainable parameters. Alex et al. [15] use 5 layers deep Stacked Denoising Auto-Encoder (SDAE) and Randhawa et al. [16] use 8 layers CNN and Pereira et al. [17] use deeper CNN architecture with small kernel for segmenting gliomas from MRI. Shen et al. [32] introduce boundary-aware FCN for brain tumor segmentation which extracts multi-level contextual information by concatenating hierarchical features from multi-modal MRI and their symmetric-difference images. However, most of the above models either 2D or 3D patch wise segmentation which are unable to carry all the contextual information in training time.

In spatially-invariant label prediction problem like semantic segmentation, every separate label per pixel predicts using a convolutional architecture. As a result, gradient based learning like Stochastic gradient descent (SGD) treats training data as sampled independently and form an identical distribution [18]. Hyvärinen et al. [19] demonstrate that pixel in a given image is highly correlated and neighbouring pixels are not independent. To capture the high-level global context and minimize the loss of the contextual information in higher convolutional layers, many predictors have been built based on multiscale feature extraction from multiple layers of a CNN [20]. Hariharan et al. [21] extract features of the same pixels from multiple layers and accumulate in a feature vector called "Hypercolumns". To extract feature, an FCN model [22] efficiently implements linear prediction in a coarse to fine manner. To reduce memory footprint, DeepLab [23] incorporates filter dilation and linear-weighted fusion in fully connected layers. ParseNet [24] averages the pooling feature by normalization and concatenation to add spatial context for a layer response. PixelNet [25] adopt both Hariharan et al. [21] and ParseNet [24] to build hypercolumn and concatenate spatial context in the layer with the tradeoff between statistical and computational efficiency for convolutional learning. In this work, we use PixelNet with multimodal MRI for brain tumor segmentation. Three modalities of MRI utilize as 3 channels in PixelNet for training. PixelNet shows state of art performance for in BRATS 2017 [27–30] training, validation and testing dataset.

2 Methodology

PixelNet extracts multi-scale convolution and feature and concatenate them as hyper-column to ensure all local and global contextual information in the learning phase (Fig. 1). It forms of 15 convolutional layers where first 13 convolutional layers follow as convolutional layers of VGG-16 [26] architecture and remaining 2 convolutional filters as [22]. The convolutional layers can be denoted as $\{C_{11}, C_{12}, C_{21}, C_{22}, C_{31}, C_{32}, C_{33}, C_{41}, C_{41}, C_{43}, C_{51}, C_{52}, C_{53}, C_6, C_7\}$. Convolutional features from 5 layers such as $\{C_{12}, C_{22}, C_{33}, C_{43}, C_{53}, C_7\}$ have been extracted to form hypercolumn. A hypercolumn descriptor can be written as:

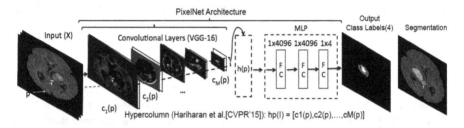

Fig. 1. Three modalities (Flair, T1c, T2) input in a CNN and extract hypercolumn descriptor for a sample pixel from multiple convolutional layers. The hypercolumn descriptor is then fed to a multi-layer perceptron for non-linear optimization.

$$h_p = [c_1(p), c_2(p), \ldots, c_M(p)] \tag{1}$$

where h_p denote the multiscale hypercolumn features for the pixel p, and $c_i(p)$ denote the feature vector from layer i. PixelNet considers pixel wise prediction as operating over hypercolumn features. Later, hypercolumn features feed to a multi-layer perceptron (MLP) with three fully connected (FC1, FC2, FC3) layers of size 4096 followed by ReLU activation layer. Finally, it predicts the output of K (4) classes. The final prediction for pixel p can be written as,

$$f_{\theta,p}(X) = g(h_p(X)) \tag{2}$$

where θ represent both hypercolumn features h and pixel wise predictor g. θ updates by using SGD training. We use a series of fully connected layers followed by ReLU activation function similar to VGG-16 [26] to implement non-linear predictor. We adopt sparse pixel prediction at training time for efficient mini-batch generation. In sparse prediction, hypercolumn features h_p choose from dense convolutional responses at all layers by computing the 4 discrete locations in the feature map c_i (for i^{th} layer) closest to sampled pixel $p \in P$ and finally apply bilinear interpolation to get i^{th} layer response in hypercolumn. In training phase, N modest number of random pixels utilize for the optimization where N constructs as a layer with number of pixels and coordinates of corresponding pixels in the input image in PixelNet architecture. All the pixels are considered as N in testing phase to predict whole image.

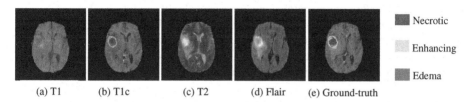

Fig. 2. A slice of BraTS 2017 training data with four modalities such as (a) T1, (b) T1c, (c) T2, (d) Flair. (e) Ground-truth with experts' segmentation.

3   Experiment and Evaluation

We use depth slicing to extract images from MRI to train our FCN model. To evaluate our predicted segmentation, we use online evaluation portal of BraTS 2017 challenge.

3.1   Dataset

BRATS 2017 (Brain Tumor Image Segmentation Benchmark) [27–30] database consists 285 cases of training, 46 cases of validation and 146 cases of testing MRI scans (Table 1). It is a multi-modal MRI scans of both high-grade glioma (HGG) and low-grade glioma (LGG) and 4 different modalities including T1 (spin- lattice relaxation), T1c (T1-contrasted), T2 (spin-spin relaxation) and FLAIR (fluid attenuation inversion recovery). Each scan is a continuous 3D volume of 155 2D slices of size 240 × 240. The volume of the various modalities is already skull-stripped, aligned with T1c and interpolated to 1 mm voxel resolution. The provided ground truth with manual (expert) segmentation includes three labels such as GD-enhancing tumor (ET — label 4), the peritumoral edema (ED — label 2), and the necrotic and non-enhancing tumor (NCR/NET — label 1) where background (label 0) covers healthy tissue and padding. The predicted labels are evaluated by merging three regions: whole tumor (WT: all four labels), tumor core (TC: 1,2) and enhancing tumor (ET: 4). Table 1 shows short description of dataset and Fig. 2 visualizes a slice of the training data.

Table 1. BRATS 2017 dataset

Data	Cases
Training	285
Validation	46
Testing	146

3.2   Training

We use depth slicing images on axial orientation on the mixed HGG and LGG data (285 MRI cases in total). We use VGG-16 [26] pre-trained model to initialize our model parameters. During training phase, N (2000) pixels have been randomly sampled and multi-scale convolutional features have been extracted to form hypercolumn. However, this dataset is highly imbalance where ground-truth contains 98% pixel are healthy tissue (label 0) and remaining are also unequal ratios of four ROI labels such as edema, enhancing, necrotic and non-enhancing. We deal this issue by ignoring all the blank slices in groundtruth (both background and healthy issue) and train PixelNet with corresponding 3 modalities such as flair, T1C and T2. So, we ignore T1 scan as [31] to reduce the cost of data acquisition and storage (Table 2).

Table 2. PixelNet parameters with dimension at training

Layer	Name	Dimension
1	Data	$3 \times 240 \times 240$
2	Pixels	2000
3	Labels	2000
4	C_{11}	$64 \times 240 \times 240$
5	C_{12}	$64 \times 240 \times 240$
6	Pool1	$64 \times 120 \times 120$
7	C_{21}	$128 \times 120 \times 120$
8	C_{22}	$128 \times 120 \times 120$
9	Pool2	$28 \times 60 \times 60$
10	C_{31}	$256 \times 60 \times 60$
11	C_{32}	$256 \times 60 \times 60$
12	C_{33}	$256 \times 60 \times 60$
13	Pool3	$256 \times 30 \times 30$
14	C_{41}	$512 \times 30 \times 30$
15	C_{42}	$512 \times 30 \times 30$
16	C_{43}	$512 \times 30 \times 30$
17	Pool4	$512 \times 15 \times 15$
18	C_{51}	$512 \times 15 \times 15$
19	C_{52}	$512 \times 15 \times 15$
20	C_{53}	$512 \times 15 \times 15$
21	Pool5	$512 \times 8 \times 8$
22	C_6	$4096 \times 2 \times 2$
23	C_7	$4096 \times 2 \times 2$
24	Hypercolumn	2000×5568
25	FC1	2000×4096
26	FC2	2000×4096
27	FC3	2000×4

Though BRATS 2017 has in total 44175 (285 × 155) slices in axial view, we utilize only 18924 (43% data) slices corresponding to ground-truth with non-zero class (contains at least one class 1 or 2 or 4). In testing phase, entire image feed-forwards to predict segmentation from last layer. We use Caffe deep learning platform with Nvidia GPU 1080 Ti to perform all of our experiments.

3.3 Evaluation

To get most accurate and proper performance, there are 4 metrics use to evaluate segmentation task of BraTS 2017 challenge. These are Dice, Hausdorff, Sensitivity and Specificity.

Dice Coefficient. It is a statistical measurement, uses for comparing similarity between clinical ground-truth (T) and predicted segmentation of the model (P). Equation (3) represent the formula of dice coefficient calculation. Finally, calculate the mean of all the cases to get final dice score.

$$Dice = \frac{2|T \cap P|}{|T| + |P|} \tag{3}$$

Hausdorff Distance. It measures the closeness of two subsets such as the ground-truth and the predicted output of a metric space mathematically. Equation (4) shows the calculation of Hausdorff distance.

$$Hausdorff(T, P) = max\{min\{d(T, P)\}\} \tag{4}$$

Sensitivity and Specificity. These are measurement tools to evaluate the rate of true positive (TP) and true negative (TN) for the predicted segmentation. Sensitivity is the ratio of true positive (TP) to sum of true positive (TP) and false negative (FN). The ratio of true negative (TN) to the sum of true negative (TN) and false positive (FP) is defined as Specificity. Equation (5) and (6) represent the formula for Sensitivity and Specificity respectively.

$$Sensitivity = \frac{TP}{TP + FN} \tag{5}$$

$$Specificity = \frac{TN}{TN + FP} \tag{6}$$

Experimental Results. After PixelNet prediction, we evaluate all the cases for training set (285 cases), validation set (46 cases) and testing set (146 cases) using online evaluation portal of BRATS 2017 challenge. Table 3 represents the training set evaluation results using simply same training data (not cross validation) where whole tumor average Dice accuracy is 90.9% and Hausdorff distance is 7.3. Table 4 shows the evaluation results of validation set where average 87.6% dice accuracy and 9.8 Hausdorff distance which is quite promising. The Dice and Hausdorff score for testing data have been shown in Table 5. The final testing score for Dice and Hausdorff distance are 85.8% and 11.96 for whole tumor region. Though enhance tumor and tumor core region have lower accuracy than whole tumor, the individual accuracy can be considered as state of art performance. Additionally, PixelNet obtains Specificity of 99% in all the evaluated tasks. Figure 3 shows some visualized examples of PixelNet prediction with comparing ground-truth. Some predicted segmentation from testing data have been shown in Fig. 4.

Table 3. Dice and Sensitivity for BRATS 2017 training dataset

	ET	WT	TC
Dice	0.711	**0.909**	0.866
Sensitivity	0.771	0.897	0.831
Specificity	0.998	0.995	0.998
Hausdorff95	6.946	**7.275**	6.103

Table 4. Dice and Sensitivity for BRATS 2017 validation dataset

	ET	WT	TC
Dice	0.689	**0.876**	0.761
Sensitivity	0.706	0.837	0.711
Specificity	0.999	0.996	0.998
Hausdorff95	12.938	**9.820**	12.361

Table 5. Dice and Hausdorff95 for BRATS 2017 testing dataset

Level	Dice			Hausdorff95		
	ET	WT	TC	ET	WT	TC
Mean	0.619	**0.858**	0.704	57.456	**11.961**	30.116
StdDev	0.325	0.123	0.296	127.442	19.139	84.619
Median	0.772	0.896	0.848	2.828	4.347	4.949
25quantile	0.501	0.844	0.610	1.799	2.828	3.162
75quantile	0.839	0.925	0.899	9.641	8.957	10.486

MRI (T1c)

Ground-Truth

PixelNet
prediction

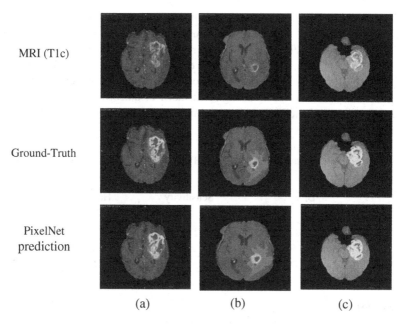

(a)   (b)   (c)

Fig. 3. PixelNet prediction for BRATS 2017 training data. Randomly visualize three cases (a, b, c) with T1c modality.

Input
(T1c)

PixelNet
Prediction

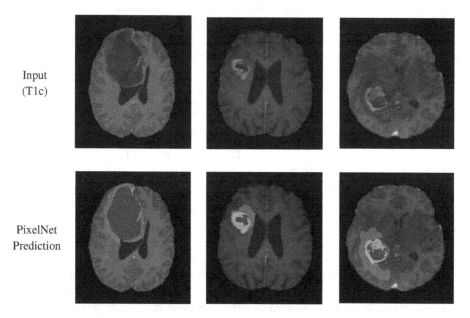

Fig. 4. PixelNet prediction for BRATS 2017 testing data. Randomly visualize three cases with T1c modality.

Experiments with Different Categories of Data. To see the effect of different combination of data with PixelNet, we train our model with all the slices (without blank) and only 12930 (29% data) slices corresponding to ground-truth consisting all three classes (1, 2, 4) and 18924 slices (43% data) non-zero slices or at least one class slices. Table 6 shows the Dice and Hausdorff evaluation for validation dataset by varying amount of training data. Though Hausdorff distance for all data have significant better accuracy, PixelNet achieves almost same performance for less dataset consisting all the classes.

Table 6. Dice, sensitivity and Hausdorff95 for BRATS 2017 validation dataset with different categories of training data.

	Dice			Sensitivity			Hausdorff95		
	ET	WT	TC	ET	WT	TC	ET	WT	TC
PixelNet (all data)	0.703	0.864	0.745	0.710	0.819	0.690	5.686	5.346	8.310
PixelNet (43% data)	0.689	0.876	0.761	0.720	0.861	0.710	12.938	9.820	12.361
PixelNet (29% data)	0.677	0.861	0.775	0.722	0.818	0.776	14.675	11.808	23.726

4   Discussion

As a pixel-level segmentation model, the main different with PixelNet and other FCN models is that PixelNet utilizes small number of pixel where conventional FCNs use either patch or whole image in training period. This is why PixelNet has less chance to converge to certain classes with imbalance dataset like BraTS. Though PixelNet tradeoff with statistical and computational efficiency, it has almost similar performance with 3 and 4 modalities of MRI cases. All of our experiments have been conducted with 3 modalities (Flair, T1c, T2) of MRI scan. Table 7 shows the comparative experimental results using 3 and 4 modalities.

Table 7. Dice, Hausdorff95 for BRATS 2017 validation dataset with 3 and 4 modalities of training data.

	Dice			Hausdorff95		
	ET	WT	TC	ET	WT	TC
PixelNet 3 channels (Flair, T1C & T2)	0.689	0.876	0.761	12.938	9.820	12.361
PixelNet 4 channels (Flair, T1, T1C & T2)	0.682	0.865	0.776	12.544	12.614	15.968

5   Conclusion

We presented an automatic brain tumor segmentation method based on pixel level semantic segmentation. We choose PixelNet which extracts multi layers convolutional feature and form hypercolumn. Hypercolumn contains useful contextual information and use sparse pixel prediction to generate efficient mini-batch which produces promising results for Brain tumor segmentation. Though the preliminary results of the ET and TC are not good as WT however we are still working on this model to achieve better accuracy in all the regions of the tumor.

Acknowledgments. This work is supported by the Singapore Academic Research Fund under Grant R-397-000-227-112, NUSRI China Jiangsu Provincial Grant BK20150386 & BE2016077 and NMRC Bedside & Bench under grant R-397-000-245-511 awarded to Dr. Hongliang Ren. I would like to thank Aayush Bansal, the author of PixelNet [25], for the assistance to implement PixelNet for this project.

References

1. Nyul, L.G., Udupa, J.K., Zhang, X.: New variants of a method of MRI scale standardization. IEEE Trans. Med. Imaging **19**(2), 143–150 (2000)
2. Ellwaa, A., et al.: Brain tumor segmantation using random forest trained on iterative selected patients. In: Proceedings of BRATS-MICCAI (2016)
3. Omuro, A., DeAngelis, L.M.: Glioblastoma and other malignant gliomas: a clinical review. JAMA **310**, 1842–1850 (2013)
4. Bauer, S., et al.: A survey of MRI-based medical image analysis for brain tumor studies. Phys. Med. Biol. **58**, R97 (2013)
5. Inda, M.M., Bonavia, R., Seoane, J.: Glioblastoma multiforme: a look inside its heterogeneous nature. Cancers **6**(1), 226–239 (2014)
6. Baumgartner, C.F., Kamnitsas, K., Matthew, J., Smith, S., Kainz, B., Rueckert, D.: Real-time standard scan plane detection and localisation in fetal ultrasound using fully convolutional neural networks. In: Ourselin, S., Joskowicz, L., Sabuncu, M.R., Unal, G., Wells, W. (eds.) MICCAI 2016. LNCS, vol. 9901, pp. 203–211. Springer, Cham (2016). https://doi.org/10.1007/978-3-319-46723-8_24
7. Azizi, S., Imani, F., Ghavidel, S., Tahmasebi, A., Kwak, J.T., Xu, S., Turkbey, B., Choyke, P., Pinto, P., Wood, B., Mousavi, P., Abolmaesumi, P.: Detection of prostate cancer using temporal sequences of ultrasound data: a large clinical feasibility study. Int. J. Comput. Assist. Radiol. Surg. **11**(6), 947–956 (2016)
8. Ronneberger, O., Fischer, P., Brox, T.: U-net: convolutional networks for biomedical image segmentation. arXiv:1505.04597v1 (2015)
9. Milletari, F., Navab, N., Ahmadi, S.A.: V-Net: fully convolutional neural networks for volumetric medical image segmentation. arXiv:1606.04797v1 (2016)
10. Havaei, M., Davy, A., Warde-Farley, D.: Brain tumor segmentation with deep neural networks. Med. Image Anal. **35**, 18–31 (2017)
11. Kamnitsas, K., et al.: Efficient multi-scale 3D CNN with fully connected CRF for accurate brain lesion segmentation. Med. Image Anal. **36**, 61–78 (2017)
12. Kamnitsas, K., et al: DeepMedic on brain tumor segmentation. In: Proceedings of BRATS-MICCAI (2016)
13. Pandian1, B., Boyle1, J., Orringer, D. A.: Multimodal tumor segmentation with 3D volumetric convolutional neural networks. In: Proceedings of BRATS-MICCAI (2016)
14. Casamitjana, A., et al.: 3D convolutional networks for brain tumor segmentation. In: Proceedings of BRATS-MICCAI (2016)
15. Alex, V., Krishnamurthi, G.: Brain tumor segmentation from multi modal MR images using stacked denoising autoencoders. In: Proceedings of BRATS-MICCAI (2016)
16. Randhawa, R., Modi, A., Jain, P., Warier, P.: Improving segment boundary classification for brain tumor segmentation and longitudinal disease progression. In: Proceedings of BRATS-MICCAI (2016)
17. Pereira, S., et al.: Brain tumor segmentation using convolutional neural networks in MRI images. IEEE Trans. Med. Imaging **35**, 1240–1251 (2016)

18. Bottou, L.: Large-scale machine learning with stochastic gradient descent. In: Lechevallier, Y., Saporta, G. (eds.) Proceedings of COMPSTAT 2010, pp. 177–186. Springer, Heidelberg (2010)

19. Hyvärinen, A., Hurri, J., Hoyer, P. O.: Natural Image Statistics: A Probabilistic Approach to Early Computational Vision, vol. 39 (2009). https://doi.org/10.1007/978-1-84882-491-1. (1. Aufl. ed.)

20. Denton, E.L., Chintala, S., Fergus, R., et al.: Deep generative image models using a Laplacian pyramid of adversarial networks. In: NIPS (2015)

21. Hariharan, B., Arbelaez, P., Girshick, R., Malik, J.: Hypercolumns for object segmentation and fine-grained localization. In: CVPR (2015)

22. Long, J., Shelhamer, E., Darrell, T.: Fully convolutional models for semantic segmentation. In: CVPR (2015)

23. Chen, L.-C., Papandreou, G., Kokkinos, I., Murphy, K., Yuille, A. L.: Semantic image segmentation with deep convolutional nets and fully connected CRFs. In: ICLR (2015)

24. Liu, W., Rabinovich, A., Berg, A. C.: Parsenet: looking wider to see better. arXiv preprint arXiv:1506.04579 (2015)

25. Bansal, A., et al: PixelNet: Representation of the pixels, by the pixels, and for the pixels. arXiv:1702.06506v1 (2017)

26. Simonyan, K., Zisserman, A.: Very deep convolutional networks for large-scale image recognition. arXiv preprint arXiv:1409.1556 (2014)

27. Menze, B., et al.: The multimodal brain tumor image segmentation benchmark (brats). IEEE Trans. Med. Imaging **34**, 1993–2024 (2015)

28. Bakas, S., Akbari, H., Sotiras, A., Bilello, M., Rozycki, M., Kirby J. S., Freymann, J. B., Farahani, K., Davatzikos, C.: Advancing the cancer genome atlas glioma MRI collections with expert segmentation labels and radiomic features. Nat. Sci. Data (2017, in Press)

29. Bakas, S., Akbari, H., Sotiras, A., Bilello, M., Rozycki, M., Kirby, J., Freymann, J., Farahani, K., Davatzikos, C.: Segmentation labels and radiomic features for the pre-operative scans of the TCGA-GBM collection. Cancer Imaging Arch. (2017). https://doi.org/10.7937/K9/TCIA.2017.KLXWJJ1Q

30. Bakas, S., Akbari, H., Sotiras, A., Bilello, M., Rozycki, M., Kirby, J., Freymann, J., Fara-hani, K., Davatzikos, C.: Segmentation labels and radiomic features for the pre-operative scans of the TCGA-LGG collection. Cancer Imaging Arch. (2017). https://doi.org/10.7937/K9/TCIA.2017.GJQ7R0EF

31. Zhao, X., Wu, Y., Song, G., Li, Z., Fan, Y., Zhang, Y.: Brain tumor segmentation using a fully convolutional neural network with conditional random fields. In: Proceedings of BRATS-MICCAI (2016)

32. Shen, H., Wang, R., Zhang, J., McKenna, S.J.: Boundary-aware fully convolutional network for brain tumor segmentation. In: Descoteaux, M., Maier-Hein, L., Franz, A., Jannin, P., Collins, D.L., Duchesne, S. (eds.) MICCAI 2017. LNCS, vol. 10434, pp. 433–441. Springer, Cham (2017). https://doi.org/10.1007/978-3-319-66185-8_49

33. Chen, H., Qi, X.J., Cheng, J.Z., Heng, P.A.: Deep contextual networks for neuronal structure segmentation. In: AAAI (2016)

34. Chen, H., Qi, X., Yu, L., Heng, P.A.: DCAN: deep contour-aware networks for accurate gland segmentation. In: CVPR, pp. 2487–2496 (2016)

35. Ronneberger, O., Fischer, P., Brox, T.: U-net: convolutional networks for biomedical image segmentation. CoRR, vol. abs/1505.04597 (2015)

Brain Tumor Segmentation Using Dense Fully Convolutional Neural Network

Mazhar Shaikh, Ganesh Anand, Gagan Acharya, Abhijit Amrutkar,
Varghese Alex, and Ganapathy Krishnamurthi[✉]

Medical Imaging and Reconstruction Lab, Department of Engineering Design,
Indian Institute of Technology Madras, Chennai, India
gankrish@iitm.ac.in

Abstract. Manual segmentation of brain tumor is often time consuming and the performance of the segmentation varies based on the operators experience. This leads to the requisition of a fully automatic method for brain tumor segmentation. In this paper, we propose the usage of the 100 layer Tiramisu architecture for the segmentation of brain tumor from multi modal MR images, which is evolved by integrating a densely connected fully convolutional neural network (FCNN), followed by post-processing using a Dense Conditional Random Field (DCRF). The network consists of blocks of densely connected layers, transition down layers in down-sampling path and transition up layers in up-sampling path. The method was tested on dataset provided by Multi modal Brain Tumor Segmentation Challenge (BraTS) 2017. The training data is composed of 210 high-grade brain tumor and 74 low-grade brain tumor cases. The proposed network achieves a mean whole tumor, tumor core & active tumor dice score of 0.87, 0.68 & 0.65. Respectively on the BraTS '17 validation set and 0.83, 0.65 & 0.65 on the Brats '17 test set.

Keywords: Fully convolutional neural networks
Multi modal mri segmentation · Conditional random fields · Tiramisu

1 Introduction

Accurate tumor segmentation is crucial for treatment and survival prediction of cancer patients. Segmentation of the gliomas from MR images is the preliminary step for treatment and surgical planning. Generally, manual segmentation of gliomas is known to be tedious and can often results in inter rater variability. In order to automate this process, we adopt a 103 layer deep fully convolution neural network (FCNN) for tumor segmentation. Originally proposed in [6], the Tiramisu model has significantly outperformed most state-of-the-art techniques like [7,8] on the CamVid [20] and Gatech [21] datasets. The architecture uses a characteristic upsampling path to overcome the problem of memory demand as a result of feature map explosion and allows the network to be very deep.

© Springer International Publishing AG, part of Springer Nature 2018
A. Crimi et al. (Eds.): BrainLes 2017, LNCS 10670, pp. 309–319, 2018.
https://doi.org/10.1007/978-3-319-75238-9_27

In this paper, we demonstrate the adaptation of this model for slice based biomedical image segmentation purposes. The network is further supplemented by post processing techniques like CRF and connected components analysis to remove false positives generated by the network.

2 Related Work

Most of the work on brain tumor segmentation using convolutional neural networks(CNN) can be classified as either patch based including volumetric patches or slice based on the basis of the input and the corresponding output. In patch based techniques, we input a 2D/3D patch and output the center voxel class. While in slice based methods, the network inputs the entire slice/volume and gives a segmentation map having the same size as the input.

2.1   Patch Based Techniques

Patch Based Techniques such as by Pereira et al. [12] make use of a CNN which takes a patch from the image and predicts the class for the center voxel. These techniques allow for using information from the immediate surrounding region for prediction. The main drawback of such techniques is that, being local, the predictions for voxels are independent of each other and as such there can be inconsistencies between nearby predictions which need to be corrected with post-processing. However, patch based models can address the issue of class imbalance by selective sampling of patches from the MRI data during training, like in [19]. Extending patch based techniques which use 2D image patches to 3D volumes (*DeepMedic* [9]) involves predicting the classes for a subset of the volume given as input to a 3D CNN.

2.2   Slice Based Techniques

Slice based techniques refer to networks which predict the classes for all the pixels or voxels for a given input. These techniques generally use convolutional layers along with pooling layers to capture high level information about the input in the downsampling path and then use transposed convolutions or unparametrized upsampling methods such as bilinear upsampling in the upsampling path to predict the classes for the whole input. They make use of skip connections [17] to preserve low level feature information in the upsampling[1] path for sharper predictions. Prediction of classes for the whole input is generally quicker and uses more information than patch based techniques as the inputs are usually larger. FCNNs for 3D volumes, [11] and Unet-3D [18] offer better performance but have greater computational and memory requirements. The inherent problem in any of these techniques is handling class imbalance.

---

[1] Upsampling here refers to increasing the resolution of the feature maps back to the input size.

3   Materials and Method

3.1   Data

The images used to train and validate this model were obtained from the BraTS 2017 challenge dataset [1–4]. The training dataset consisted of multi modal MR images of 284 patients, with 210 patients from the high grade gliomas category (HGG) and 74 patients from the low grade gliomas (LGG) category. The following MRI modalities were provided for each patient: T2-weighted fluid attenuated inversion recovery (FLAIR), T1-weighted (T1), T1-weighted contrast-enhanced (T1ce), and T2-weighted (T2). The provided sequences were co-registered to the same anatomical template, interpolated to the same resolution ($1\,\text{mm}^3$) and skull-stripped. The image dimensions were $240 \times 240 \times 155$, with 155 being the number of slices in the axial direction. Manually annotated ground truth segmentations were provided for three classes: GD-enhancing tumor (ET label 4), the peritumoral edema (ED label 2), and the necrotic and non-enhancing tumor (NCR/NET label 1). The network was trained on slices extracted from the axial plane.

3.2   Pre-processing

Multi modal scans can vary between patients depending on several factors including the instrument used, image acquisition axis, etc. In order to account for the patient-to-patient variation in the MR images, we adopted z-score normalization, Eq. 1, where we subtract the mean and divide by the standard deviation of the entire volume for each of the four sequences of an individual's scan.

$$I_{norm} = \frac{I - \mu}{\sigma} \tag{1}$$

3.3   Densely Connected FCNN Model

Our segmentation technique is based on the One Hundred Layers Tiramisu model originally proposed by Jégou et al. [6]. Like most state-of-the-art models like [17], the Tiramisu model involves a down-sampling path and up-sampling path, where a single slice of the brain is provided as input at the beginning of the model and class-wise probabilities for every pixel is output at the end of the up-sampling path.

The Tiramisu model, shown in Fig. 1, consists of dense blocks(DB) used in DenseNet [5], which are made up of repeated Batch Normalization layers [14], ReLU [15], 3×3 convolutions and short skip connections. The dense blocks are paired with transition down layers(TD) in the down-sampling path and transition up layers(TU) in the up-sampling path with long skip connections [16]. Skip Connections here refer to concatenation of the feature maps. The transition down layer consists of 1×1 convolutions followed by 2×2 max-pool layer with stride 2. Transition up layer is composed of 3×3 transpose convolutions with stride 2. The various blocks used in the model as well as the number of layers per dense block are shown in Fig. 2.

3.4 Post-processing Using Dense-CRFs and Connected Components Analysis

To smoothen the segmentation predicted by the above model, we used fully connected conditional random fields with Gaussian edge potentials as proposed by Krähenbühl et al. [10]. The unary potentials used by the CRF was computed

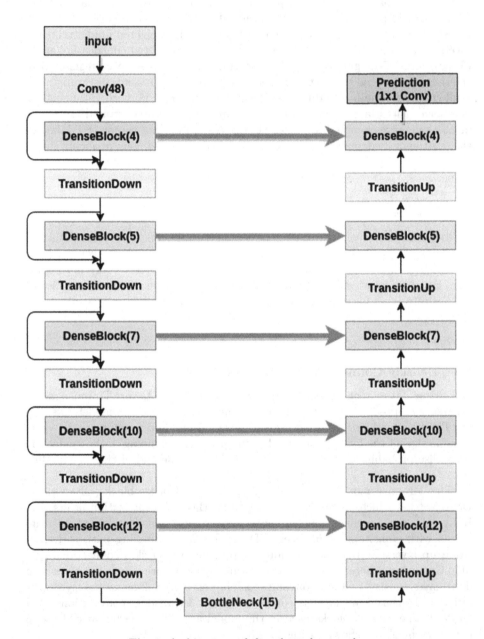

Fig. 1. Architecture of the adopted network

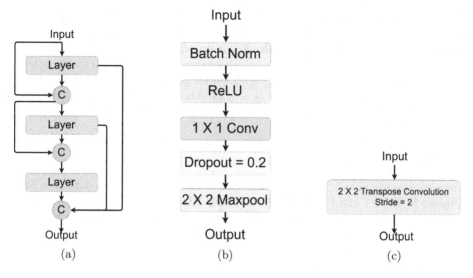

Fig. 2. Blocks used in the model. (a) Dense block. (b) Transition down. (c) Transition up

using the predicted softmax probabilities. Further, the MR brain slice (all four modalities) along with the computed unary potentials was used for inferring the pixel labels. CRF was implemented using open source code from the pydenscrf[2] repository was used for this purpose. The false positives in the prediction were further reduced by using connected component analysis, wherein only the largest component of the segmentation predicted is retained.

4   Implementation

The network was developed using TensorFlow [22] framework. Nvidia Titan X Maxwell GPU was used for training the model. The model was trained separately using cross entropy cost function, soft dice loss and cross entropy with soft dice score (2) as a regularizer. We observed that the soft dice loss gave a higher mean dice score and hence proceeded to train the network using the same. The soft dice score for binary classification [11] is given as

$$D = \frac{2\sum_i^N p_i g_i}{\sum_i^N p_i^2 + \sum_i^N g_i^2} \tag{2}$$

ADAM [13] optimizer was used with $\beta_1 = 0.99$ and $\beta_2 = 0.995$ and an exponential decay rate of 0.9 every 1000 minibatches. Because of memory limitations, the batch size used during the training phase was 6 slices.

---

[2] Pydensecrf: https://github.com/lucasb-eyer/pydensecrf.

Class Imbalance. As the employed network is slice based, the data is prone to have class imbalance owing to the fact that tumor comprises only a small fraction of the slice. In order to address this imbalance, we assign the following class weights in the loss function; 1 for the background class and 100 for the other classes. Also, only those image slices with tumor pixels in them were passed for training. We acknowledge that this is a run-of-the-mill technique and could be handled more effectively using data augmentation and patch based techniques.

5 Results

The performance of the proposed technique on the local HGG test data $(n = 21)$ is shown in Table 1 and Fig. 3. On the local test HGG data, the network achieved as mean whole tumor, tumor core and active tumor dice score of 0.84, 0.83, 0.80 respectively. The proposed post processing technique (CRF+connected component analysis) yield a 1% improvement in the whole tumor dice score, 1% in tumor core and 0.5% in active tumor respectively.

On the local LGG test data (n = 8), the model under performs on Tumor core segmentation, while maintaining good performance on the whole tumor segmentation. The overall performance (LGG+HGG) is given in Table 2.

Table 1. Results of local test data

	HGG $(n = 21)$			LGG $(n = 8)$	
	Whole tumor	Tumor core	Active tumor	Whole tumor	Tumor core
Mean	0.84	0.83	0.80	0.82	0.43
Std	0.16	0.18	0.14	0.11	0.29
Median	0.89	0.87	0.84	0.85	0.44

Table 2. Overall performance on local test data (number of cases $= 29$)

	Whole tumor	Tumor core	Active tumor
Mean	0.83	0.72	0.69
Std. deviation	0.14	0.21	0.18

The performance of the proposed technique on the BraTS 2017 validation data (mixture of HGG and LGG) is given in Table 3. For whole tumor segmentation, the network maintains its performance on the validation data. The poor performance of the proposed technique on LGG tumor core segmentation negatively skews the performance statistics of our method on the validation data. We attribute this relatively lower performance to the lesser number of images for

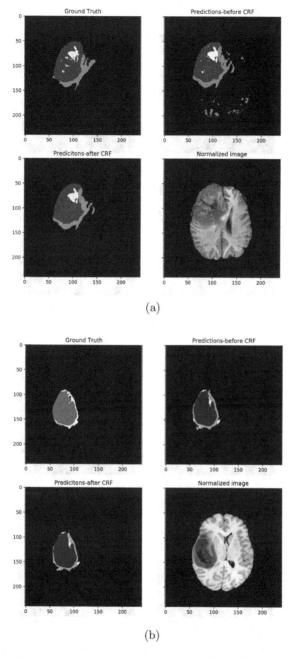

Fig. 3. Results of the proposed network on local test data. For each sub-figure (Left to Right, Top to Bottom), Ground truth, Prediction(before post-processing), Prediction(after post-processing), and the normalized FLAIR image slice, in that order.

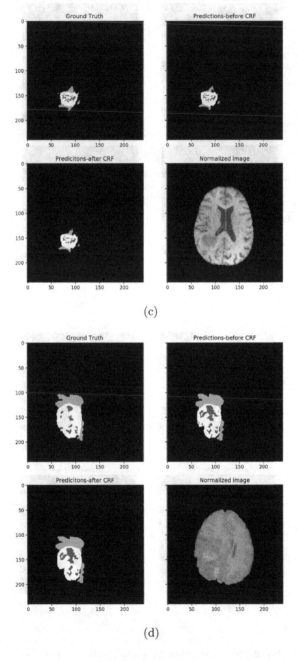

Fig. 3. (*continued*)

LGG cases compared to HGG and the poor data augmentation scheme employed to address this issue.

The performance on the BraTS 2017 test data is given in Table 4. We find the whole tumor dice score to be similar to that of the local data. Overall, we observe that the training performance is similar to the test performance which means that the network has not been over-fitted to the training data.

Table 3. Results of BraTS 2017 validation data (number of cases = 46)

	Whole tumor	Tumor core	Active tumor
Mean	0.87	0.68	0.65
Std. deviation	0.11	0.34	0.32
Median	0.91	0.82	0.78

Table 4. Results of BraTS 2017 test data (number of cases = 147)

	Whole tumor	Tumor core	Active tumor
Mean	0.83	0.65	0.65
Std. deviation	0.17	0.33	0.31
Median	0.89	0.84	0.78

In order to reduce the false negative occurrences in the predictions caused by the class imbalance, we utilized hard negative mining i.e. repeated retraining of the network with slices that have large false negative outputs. However, it was observed that this did not yield significant improvement in the local validation set.

6 Conclusion

In this paper, we propose an automatic technique to segment gliomas from MR scans.

- A 103 layer deep network was implemented for segmentation of the gliomas from MR scans.
- A single network was used for the segmentation task, irrespective of the grade of the glioma.
- The Dense CRF improved the performance of the network in all compartments. Further connected component analysis removed grainy segments from the prediction. While reducing false positives, this technique will however result in removal of smaller tumor clusters.
- The proposed network completes the entire pipeline (preprocessing, prediction & post processing) under 30 s.

As visible from the results the network performs well on whole Tumor but faces difficulty distinguishing between tumor core and enhancing tumor. This disparity is possibly due the inherent class imbalance and poor data augmentation. Regardless of this, the network achieves good results and is able to generalize well between the training set and test set.

This work only uses a 2D FCNN model. 2D models have to make predictions for a region with less information than 3D FCNNs. Going forward 3D FCNNs will be used to improve performance. An exploration of the design space for 3D FCNNs will be done to find architectures which improve performance from 2D while still being able to run on a single GPU.

References

1. Bakas, S., Akbari, H., Sotiras, A., Bilello, M., Rozycki, M., Kirby, J.S., Freymann, J.B., Farahani, K., Davatzikos, C.: Advancing the cancer genome Atlas glioma MRI collections with expert segmentation labels and radiomic features. Nat. Sci. Data (2017, in Press)
2. Menze, B.H., et al.: The multimodal brain tumor image segmentation benchmark (BRATS). IEEE Trans. Med. Imaging **34**(10), 1993–2024 (2015)
3. Bakas, S., Akbari, H., Sotiras, A., Bilello, M., Rozycki, M., Kirby, J., Freymann, J., Farahani, K., Davatzikos, C.: Segmentation labels and radiomic features for the pre-operative scans of the TCGA-GBM collection. Cancer Imaging Arch. (2017). https://doi.org/10.7937/K9/TCIA.2017.KLXWJJ1Q
4. Bakas, S., Akbari, H., Sotiras, A., Bilello, M., Rozycki, M., Kirby, J., Freymann, J., Farahani, K., Davatzikos, C.: Segmentation labels and radiomic features for the pre-operative scans of the TCGA-LGG collection. Cancer Imaging Arch. (2017). https://doi.org/10.7937/K9/TCIA.2017.GJQ7R0EF
5. Huang, G., Liu, Z., Weinberger, K.Q., van der Maaten, L.: Densely connected convolutional networks. arXiv preprint arXiv:1608.06993, 25 August 2016
6. Jégou, S., Drozdzal, M., Vazquez, D., Romero, A., Bengio, Y.: The one hundred layers Tiramisu: fully convolutional DenseNets for semantic segmentation. arXiv preprint arXiv:1611.09326, 28 November 2016
7. Badrinarayanan, V., Kendall, A., Cipolla, R.: Segnet: a deep convolutional encoder-decoder architecture for image segmentation. CoRR, abs/1511.00561 (2015)
8. Long, J., Shelhamer, E., Darrell, T.: Fully convolutional networks for semantic segmentation. In: IEEE Conference on Computer Vision and Pattern Recognition (CVPR) (2015)
9. Sadowská, M.: Analysis. Scalable Algorithms for Contact Problems. AMM, vol. 36, pp. 59–66. Springer, New York (2016). https://doi.org/10.1007/978-1-4939-6834-3_4
10. Krhenbhl, P., Koltun, V.: Efficient inference in fully connected CRFs with Gaussian edge potentials. In: Advances in Neural Information Processing Systems (2011)
11. Milletari, F., Navab, N., Ahmadi, S.-A.: V-Net: fully convolutional neural networks for volumetric medical image segmentation. arXiv preprint arXiv:1606.04797, 15 June 2016
12. Pereira, S., Pinto, A., Alves, V., Silva, C.A.: Deep convolutional neural networks for the segmentation of gliomas in multi-sequence MRI. In: Crimi, A., Menze, B., Maier, O., Reyes, M., Handels, H. (eds.) BrainLes 2015. LNCS, vol. 9556, pp. 131–143. Springer, Cham (2016). https://doi.org/10.1007/978-3-319-30858-6_12

13. Kingma, D.P., Ba, J.: Adam: a method for stochastic optimization. arXiv:1412.6980, 30 January 2017
14. Ioffe, S., Szegedy, C.: Batch normalization: accelerating deep network training by reducing internal covariate shift. CoRR, abs/1502.03167 (2015)
15. Nair, V., Hinton, G.E.: Rectified linear units improve restricted Boltzmann machines
16. Drozdzal, M., Vorontsov, E., Chartrand, G., Kadoury, S., Pal, C.: The importance of skip connections in biomedical image segmentation. arXiv:1608.04117
17. Ronneberger, O., Fischer, P., Brox, T.: U-Net: convolutional networks for biomedical image segmentation. In: Navab, N., Hornegger, J., Wells, W.M., Frangi, A.F. (eds.) MICCAI 2015. LNCS, vol. 9351, pp. 234–241. Springer, Cham (2015). https://doi.org/10.1007/978-3-319-24574-4_28
18. Çiçek, Ö., Abdulkadir, A., Lienkamp, S.S., Brox, T., Ronneberger, O.: 3D U-Net: learning dense volumetric segmentation from sparse annotation. arXiv:1502.03240
19. Zhao, X., et al.: A deep learning model integrating FCNNs and CRFs for brain tumor segmentation
20. Brostow, G.J., Shotton, J., Fauqueur, J., Cipolla, R.: Segmentation and recognition using structure from motion point clouds. In: Forsyth, D., Torr, P., Zisserman, A. (eds.) ECCV 2008. LNCS, vol. 5302, pp. 44–57. Springer, Heidelberg (2008). https://doi.org/10.1007/978-3-540-88682-2_5
21. Raza, S.H., Grundmann, M., Essa, I.: Geometric context from video. In: IEEE Conference on Computer Vision and Pattern Recognition (CVPR) (2013)
22. Abadi, M., Agarwal, A., Barham, P., Brevdo, E., Chen, Z., Citro, C., Corrado, G.S., Davis, A., Dean, J., Devin, M., Ghemawat, S., Goodfellow, I., Harp, A., Irving, G., Isard, M., Jozefowicz, R., Jia, Y., Kaiser, L., Kudlur, M., Levenberg, J., Man, D., Schuster, M., Monga, R., Moore, S., Murray, D., Olah, C., Shlens, J., Steiner, B., Sutskever, I., Talwar, K., Tucker, P., Vanhoucke, V., Vasudevan, V., Vigas, F., Vinyals, O., Warden, P., Wattenberg, M., Wicke, M., Yu, Y., Zheng, X.: TensorFlow: large-scale machine learning on heterogeneous systems (2015). Software available from tensorflow.org

Brain Tumor Segmentation in MRI Scans Using Deeply-Supervised Neural Networks

Reza Pourreza, Ying Zhuge$^{(\boxtimes)}$, Holly Ning, and Robert Miller

Radiation Oncology Branch, National Cancer Institute,
National Institute of Health, Bethesda, MD 20814, USA
zhugey@nih.gov

Abstract. Gliomas are the most frequent primary brain tumors in adults. Improved quantification of the various aspects of a glioma requires accurate segmentation of the tumor in magnetic resonance images (MRI). Since the manual segmentation is time-consuming and subject to human error and irreproducibility, automatic segmentation has received a lot of attention in recent years. This paper presents a fully automated segmentation method which is capable of automatic segmentation of brain tumor from multi-modal MRI scans. The proposed method is comprised of a deeply-supervised neural network based on Holistically-Nested Edge Detection (HED) network. The HED method, which is originally developed for the binary classification task of image edge detection, is extended for multiple-class segmentation. The classes of interest include the whole tumor, tumor core, and enhancing tumor. The dataset provided by 2017 Multimodal Brain Tumor Image Segmentation Benchmark (BraTS) challenge is used in this work for training the neural network and performance evaluations. Experiments on BraTS 2017 challenge datasets demonstrate that the method performs well compared to the existing works. The assessments revealed the Dice scores of 0.86, 0.60, and 0.69 for whole tumor, tumor core, and enhancing tumor classes, respectively.

Keywords: HED · Brain tumor · MRI · BraTS

1 Introduction

Glioma is the most common type of primary brain tumor arising from glial cells. Gliomas may have different degrees of aggressiveness, variable prognosis and several heterogeneous histological sub-regions [1]. Treatment for a glioma is customized to the individual patient and may include surgery, radiation therapy, chemotherapy, or observation. Magnetic resonance imaging (MRI) is a widely used technique employed in the diagnosis, management, and follow-up of gliomas in clinical practice. In radiation therapy treatment planning, a CT scan is often the primary image set while MRI provides excellent secondary image set for soft tissue contouring. Accurate segmentation and measurement of the different tumor sub-regions is critical for monitoring progression, surgery or radiotherapy planning and follow-up studies. However, computational brain tumor segmentation in MRI is still a challenging task due to fuzzy border between tumor and normal tissues, high variation in brain tumor shape, size, and

© Springer International Publishing AG, part of Springer Nature 2018
A. Crimi et al. (Eds.): BrainLes 2017, LNCS 10670, pp. 320–331, 2018.
https://doi.org/10.1007/978-3-319-75238-9_28

location, despite long history of research and development [1, 2]. Currently, brain tumors are usually delineated manually by medical professionals, which requires a high degree of skill and concentration, and is time-consuming, expensive, and prone to operator bias. Computer-aided brain tumor segmentation using MRI would overcome these issues and provide medical professionals an unprecedented tool for efficient and reliable diagnosis, treatment and prognosis of brain tumors and could allow for the inclusion of advanced imaging techniques that are more challenging to human interpretation, e.g., diffusion-weighted imaging, attenuated diffusion coefficient maps, magnetic resonance spectroscopy, etc.

Brain tumor segmentation methods can roughly be grouped into semiautomatic and fully automatic categories. Instances of the semiautomatic methods include yet not limited to the followings. A graph cut distribution matching approach for glioma and edema segmentation in 3D multimodal MRI images is presented in [6]. A so-called "tumor-cut" method is proposed in [5] that combines graph-oriented and cellular automata-based segmentation methods. Initially, maximum tumor diameter is drawn by an expert to initialize the segmentation. The basic set operations are then utilized to combine the segmented volumes from different modalities. A latent atlas-based approach for image ensembles segmentation is presented in [4] where a manual segmentation is required to initialize level-set propagation. Active contours are used in [3] where initially an approximate contour surrounding the tumor mass is manually drawn. Then the hyperintense tumor is segmented by using a combination of global and local active contour models.

Fully automatic MRI-based brain tumor segmentation further falls into several categories including Bayesian and Markov random field (MRF) [7], atlas-based registration and combination of segmentation with registration [8, 9], statistical model of deformation [10], support vector machine (SVM) [11], random forests (RF) [12–14], and convolutional neural networks (CNN) [15–18], amongst which RFs and CNNs have received a lot of attention recently. RFs are an ensemble learning method that operate by constructing a multitude of decision trees at training time and outputting the class that is the mode of the classes of the individual trees. RFs are capable of naturally handling multi-class tasks and utilizing large number of different input features. Moreover, they correct for decision trees' habit of overfitting to their training set. While the input feature vectors to the RF approaches are mostly engineered, CNN-based methods have shown the advantages in automatic learning of the hierarchy of complex features from in-domain data [19]. Numerous CNN-based methods have been presented in Multimodal Brain Tumor Image Segmentation Benchmark (BraTS) challenges in years of 2014, 2015, and 2016 [2, 18, 20–28].

Traditional standard CNN-based methods are typically patch-based. They predict the class of a pixel by processing a square patch centered on that pixel and mainly focus on local features. In this paper, a fully automatic brain tumor segmentation method is presented which consists of a deeply supervised neural network [29] based on a modified a modified Holistically-Nested Edge Detection (HED) neural network [30]. HED was initially developed for edge detection using deep CNNs. However, it has also been shown to be effective in object segmentation [31]. The HED-based method has three advantages over traditional CNNs: (a) holistic image training and prediction in an image-to-image fashion, rather than patch-based, where each pixel has a cost function; (b) nested multiscale and multilevel image feature learning inspired by deeply-supervised, (c) enables to classify all the voxels in a slice using a single forward pass thereby reducing the time required for prediction considerably as opposed to a patch based technique. In this paper, the HED-based object segmentation method [31] has been extended for multiple-class segmentation.

2 Material

The MRI scans used in this study are the data from the BraTS 2017 challenge including 210 high grade glioma (HGG) and 75 lower grade glioma (LGG) cases. The image datasets share the following four MRI contrasts: T1, post-contrast T1-weighted (T1c), T2-weighted (T2), and T2 Fluid Attenuated Inversion Recovery (FLAIR). All the images are co-registered and resampled to the same voxel resolution: 155 slices of 240 × 240 pixels. The scans are annotated by domain experts and four labels are used: edema, non-enhancing (solid) core, necrotic (or fluid-filled) core, and enhancing core. In this study, T1 modality is discarded based on our preliminary experiments that it does not help in improving the final prediction, and the remaining three modalities are used. The target classes in this study are the whole tumor (WT), tumor core (TC), and enhancing tumor (ET). The WT class includes all the mentioned annotated labels, the TC class includes all the labels but edema, and the ET class includes only enhancing core label.

3 Proposed Method

The proposed method consists of three steps: preprocessing, classification, and postprocessing. The MRI scans are initially processed in the preprocessing step to remove the artifacts and normalize the voxel intensities. The preprocessed MRI scans are then further processed in the classification step to determine the class label per voxel. The classification core is a deep neural network that receives the MRI scans slice by slice and generates the classification results for the input slice. The classification results for all the slices are then put together to reconstruct the volumetric data. The volumetric classification outcomes are finally processed in the postprocessing step to get more consistent results and reduce the false alarms. These steps are explained in more details in the next subsections.

3.1 Preprocessing

There are two major types of artifacts in MRI scans that affect the performance of the tumor segmentation algorithms. The first artifact is bias field distortion that causes a slowly varying, inhomogeneous background in an MRI image. This problem has been studied extensively and many effective methods have been developed [32, 33]. The second artifact is the nonphysical meaning of the MRI intensities. Unlike computed tomography (CT) where the measurements are done in absolute units, MRI scans are expressed in arbitrary units that differ between study visits and subjects. The importance of handling such MRI intensity normalization has been emphasized the literature [2, 34, 35].

The well-known N4ITK filter is employed in this work to remove the bias field distortion. A sample outcome is shown in Fig. 1.

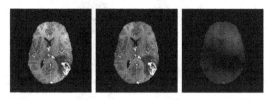

Fig. 1. Sample N4ITK filtering result, left: input (range: [0,600]), middle: output (range: [0,600]), right: difference between input and output (range: range [0,300]).

Then, voxel intensities are normalized using a histogram-based method [31, 35] to make the histograms of all MRI modalities consistent across different subjects. In this work, the median of the histogram (the index of the highest bin) is chosen as the landmark. That is because histogram median typically corresponds to the white matter tissue since it occupies the largest volume of the brain. It is worth to mention that the background voxels are excluded from the histogram. The background is identified as the largest connected component of all zero-value voxels. Once the landmark is generated for each MRI scan, a piecewise linear transform is performed by mapping the landmark intensity to the normalized intensity scale, as illustrated in Fig. 2. Here, the segment linear transformation is chosen due to its simplicity and effectiveness in producing similar histograms of MRI images across different subjects. As mentioned in the original intensity normalization paper [35], other non-linear transformation to stretch histogram segments may also be used.

As can be seen from Fig. 2, there are 4 linear transformations in histogram normalization: (i) the intensities below I_1 are mapped to O_1, (ii) the intensities between I_1 and I_2 are linearly mapped to $[O_1, O_2]$, (iii) the intensities between I_2 and I_3 are linearly mapped to $[O_2, O_3]$, (iv) the intensities above I_3 are mapped to O_3. Here, I_2 is the histogram median and I_1 and I_3 are 0.1 and 99.9 percentiles, respectively. In this work, O_1 and O_3 are chosen as 0 and 255 to be consistent with gray-level images and O_2 is set to 100 empirically. A sample histogram normalization result is shown in Fig. 3.

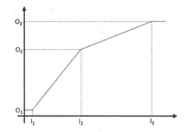

Fig. 2. Output intensities (vertical) versus input intensities (horizontal)

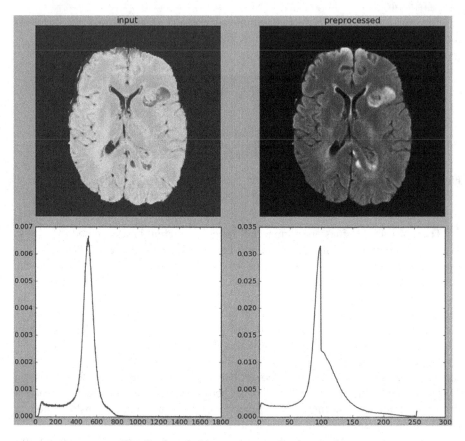

Fig. 3. Sample histogram normalization result

3.2 Classification

The classification is done via a HED-based neural network [30]. Unlike traditional CNNs that perform a pixel classification prediction using patch-based approaches, the HED-based method performs learning and prediction in an image-to-image fashion, by combining multiscale and multilevel hierarchical intensity representations of the image. HED is an extension of the traditional Fully Convolutional Networks (FCNs) and is able to produce predictions from multiple scales. HED consists of a single-stream deep network with multiple side outputs, and each corresponds to one image scale. Each side output is associated with one side-output layer, which has a separate classifier. An additional weighted fusion layer is added to unify the multiple side outputs. The side outputs as well as the fusion output are compared to the ground truth during the training and this deep supervision makes the network to be trained more effectively compared to the FCNs.

Although HED is introduced for binary classification (edge/non-edge), the architecture is changed in this work for multiple-class classification tasks. The modified network structure is shown in Fig. 4. The original HED receives an RGB image of size

$M \times M \times 3$ (three $M \times M$ planes) as the input and generates K side-outputs and one fusion output. In the modified HED, MRI scans are processed slice by slice. In other words, for every slice, T1c, T2, and FLAIR modalities are put together and fed to the network as an $M \times M \times 3$ input. This part is similar to the original HED. And the modified HED still generates K ($K = 5$ in this paper) side-outputs, but each side-output consists of three planes, each with size of $M \times M$, which correspond to prediction maps of WT, TC, and ET classes, respectively. In order to generate higher dimension outputs ($M \times M \times 3$), the convolutions and the deconvolutions in all the side-output layers are modified while the main single stream is remained the same. Note that each output is a prediction probability map of one class corresponding to a particular image scale. The weighed fusion layer is used to combine all side-output predictions.

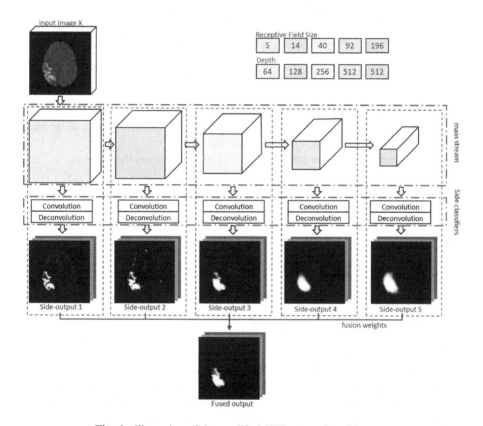

Fig. 4. Illustration of the modified HED network architecture

In this work, the training data are denoted by $S = \{(X_n, Y_n), n = 1, \ldots, N\}$ where X_n denotes the $M \times M \times 3$ input (the three modalities of one slice) and Y_n denotes the corresponding $M \times M \times 3$ binary ground truth for input X_n. In Y_n, 0 and 1 values represent normal and tumor tissues, respectively. Suppose the collection of all parameters in the single main stream, the side output classifiers, and the fusion part are denoted by W_m, W_s and W_f, respectively, then the objective functions can be defined as follows:

$$\left(W_m + W_s + W_f\right)^* = \mathrm{argmin}\left(L_{side}(W_m + W_s) + L_{fuse}\left(W_m + W_s + W_f\right)\right) \tag{1}$$

$$L_{side}(W_m + W_s) = \sum_{k=1}^{K} \alpha_k l_{side}^{(k)}\left(W_m + W_s^{(k)}\right) \tag{2}$$

where L_{side} and L_{fuse} are the total side and fusion loss functions, K is the number of side outputs which is 5 in this paper, and $l_{side}^{(k)}$ denotes the image level loss function for k^{th} side output. Suppose $\hat{Y}_{side}^{(k)}$ and $\hat{Y}_{fuse}$ denote the network-generated side outputs and the fusion output, respectively, then L_{fuse} and $l_{side}^{(k)}$ are defined as follows:

$$L_{fuse}\left(W_m + W_s + W_f\right) = cross\_entropy(Y, \hat{Y}_{fuse}) \tag{3}$$

$$l_{side}^{(k)}(W_m + W_s) = cross\_entropy(Y, \hat{Y}_{side}^{(k)}) \tag{4}$$

where $cross\_entropy$ is the sum of the pixel-wise cross entropies over the three output planes (WT, TC, and ET). Putting everything together, the optimal network parameters are found via standard stochastic gradient descent.

For an unseen input X, the trained network (*NET*) generates the outputs:

$$(\hat{Y}_{fuse}, \hat{Y}_{side}^{(1)}, \ldots, \hat{Y}_{side}^{(K)}) = NET(X, (W_m + W_s + W_f)^*) \tag{5}$$

and the network unified output can be obtained by further aggregating these generated outputs:

$$\hat{Y}_{net} = average(\hat{Y}_{fuse}, \hat{Y}_{side}^{(1)}, \ldots, \hat{Y}_{side}^{(K)}) \tag{6}$$

3.3 Postprocessing

Once all the slices of an MRI scan are processed by the network, all the $\hat{Y}_{net}$s corresponding to all the slices are aggregated to generate the 3d output $\hat{Y}_{3d}$. The 3d output is thresholded to generate binary output $\hat{Y}_{bin}$ and then postprocessed to produce the final output $\hat{Y}_{final}$. The optimal thresholds are found by maximizing Dice score over the training samples. Dice score for two binary sets A and B is defined below:

$$Dice(A, B) = \frac{2|A \cap B|}{|A| + |B|} \tag{7}$$

where $|.|$ operator denotes the number of voxels with value 1.

The binary output suffers from false alarms. Postprocessings for the three classes are conducted individually to reduce the false alarms and improve the accuracy. For the

WT class, postprocessing includes maintaining the largest connected object and getting rid of the other objects. But before applying this, a morphological binary opening operator ($3 \times 3 \times 3$) is applied to the binary map to separate those false alarms that are connected using weak connections and subsequently reduced their sizes. Postprocessing for TC class includes multiplying its binary map by the postprocessed WT binary map. By doing this, all the false alarms outside the whole tumor segment are removed. Similar to the CT class, postprocessing for ET class includes multiplying its binary map by both the postprocessed WT and CT binary maps. as illustrated in Fig. 5.

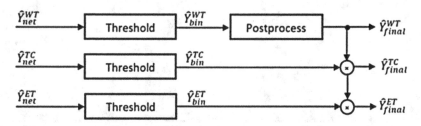

Fig. 5. Postprocessing illustration

3.4 Results and Discussions

The original HED has been implemented in a slightly modified version of the publicly available *Caffe* library. In this work, the original HED Caffe model was modified to adapt to the current problem by adding the extra weights in the side output classifiers. The rest of the pipeline including the preprocessing, data preparation, postprocessing, train and test controls were implemented in Python.

All the available training data from BraTS 2017 were used in training the neural network. However, since the number of normal voxels was much higher than the number of tumor voxels in the dataset, the classes were highly skewed. Two simple solutions were sought in this work to reduce the class skewness. First, those slices with no signals were excluded from training. Second, a 200×200 window was cropped from the center of the 240×240 slice for training and the border pixels were discarded. The removed pixels corresponded to the background area around the skull. This simple solution reduced the number of background pixels at least by 30% and consequently lowered the class skewness. Moreover, transfer learning was used in this work since the number of the training samples was not enough to train the network initialized with random weights. In other words, the network weights were initialized with those of the trained HED rather than random values.

The training was carried out via a Stochastic Gradient Descent strategy with a batch size of 30 on a NVIDIA Titan Xp graphic card. The program took around 48 h for training, and took around 30 s per scan for the inference and postprocessing.

The performance was measured using BraTS online evaluation system for the training, validation, and testing datasets. The achieved Dice scores are reported in Table 1. A sample segmentation outcome together with the ground truth is shown in Fig. 6.

Table 1. Dice scores for the training, validation, and testing datasets

Dataset	WT	TC	ET
Training	0.86	0.65	0.58
Validation	0.86	0.60	0.69
Testing	0.80	0.55	0.55

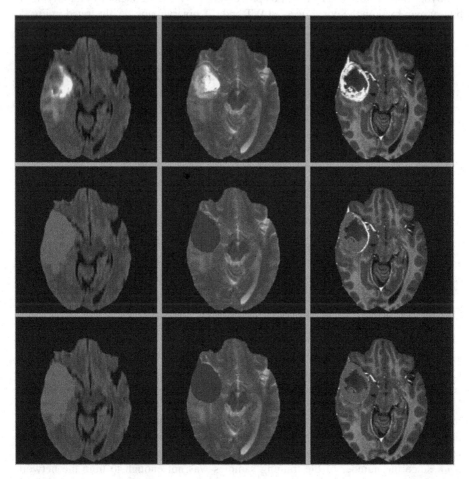

Fig. 6. Sample segmentation results. Top row from left to right: FLAIR, T2, and T1c. Middle row: segmented WT, TC, and ET. Bottom row: ground truth WT, TC, and ET.

4   Conclusions

An automatic method for brain tumor segmentation method in MRI scans was presented in this paper. The classification core of the presented method is a deeply supervised neural network based on HED. Low computational, yet very effective preprocessing and postprocessing steps were added to the pipeline that highly improved the accuracy of the segmentation. The achieved results are very promising and demonstrate the effectiveness of the presented method in terms of the segmentation accuracy. Moreover, the method has very low computational burden as the neural network as well as the preprocessing and postprocessing steps are very computationally efficient.

Acknowledgements. This research was supported by the Intramural Research Program of the National Cancer Institute, NIH.

References

1. Holland, E.C.: Progenitor cells and glioma formation. Curr. Opin. Neurol. **14**(6), 683–688 (2001)
2. Pereira, S., Pinto, A., Alves, V., Silva, C.A.: Brain tumor segmentation using convolutional neural networks in MRI images. IEEE Trans. Med. Imaging **35**, 1240–1251 (2016)
3. Njeh, I., Sallemi, L., Ayed, I.B., et al.: 3D multimodal MRI brain glioma tumor and edema segmentation: a graph cut distribution matching approach. Comput. Med. Imaging Graph. **40**, 108–119 (2015)
4. Hamamci, A., Kucuk, N., Karaman, K., Engin, K., Unal, G.: Tumor-Cut: segmentation of brain tumors on contrast enhanced MR images for radiosurgery applications. IEEE Trans. Med. Imaging **31**, 790–804 (2012)
5. Raviv, T.R., Van Leemput, K., Menze, B.H., Wells 3rd, W.M., Golland, P.: Segmentation of image ensembles via latent atlases. Med. Image Anal. **14**, 654–665 (2010)
6. Guo, X.G., Schwartz, L., Zhao, B.: Semi-automatic segmentation of multimodal brain tumor using active contours. In: Medical Image Computing and Computer Assisted Intervention, pp. 27–30 (2013)
7. Prastawa, M., Bullitt, E., Ho, S., Gerig, G.: A brain tumor segmentation framework based on outlier detection. Med. Image Anal. **8**, 275–283 (2004)
8. Prastawa, M., Bullitt, E., Moon, N., Van Leemput, K., Gerig, G.: Automatic brain tumor segmentation by subject specific modification of atlas priors. Acad. Radiol. **10**, 1341–1348 (2003)
9. Cuadra, M.B., Pollo, C., Bardera, A., Cuisenaire, O., Villemure, J.G., Thiran, J.P.: Atlas-based segmentation of pathological MR brain images using a model of lesion growth. IEEE Trans. Med. Imaging **23**, 1301–1314 (2004)
10. Mohamed, A., Zacharaki, E.I., Shen, D., Davatzikos, C.: Deformable registration of brain tumor images via a statistical model of tumor-induced deformation. Med. Image Anal. **10**, 752–763 (2006)
11. Zhang, N., Ruan, S., Lebonvallet, S., Liao, Q., Zhu, Y.: Kernel feature selection to fuse multi-spectral MRI images for brain tumor segmentation. Comput. Vis. Image Underst. **115**, 256–259 (2011)
12. Breiman, L.: Random forests. Mach. Learn. **45**, 5–32 (2001)
13. Tustison, N.J., Shrinidhi, K.L., Wintermark, M., et al.: Optimal symmetric multimodal templates and concatenated random forests for supervised brain tumor segmentation (simplified) with ANTsR. Neuroinformatics **13**, 209–225 (2015)
14. Pinto, A., Pereira, S., Correia, H., Oliveira, J., Rasteiro, D.M., Silva, C.A.: Brain tumour segmentation based on extremely randomized forest with highlevel features. In: Conference Proceedings IEEE Engineering in Medicine and Biology Society 2015, pp. 3037–3040 (2015)

15. LeCun, Y., Bengio, Y., Hinton, G.: Deep learning. Nature **521**, 436–444 (2015)
16. Krizhevsky, A., Sutskever, I., Hinton, G.E.: ImageNet classification with deep convolutional neural networks. Adv. Neural. Inf. Process. Syst. **1**, 1097–1115 (2012)
17. Zhao, L., Jia, K.: Multiscale CNNs for brain tumor segmentation and diagnosis. Comput. Math. Methods Med. **2016**, 8356291–8356297 (2016)
18. Havaei, M., Dutil, F., Pal, C., Larochelle, H., Jodoin, P.-M.: A convolutional neural network approach to brain tumor segmentation. In: Proceeding of the Multimodal Brain Tumor Segmentation Challenge, pp. 29–33 (2015)
19. Bengio, Y., Courville, A., Vincent, P.: Representation learning: a review and new perspectives. IEEE Trans. Pattern Anal. Mach. Intell. **35**, 1798–1828 (2013)
20. Menze, B.H., Jakab, A., Bauer, S., Kalpathy-Cramer, J., Farahani, K., Kirby, J., Burren, Y., Porz, N., Slotboom, J., Wiest, R., Lanczi, L., Gerstner, E., Weber, M.A., Arbel, T., Avants, B.B., Ayache, N., Buendia, P., Collins, D.L., Cordier, N., Corso, J.J., Criminisi, A., Das, T., Delingette, H., Demiralp, Ç., Durst, C.R., Dojat, M., Doyle, S., Festa, J., Forbes, F., Geremia, E., Glocker, B., Golland, P., Guo, X., Hamamci, A., Iftekharuddin, K.M., Jena, R., John, N.M., Konukoglu, E., Lashkari, D., Mariz, J.A., Meier, R., Pereira, S., Precup, D., Price, S.J., Raviv, T.R., Reza, S.M., Ryan, M., Sarikaya, D., Schwartz, L., Shin, H.C., Shotton, J., Silva, C.A., Sousa, N., Subbanna, N.K., Szekely, G., Taylor, T.J., Thomas, O. M., Tustison, N.J., Unal, G., Vasseur, F., Wintermark, M., Ye, D.H., Zhao, L., Zhao, B., Zikic, D., Prastawa, M., Reyes, M., Van Leemput, K.: The multimodal brain tumor image segmentation benchmark (BraTS). IEEE Trans. Med. Imaging **34**(10), 1993–2024 (2015)
21. Bakas, S., Akbari, H., Sotiras, A., Bilello, M., Rozycki, M., Kirby, J.S., Freymann, J.B., Farahani, K., Davatzikos, C.: Advancing the cancer genome atlas glioma MRI collections with expert segmentation labels and radiomic features. Nat. Sci. Data (2017, in press)
22. Bakas, S., Akbari, H., Sotiras, A., Bilello, M., Rozycki, M., Kirby, J., Freymann, J., Farahani, K., Davatzikos, C.: Segmentation labels and radiomic features for the pre-operative scans of the TCGA-GBM collection. The Cancer Imaging Archive (2017). https://doi.org/10.7937/k9/tcia.2017.klxwjj1q
23. Bakas, S., Akbari, H., Sotiras, A., Bilello, M., Rozycki, M., Kirby, J., Freymann, J., Farahani, K., Davatzikos, C.: Segmentation labels and radiomic features for the pre-operative scans of the TCGA-LGG collection. The Cancer Imaging Archive (2017). https://doi.org/10.7937/k9/tcia.2017.gjq7r0ef
24. Urban, G., Bendszus, M., Hamprecht, F., Kleesiek, J.: Multi-modal brain tumor segmentation using deep convolutional neural networks. In: Proceeding of the Multimodal Brain Tumor Segmentation Challenge, pp. 31–35 (2014)
25. Davy, A., Havaei, M., Warde-farley, D., et al.: Brain tumor segmentation with deep neural networks. In: Proceeding of the Multimodal Brain Tumor Segmentation Challenge, pp. 1–5 (2014)
26. Rao, V., Sarabi, M.S., Jaiswal, A.: Brain tumor segmentation with deep learning. In: Proceeding of the Multimodal Brain Tumor Segmentation Challenge, pp. 56–59 (2015)
27. Lun, T.K., Hsu, W.: Brain tumor segmentation using deep convolutional neural network. In: Proceeding of the Multimodal Brain Tumor Image Segmentation Challenge, pp. 26–29 (2016)
28. Zhao, X., Wu, Y., Song, G., Li, Z., Fan, Y., Zhang, Y.: Brain tumor segmentation using a fully convolutional neural network with conditional random fields. In: Proceeding of the Multimodal Brain Tumor Image Segmentation Challenge, pp. 77–80 (2016)
29. Lee, C.Y., Xie, S., Gallagher, P., Zhang, Z., Tu, Z.: Deeply-supervised nets. In: Proceedings of AISTATS, pp. 562–570 (2015)
30. Xie, S., Tu, Z.: Holistically-nested edge detection. Int. J. Comput. Vision, 1–16 (2017)

31. Zhuge, Y., Krauze, A.V., Ning, H., Cheng, J.C., Arora, B.C., Camphausen, K., Miller, R.W.: Brain tumor segmentation using holistically nested neural networks in MRI images. Med. Phys. **44**, 5234–5243 (2017)
32. Guillemaud, R., Brady, M.: Estimating the bias field of MR images. IEEE Trans. Med. Imaging **16**, 238–251 (1997)
33. Tustison, N.J., Avants, B.B., Cook, P.A., et al.: N4ITK: improved N3 bias correction. IEEE Trans. Med. Imaging **29**, 1310–1320 (2010)
34. Zhuge, Y., Udupa, J.K.: Intensity standardization simplifies brain MR image segmentation. Comput. Vis. Image Underst. **113**, 1095–1103 (2009)
35. Nyul, L.G., Udupa, J.K., Zhang, X.: New variants of a method of MRI scale standardization. IEEE Trans. Med. Imaging **19**, 143–150 (2000)

Brain Tumor Segmentation and Parsing on MRIs Using Multiresolution Neural Networks

Laura Silvana Castillo$^{(\boxtimes)}$(iD), Laura Alexandra Daza$^{(\boxtimes)}$(iD),
Luis Carlos Rivera$^{(\boxtimes)}$(iD), and Pablo Arbeláez(iD)

Department of Biomedical Engineering, Universidad de los Andes, Bogotá, Colombia
{ls.castillo332,la.daza10,lc.rivera10}@uniandes.edu.co

Abstract. Brain lesion segmentation is a critical application of computer vision to the biomedical image analysis. The difficulty is derived from the great variance between instances, and the high computational cost of processing three dimensional data. We introduce a neural network for brain tumor semantic segmentation that parses their internal structures and is capable of processing volumetric data from multiple MRI modalities simultaneously. As a result, the method is able to learn from small training datasets. We develop an architecture that has four parallel pathways with residual connections. It receives patches from images with different spatial resolutions and analyzes them independently. The results are then combined using fully-connected layers to obtain a semantic segmentation of the brain tumor. We evaluated our method using the 2017 BraTS Challenge dataset, reaching average dice coefficients of 89%, 88% and 86% over the training, validation and test images, respectively.

Keywords: Semantic segmentation · Brain tumors
Machine learning · Deep learning · MRI

1 Introduction

Brain tumors are abnormal formations of mass that apply pressure to the surrounding tissues, causing several health problems such as unexplained nausea, seizures, personality changes or even death [1]. They have different shapes, sizes and internal structures, which makes the task of detection and classification difficult and highly dependent on the experience of the specialist, even for experts. These lesions can be classified into Low-Grade Gliomas (LGG) and High-Grade Gliomas (HGG). LGGs are benign, slowly growing tumors that can become life-threatening in the course of disease. HGGs are malignant, fast growing tumors capable of inducing the development of new tumors in different parts of the central nervous system. Without an appropriate treatment, HGGs can be lethal in just a few months [2,3]. Even after a diagnosis had been made there is a high probability that the treatment could not be the best one for that specific case.

L.S. Castillo, L.A, Daza, L.C. Rivera—Authors with equal contribution.

© Springer International Publishing AG, part of Springer Nature 2018
A. Crimi et al. (Eds.): BrainLes 2017, LNCS 10670, pp. 332–343, 2018.
https://doi.org/10.1007/978-3-319-75238-9_29

Nowadays, doctors make use of Magnetic Resonance Imaging (MRI) to visualize the brain of a patient to look for any life-threatening abnormality. However, finding those structures in a 3D medical image is a complicated task, highly prone to error [4]. In spite of the fact that the treatment selection is based directly on the diagnosis, these days that process is made manually, which causes it to be inefficient and observer-dependent. The responsibility to find whether there is an abnormality or not in the exam lies on the neurologist's hands, who decides, based on his own experience, if there is a lesion and what is the best way to proceed. As a consequence, the uncertainty of the patient's outcome is significant.

For more than a decade, automatic brain lesion segmentation has been a topic of interest. Initial approaches to solve this problem were based on the detection of abnormalities using healthy-brain atlases and probabilistic models [5]. Later, results were improved using deformable registration fields along with Markov Random Fields (MRF) [6]. Subsequent approaches using machine learning techniques, such as Random Forests [7,8], yielded better results, reaching an average dice coefficient of 60% in the 2012 BraTS Challenge.

In the last years, Convolutional Neural Networks (CNN) have shown outstanding results in detection, classification and segmentation tasks, matching humans. Part of this success is due to the rapid improvement of machine's computational power and to the CNNs ability of abstracting features in different hierarchical representations of an image [9]. Fully convolutional networks (FCN) proved to be an effective way to perform pixel-by-pixel classification [10], obtaining a mean Intersection over Union (IoU) of 67% in the PASCAL-VOC dataset in 2012, where the task was to produce an accurate segmentation of 20 different categories in natural images. This method offers the advantage of combining coarse and shallow semantic information from images with an arbitrary input size [10]. In 2015, U-Net, an architecture based on FCN and specialized in the task of segmenting medical images, was developed. U-Net's architecture has a contracting path to extract local information and an expanding path to locate the object within the whole image [11]. Recently V-Net, an expansion of this method to process three-dimensional data, was presented. V-Net demonstrated a remarkable behavior in the MICCAI 2012 PROMISE Challenge dataset for prostate segmentation in computerized tomography (CT), obtaining an average dice coefficient of 82% [12]. Another method to process medical images is Deepmedic, a neural network that segments brain tumors using information from different MRI modalities. It takes as inputs 3D patches (small volumetric cuts) extracted from MRIs at different modalities, and analyzes the information using two pathways. It then uses fully connected layers to obtain a segmentation of each category [13].

In this paper, we aim at providing an efficient, accurate and objective way of automatically estimating the volume and location of a brain tumor. For this purpose, we use the 2017 BraTS Challenge dataset, which utilizes multi-institutional pre-operative MRI scans and focuses on the segmentation of intrinsically heterogeneous (in appearance, shape, and histology) brain tumors, namely gliomas [4,14–16]. This open source dataset has MRIs from 210 patients with

HGG and 75 patients with LGG tumors for training; there are four different MRI modalities per patient and annotations made by several specialists. In terms of methodology, inspired by DeepMedic's [13] success on modeling multisacale information, we developed a neural network with four contracting pathways and residual connections that receive patches centered on the same voxel, but with different spatial resolutions. During the testing stage, the average dice coefficient and the Hausdorff distance were calculated to measure the performance of the methods.

2   Methodology

2.1   Multimodality Volumetric Neural Network

Multiple Resolutions: different architectures for semantic segmentation, such as VGG [17] and FCN [10], take advantage of multiple image resolutions to simultaneously extract fine details and coarse structures from the input data. This is done using groups of convolutional layers and non-linearities, usually Rectified Linear Units (ReLU), followed by pooling operations. However, as the image resolution is reduced, so is the accuracy in the segmentation location. To overcome this drawback, we designed a network that extracts features from different input resolutions in a parallel and independent manner. This allows us to retrieve detailed appearance data along with accurate semantic information. After that, we can combine those results to obtain the final segmentation.

Figure 1 shows an overview of our approach. Our method has four identical parallel pathways, each one with six convolutional layers and two residual connections. All the paths receive patches centered at the same voxel, but extracted from different versions of the image (original and downsampled by factors of three, six and eight). The patches have input sizes of 36^3, 20^3, 18^3 and 15^3 for the different resolution pathways. We tested different downsample factors and input sizes, and the best result was chosen empirically on the validation set. In addition, deconvolutional layers are used to upsample the outputs when necessary. Finally, the results are concatenated and introduced in the fully connected layers to be combined and then classified. The classification layer is a convolution with kernel size of 1^3 and the final output is predicted using a softmax classifier.

Patch-Wise Approach: given the amount of data in a MRI, the memory requirements to process each image are substantial. Furthermore, the use of multiple modalities increases the input size even more, resulting in considerable memory consumption. On the other hand, segmenting brain tumors is a highly imbalanced problem, in which the background voxels cover over 90% of the images, while the remaining elements can belong to any of the three internal structures of the tumor. Nonetheless, both of these problems can be addressed by analyzing small patches rather than the whole image. This is because patches do not only reduce the input data size, but can also be used to balance the number of instances per category that the model will see. With this in mind, we trained our method using patches extracted randomly from the training images. The only constraints imposed were that 50% of the patches must be centered on a foreground voxel, and no patches centered on background voxels that don't belong to the brain were extracted.

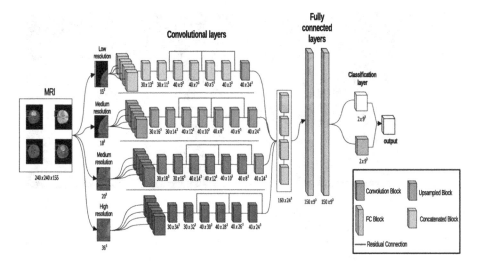

Fig. 1. Proposed Architecture. The kernels of the convolutions in the four pathways are 3^3 and no padding was made in those operations. The input of the four paths are 3D patches of each modality centered in the same voxel, but the lower resolution patches are obtained from downsampled versions of the image by factors of 3, 6 and 8, respectively.

2.2   Data

The method was trained, validated and tested using the BraTS challenge 2017 datasets. The training dataset includes 210 different MRI files from high grade glioma (HGG) cases, and 75 MRIs from low grade gliomas (LGG). The validation and test datasets include 46 and 146 different MRI files, respectively. Every image has four modalities: T1, T1 contrast-enhanced, T2 and FLAIR. The ground truth annotations were made by experts and manually-revised by board-certified neuroradiologists, and were made publicly available only for the training dataset. The annotations contain four different categories representing the background and the internal structures of the tumor as shown in Fig. 2 and listed below [4,14–16]:

0. Everything Else.
1. Necrosis and Non-Enhancing tumor.
2. Edema.
4. Enhancing tumor.

The internal structures are used to obtain the segmentations of the three glioma sub-regions evaluated in the challenge: The enhancing tumor (ET); the tumor core (TC), that includes the necrotic area, the non-enhancing and enhancing tumors; and the whole tumor (WT), represented by the edema.

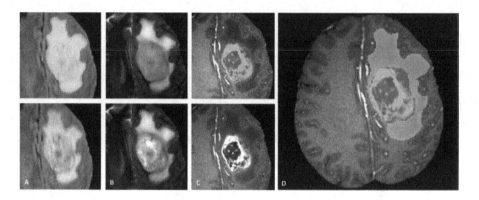

Fig. 2. Manual annotation through expert raters. Shown are image patches with the tumor structures that are annotated in the different modalities (top left) and the final labels for the whole dataset (right). Image patches show from left to right: the whole tumor visible in FLAIR (a), the tumor core visible in T2 (b), the enhancing tumor structures visible in T1c (blue), surrounding the cystic/necrotic components of the core (green) (c). Segmentations are combined to generate the final labels of the tumor structures (d): edema (yellow), non-enhancing solid core (red), necrotic/cystic core (green), enhancing core(blue). (Figure taken from the BraTS IEEE TMI paper [4]) (Color figure online)

2.3   Training

The architecture was trained using the 285 cases from the training dataset, without discriminating between the two categories of glioma, seeking to obtain a robust model that could segment both lesions without difficulty. Our method's inputs are patches of size 36^3 that are extracted randomly, making sure that 50% of them are centered at a voxel labeled as tumor, as explained in Sect. 2.1. The data is normalized individually per MRI volume by setting the mean to 0 and the variance to 1. Data augmentation is made to avoid overfitting of the model due to the small size of the training dataset, and it is performed on the fly to prevent memory issues. The process is made by reflecting randomly chosen volumes along the sagittal axis. To train the method, the learning rate was set to $1e-4$ and it remained constant during the 35 epochs. We use sparse softmax cross entropy loss and minimize it using the Adam optimizer with $\beta_1 = 0.9$, $\beta_2 = 0.999$ and $\epsilon = 1e-8$.

2.4   Validation and Test

To test the model, the 46 volumes from the validation dataset and the 146 from the test dataset were evaluated with the network. The only pre-processing step applied to the data is the individual normalization per MRI described in Sect. 2.3. In these stages, the patches are extracted at uniform intervals in the images. No additional post-processing was done to the volumes. Lastly, the whole volume was reconstructed using the segmented patches. In this testing stage a new MRI takes less than 15 seconds in producing the prediction.

2.5   Evaluation Metrics

We consider the four complementary performance metrics proposed in the challenge for quantitative evaluation.

Dice Coefficient: for every model, the Dice-Coefficient (Eq. 1) is calculated as performance metric. This measure states the similarity between clinical ground truth annotations and the output segmentation of the model. Afterwards, we calculate the average of the results to obtain the overall dice coefficient of the models.

$$DC = \frac{2|A \cap B|}{|A| + |B|} \tag{1}$$

Hausdorff Distance: the Hausdorff Distance (Eq. 2) is mathematically defined as the maximum distance of a set to the nearest point in the other set [18]. In other words, it measures how close are the segmentation's and the expected output's boundaries. This metric is used to assess the alignment between the contours of the segmentations.

$$H(A, B) = max\{min\{d(A, B)\}\} \tag{2}$$

Sensitivity and Specificity: are statistical measures used to evaluate the behavior of the predictions and the proportions of True Positives (TP), False Negatives (FN), False Positives (FP) and True Negatives (TN). The Sensitivity (Eq. 3), also known as True Positive Rate, gives the proportion of true positives predicted correctly. The specificity (Eq. 4), also known as True Negative Rate, measures how well the true negatives are predicted.

$$Sensitivity = TPR = \frac{TP}{TP + FN} \tag{3}$$

$$Specificity = TNR = \frac{TN}{TN + FP} \tag{4}$$

3   Experimental Results

We performed extensive experiments to find the optimal number of paths needed to solve this task. We tested the architecture for three, four and five pathways with multiple resolutions in the validation dataset. In Table 1 we present the results:

Table 1. Dice coefficient, sensitivity, specificity and Hausdorff distance of our neural network for Enhanced Tumor, Whole Tumor and Core Tumor; evaluated over the validation dataset from BraTS 2017.

	Dice			Sensitivity			Specificity			Hausdorff		
	Enh.	Wh.	Core	Enh.	Wh.	Core	Enh.	Wh.	Core	Enh.	Wh.	Core
3 paths	0,68	0,86	0,69	0.74	0.87	0.69	0.99	0.99	0.99	10.34	14.74	14.12
4 paths	0,71	0,88	0,68	0.72	0.86	0.68	0.99	0.99	0.99	6,12	9,63	11,38
5 paths	0,68	0,88	0,69	0.74	0.86	0.69	0.99	0.99	0.99	7.43	7.99	12.86

As demonstrated by Table 1, the four-pathway architecture obtains the best results in the previous experiment. The 5 path approach (with additional downsamples of three, four, six and eight) gets a similar performance with a minimal decrease. However, this method uses more trainable parameters and therefore takes longer to train. For this reason, we choose the four-pathway architecture that takes advantage of a multi-resolution approach, in order to get information of the location of the tumor and, at the same time, acquire local data that helps to differentiate the structures of the lesions in a reasonable time. In Table 2 we present the results on the training, validation and test datasets using the evaluation metrics explained in 2.5:

Table 2. Dice coefficient, sensitivity, specificity and Hausdorff distance of our neural network for Enhanced Tumor, Whole Tumor and Core Tumor; evaluated over the training, validation and test datasets from BraTS 2017. Note: Sensitivity and specificity measures were not provided for the evaluation in test dataset.

	Dice			Sensitivity			Specificity			Hausdorff		
	Enh.	Wh.	Core	Enh.	Wh.	Core	Enh.	Wh.	Core	Enh.	Wh.	Core
Train	0,74	0,89	0,87	0.83	0.91	0.89	0.99	0.99	0.99	5,85	15,99	11,18
Val	0,71	0,88	0,68	0.72	0.86	0.68	0.99	0.99	0.99	6,12	9,63	11,38
Test	0,65	0,86	0,67	–	–	–	–	–	–	51,70	10,39	36,20

Overall, our approach reached a competitive result. The usage of different levels of resolution and fully connected layers proved to be an effective way to obtain a detailed and accurately located segmentation of brain tumors in MRIs.

This behavior is exhibited in the average dice coefficients obtained for the whole tumor segmentation task, as shown on Table 2. Our method reached a result of 89% in the training phase. Furthermore, when introducing completely new data we get a similar performance (88% in validation and 86% in test). The minimal change between these results demonstrates the robustness of the model.

Table 3. Visual comparison between the ground truth against some results obtained by our neural network

Ground truth	Our segmentation

The sensitivity and specificity were also measured for the train and validation datasets. We obtain high sensitivity results, ranging between 68% and 91% for all the evaluated tasks. Therefore, the method has a good recall. In medical problems, this is a specially important measure due to the interest in finding every ailment affecting the patient, in order to prevent any complication. Additionally, our neural network obtains a specificity of 99% for all the evaluated tasks in both training and validation, which shows that the method is able to predict with great certainty which parts of the brain are healthy. Another strong point of our network is the ability to produce fast segmentations, as it takes around fifteen seconds to process the four modalities and produce the new segmentation. In critical and time-sensitive clinical situations, the efficiency of our approach represents a faster diagnosis and a higher probability of survival for the patient.

Table 4. Dice coefficient, sensitivity, specificity and Hausdorff distance of our neural network and the Deepmedic implementation for Enhanced Tumor, Whole Tumor and Core Tumor; evaluated over validation datasets from BraTS 2017.

	Dice			Sensitivity			Specificity			Hausdorff		
	Enh.	Wh.	Cor.	Enh.	Wh.	Cor.	Enh.	Wh.	Cor.	Enh.	Wh.	Cor.
Deepmedic	0.69	0.86	0.68	0.72	0.86	0.64	0.99	0.99	0.99	10.1	25.0	17.5
Ours	**0,71**	**0,88**	**0,68**	**0.72**	**0.86**	**0.68**	**0.99**	**0.99**	**0.99**	**6,12**	**9,63**	**11,38**

Table 4 shows a comparison between the results of our architecture against the implementation of Deepmedic (available in [13]) over the validation dataset of BraTS 2017. Our method reached a better performance in all the evaluated metrics, the high improvement in the Enhancing tumor and Whole tumor tasks (2 points in Dice coefficient measure) demonstrates that our approach is not only able to locate the area of the tumor better, but also has a greater capacity to identify correctly the internal structures of the lesion, information that can be vital when performing a diagnosis and treatment of a patient.

In Table 3, we present some examples of the predictions against the ground truth. It is important to emphasize the precision with which our method differentiates the structures that compose the tumor. We can see its capability to predict the exact area where the patient's tumor occurs with minimal noisy activations in other areas. In Table 5, we present some examples of the predictions against the ground truth that show the limitations of our method. We found that it can identify and locate the tumor with a high degree of precision in all the evaluated cases. However, when differentiating between the inner parts of the tumor, it falls short in some examples. In general, as can be seen in Table 5, the prediction is correct for the location of the affected region, but it predicts false positives in the contours of the specific structures. Taking into account the difficulty of the problem, where even for the experts it is complicated to locate the tumor accurately and even more to identify their internal parts, our method obtains an robust performance in a reduced period time.

Table 5. Visual comparison between the ground truth against the worst results obtained by our neural network

4   Conclusion

We propose a volumetric multimodality neural network. Our method receives as input 3D patches extracted from the dataset images. The architecture consist of four identical parallel pathways, to extract features on four specific resolution levels, each one with six convolutional layers and two residual connections. We then combine their results using fully connected layers. Finally, every pixel is classified into background or one of the three categories belonging to the tumor. In this paper, we have presented results in the 2017 BraTS Challenge dataset

(Training, Validation and Test) reaching an average dice coefficient of 89% over training dataset, 88% over validation dataset and 86% over test dataset for the whole tumor segmentation task (Table 2).

The use of multiple resolutions has proven to be an effective way to extract detailed information and coarse, semantic data from the images. However, most methods use a series of consecutive blocks and pooling operations for that purpose. As a consequence, deeper blocks lose some of the fine information obtained in early stages. In this paper, we showed that the use of parallel independent blocks to extract different levels of features allows us to obtain accurate and detailed results. Additionally, the use of a patch-wise approach has proven to be useful to deal with large amounts of data, which are highly imbalanced and need to be processed simultaneously to avoid the loss of 3D and multimodality information.

References

1. Mayo Clinic: Brain tumor - Symptoms and causes. http://www.mayoclinic.org/diseases-conditions/brain-tumor/symptoms-causes/dxc-20117134. Accessed 19 July 2017
2. kinderkrebsinfo.de: Brain tumours - tumours of the central nervous system. https://www.kinderkrebsinfo.de/diseases/brain_tumours/index_eng.html. Accessed 24 Aug 2017
3. The Royal Marsden NHS Foundation Trust: Glioma. https://www.royalmarsden.nhs.uk/your-care/cancer-types/paediatric-cancers/glioma. Accessed 24 Aug 2017
4. Menze, B., Jakab, A., Bauer, S., Kalpathy-Cramer, J., Farahani, K., Kirby, J., Burren, Y., Porz, N., Slotboom, J., Wiest, R., Lanczi, L., Gerstner, E., Weber, M.A., Arbel, T., Avants, B., Ayache, N., Buendia, P., Collins, L., Cordier, N., Corso, J., Criminisi, A., Das, T., Delingette, H., Demiralp, C., Durst, C., Dojat, M., Doyle, S., Festa, J., Forbes, F., Geremia, E., Glocker, B., Golland, P., Guo, X., Hamamci, A., Iftekharuddin, K., Jena, R., John, N., Konukoglu, E., Lashkari, D., Antonio Mariz, J., Meier, R., Pereira, S., Precup, D., Price, S.J., Riklin-Raviv, T., Reza, S., Ryan, M., Schwartz, L., Shin, H.C., Shotton, J., Silva, C., Sousa, N., Subbanna, N., Szekely, G., Taylor, T., Thomas, O., Tustison, N., Unal, G., Vasseur, F., Wintermark, M., Hye Ye, D., Zhao, L., Zhao, B., Zikic, D., Prastawa, M., Reyes, M., Van Leemput, K.: The multimodal brain tumor image segmentation benchmark (BRATS). IEEE Trans. Med. Imaging **34**(10), 1993–2024 (2015)
5. Prastawa, M., Bullitt, E., Ho, S., Gerig, G.: A brain tumor segmentation framework based on outlier detection. Med. Image Anal. **8**(3), 275–283 (2004)
6. Parisot, S., Duffau, H., Chemouny, S., Paragios, N.: Joint tumor segmentation and dense deformable registration of brain MR images. In: Ayache, N., Delingette, H., Golland, P., Mori, K. (eds.) MICCAI 2012. LNCS, vol. 7511, pp. 651–658. Springer, Heidelberg (2012). https://doi.org/10.1007/978-3-642-33418-4_80
7. Bauer, S., Fejes, T., Slotboom, J., Wiest, R., Nolte, L.P., Reyes, M.: Segmentation of brain tumor images based on integrated hierarchical classification and regularization. In: Proceedings MICCAI-BRATS (2012)
8. Menze, B.H., Geremia, E., Ayache, N., Szekely, G.: Segmenting glioma in multimodal images using a generative-discriminative model for brain lesion segmentation. In: Proceedings MICCAI-BRATS (2012)

9. Zeiler, M.D., Fergus, R.: Visualizing and understanding convolutional networks. In: Fleet, D., Pajdla, T., Schiele, B., Tuytelaars, T. (eds.) ECCV 2014. LNCS, vol. 8689, pp. 818–833. Springer, Cham (2014). https://doi.org/10.1007/978-3-319-10590-1_53

10. Shelhamer, E., Long, J., Darrell, T.: Fully convolutional networks for semantic segmentation. CoRR abs/1605.06211 (2016)

11. Ronneberger, O., Fischer, P., Brox, T.: U-net: convolutional networks for biomedical image segmentation. CoRR abs/1505.04597 (2015)

12. Milletari, F., Navab, N., Ahmadi, S.: V-net: fully convolutional neural networks for volumetric medical image segmentation. CoRR abs/1606.04797 (2016)

13. Kamnitsas, K., Ferrante, E., Parisot, S., Ledig, C., Nori, A., Criminisi, A., Rueckert, D., Glocker, B.: Deepmedic on brain tumor segmentation. In: Proceedings of BRATS-MICCAI code, Athens, Greece. https://github.com/Kamnitsask/deepmedic

14. Bakas, S., Akbari, H., Sotiras, A., Bilello, M., Rozycki, M., Kirby, J., Freymann, J., Farahani, K., Davatzikos, C.: Advancing the cancer genome atlas glioma MRI collections with expert segmentation labels and radiomic features. Nat. Sci. Data **4**, 170117 (2017)

15. Bakas, S., Akbari, H., Sotiras, A., Bilello, M., Rozycki, M., Kirby, J., Freymann, J., Farahani, K., Davatzikos, C.: Segmentation labels and radiomic features for the pre-operative scans of the TCGA-GBM collection. The Cancer Imaging Archive (2017). https://doi.org/10.7937/K9/TCIA.2017.KLXWJJ1Q

16. Bakas, S., Akbari, H., Sotiras, A., Bilello, M., Rozycki, M., Kirby, J., Freymann, J., Farahani, K., Davatzikos, C.: Segmentation labels and radiomic features for the pre-operative scans of the TCGA-IGG collection. The Cancer Imaging Archive (2017). https://doi.org/10.7937/K9/TCIA.2017.GJQ7R0EF

17. Simonyan, K., Zisserman, A.: Very deep convolutional networks for large-scale image recognition. arXiv preprint arXiv:1409.1556 (2014)

18. Rote, G.: Computing the minimum hausdorff distance between two point sets on a line under translation. Inf. Process. Lett. **38**(3), 123–127 (1991)

Brain Tumor Segmentation Using Deep Fully Convolutional Neural Networks

Geena Kim[(✉)] [ID]

College of Computer and Information Sciences,
Regis University, Denver, CO, USA
geenakim@regis.edu

Abstract. In this study, brain tumor substructures are segmented using 2D fully convolutional neural networks. A number of modifications such as double convolution layers, inception modules, and dense modules were added to a U-Net to achieve a deep architecture and test if the increased depth improves the performance. The experiments show that the deep architectures improve the performance. Also, the performance is enhanced from ensembling across the models trained on images in different orientations and ensembling across the models with different architectures. Even without any data augmentation, the ensembled model achieves a competitive performance and generalizes well on a new dataset. The resulting mean 3D Dice scores (ET/WT/TC) on the BRATS17 validation and test sets are 0.75/0.88/0.73 and 0.72/0.86/0.73.

Keywords: Brain Tumor Segmentation
Fully convolutional neural networks
Deep convolutional neural networks

1 Introduction

Though developed long ago, convolutional neural network (CNN) has recently become the most popular approach in the field of computer vision after the AlexNet won by a large margin in the Large Scale Visual Recognition Challenge (LSVRC), a computer vision challenge with a task of classifying objects in natural images [6]. In following studies, deep CNN models such as VGGNet, GoogLeNet (also called InceptionNet) and ResNet improved the classification accuracy further and showed that CNNs with deep-layer architectures can learn more complicated features from images [7–9]. Since then, the CNN approach has improved the accuracy beyond the human-level [10].

A deep CNN model has typically millions of parameters, thus requires a large amount of training images. The success of CNNs in recognizing natural images was largely due to the large public datasets such as the ImageNet, a massive dataset with 14 million images which annotation was crowd-sourced inexpensively [5].

© Springer International Publishing AG, part of Springer Nature 2018
A. Crimi et al. (Eds.): BrainLes 2017, LNCS 10670, pp. 344–357, 2018.
https://doi.org/10.1007/978-3-319-75238-9_30

Analyzing medical images is more challenging than natural images by nature and it is also costly to obtain annotated data. Recent efforts organizing challenges on automated medical image analysis and creating annotated datasets such as the Brain Tumor Segmentation (BRATS) challenge and its image collections [1–4] helped improving automated medical image analysis algorithms. Thanks to the considerable size and quality of the annotated data in BRATS, a number of deep CNN architectures have been developed and showed good performances [16–20]. With performances comparable to the top-performing non-neural network algorithms [11–15], the CNN-based algorithms have been steadily increasing their popularity in the challenge leaderboard, yet there are still rooms to improve.

Different from image classification tasks, the final output is 2D (or higher) in image segmentation tasks. Therefore, in segmentation, the classification of one pixel is highly correlated with that of adjacent pixels. One popular method to predict the label is the patch-based method, which a model classifies the center pixel based on the information from surrounding pixels (patch) [23]. Many CNN architectures previously implemented in BRATS use the patch-based approach which has an added benefit that it can help mitigating severe class imbalance by oversampling more patches from the tumor region. Recently, the fully convolutional neural network (FCN) approach showed that it can produce labels more time-efficiently than the patch-based approach [24] and was also implemented in BRATS [18,20]. Other good examples of FCN-based models in medical images are the U-Net and the V-Net which have symmetric contracting and expanding paths and feature map concatenations between the two paths to preserve local features [25,26].

In this paper, with an assumption that deep-layer architectures and the modules from the successful deep CNN models such as VGGNet, InceptionNet, ResNet, and DenseNet developed for recognizing natural images are also useful in medical images, modifications such as double convolution, inception modules and dense modules are implemented to the U-Net architecture to segment brain tumor substructures. Also ensembling across models trained on 2D images with axial, coronal and sagittal views as well as across the model architectures are implemented to enhance the performance.

2 Method

2.1 Data Preparation

The BRATS 17 Training data is normalized per MR image volume and per modality using the median pixel value X_m from the histogram.

$$X_n = \frac{X - X_m}{wX_m} \tag{1}$$

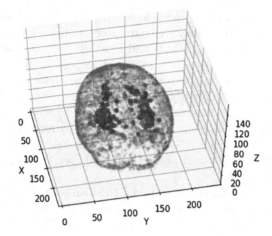

Fig. 1. 3D plot of tumor center locations (aggregated). Blue: Tumor centers, Red: brain contour. (Color figure online)

The constant w can be arbitrary, but was chosen to be 4 to approximate the histogram width. Using the training dataset's segmentation label, each case is categorized based on tumor location-size pair. Tumor location (simple mean x, y, z-coordinates of whole tumor pixels) is categorized to x: Anterior, Center, Posterior, y: Left, Center, Right, z: Top, Center, Bottom, and the size is categorized to Small, Medium and Large based on the tumor volume histograms (Fig. 2). Usually the tumor centers are found mostly in the middle part of the cerebrum and left and right outside to the ventricles (Fig. 1), but there are also less frequent cases found on the top or bottom parts of the brain.

After each scan is categorized, the training data is split into training, validation, and test subsets such that location-size pair categories are well mixed among those subsets. The 2D image slices are then shuffled within each subset. Though it may be useful, N4 biasfield correction was omitted in the preprocessing as it is time consuming. Also, no data augmentation such as translation, rotation, mirroring and warping was used in data preparation. About 30% of slices without any tumor or brain pixels were randomly discarded to make the training faster. Also, coronal- and sagittal-view 2D images were prepared in the same manner.

2.2   Architecture

Model A: Mini U-Net. Figure 3 shows the base model (mini U-Net). It has total 11 2d-convolution layers. Except the last convolution layer (1×1 convolution layer) for the output, all other convolution layers have 3×3 filters. After each convolution, batch normalization and ReLU activation are applied. Maxpooling is used to contract and upsampling is used to expand spatially. An upsampling layer uses simple resizing by nearest neighbor interpolation. As shown in Fig. 3, a feature map from the last layer of each downsampling step is concatenated depth-wise with the upsampled layer.

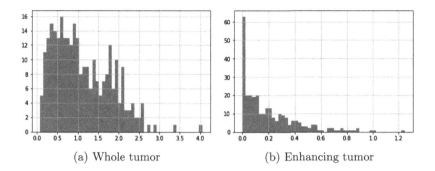

(a) Whole tumor   (b) Enhancing tumor

Fig. 2. Tumor volume histogram. Total pixels divided by the total pixels × 100.

Model B: Mini U-Net with Double Convolution Layers. This model has the same structure with the model A except that there are two 3×3 convolution layers before an activation to increase the receptive field (field of view). Having two successive 3×3 convolution layers is equivalent to having one 5×5 convolution but is computationally less expensive by factor of $25/9$.

Model C: Mini U-Net with Inception Modules. Another variant of U-Net tested in this work uses modified inception modules. Typically, an inception module consists of 1×1, $1 \times 1 - 3 \times 3$, $1 \times 1 - 5 \times 5$ and 3×3 maxpool-1×1 paths running in parallel then merging depth-wise. In the InceptionNet, 1×1 convolutions before the other convolutions make it computationally less expensive, thus help obtaining a deep layer architecture with less number of parameters. Inception-like modules which replace 5×5 convolutions with two 3×3 convolutions as mentioned above are added to the mini U-Net. Figure 5 shows the overall architecture of the model C. A module A has 1×1, $1 \times 1 - 3 \times 3$, and $1 \times 1 - 3 \times 3 - 3 \times 3$ convolution paths with stride $= 1$ and padding. A module B has a 3×3 max pooling layer with stride 2 (denoted as /2 by convention), 1×1-$3 \times 3/2$, and $1 \times 1 - 3 \times 3 - 3 \times 3/2$ convolution layers. A module C is a reverse of a module B and consists of an upsampling layer, $1 \times 1 - 3 \times 3/2$, and $1 \times 1 - 3 \times 3 - 3 \times 3/2$ deconvolution (transpose convolution) layers.

Model D: Mini U-Net with Dense Modules. This model incorporates Dense modules from a DenseNet architecture into a U-net. Like ResNet [9], DenseNet [27] has bypass connections where information from early layers can reach to the end without being lost by a series of activations. An important architectural difference is that ResNet achieves the bypass using element-wise addition known as residual connection while DenseNet uses depthwise concatenation after a convolution layer. DenseNet requires less number of parameters due to dense connections each of which adds a small number of feature maps

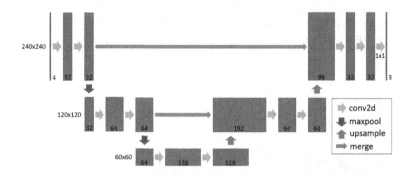

Fig. 3. Model A: mini U-Net architecture.

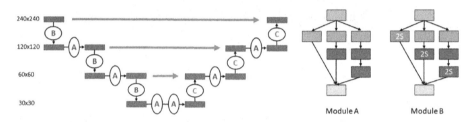

Fig. 4. Model C: mini U-Net architecture with inception-like modules. In the diagrams of Module A and B-orange squares represent the input layers to the modules, green squares represent 1×1 convolution layers, blue squares represent 3×3 convolution layers, and yellow squares represent depth-wise concatenation. (Color figure online)

to the concatenation and uses smaller number of weights rather than changing the weights for all the feature maps. As the depth of a network increases, even a small growth rate k, a hyper parameter (number of filters) of a dense module, can make the feature map size grow quickly. To reduce the number of feature maps, it is useful to use bottle neck and compression by using 1×1 convolutions. In this work, the DenseNet parameters were limited to $N = 4$ and $k = 8$ to fit the model in one GPU (Fig. 4).

2.3   Training

The models are trained using Keras and TensorFlow python libraries on a NVIDIA TitanX GPU. Models A, B, C, and D have roughly 0.5 M, 1 M, 0.5 M, and 0.2 M parameters and the training for 100–150 epochs takes 0.5–2 days on about 20 k images. All models use an Adam optimizer with a learning rate between 0.001 to 0.01, and the categorical cross-entropy for the loss function. Batch normalization is applied before every ReLU activation to reduce overfitting and to use a higher learning rate.

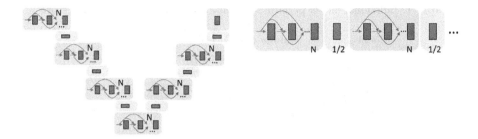

Fig. 5. Model D: mini U-Net architecture with dense modules. Left: the overall model architecture, Right: Zoomed-in view of dense modules. The blue squares represent convolution layers and the green squares are pooling and unpolling layers. Blue arrows represent feature maps concatenation. In a dense module (light blue block), 3×3 convolution layers are repeated N times and at the end of each convolution layer, feature maps from previous layers are concatenated. (Color figure online)

3 Result

3.1 Individual vs. Ensemble

A summary of individual model performances on axial view images is shown in Table 1. It shows that having more layers helps and increases the Dice score on both Training and Validation datasets. The models also generalize well on the Validation set. Training on the axial view images was a natural choice because most of the images in the dataset have been obtained in axial view, as well as the image shape is square (240×240), yet it is beneficial to combine information from side views (coronal and sagittal). Table 2 shows the performance boost when it is ensembled across all views for an individual model. Ensembling is done by averaging the probabilities on each pixel, then rounding up to create labels. There can be other ways to combine all views: for example, instead of averaging probabilities then rounding up, the label can be generated by voting after rounding up individual views. The latter might be a more strict way to eliminate a false positive label with a high probability from one orientation and low probabilities from other orientations, however, was not tested in this study. Table 3 shows the results from ensembling across all views and models. Ensembling across models still contributes to a higher Dice score although the effect is not as big as when ensembling across views. The ensembled model also generalizes well on the validation and the test set.

3.2 Dice Score by Labels

Figure 6 shows individual model Dice scores by segmentation labels and tumor substructures tested on the test subset of the training dataset. Dice score for necrosis and non-enhancing tumor has the largest spread and lowest mean, which may attribute to the small size and low frequency of necrosis in general. Each model performs similar on enhancing tumor with mean Dice scores between

Table 1. Individual model performances on axial images: mean 3D Dice score

Model	Train hours	Dice score (ET/WT/TC) Test data	
		Train17	Val17
A. Baseline	20	63/83/75	64/83/68
B. Double-conv	27	64/85/77	68/86/70
C. Inception	54	66/86/77	66/87/72
D. Dense	20	66/85/78	68/86/72

Table 2. Ensembling across views: mean 3D Dice score

Model	View	Dice score (ET/WT/TC) Tested on Train17	
		Individual	Ensemble
B. Double-conv	Axial	64/85/77	69/87/80
B. Double-conv	Coronal	65/81/76	
B. Double-conv	Sagittal	65/85/78	
D. Dense	Axial	66/85/78	70/85/78
D. Dense	Coronal	64/84/75	
D. Dense	Sagittal	64/82/77	

Table 3. Ensembling across views and models: mean 3D Dice score.

Model	View	Dice score (ET/WT/TC)				
		Train17		Val17		Test17
		Individual	Ensemble	Individual	Ensemble	Ensemble
B. Double-conv	Axial	64/85/77	71/87/81	68/86/70	75/88/73	72/86/73
C. Inception	Axial	66/86/77		66/87/72		
D. Dense	Axial	66/85/78		68/86/72		
B. Double-conv	Coronal	65/81/76		–		
C. Inception	Coronal	63/85/76		–		
D. Dense	Coronal	64/84/75		–		
B. Double-conv	Sagittal	65/85/78		–		
C. Inception	Sagittal	65/84/78		–		
D. Dense	Sagittal	64/82/77		–		

0.64–0.66. The outliers with low ET Dice scores are usually from the ones with little to no enhancing tumor region while the whole tumor size is big, or from the rare cases.

Table 4. Model performances on various data subsets in axial view: mean 3D Dice score. In the Val17 column, the † symbol means that the Dice scores are obtained using a subset (HGG) of the Val17 dataset.

Experiment	Model	Trained on	Dice score (ET/WT/TC)				
			Test data				
			TR15HGG	TR17HGG	TR17LGG	TR17ALL	Val17
1	A	TR15HGG	83/89/82	77/80/78	26/77/40	63/80/68	–
2	A	TR17HGG	–	79/84/83	20/66/32	64/81/72	80/83.5/81†
3	A	TR17ALL	–	79/83/81	–	63/83/75	64/83/68
4	A	TR17HGG	–	79/84/85	22/72/32	64/82/71	–
5	B	TR17HGG	–	80/85/86	32/76/31	65/83/71	–
6	A	TR17LGG	–	62/72/50	24/82/66	52/75/54	–
7	B	TR17LGG	–	67/76/52	20/82/63	54/78/56	–
8	C	TR17LGG	–	66/77/49	24/82/66	55/79/54	–
9	B	TR17ALL	–	79/85/82	22/83/65	64/85/77	68/86/70
10	C	TR17ALL	–	80/87/82	25/83/60	65/86/77	66/87/72

3.3   Performance Comparison on HGG, LGG and HGG+LGG

Table 4 shows the individual model performance on various datasets in axial view. The performance of the model A (Baseline model: mini U-Net with a single convolution per layer) trained on the BRATS15 training dataset versus on the BRATS17 training dataset is shown in the experiments 1 and 2. The model trained on BRATS15 data has decreased Dice scores on BRATS17 data but is still comparable to when it was trained on BRATS17 data.

Also, models A, B, and C were trained and tested on different subsets of BRATS17 training data (HGG, LGG, and ALL). In general, the performances of models trained on HGG vs. HGG+LGG (ALL) data make little difference on ET and WT, but there is an improvement for TC Dice score when trained with HGG+LGG data. Also, usually models perform better when inferencing over HGG data than HGG+LGG or LGG alone. Inferencing enhancing tumor on LGG seems more challenging no matter which dataset a model was trained on, which might be because there are cases with a large whole tumor region without any enhancing tumor pixels (Fig. 7).

Experiments 1–3 and 4–10 use different normalization methods for preprocessing the images. The method used in experiments 4–10 uses the median pixel value in the brain pixels histogram instead of the 1–99 percentile pixel values to normalize. The previous method (1–99) used in experiments 1–3 was considered mainly to mitigate an effect of outlier pixel values. However, it has a drawback of

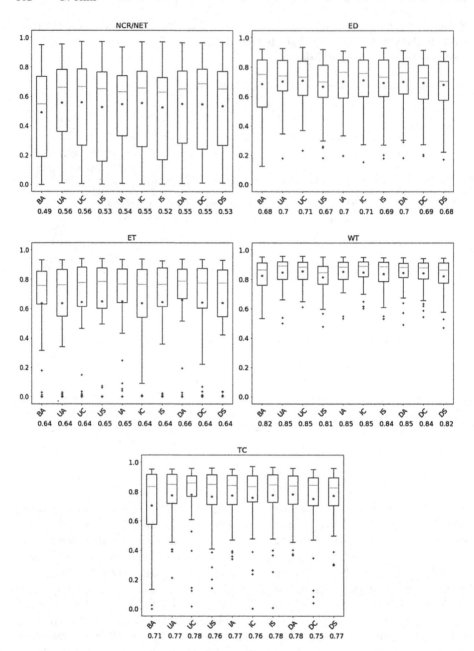

Fig. 6. Box plots of 3D Dice score for tumor substructures. Tested on the test-subset of the BRATS17 Training set. Top Left: Necrosis (NEC) and non-enhancing tumor (NET), Top Right: Edema (ED), Middle Left: Enhancing tumor (ET), Middle Right: Whole tumor (WT), Bottom: Tumor core (TC). The x-labels represent the models and training image orientation. For example, the first letters B, U, I, D mean baseline model, Unet with double convolutions, with Inception modules, with Dense modules. The second letters A, C, S are the orientations: axial, coronal and sagittal. Numbers below x-labels are the mean 3D Dice scores, also marked by blue star symbol on the plot. The y-axis is the 3d Dice score. The + symbols are the outliers. (Color figure online)

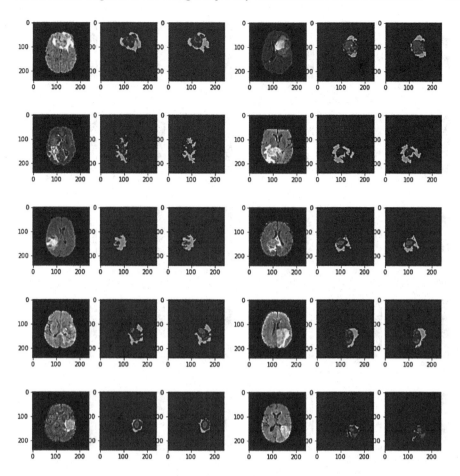

Fig. 7. Visualization of 10 random cases. For visualization purpose, ones with all three labels were selected. Each case is a set of three displays, which the left is the image (X) of the FLAIR modality, the middle is the prediction labels (Yp), and the right is the manual segmentation labels (Yt). For the label colors, Green: Necrosis+Non-enhancing Tumor, Yellow: Edema, Red: Enhancing Tumor. (Color figure online)

pushing the brightest 1% pixels to the same larger pixel values regardless of its original brightness, which makes more false positives for enhancing tumor. The second method (normalized by median) performs slightly better on the LGG data but shows little to no difference on the HGG+LGG data (Fig. 8).

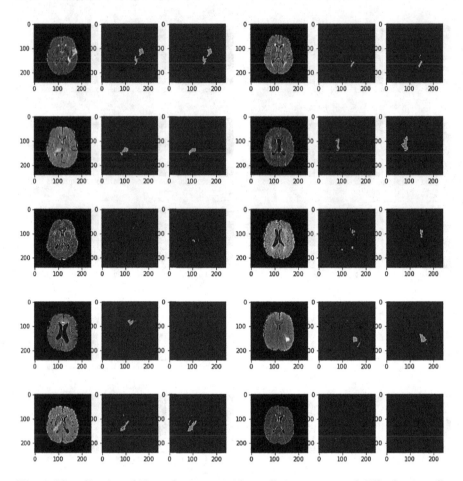

Fig. 8. Visualization of 10 random cases with small size tumors and difficult cases. Some cases with small tumors and slices without tumor may be prone to false positives. Each case consists of visualizations of the image X (FLAIR), prediction labels Yp, target labels Yt. Green: Necrosis+Non-enhancing Tumor, Yellow: Edema, Red: Enhancing Tumor. (Color figure online)

4   Conclusion

In this study, 2D fully convolutional neural networks were used to segment brain tumor substructures and address these questions: 1. Do models with deeper layers perform better? 2. How much a performance increases by ensembling models across views and across different architectures. In conclusion, a deeper layer architecture improves the performance. Ensembling can greatly enhance the performance especially when information from different views are combined. Perhaps is it due to that these models are based on 2D images and the information from other views help inferencing in 3D. An ensemble of the three models (modified U-Nets with double convolution, Inception and Dense modules) trained on images in each of the three views (axial, coronal, and sagittal) gives 3D mean Dice scores 0.71/0.87/0.81 on the training set and generalizes well to similar values of 0.75/0.88/0.73 on the validation and 0.72/0.86/0.73 on the test set. Considering that the cases with the lowest scores are usually the rare cases (very small or unusual locations) or confusing cases (large whole tumor with little to no enhancing tumor), training with minority-oversampled and augmented data or curriculum learning may improve the result.

Acknowledgement. We thank NVIDIA for their kind donation of a TitanX GPU.

References

1. Menze, B.H., Jakab, A., Bauer, S., Kalpathy-Cramer, J., Farahani, K., Kirby, J., Burren, Y., Porz, N., Slotboom, J., Wiest, R., Lanczi, L., Gerstner, E., Weber, M.A., Arbel, T., Avants, B.B., Ayache, N., Buendia, P., Collins, D.L., Cordier, N., Corso, J.J., Criminisi, A., Das, T., Delingette, H.: Demiralp, Ç., Durst, C.R., Dojat, M., Doyle, S., Festa, J., Forbes, F., Geremia, E., Glocker, B., Golland, P., Guo, X., Hamamci, A., Iftekharuddin, K.M., Jena, R., John, N.M., Konukoglu, E., Lashkari, D., Mariz, J.A., Meier, R., Pereira, S., Precup, D., Price, S.J., Raviv, T.R., Reza, S.M.S., Ryan, M., Sarikaya, D., Schwartz, L., Shin, H.C., Shotton, J., Silva, C.A., Sousa, N., Subbanna, N.K., Szekely, G., Taylor, T.J., Thomas, O.M., Tustison, N.J., Unal, G., Vasseur, F., Wintermark, M., Ye, D.H., Zhao, L., Zhao, B., Zikic, D., Prastawa, M., Reyes, M., Leemput, K.V.: The multimodal brain tumor image segmentation benchmark (BRATS). IEEE Trans. Med. Imaging. **34**, 1993–2024 (2015)
2. Bakas, S., Akbari, H., Sotiras, A., Bilello, M., Rozycki, M., Kirby, J., Freymann, J., Farahani, K., Davatzikos, C.: Advancing the cancer genome atlas glioma MRI collections with expert segmentation labels and radiomic features. Nature Sci. Data **4**, 170117 (2017)
3. Bakas, S., Akbari, H., Sotiras, A., Bilello, M., Rozycki, M., Kirby, J., Freymann, J., Farahani, K., Davatzikos, C.: Segmentation labels for the pre-operative scans of the TCGA-GBM collection. Cancer Imaging Arch. (2017)
4. Bakas, S., Akbari, H., Sotiras, A., Bilello, M., Rozycki, M., Kirby, J., Freymann, J., Farahani, K., Davatzikos, C.: Segmentation labels for the pre-operative scans of the TCGA-LGG collection. Cancer Imaging Arch. (2017)
5. Russakovsky, O., Deng, J., Su, H., Krause, J., Satheesh, S., Ma, S., Huang, Z., Karpathy, A., Khosla, A., Bernstein, M., Berg, A.C., Fei-Fei, L.: ImageNet large scale visual recognition challenge. Int. J. Comput. Vis. **115**, 211–252 (2015)
6. Krizhevsky, A., Sutskever, I., Hinton, G.E.: Imagenet classification with deep convolutional neural networks. In: Advances in Neural Information Processing Systems, pp. 1097–1105 (2012)
7. Simonyan, K., Zisserman, A.: Very deep convolutional networks for large-scale image recognition. arXiv preprint arXiv:1409.1556 (2014)
8. Szegedy, C., Liu, W., Jia, Y., Sermanet, P., Reed, S., Anguelov, D., Erhan, D., Vanhoucke, V., Rabinovich, A.: Going deeper with convolutions. In: Proceedings of the IEEE Conference on Computer Vision and Pattern Recognition, pp. 1–9 (2015)

9. He, K., Zhang, X., Ren, S., Sun, J.: Deep residual learning for image recognition. In: Proceedings of the IEEE Conference on Computer Vision and Pattern Recognition, pp. 770–778 (2016)
10. He, K., Zhang, X., Ren, S., Sun, J.: Delving deep into rectifiers: surpassing human-level performance on ImageNet classification. In: Proceedings of the IEEE International Conference on Computer Vision, pp. 1026–1034 (2015)
11. Bakas, S., et al.: GLISTRboost: combining multimodal MRI segmentation, registration, and biophysical tumor growth modeling with gradient boosting machines for glioma segmentation. In: Crimi, A., Menze, B., Maier, O., Reyes, M., Handels, H. (eds.) BrainLes 2015. LNCS, vol. 9556, pp. 144–155. Springer, Cham (2016). https://doi.org/10.1007/978-3-319-30858-6_13
12. Maier, O., Wilms, M., Handels, H.: Image features for brain lesion segmentation using random forests. In: Crimi, A., Menze, B., Maier, O., Reyes, M., Handels, H. (eds.) BrainLes 2015. LNCS, vol. 9556, pp. 119–130. Springer, Cham (2016). https://doi.org/10.1007/978-3-319-30858-6_11
13. Meier, R., Karamitsou, V., Habegger, S., Wiest, R., Reyes, M.: Parameter learning for CRF-based tissue segmentation of brain tumors. In: Crimi, A., Menze, B., Maier, O., Reyes, M., Handels, H. (eds.) BrainLes 2015. LNCS, vol. 9556, pp. 156–167. Springer, Cham (2016). https://doi.org/10.1007/978-3-319-30858-6_14
14. Song, B., Chou, C.-R., Chen, X., Huang, A., Liu, M.-C.: Anatomy-guided brain tumor segmentation and classification. In: Crimi, A., Menze, B., Reyes, M., Winzeck, S., Handels, H. (eds.) BrainLes 2016. LNCS, vol. 10154, pp. 162–170. Springer, Cham (2016). https://doi.org/10.1007/978-3-319-55524-9_16
15. Zeng, K., et al.: Segmentation of gliomas in pre-operative and post-operative multimodal magnetic resonance imaging volumes based on a hybrid generative-discriminative framework. In: Crimi, A., Menze, B., Maier, O., Reyes, M., Winzeck, S., Handels, H. (eds.) BrainLes 2016. LNCS, vol. 10154, pp. 184–194. Springer, Cham (2016). https://doi.org/10.1007/978-3-319-55524-9_18
16. Havaei, M., Dutil, F., Pal, C., Larochelle, H., Jodoin, P.-M.: A convolutional neural network approach to brain tumor segmentation. In: Crimi, A., Menze, B., Maier, O., Reyes, M., Handels, H. (eds.) BrainLes 2015. LNCS, vol. 9556, pp. 195–208. Springer, Cham (2016). https://doi.org/10.1007/978-3-319-30858-6_17
17. Pereira, S., Pinto, A., Alves, V., Silva, C.A.: Deep convolutional neural networks for the segmentation of gliomas in multi-sequence MRI. In: Crimi, A., Menze, B., Maier, O., Reyes, M., Handels, H. (eds.) BrainLes 2015. LNCS, vol. 9556, pp. 131–143. Springer, Cham (2016). https://doi.org/10.1007/978-3-319-30858-6_12
18. Chang, P.D.: Fully convolutional deep residual neural networks for brain tumor segmentation. In: Crimi, A., Menze, B., Maier, O., Reyes, M., Winzeck, S., Handels, H. (eds.) BrainLes 2016. LNCS, vol. 10154, pp. 108–118. Springer, Cham (2016). https://doi.org/10.1007/978-3-319-55524-9_11
19. Kamnitsas, K., et al.: DeepMedic for brain tumor segmentation. In: Crimi, A., Menze, B., Maier, O., Reyes, M., Winzeck, S., Handels, H. (eds.) BrainLes 2016. LNCS, vol. 10154, pp. 138–149. Springer, Cham (2016). https://doi.org/10.1007/978-3-319-55524-9_14
20. Zhao, X., Wu, Y., Song, G., Li, Z., Fan, Y., Zhang, Y.: Brain tumor segmentation using a fully convolutional neural network with conditional random fields. In: Crimi, A., Menze, B., Maier, O., Reyes, M., Winzeck, S., Handels, H. (eds.) BrainLes 2016. LNCS, vol. 10154, pp. 75–87. Springer, Cham (2016). https://doi.org/10.1007/978-3-319-55524-9_8

21. Havaei, M., Davy, A., Warde-Farley, D., Biard, A., Courville, A., Bengio, Y., Pal, C., Jodoin, P.-M., Larochelle, H.: Brain tumor segmentation with deep neural networks. Med. Image Anal. **35**, 18–31 (2016)
22. Kamnitsas, K., Ledig, C., Newcombe, V.F.J., Simpson, J.P., Kane, A.D., Menon, D.K., Rueckert, D., Glocker, B.: Efficient multi-scale 3D CNN with fully connected CRF for accurate brain lesion segmentation. Med. Image Anal. **36**, 61–78 (2017)
23. Ciresan, D., Giusti, A., Gambardella, L.M., Schmidhuber, J.: Deep neural networks segment neuronal membranes in electron microscopy images. In: Advances in Neural Information Processing Systems, pp. 2843–2851 (2012)
24. Long, J., Shelhamer, E., Darrell, T.: Fully convolutional networks for semantic segmentation. In: Proceedings of the IEEE Conference on Computer Vision and Pattern Recognition, pp. 3431–3440 (2015)
25. Ronneberger, O., Fischer, P., Brox, T.: U-Net: convolutional networks for biomedical image segmentation. In: Navab, N., Hornegger, J., Wells, W.M., Frangi, A.F. (eds.) MICCAI 2015. LNCS, vol. 9351, pp. 234–241. Springer, Cham (2015). https://doi.org/10.1007/978-3-319-24574-4_28
26. Milletari, F., Navab, N., Ahmadi, S.-A.: V-Net: fully convolutional neural networks for volumetric medical image segmentation. arXiv:1606.04797 [cs] (2016)
27. Huang, G., Liu, Z., Weinberger, K.Q., van der Maaten, L.: Densely connected convolutional networks. arXiv:1608.06993 [cs] (2016)

Glioblastoma and Survival Prediction

Zeina A. Shboul$^{(\boxtimes)}$, Lasitha Vidyaratne, Mahbubul Alam,
and Khan M. Iftekharuddin

Vision Lab, Electrical & Computer Engineering,
Old Dominion University, Norfolk, USA
{zshbo001,lvidy001,malam001,kiftekha}@odu.edu

Abstract. Glioblastoma is a stage IV highly invasive astrocytoma tumor. Its heterogeneous appearance in MRI poses a critical challenge in diagnosis, prognosis and survival prediction. This work proposes an automated survival prediction method by utilizing different types of texture and other features. The method tests feature significance and prognostic values, and then utilizes the most significant features with a Random Forest regression model to perform survival prediction. We use 163 cases from BraTS17 training dataset for evaluation of the proposed model. A 10-fold cross validation offers normalized root mean square error of 30% for the training dataset and the cross-validated accuracy of 67%, respectively. Finally, the proposed model ranked first in the Survival Prediction task for global Brain Tumor Segmentation Challenge (BraTS) 2017 and an accuracy of 57.9% is achieved.

Keywords: Glioblastoma · Survival prediction · Random forest

1 Introduction

Glioblastoma (GB) is categorized as a World Health Organization (WHO) stage IV brain cancer that originates in star-shaped brain cells in the cerebrum called astrocytes [1, 2]. GB is the most invasive brain tumor and its highly diffusive infiltrative characteristics make glioma a lethal disease [3] with a median survival of 14.6 months with radiotherapy and temozolomide, and 12.1 months with radiotherapy alone [4]. In addition, heterogeneity in GBM [5] poses a further challenge not just for diagnosis, but also for prognosis and survival prediction using MR imaging.

Several studies [6, 7, 9] have proposed different methods for predicting the survivability of patients with brain tumors. In [6], the authors use the different subtype tumor volumes, the extent of resection, location, size and other imaging features in order to evaluate the capability of these features in predicting survival.

The authors in [7] use comprehensive visual features set known as VASARI (Visually AcceSAble Rembrandt Images) [8] in order to predict survival and correlate these features for genetic alterations and molecular subtypes.

L. Vidyaratne and M. Alam—The two authors have similar contributions.

In [9], the authors quantify a large number of radiomic image features including shape and texture in computed tomography images of lung and head-and-neck cancer patients. However, most of the survival prediction studies utilize traditional regression survival models such as the proportional hazard method and only a few utilize machine learning methods to predict survival.

Consequently, this work proposes an overall survival prediction method using Random forest regression model based on different structural multiresolution texture features, volumetric, and histogram features.

However, accurate representative tumor features require accurate tumor segmentation. The recent developments in deep learning domain have opened up new avenues in various medical image processing research. Several recent studies [10, 11] apply Convolutional Neural Network (CNN) based deep learning methods to solve brain tumor segmentation problem successfully. Consequently, this work implements a state-of-the-art CNN architecture following [10] to enhance brain tumor segmentation task. We used the proposed pipeline to participate in the Brain Tumor Segmentation Challenge (BraTS) 2017 – Task of Survival Prediction and the method ranked first.

2 Dataset

In this study, we use MR images of 163 high grade GBM patients from BtaTS17 training dataset [12–15]. The dataset provides the ground truth segmentation of tumor tissues which comprises of enhancing tumor (ET), edema (ED), and the necrosis and non-enhancing tumor (NCR/NET). In addition, the training dataset provides age (median age, 61.167 years; range, 18.975–78.762 years), and overall survival (in days) data. The available scans of the MRI are native (T1), post-contrast T1-weighted (T1Gd), T2-weighted (T2), and T2 Fluid Attenuated Inversion Recovery (FLAIR) volumes. The dataset is co-registered, re-sampled to $1 \, mm^3$ and skull-stripped.

3 Methodology

3.1 Brain Tumor Segmentation

Accurate segmentation of tumor from the MRI is pre-requisite for survival prediction as most potent features are derived from the affected region. The complete pipeline for survival prediction is shown in Fig. 1. Note this paper primarily explains the proposed survival model.

Features-Based Brain Tumor Segmentation. Our previous works on multiclass MRI brain tumor segmentation using texture based features [16, 17] ranked third in the BraTS 2013 challenge [12] in which the results were presented. The results indicate that using Dice overlap metric for tumor core and complete tumor ranged from 63% to 76%. A detailed description of multiclass abnormal brain tumor segmentation is found in [16, 17]. A general flow diagram of our multiclass MRI brain tumor segmentation is illustrated in Fig. 2. Our texture features are extracted from raw (T1, T1Gd, T2, and Flair) modalities tumor volumes. The texture representations are piecewise triangular prism surface area (PTPSA) [18], multifractional Brownian motion (mBm) [19–21], Generalized multifractional Brownian motion (GmBm) [22, 23], and five representations of Texton filters [24], respectively.

Along with the texture features, non-local intensity features are extracted, such as normalized intensity and the difference in normalized intensity between the different modalities. Normalization of MR volumes is done as suggested in [25].

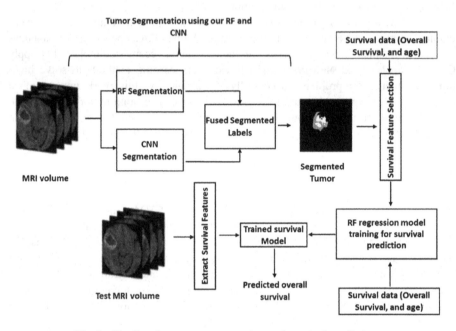

Fig. 1. Pipeline for tumor segmentation and survival prediction.

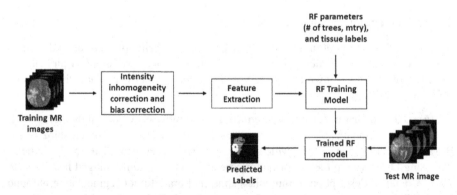

Fig. 2. General flow diagram of Random forest multiclass abnormal brain tissue segmentation.

Then, the extracted features are combined with the tumor tissue labels into a 3D features matrix and fed to a Random Forest (RF) classifier. The RF trained model is subsequently used on the test dataset.

This work further improves the segmentation performance by employing a two-stage process in which the outcomes from the deep learning based method are fused with that of a handcrafted feature based method that utilizes Random Forest (RF) for the classification task.

Deep Learning Based Tumor Segmentation. The input to the CNN is image patches of size ($33 \times 33 \times 4$) where the 3rd dimension is comprised of the four MRI modalities: T1, T1Gd, T2, and FLAIR. The CNN classifies the middle pixel of each patch based on the five tissues such as background, enhanced tumor, edema, necrosis and non-enhanced tumor, respectively.

The CNN architecture is implemented following the work in [10]. Consequently, the network consists of total 6 convolutional layers, 2 pooling layers, 3 fully connected layers including the classification layer that utilizes soft-max activation. All convolutional layers utilizes small 3×3 convolutional kernels, which allows for a deeper architecture.

The convolutional and fully connected layers (except for the classification layer) applies leaky rectified linear activation with a leak factor of 0.3. Dropout regularization is utilized exclusively for the fully connected layers with a dropout rate of 0.1. All the inputs to the CNN are pre-processed with N4-ITK bias correction, and intensity normalization for inter-volume consistency [10].

The training set consist of 900,000 image patches randomly obtained from the BRATS 2017 training MRI volume set, with 500,000 representing the normal tissue, and 100,000 patches each representing the abnormal tissue types mentioned above. The large number of background tissue samples are obtained to adequately represent the inherent imbalance in the tissue types available in MRI. The training set is further augmented by applying affine rotation using 4 representative parameters (0^0, 90^0, 180^0, 270^0), obtaining a final training set of size 3,600,000. The sufficiently trained CNN is subsequently used for the segmentation of testing data as shown in Fig. 3.

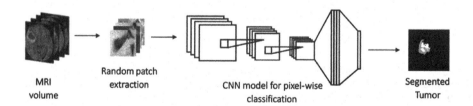

Fig. 3. Brain tumor segmentation from MRI images using convolutional neural networks (CNNs).

Finally, the segmented RF labels are masked with the outcomes of the deep learning based method to obtain the final tumor segmentation result. Figure 4 shows examples of segmented results using RF segmentation method, CNN based segmentation method and the fused outcome.

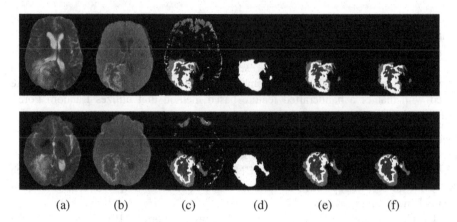

(a)   (b)   (c)   (d)   (e)   (f)

Fig. 4. Examples of segmentation results from BraTS'17 training dataset. (a) Input T2 scan (b) T1_Gd, (c) RF segmented labels, (d) binary mask of CNN outcome, (e) fused segmented outcome, and (f) ground truth.

3.2 Survival Prediction

In this study, we address the association between structural multiresolution texture features and overall survival data.

Feature Extraction. A total of one thousand, three hundred sixty-six (1366) features characterize the tumor and the sub-regions (edema, enhancing tumor, and tumor core). We extract 42 features [26] from the raw MRI modality (T1Gd, T2, and Flair) and eight texture representation of the whole tumor volume. The texture representations are PTPSA, fractal dimension computed as suggested in [19–21], Holder exponent computed as explained in [23], and five representations of Texton filters [24].

The 42 features [26] are described by the histogram, the co-occurrence matrix (measure the texture of image), the neighborhood gray tone difference matrix (measure a grayscale difference between pixels with certain grayscale and their neighboring pixels) Size Zone Matrix. In addition, we extract 7 volumetric; the volume of the whole tumor (WT), the volume of the whole tumor with respect to the brain, the volume of sub-regions (ED, ET, and NCR/NET) with respect to the whole tumor and the volumes of the ET and NCR/NET with respect to the ED are computed. In addition, 6 histogram-based statistics (mean, variance, skewness, kurtosis, energy, and entropy) features are extracted from the tumor and the different tumor sub-regions (ED, ET, and NCR/NET).

Further, the tumor locations and the spread of the tumor in the brain are also considered. Features extracted from the histogram of the four modalities of the whole tumor and its subregions are also considered. These features represent the frequency at different intensity bins (number of bins = 11, 23), and the bins of the max frequency.

Finally, 9 area properties (area, centroid, perimeter, major axis length, minor axis length, eccentricity, orientation, solidity, extent) are extracted from the whole tumor from three viewpoints (view are set along x, y and z axis).

Feature Selection. Feature selection is performed in three steps; first, the significant features are selected by fitting a univariate Cox regression model on extracted features. Then, another univariate Cox regression is applied to the quantified significant features. This ensures that these features are able to split the dataset into short vs. long survival. Figure 5 shows the Kaplan-Meier of three significant features that are able to split the dataset.

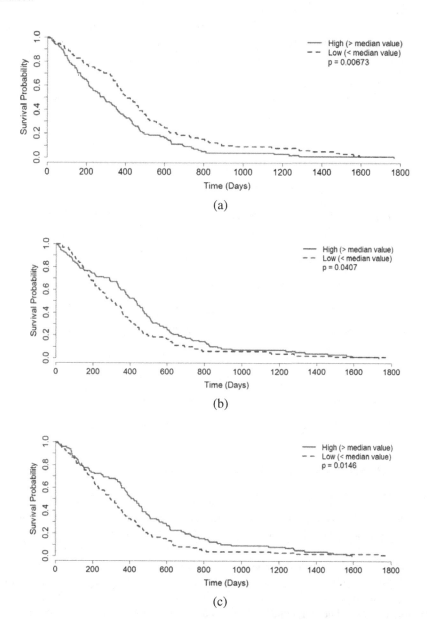

Fig. 5. Kaplan-Meier overall survival (OS) curves based (a) Area feature value (major axis value) in z axis, (b) Texton-cluster prominence derived from T2, (c) and texture coarseness derived from T2.

A total of two hundred and forty (240) features out of one thousand, three hundred sixty-six (1366) features ($\sim 17.5\%$ of the total extracted features) are found to be significant in the previous two feature selection steps.

Finally, the two hundred and forty features are reduced to forty significant features using a recursive feature selection algorithm. The distribution of the 40 features is as follows: eleven features portray Texton of the tumor, nine features extracted from the fractal/Holder exponent representations of the tumor, five features represent the histogram of the sub-regions, four from the raw MR modality of the tumor and sub-regions, two describes the volume of the tumor and the sub-regions, and five features are extracted from the tumor area and major axis length.

Random Forest Regression Training. The forty features are used with Random Forest regression model [27] for survival prediction. The steps of feature selection and survival prediction is shown in Fig. 6.

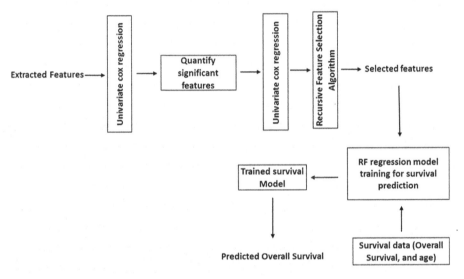

Fig. 6. Pipeline for survival prediction.

4   Experimental Results

Following the overall pipeline in Fig. 1, we first perform the CNN and RF fused tumor segmentation task. The segmentation performance (in dice similarity coefficient) of the CNN and RF fused method for the BraTS17 testing dataset is shown in Table 1. Note that the segmentation is performed only on the high-grade MRI volumes that are subsequently used for survival analysis.

The CNN and RF combined method provide adequate accuracy in identifying the abnormal tissue types within the tumor region, which is vital for the survival feature extraction process. The segmented MRI volumes are then utilized for the survival prediction segment of the overall pipeline of Fig. 1.

Table 1. Brain tumor segmentation performance of the CNN and RF fused method on BraTs17 high-grade test dataset

Label	Dice_ET	Dice_WT	Dice_TC
Mean	0.73	0.83	0.72
StdDev	0.16	0.08	0.17
Median	0.78	0.85	0.78

We first perform tenfold cross-validation on survival prediction features extracted from the ground truth, which is available with the BraTS17 training dataset (163 patients). We evaluate the performance of the proposed RF survival regression model using the normalized root mean square error (NRMSE) of the overall survival predicted values as a metric for regression evaluation. In order to evaluate the performance of the survival model based on classification, the overall survival is divided into three classes (long, medium and short) survivors corresponds to (>15 months, >10 months and <15 months, <10 months), respectively.

The cross-validated NRMSE of the training dataset is 30% with a cross-validated accuracy of 67%.

Whereas with the BraTS17 validation dataset, survival prediction features are extracted from the fused segmented tumor outcome as described in Fig. 1. Table 2 shows the online evaluation results we achieve with the BraTS'17 validation dataset and the test dataset.

Table 2. BraTS17 validation dataset and test dataset evaluation

Dataset	Accuracy	MSE	medianSE	stdSE	SpearmanR
Validation dataset	0.667	209908.43	42555.31	562296.09	0.48
Test dataset	0.579	245779.51	24944.40	726624.65	0.425

The test dataset accuracy of the proposed method is the highest among all the participants of the BraTS17 survival prediction challenge.

5   Conclusion

This work proposes an automated pipeline to perform survival prediction task using MRI images. The task is performed in two steps: (1) brain tumor segmentation and (2) patient survival prediction. The segmentation is obtained by fusing the outcomes from the deep learning based method with the handcrafted feature based RF method. Finally, the segmented tumor volumes and its' subregions along with other structural, texture, volumetric, and histogram features derived from these are used in an RF regression model for survival prediction. We use the proposed pipeline to participate in the Brain Tumor Segmentation Challenge (BraTS) 2017 – Task of Survival Prediction.

Consequently, we achieve a cross-validated NRMSE of 30% and a cross-validated accuracy of 67%, respectively on the BraTS'17 training dataset. Additionally, with

BraTS'17 validation dataset, the proposed method achieves an accuracy of %66.7. Using the test dataset, we achieved an accuracy of 57.9%. Even though the proposed method shows the best performance in the Survival prediction task (using the test validation and the test datasets), we believe that the performance may be further improved by integrating more clinical, and molecular information with MRI-based features as input.

Acknowledgements. This work was funded by NIBIB/NIH grant# R01 EB020683.

References

1. Louis, D.N., Ohgaki, H., Wiestler, O.D., Cavenee, W.K., Burger, P.C., Jouvet, A., Scheithauer, B.W., Kleihues, P.: The 2007 WHO classification of tumours of the central nervous system. Acta Neuropathol. **114**(2), 97–109 (2007)
2. Kliehues, P., Burger, P.C., Collins, V.P., Newcombe, E.W., Ohgaki, H., Cavenee, W.K.: Glioblastoma. In: WHO Classification of Tumours: Pathology and Genetics of Tumours of the Nervous System, Lyon, France, pp. 29–39. International Agency for Research on Cancer (2000)
3. Claes, A., Idema, A.J., Wesseling, P.: Diffuse glioma growth: a guerilla war. Acta Neuropathol. **114**(5), 443–458 (2007)
4. Stupp, R., Mason, W.P., van den Bent, M.J., Weller, M., Fisher, B., Taphoorn, M.J.B., Belanger, K., Brandes, A.A., Marosi, C., Bogdahn, U., Curschmann, J., Janzer, R.C., Ludwin, S.K., Gorlia, T., Allgeier, A., Lacombe, D., Cairncross, J.G., Eisenhauer, E., Mirimanoff, R.O.: Radiotherapy plus concomitant and adjuvant temozolomide for glioblastoma. N. Engl. J. Med. **352**(10), 987–996 (2005)
5. Soeda, A., Hara, A., Kunisada, T., Yoshimura, S., Iwama, T., Park, D.M.: The evidence of glioblastoma heterogeneity. Sci. Rep. **5**, 9630 (2015)
6. Pope, W.B., Sayre, J., Perlina, A., Villablanca, J.P., Mischel, P.S., Cloughesy, T.F.: MR imaging correlates of survival in patients with high-grade gliomas. Am. J. Neuroradiol. **26**(10), 2466–2474 (2005)
7. Gutman, D.A., Cooper, L.A., Hwang, S.N., Holder, C.A., Gao, J., Aurora, T.D., Dunn Jr., W.D., Scarpace, L., Mikkelsen, T., Jain, R., Wintermark, M., Jilwan, M., Raghavan, P., Huang, E., Clifford, R.J., Mongkolwat, P., Kleper, V., Freymann, J., Kirby, J., Zinn, P.O., Moreno, C.S., Jaffe, C., Colen, R., Rubin, D.L., Saltz, J., Flanders, A., Brat, D.J.: MR imaging predictors of molecular profile and survival: multi-institutional study of the TCGA glioblastoma data set. Radiology **267**(2), 560–569 (2013)
8. VASARI Research Project - Cancer Imaging Archive Wiki. https://wiki.cancerimagingarchive.net/display/Public/VASARI+Research+Project
9. Aerts, H.J., Velazquez, E.R., Leijenaar, R.T., Parmar, C., Grossmann, P., Carvalho, S., Bussink, J., Monshouwer, R., Haibe-Kains, B., Rietveld, D., Hoebers, F., Rietbergen, M.M., Leemans, C.R., Dekker, A., Quackenbush, J., Gillies, R.J., Lambin, P.: Decoding tumor phenotype by noninvasive imaging using a quantitative radiomics approach. Nat. Commun. **5**, 4006 (2014)
10. Pereira, S., Pinto, A., Alves, V., Silva, C.A.: Brain tumor segmentation using convolutional neural networks in MRI images. IEEE Trans. Med. Imaging **35**, 1240–1251 (2016)
11. Havaei, M., Davy, A., Warde-Farley, D., Biard, A., Courville, A., Bengio, Y., Pal, C., Jordoin, P.M., Larochelle, H.: Brain tumor segmentation with deep neural networks. Med. Image Anal. **35**, 18–31 (2016)

12. Menze, B.H., Jakab, A., Bauer, S., Kalpathy-Cramer, J., Farahani, K., Kirby, J., Burren, Y., Porz, N., Slotboom, J., Wiest, R., Lanczi, L., Gerstner, E., Weber, M.A., Arbel, T., Avants, B.B., Ayache, N., Buendia, P., Collins, D.L., Cordier, N., Corso, J.J., Criminisi, A., Das, T., Delingette, H., Demiralp, Ç., Durst, C.R., Dojat, M., Doyle, S., Festa, J., Forbes, F., Geremia, E., Glocker, B., Golland, P., Guo, X., Hamamci, A., Iftekharuddin, K.M., Jena, R., John, N.M., Konukoglu, E., Lashkari, D., Mariz, J.A., Meier, R., Pereira, S., Precup, D., Price, S.J., Raviv, T.R., Reza, S.M., Ryan, M., Sarikaya, D., Schwartz, L., Shin, H.C., Shotton, J., Silva, C.A., Sousa, N., Subbanna, N.K., Szekely, G., Taylor, T.J., Thomas, O. M., Tustison, N.J., Unal, G., Vasseur, F., Wintermark, M., Ye, D.H., Zhao, L., Zhao, B., Zikic, D., Prastawa, M., Reyes, M., Van Leemput, K.: The multimodal brain tumor image segmentation benchmark (BRATS). IEEE Trans. Med. Imaging 34(10), 1993–2024 (2015)
13. Bakas, S., Akbari, H., Sotiras, A., Bilello, M., Rozycki, M., Kirby, J.S., Freymann, J.B., Farahani, K., Davatzikos, C.: Advancing the cancer genome atlas glioma MRI collections with expert segmentation labels and radiomic features. Nat. Sci. Data 4, 170117 (2017)
14. Bakas, S., Akbari, H., Sotiras, A., Bilello, M., Rozycki, M., Kirby, J., Freymann, J., Farahani, K., Davatzikos, C.: Segmentation labels and radiomic features for the pre-operative scans of the TCGA-GBM collection. The Cancer Imaging Archive (2017). https://doi.org/10.7937/k9/tcia.2017.klxwjj1q
15. Bakas, S., Akbari, H., Sotiras, A., Bilello, M., Rozycki, M., Kirby, J., Freymann, J., Farahani, K., Davatzikos, C.: Segmentation labels and radiomic features for the pre-operative scans of the TCGA-LGG collection. The Cancer Imaging Archive (2017). https://doi.org/10.7937/k9/tcia.2017.gjq7r0ef
16. Ahmed, S., Iftekharuddin, K.M., Vossough, A.: Efficacy of texture, shape, and intensity feature fusion for posterior-fossa tumor segmentation in MRI. IEEE Trans. Inf. Technol. Biomed. 15, 206–213 (2011)
17. Reza, S., Iftekharuddin, K.M.: Multi-fractal texture features for brain tumor and edema segmentation. In: SPIE, Medical Imaging 2014: Computer-Aided Diagnosis, San Diego, California (2014)
18. Iftekharuddin, K.M., Jia, W., Marsh, R.: Fractal analysis of tumor in brain images. Mach. Vis. Appl. 13, 352–362 (2003)
19. Islam, A., Reza, S.M.S., Iftekharuddin, K.M.: Multifractal texture estimation for detection and segmentation of brain tumors. IEEE Trans. Biomed. Eng. 60(11), 3204–3215 (2013)
20. Islam, A., Iftekharuddin, K.M., Ogg, R., Laningham, F.H., Sivakumar, B.: Multifractal modeling, segmentation, prediction, and statistical validation of posterior fossa tumors. In: SPIE Medical Imaging (2008)
21. Ahmed, S., Iftekharuddin, K.M., Vossough, A.: Efficacy of texture, shape, and intensity feature fusion for posterior-fossa tumor segmentation in MRI. IEEE Trans. Inf Technol. Biomed. 15(2), 206–213 (2011)
22. Ayache, A., Vehel, J.L.: On the identification of the pointwise holder exponent of the generalized multifractional Brownian motion. Stoch. Process Appl. 111, 119–156 (2004)
23. Ayache, A., Véhel, J.L.: Generalized multifractional Brownian motion: definition and preliminary results. In: Dekking, M., Véhel, J.L., Lutton, E., Tricot, C. (eds.) Fractals: Theory and Applications in Engineering, pp. 17–32. Springer, London (1999). https://doi.org/10.1007/978-1-4471-0873-3_2
24. Leung, T., Jitendra, M.: Representing and recognizing the visual appearance of materials using three-dimensional textons. Int. J. Comput. Vis. 43, 29–44 (2001)

25. Kleesiek, J., Biller, A., Urban, G., Köthe, U., Bendszus, M., Hamprecht, F.A.: Ilastik for multi-modal brain tumor segmentation. In: MICCAI BraTS (Brain Tumor Segmentation Challenge) (2014)
26. Vallières, M., Freeman, C.R., Skamene, S.R., El Naqa, I.: A radiomics model from Joint FDG-PET and MRI texture features for the prediction of lung metastases in soft-tissue sarcomas of the extremities. Phys. Med. Biol. **60**(14), 5471–5496 (2015)
27. Caret: classification and regression training. https://CRAN.R-project.org/package=caret

MRI Augmentation via Elastic Registration for Brain Lesions Segmentation

Egor Krivov[1,2,3], Maxim Pisov[1,3], and Mikhail Belyaev[2,1(✉)]

[1] Kharkevich Institute for Information Transmission Problems, Moscow, Russia
[2] Skolkovo Institute of Science and Technology, Moscow, Russia
m.belyaev@skoltech.ru
[3] Moscow Institute of Physics and Technology, Dolgoprudny, Russia

Abstract. Datasets for medical image segmentation usually contain a very limited number of training examples. However, deep learning methods prove to be very competitive for such data analysis problems. Surprisingly, quite limited data augmentation is used during training. We presume that it's due to historical reasons: standardization and normalization of medical images dominate over methods for increasing the size of a training set by artificial transformation of images. We assume that it is partly caused by the absence of methods which preserve properties of adequately preprocessed medical images. In this paper, we propose a new method for brain MRI augmentation, which allows us to map a lesion from an original image to a healthy brain. We compare the performance of U-Net and DeepMedic, two popular deep learning architectures, using the proposed method, a set of classical image augmentation methods, and a combination of both approaches. Our results suggest that at least one of the individual strategies, as well as their combination, provide an increase in accuracy of brain lesions segmentation if the training sample is relatively small.

Keywords: Image augmentation · CNN · Segmentation · MRI
BraTS

1 Introduction

Medical image segmentation is a popular data analysis problem. Various examples include pulmonary nodules detection [20], brain tumor segmentation [17] and multiple sclerosis segmentation [10] among others. One of the core ideas is to use imaging data to construct quantitative noninvasive biomarkers which can be used to detect and track disease progression or to predict the treatment outcome [17]. In case of brain lesions, a set of candidates consists of various geometrical characteristics such as total volume of a lesion or its substructures, localization, some other geometrical attributes like length or radius.

Well-developed methods for brain tissue segmentation are usually built upon a set of pre-segmented atlases and strict geometrical prior assumptions [8]. However, application of these methods to brain lesion segmentation is limited due

© Springer International Publishing AG, part of Springer Nature 2018
A. Crimi et al. (Eds.): BrainLes 2017, LNCS 10670, pp. 369–380, 2018.
https://doi.org/10.1007/978-3-319-75238-9_32

to the absence of strong prior assumptions on lesions localizations and shapes due to high heterogeneity of lesions localization and shape. Even simpler segmentation problems like skull stripping still severely affected by the presence of lesions [19]. Instead, a machine learning method can be used to segment lesions by catching local differences in image intensities. Until recently, random forests was the method of choice for the brain lesion segmentation [16].

It's worth mentioning that only a limited amount of training images is available. There are various reasons for that including issues with privacy and costly procedures of images collection and annotation. A typical dataset consists of images with up to a couple of hundreds of patients (e.g., see [3]). Moreover, images are three-dimensional, and each image can contain up to 10 million voxels. At the same time, sets of 2D non-medical images usually contain up to millions of images and each image typically contains less than 100 thousands of pixels [7].

Surprisingly, deep learning methods dominate medical image segmentation even in such tough conditions by now. Two of the most popular network architectures are U-Net [18] and DeepMedic [13]. U-Net was originally developed for neuronal structures segmentation in electron microscopic stacks, but during the last two years a lot of modifications for medical images segmentation were proposed including a 3D version of the network [6] and applications to various domains (e.g., prostate cancer [22]). One of the major points of the original U-Net paper is very intensive data augmentation. However, methods for medical image segmentation (even U-Net-based ones) use a very limited augmentation. Usually, the data transformations are restricted to variations of intensities, a simple mirroring across the central sagittal plane (i.e. exchange of hemispheres in case of brain MRI) [13], or simple rotations [6].

We suppose that traditionally medical image community preprocess data intensively, so images become highly standardized. At the same time, non-medical images usually cannot be normalized to that extent. To compensate this, researchers apply random transformation such as cropping and rotating. It allows increasing training samples by artificial images which have the same "distribution" as the original data. However, the same set of methods destroys the normalization of medical images. We believe that this fact limits the usage of classical data augmentation methods for medical image analysis problems.

In this paper, we propose a new registration-based augmentation method that preserve all the desired properties of a processed MR image while also significantly increase the size of the training set. The core idea of the method is to "map" a lesion from a training set to an external healthy brain using elastic registration. To prevent a failure of a registration algorithm, we propose to exclude invaded tissues from the registration cost function. To evaluate the proposed approach as well as the classical image augmentation techniques, we performed an intensive set of deep learning experiments using the Multimodal Brain Tumor Segmentation Challenge 2017 dataset (BraTS) [4,5] and the Ischemic Stroke Lesion Segmentation Challenge 2015, the sub-acute ischemic stroke dataset (ISLES) [15]. As segmentation methods, we used U-Net and DeepMedic architectures.

2   Data Augmentation

As we stated in the introduction, the usage of data augmentation methods for medical image segmentation is limited. We suppose that there are two reasons for this. First, medical images are way more standardized than other images. The target body organs are usually located in the center of the image, and there is a predefined number of their instances in each image (i.e., there is one, and only one brain that can be present in a head MRI). Second, we deem that there are two opposite strategies to deal with data variability: decrease variability in all data by some data preprocessing or use extensive data augmentation, increasing data variability and the size of the training set.

The medical image computing community historically prefers preprocessing. Various tools were developed and implemented to normalize images, reduce variability and remove irrelevant information from MRI (ANTs [2], FSL [11] to name a few). Indeed, a typical brain MRI preprocessing pipeline includes, bias field correction [21], image alignment, brain extraction [19], resampling to isotropic resolution. Conversely, some of the classical data augmentation methods such as random rotations can break the alignment; too aggressive elastic deformations may lead to non-physiological shapes of a brain.

In this work, we propose a coregistration-based data augmentation method which preserves the normalization of medical images and compares it with the traditional image augmentation such as random elastic transformations and affine transformations: scaling, rotation, and reflection. We ignore the spatial translation because convolutional neural networks are invariant to this type of transformations. Also, we estimated the effect of joint usage of both types of data augmentation techniques. The following subsections provide details of these two approaches.

2.1   Affine Transformations

Let $x = (x_1, x_2, x_3)^T$ be the coordinates of every voxel in a 3D image and $\mathcal{N}(m, \sigma^2)$ be a univariate Gaussian distribution with mean m and variance σ^2.

Then the traditional set of the data augmentation techniques includes the following transformations:

1. Scale: $x_i \mapsto x_i \cdot s_i$, where $s_i \sim \mathcal{N}(1, \sigma_s^2)$ is a random scaling factor.
2. Reflection: $x_2 \mapsto x_2 \cdot f$, where $f = \begin{cases} 1, p = \frac{1}{2} \\ -1, p = \frac{1}{2} \end{cases}$ is a random multiplier.
3. Rotation by α degrees along the OZ axis and θ degrees along the OY axis, where $\alpha, \theta \sim \mathcal{N}(0, \sigma_r^2)$ are random angles.

In our experiments we independently scaled the image along each axis by a random factor, then we performed random rotations, and finally we flipped the image with a probability of 1/2. The flip was made only by one axis and was intended to "swap the hemispheres" of the brain. For the random scaling and rotating we used the following values of standard deviations $\sigma_s = 0.15, \sigma_r = 5$.

2.2 Coregistration

Coregistration is a procedure of alignment of two MR images [14]. Usually, coregistration is used for two purposes. First, an intra-subject analysis of functional MRI data requires the alignment of all scans from the series. Technically it can be done by coregistration of these images with a structural image for the same subject. Second, inter-subject analysis (e.g., a search of specific activation patterns) requires the voxel-to-voxel correspondence for all subjects. In that case, coregistration with a template MRI is used.

From mathematical points of view, coregistration is the following optimization problem [1]:

$$\phi^* = argmin_{\phi \in \Phi}\Big(\mathcal{Q}\big(\phi(\mathbf{X}), \mathbf{Z}\big) + \lambda\mathcal{L}(\phi)\Big),$$

where

- Φ is a set of transformations and ϕ is an element of this set,
- $\mathbf{Z}$ is the template image, $\mathbf{X}$ is the moving image,
- $\mathcal{Q}$ is a measure of similarity of two images (e.g., mutual information),
- λ is a regularization parameter and $\mathcal{L}$ is a regularization functional which controls the smoothness of the transformation ϕ.

There are two main options for selecting Φ. Linear coregistration is used for intra-subject analysis, whereas nonlinear transformations are required for inter-subject studies.

In this paper we aim to investigate the potential of coregistration as a data augmentation strategy. Let $\{\mathbf{X}_i\}_{i=1}^{N}$ be a dataset of MRI scans with some lesions and $\{\mathbf{Z}_i\}_{i=1}^{K}$ - another set of MRI images of healthy patients, then for each pair $(\mathbf{X}_i, \mathbf{Z}_j)$ we apply coregistration using $\mathbf{Z}_i$ as a template. In that case we need to use a special version of $\mathcal{Q}$ since voxel intensities for lesions differ dramatically from healthy tissues and should be removed from optimization process. We excluded voxels marked as a part of a lesion from functional $\mathcal{Q}$.

Figure 1 shows an example of this procedure. Note how the lesioned region adjusts its shape to match the new brain geometry. If the initial dataset has several modalities, we apply the mapping, obtained during the coregistration step, to other modalities and binary masks (if any).

As a result, this approach yields $N \cdot K$ brain images that slightly differ from the original N, which effectively increases the dataset size by a factor of $K + 1$. However, caution is advised during the model evaluation step: because the images originating from the same brain x_i differ only slightly, all of them must be present either in train, validation or test set, otherwise model performance overestimation is inevitable.

In our experiments we used MRI images of 8 healthy patients from the ADNI dataset aged under 65 years. During the coregistration step the T1 modality was used to create the mapping, and in case of BRATS-17 the "Whole Tumor" mask was interpreted as "the lesioned region". This step was performed with the "Advanced Normalization Tools" (ANTs) toolkit [1].

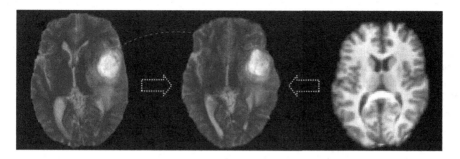

Fig. 1. Schematic representation of coregistration in presence of lesions: a brain image from BRATS-17 (T2, left), a brain image from ADNI (T1, right), coregistration result (center). Informally speaking, this operation answers the question: How would this lesion (left, red) look on this healthy patient (right)?

3   Models

For our computational experiments we used the two most popular architectures for brain lesions segmentation: U-net [18] and DeepMedic [13]. U-net is a 2D Fully-Convolutional Network (FCN) which consists of two major paths: the contracting path, that finds useful low-dimensional patterns and the expanding path, that obtains the final segmentation. A key addition to a standard FCN is a set of additional connections between the paths. These additional links could take into account locations of patterns in slightly processed images from the contracting path and combine it with highly processed images from the expanding path to improve localization of regions of interests. DeepMedic is a 3D FCN network with two input branches. The first one uses an image patch with an original resolution, which could help in locating lesion borders, while the second branch starts with a coarser image path which covers a larger area of the full image, which could help by providing information about more global picture. The following two subsections provide some additional details.

3.1   DeepMedic

The DeepMedic architecture (Fig. 2) has proven to be one of the best solutions for medical image segmentation. It is based on volumetric 3-dimensional

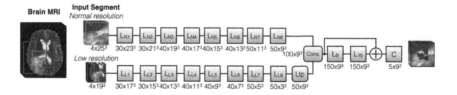

Fig. 2. Original DeepMedic architecture from [13]

convolutional layers which allow the network to use information from all three spatial dimensions. The architecture is split up into two pathways: a detailed pathway, that allows the network to provide accurate segmentation on object's boundaries, and a context pathway, which extracts contextual information about the image region, supposedly improving general understanding of this region. DeepMedic is a fully convolutional network, allowing fast and effective evaluation on large images.

We wanted to reproduce the architecture and the training procedure as close as possible to the original, so in our experiments we use the architecture from [13], since this paper has more details than more recent [12]. The difference between these two is that the more recent version uses residual connections, which slightly improves accuracy. We also use the same training procedure as [13], to be more specific, we employ the same patch sampling procedure, when half of the batch consists of patches, centered on background (healthy tissue) and the other half – on the foreground (unhealthy tissue).

During training we use batch size of 64. We consider one training epoch to be 100 train steps, so during one epoch our model sees 100×64 patches We trained the models for 120 epochs since both training and validation losses stopped changing at this point for all cases.

3.2   U-Net

We use the two-dimensional U-Net architecture, proposed in [18], which is a state-of-the-art solution for 2D image segmentation. We apply it to scan slices across the OZ axis, therefore the network can only see one slice during the

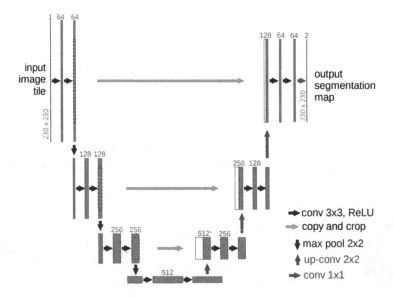

Fig. 3. Slight modification of the U-Net architecture from [18]

inference step. We use original U-Net architecture with two modifications: firstly, we use a different depth of the model in order to adapt it to the spatial size of our images, and secondly, we use zero-padding on all the layers to keep the spatial size of the output equal to the input (Fig. 3).

During training we use batches of size 20, filling them with samples as follows:

1. Shuffle the training set.
2. For each 3D MRI image extract the slices along the OZ axis containing at least one foreground pixel.
3. Fill the batch with samples.

This whole procedure corresponds to one training epoch. Therefore, during one training epoch, the model observes all the slices that have at least one foreground pixel in all the scans. U-Net was trained for 60 epochs in case if the augmentation strategy contained coregistration and for 150 epochs if it did not. In both cases, the learning was stopped due to the fact that the loss function plateaued on both training and validation set.

4   Data

In this paper we use three different datasets: Brain Tumor Segmentation Challenge 2017 (BraTS-17), Ischemic Stroke Lesion Segmentation 2015 (ISLES-15) and Alzheimer's Disease Neuroimaging Initiative (ADNI). The latter was not used directly during the training, but implicitly during the proposed data augmentation procedure, see Sect. 2.

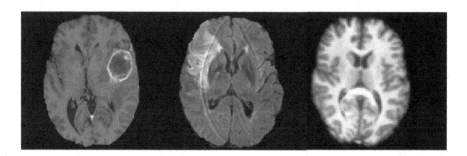

Fig. 4. Samples from each dataset: BraTS-17 (T1Gd, left), ISLES-15 (FLAIR, center), ADNI (T1, right)

4.1   BraTS

BraTS is a dataset from Multimodal Brain Tumor Segmentation Challenge 2017 [3–5,17]. This competition utilizes pre-operative MRI scans from different institutions and focuses on the segmentation of brain tumors. The dataset has 285

3-dimensional scans of 4 modalities (native (T1); post-contrast T1-weighted (T1Gd); T2-weighted; T2 Fluid Attenuated Inversion Recovery (FLAIR)) as well as segmentation masks describing the tumor type for each voxel. There are 3 masks for each scan: Whole Tumor (WT), Tumor Core (TC) and Enhancing Tumor (ET). Each MRI scans was skull-stripped, re-sampled to an isotropic spacing of 1^3 mm^3 and co-registered (Fig. 4).

BraTS Subset. Since this paper aims to study the effect of data augmentation, which is a way of increasing the effective dataset size, it is interesting to observe the effect of augmentation on a small dataset. To do this we first remove 10% of the images on which DeepMedic performed the worst according to the dice score for the "Tumor Core" mask on 5-fold CV. Then, we randomly draw 28 samples from the remaining scans, to match the ISLES-15 dataset size.

4.2   ISLES-15

ISLES is a dataset from the Ischemic Stroke Lesion Segmentation (2015) challenge [15]. In this paper we used the subset from the Sub-acute Ischemic Stroke lesion Segmentation (SISS) case, because, according to the results of the competition, this is a more challenging task, allowing us observe the effects of augmentation more clearly.

The dataset contains 28 brain MRI images with 4 modalities (DWI, Flair, T1, T2) and one binary mask (expert segmentation). Each of the 28 MRI scans was skull-stripped, re-sampled to an isotropic spacing of 1^3 mm^3 and co-registered to the FLAIR modality.

4.3   ADNI

Alzheimer's Disease Neuroimaging Initiative (ADNI)[9] is a database consisting of more than a thousand human brain MRI scans and is split into four classes: Normal Cohort (NC), Early Mild Cognitive Impairment (EMCI), Late Mild Cognitive Impairment (LMCI), and Alzheimer's Disease (AD). However, in this study we use only 8 images from this dataset to perform coregistration-based data augmentation. (See the Data augmentation Sect. 2 for details).

5   Experiments and Results

To evaluate the suggested methods, we have implemented DeepMedic and U-Net architectures as well as suggested data augmentation in our library[1]. All computations were performed on a single Nvidia Titan X GPU card.

To evaluate the segmentation quality we used the Dice score, as one of the most commonly accepted metrics. We used 5-fold cross-validation on each dataset. During training, we used six scans for big BraTS dataset, and five scans

---

[1] Code is publicly available at https://github.com/neuro-ml/deep_pipe.

Table 1. DeepMedic performance on three datasets with different augmentation strategies. Each cell contains the mean Dice Score over 5 test folds and its standard deviation.

	BRATS-17			BRATS-17 subset			ISLES-15
	WT	TC	ET	WT	TC	ET	
None	.85 ± .13	.76 ± .24	.67 ± .30	.80 ± .19	.71 ± .27	.65 ± .29	.52 ± .28
Spatial	.84 ± .14	.75 ± .23	.66 ± .30	.77 ± .20	.69 ± .28	.63 ± .28	.52 ± .28
Coregistration	.86 ± .12	.75 ± .24	.66 ± .30	.77 ± .21	.70 ± .27	.61 ± .28	.55 ± .28
Both	.85 ± .13	.75 ± .22	.66 ± .29	.79 ± .16	.69 ± .24	.62 ± .27	.55 ± .27

for small BraTS and ISLES15 as the validation set used to trace quality during training. No dropout or weight regularization was used since we didn't notice any overfitting on the validation set. Learning rate was initially set to 0.1 and was halved each time validation loss plateaued (we checked that validation loss didn't decrease significantly for five epochs).

BraTS. The segmentation problem on this dataset can be interpreted as a pixel-wise multiclass classification problem. According to this interpretation, we use the softmax layer to provide probabilities for each class in the network output, and we minimize the multiclass logarithmic loss during training. To discretize the predictions, we use the argmax function.

ISLES15. The segmentation problem on this dataset can be interpreted as a binary pixel-wise classification problem. According to this interpretation, we use the sigmoid layer to provide probabilities for each class in the network output and we minimize the binary logarithmic loss during training. To discretize the predictions, we find a threshold for the probability maps that maximize the Dice score on the validation set.

5.1 Discussion

The results of the computational experiments are presented in Tables 1 and 2 for DeepMedic and U-net architectures respectively. Interestingly, DeepMedic outperforms U-net for all three data sets.

Table 2. U-Net performance on three datasets with different augmentation strategies. Each cell contains the mean Dice Score over 5 test folds and its standard deviation.

	BRATS-17			BRATS-17 subset			ISLES-15
	WT	TC	ET	WT	TC	ET	
None	.80 ± .17	.62 ± .30	.60 ± .30	.72 ± .22	.56 ± .28	.55 ± .29	.43 ± .33
Spatial	.80 ± .17	.62 ± .29	.58 ± .29	.75 ± .20	.58 ± .27	.60 ± .27	.42 ± .34
Coregistration	.79 ± .18	.56 ± .33	.56 ± .32	.73 ± .20	.60 ± .27	.60 ± .27	.48 ± .30
Both	.78 ± .18	.63 ± .28	.58 ± .30	.72 ± .24	.62 ± .29	.61 ± .27	.51 ± .29

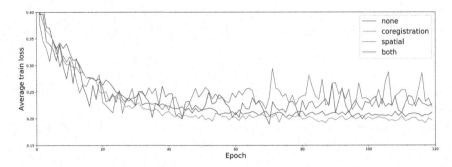

Fig. 5. Average learning curves (across 5 models) for DeepMedic model on the full BraTS-17 dataset. The cost function is multiclass logarithmic loss.

For both BraTS samples and DeepMedic model, all three types of augmentation don't affect the outcome. A deeper analysis showed that training error for these networks reach the same plateau at a value significantly higher than zero, see Fig. 5. Two factors can cause it: (1) DeepMedic architecture lacks representation power to catch more complex dependencies and (2) inter-rater variability of human annotation introduces irreducible error. We assume that the observed effect can be explained by a combination of these two factors.

For ISLES-15 dataset, augmentation via registration as well as the combination of two types of augmentation improved accuracy for both models. Moreover, the combined approach allows to significantly increase the quality of U-net models and allows to achieve performance level similar to dominating DeepMedic.

6   Conclusion

Our result suggests that data augmentation can be useful for datasets with small number of samples. For larger datasets the studied methods for data augmentation doesn't improve segmentation quality, but likely can be used to generate a set of candidates for building an ensemble of segmentation models. We assume that the proposed method can benefit if we use models with higher representational power. Also, it can be more useful in case of small lesions (e.g., Multiple Sclerosis) due to simpler cost function for registration methods. Another point which could affect the results is the selection of templates. Ideally, template T1 images should be collected using the same imaging protocol as MRI with lesions.

Acknowledgments. The data used in preparing this paper were obtained from the Alzheimer's Disease Neuroimaging Initiative (ADNI) database. A complete listing of ADNI investigators and imaging protocols may be found at adni.loni.usc.edu.

References

1. Avants, B.B., Tustison, N.J., Song, G., Cook, P.A., Klein, A., Gee, J.C.: A reproducible evaluation of ants similarity metric performance in brain image registration. Neuroimage **54**(3), 2033–2044 (2011)
2. Avants, B.B., Tustison, N.J., Stauffer, M., Song, G., Wu, B., Gee, J.C.: The insight toolkit image registration framework. Front. Neuroinformatics **8**, 44 (2014)
3. Bakas, S., Akbari, H., Sotiras, A., Bilello, M., Rozycki, M., Kirby, J., Freymann, J., Farahani, K., Davatzikos, C.: Advancing the cancer genome atlas glioma MRI collections with expert segmentation labels and radiomic features. Sci. Data **4**, 170117 (2017)
4. Bakas, S., Akbari, H., Sotiras, A., Bilello, M., Rozycki, M., Kirby, J., Freymann, J., Farahani, K., Davatzikos, C.: Segmentation labels for the pre-operative scans of the TCGA-GBM collection (2017)
5. Bakas, S., Akbari, H., Sotiras, A., Bilello, M., Rozycki, M., Kirby, J., Freymann, J., Farahani, K., Davatzikos, C.: Segmentation labels for the pre-operative scans of the TCGA-LGG collection (2017)
6. Çiçek, Ö., Abdulkadir, A., Lienkamp, S.S., Brox, T., Ronneberger, O.: 3D U-net: learning dense volumetric segmentation from sparse annotation. In: Ourselin, S., Joskowicz, L., Sabuncu, M.R., Unal, G., Wells, W. (eds.) MICCAI 2016, Part II. LNCS, vol. 9901, pp. 424–432. Springer, Cham (2016). https://doi.org/10.1007/978-3-319-46723-8_49
7. Deng, J., Dong, W., Socher, R., Li, L.J., Li, K., Fei-Fei, L.: Imagenet: a large-scale hierarchical image database. In: 2009 IEEE Conference on Computer Vision and Pattern Recognition, CVPR 2009, pp. 248–255. IEEE (2009)
8. Fischl, B., Salat, D.H., Busa, E., Albert, M., Dieterich, M., Haselgrove, C., Van Der Kouwe, A., Killiany, R., Kennedy, D., Klaveness, S., et al.: Whole brain segmentation: automated labeling of neuroanatomical structures in the human brain. Neuron **33**(3), 341–355 (2002)
9. Jack, C.R., Bernstein, M.A., Fox, N.C., Thompson, P., Alexander, G., Harvey, D., Borowski, B., Britson, P.J., Whitwell, J.L., Ward, C., et al.: The Alzheimer's disease neuroimaging initiative (ADNI): MRI methods. J. Magn. Reson. Imaging **27**(4), 685–691 (2008)
10. Jain, S., Sima, D.M., Ribbens, A., Cambron, M., Maertens, A., Van Hecke, W., De Mey, J., Barkhof, F., Steenwijk, M.D., Daams, M., et al.: Automatic segmentation and volumetry of multiple sclerosis brain lesions from MR images. NeuroImage Clin. **8**, 367–375 (2015)
11. Jenkinson, M., Beckmann, C.F., Behrens, T.E., Woolrich, M.W., Smith, S.M.: FSL. Neuroimage **62**(2), 782–790 (2012)
12. Kamnitsas, K., et al.: DeepMedic for brain tumor segmentation. In: Crimi, A., Menze, B., Maier, O., Reyes, M., Winzeck, S., Handels, H. (eds.) BrainLes 2016. LNCS, vol. 10154, pp. 138–149. Springer, Cham (2016). https://doi.org/10.1007/978-3-319-55524-9_14
13. Kamnitsas, K., Ledig, C., Newcombe, V.F., Simpson, J.P., Kane, A.D., Menon, D.K., Rueckert, D., Glocker, B.: Efficient multi-scale 3D CNN with fully connected CRF for accurate brain lesion segmentation. Med. Image Anal. **36**, 61–78 (2017)
14. Klein, A., Andersson, J., Ardekani, B.A., Ashburner, J., Avants, B., Chiang, M.C., Christensen, G.E., Collins, D.L., Gee, J., Hellier, P., et al.: Evaluation of 14 nonlinear deformation algorithms applied to human brain MRI registration. Neuroimage **46**(3), 786–802 (2009)

15. Maier, O., Menze, B.H., von der Gablentz, J., Häni, L., Heinrich, M.P., Liebrand, M., Winzeck, S., Basit, A., Bentley, P., Chen, L., et al.: Isles 2015-a public evaluation benchmark for ischemic stroke lesion segmentation from multispectral MRI. Med. Image Anal. **35**, 250–269 (2017)

16. Maier, O., Wilms, M., von der Gablentz, J., Krämer, U.M., Münte, T.F., Handels, H.: Extra tree forests for sub-acute ischemic stroke lesion segmentation in MR sequences. J. Neurosci. Methods **240**, 89–100 (2015)

17. Menze, B.H., Jakab, A., Bauer, S., Kalpathy-Cramer, J., Farahani, K., Kirby, J., Burren, Y., Porz, N., Slotboom, J., Wiest, R., et al.: The multimodal brain tumor image segmentation benchmark (brats). IEEE Trans. Med. Imaging **34**(10), 1993–2024 (2015)

18. Ronneberger, O., Fischer, P., Brox, T.: U-Net: convolutional networks for biomedical image segmentation. In: Navab, N., Hornegger, J., Wells, W.M., Frangi, A.F. (eds.) MICCAI 2015, Part III. LNCS, vol. 9351, pp. 234–241. Springer, Cham (2015). https://doi.org/10.1007/978-3-319-24574-4_28

19. Roy, S., Butman, J.A., Pham, D.L., Initiative, A.D.N., et al.: Robust skull stripping using multiple MR image contrasts insensitive to pathology. NeuroImage **146**, 132–147 (2017)

20. Setio, A.A.A., Traverso, A., De Bel, T., Berens, M.S., van den Bogaard, C., Cerello, P., Chen, H., Dou, Q., Fantacci, M.E., Geurts, B., et al.: Validation, comparison, and combination of algorithms for automatic detection of pulmonary nodules in computed tomography images: the LUNA16 challenge. Med. Image Anal. **42**, 1–13 (2017)

21. Tustison, N.J., Avants, B.B., Cook, P.A., Zheng, Y., Egan, A., Yushkevich, P.A., Gee, J.C.: N4ITK: improved N3 bias correction. IEEE Trans. Med. Imaging **29**(6), 1310–1320 (2010)

22. Yu, L., Yang, X., Chen, H., Qin, J., Heng, P.A.: Volumetric convnets with mixed residual connections for automated prostate segmentation from 3D MR images. In: AAAI, pp. 66–72 (2017)

Cascaded V-Net Using ROI Masks for Brain Tumor Segmentation

Adrià Casamitjana, Marcel Català, Irina Sánchez, Marc Combalia, and Verónica Vilaplana$^{(\boxtimes)}$

Signal Theory and Communications Department,
Universitat Politècnica de Catalunya. BarcelonaTech, Barcelona, Spain
{adria.casamitjana,veronica.vilaplana}@upc.edu

Abstract. In this work we approach the brain tumor segmentation problem with a cascade of two CNNs inspired in the V-Net architecture [13], reformulating residual connections and making use of ROI masks to constrain the networks to train only on relevant voxels. This architecture allows dense training on problems with highly skewed class distributions, such as brain tumor segmentation, by focusing training only on the vecinity of the tumor area. We report results on BraTS2017 Training and Validation sets.

1 Introduction

Accurate localization and segmentation of brain tumors in Magnetic Resonance Imaging (MRI) is crucial for monitoring progression, surgery or radiotherapy planning and follow-up studies. Since manual segmentation is time-consuming and may lead to inter-rater discrepancy, automatic or semi-automatic approaches have been a topic of interest during the last decade. Among tumors that originally develop in the brain, gliomas are the most common type. Gliomas may have different degrees of aggressiveness, variable prognosis and several heterogeneous histological sub-regions (peritumoral edema, necrotic core, enhancing and non-enhancing tumor core) that are described by varying intensity profiles across different MRI modalities, which reflect diverse tumor biological properties [1]. However, the distinction between tumor and normal tissue is difficult as tumor borders are often fuzzy and there is a high variability in shape, location and extent across patients. Despite recent advances in automated algorithms for brain tumor segmentation in multimodal MRI scans, the problem is still a challenging task in medical imaging analysis.

Many different computational methods have been proposed to solve the problem. Here we will only review some of the most recent approaches based on deep

This work has been partially supported by the projects BIGGRAPH-TEC2013-43935-R and MALEGRA TEC2016-75976-R financed by the Spanish Ministerio de Economía y Competitividad and the European Regional Development Fund (ERDF). Adrià Casamitjana is supported by the Spanish "Ministerio de Educacin, Cultura y Deporte" FPU Research Fellowship.

A. Crimi et al. (Eds.): BrainLes 2017, LNCS 10670, pp. 381–391, 2018.
https://doi.org/10.1007/978-3-319-75238-9_33

learning, which are the top-performing methods in BraTS challenge since 2014. Representative works based on other machine learning models include [2–6] and methods reviewed in [1].

As opposed to classical discriminative models based on pre-defined features, deep learning models learn a hierarchy of increasingly complex task specific features directly from data, which results in more robust features.

Some methods do not completely exploit the available volumetric information and use two-dimensional Convolutional Neural Networks (CNN), processing 2D slices independently or using three orthogonal 2D patches to incorporate contextual information [7,8]. The model in [8] consists of two pathways, a local pathway that concentrates on pixel neighborhood information, and a global pathway, which captures global context of the slice. This two-path structure is adopted in a fully 3D approach named DeepMedic [9], consisting of two parallel 3D CNN pathways producing soft segmentation maps, followed by a fully connected 3D CRF that imposes generalization constraints. The network is extended in [10] by adding residual connections between the outputs of every two layers. The work shows empirically that the residual connections give modest but consistent improvement in sensitivity over all tumor classes. In [14] we compare the performances of three 3D CNN architectures inspired in two well known 2D models used for image segmentation [11,12] and a variant of [9] showing the importance of the multi-resolution connections to obtain fine details in the segmentation of tumor sub-regions. More recently, V-Net [13] presents successful results on challenging medical imaging segmentation tasks by using both short and long skip connections that help learning finer structures and ease training.

In this paper, in the context of BraTS Challenge 2017, we present a brain tumor segmentation method based on a cascade of two convolutional neural networks. The problem is divided in two simpler tasks that can be performed independently using two 3D-CNN and a later combination of their outputs to get the final segmentation. The network architecture used for the two tasks is a modified version of V-Net consisting of convolutional blocks and residual connections that have been reformulated according to recent findings in the literature [18]. Additionally, we introduce the use of ROI masks during the learning process in order to constrain each CNN to focus only on relevant voxels or regions from each task. Hence, the first network will be trained only on brain tissue to produce raw tumor masks and the second networks will be trained on the vecinity of the tumor to predict tumor regions.

Medical images in general and brain MRI in particular contain non-informative voxels (e.g. background or non-brain tissue) and many techniques have been developed to filter out this information. We can benefit from this knowledge and focus the entire system to train only on relevant, informative voxels or regions (e.g. apply a skull-stripping method and work with the brain mask to discard background information). To do so, the loss is computed only within the mask and the outer voxels will not contribute in the learning process, blocking the backpropagated signal through them. Finally, we use a dense-training scheme with small batch sizes that avoids patch-wise training and reduces the overall training time. Moreover, the common structure of the brain across subjects may be better learned using the whole image for training.

2   Method

One of the main problems in brain lesion detection is that lesions affect a small portion of the brain, making naive training strategies biased towards the trivial decision of null detection. Brain tumors normally correspond to only 3–5% of the overall image, accounting for 5–15% of the brain tissue and being each tumor region an even smaller portion. To address this issue, we propose to divide the brain tumor segmentation problem into two simpler tasks: (i) segmentation of the overall tumor and (ii) delineation of the different tumor regions. The tasks are performed in parallel using two CNN networks, where the output of the first network is used an input to the second one. The overall system pipeline is depicted in Fig. 1.

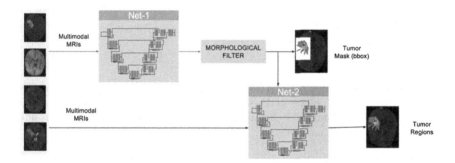

Fig. 1. The pipeline used for brain tumor segmentation

2.1   V-Net Using ROI Masks

Our network is a variant of V-Net [13] that aims at reducing the overall number of parameters by using smaller filter sizes ($3 \times 3 \times 3$ instead of $5 \times 5 \times 5$) and changing the non-linearity from PReLU to ReLU. In addition, we use batch normalization before the non-linearity to account for internal covariate shift. Based on insights from [18], we also reformulate the short residual connections in order to improve gradients flow across the network by using identity mappings as residual connections. In the case of dimensions mismatch in the addition layer, we minimally modify the residual connection with max-pooling and repeated up-sampling for spatial correspondence and $1 \times 1 \times 1$ convolutions to match the number of channels. For better understanding, we show in Fig. 2 the main changes from the original V-Net.

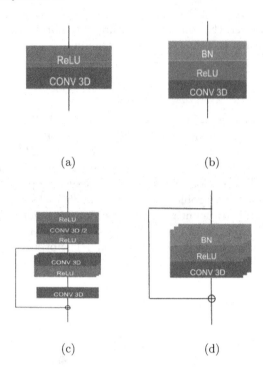

(a)   (b)

(c)   (d)

Fig. 2. Comparison between original V-Net modules and proposed modifications. First row: basic convolutional block of V-Net (a) and corresponding modification using BN (b). Second row: standard V-Net residual connections (c) and proposed residual connections (d).

We use ROI masks before the final predictions both during training and inference in order to smooth the class imbalance problem, specially for small sub-tumor regions. The ROI mask forces the outer voxels to belong to the background class with full probability by first multiplying them by 0 and turn their probability of belonging to the background class to 1. The multiplication prevents the backpropagated signal from going through the outer voxels and thus, it does not contribute in the learning process. The overall architecture is shown in Fig. 3.

2.2   Training

Each network in the pipeline performs a different task and thus, they can be independently trained. Instead of using patch-wise training and non-uniform sampling strategies to account for class imbalance, we use dense-training with a single subject per batch. The first network is trained as a binary segmentation problem with tumor/non-tumor classes and outputs a raw segmentation of the whole-tumor region. It takes the four modalities (T1, T1c, T2 and FLAIR) as inputs and uses the FLAIR intensity information in the deeper layers of the network by concatenating it with the predicted feature maps from the last level in the expanding path of the network. The network makes use of a brain mask in order to consider only brain tissue voxels for training. The loss function used is the modified dice coefficient (1) suited for binary segmentation tasks with imbalanced data:

$$L_1 = \frac{\sum_{i=1}^{N} p_i \cdot l_i}{\sum_{i=1}^{N} p_i + \sum_{i=1}^{N} l_i} \tag{1}$$

where N is the total number of voxels, p_i is the softmax output of the i-th voxel, and l_i is the i-th voxel label ($l_i = 0, 1$).

The second network is trained as a multi-class segmentation problem with four classes (non-tumor, edema, enhancing core and non-enhancing core). It also uses the four MRI modalities as input. From the ground-truth labels, we generate a rectangular mask that covers the whole tumor and it is used to train the network only in the vicinity of the tumor, avoiding to train on brain tissue far from the tumor region. As we use dense-training with a single subject per batch, the use of raw tumor masks in the training procedure helps to reduce the high class imbalance present among different classes. The loss function in the second network is a combination of cross entropy (X_E) and the dice coefficient for each tumor sub-region (whole tumor (D_{WT}), enhancing tumor (D_{ET}) and tumor core (D_{TC})). We empirically choose the values for the weights in both parts of the function:

$$L_2 = X_E + 0.5 * (D_{WT} + D_{ET} + D_{TC}) \tag{2}$$

2.3   Inference

At inference time, we first get the whole-tumor prediction from the first network. We use morphological filtering to remove small spurious detections made by the first network and we automatically find the smallest rectangular mask that covers the detected tumor. This result is then used as ROI mask in the second network to mask out the majority of false positives, since the second network is only trained to discriminate tumor regions on the vicinity of the tumor. This process can be done in parallel since one can decouple the masking process from the network prediction and thus, save inference time.

3   Results and Discussion

3.1   Data

BraTS2017 training data [15–17] consists of 210 pre-operative MRI scans of subjects with glioblastoma (GBM/HGG) and 75 scans of subjects with lower grade glioma (LGG), corresponding to the following modalities: native T1, post-contrast T1-weighted, T2-weighted and FLAIR, acquired from multiple institutions. Ground truth annotations comprise GD-enhancing tumor (ET, label 4), peritumoral edema (ED, label 2), necrotic and non-enhancing tumor

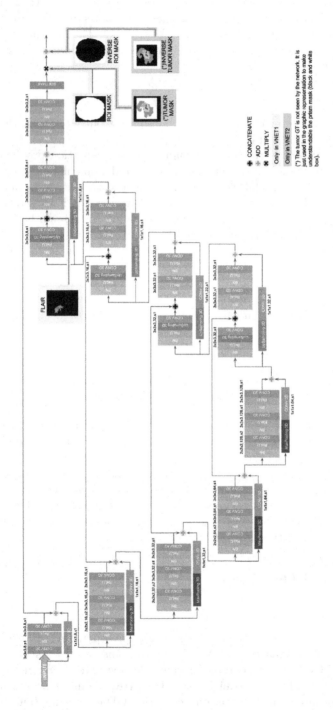

Fig. 3. V-Net architecture used in this work

(CNR/NET, label 1) as described in [1]. The data is distributed co-registered to the same anatomical template, interpolated to the same resolution ($1\,\text{mm}^3$) and skull-stripped. The validation set consists of 46 scans with no distinction between GBM/HGG and LGG.

Each scan is individually normalized in mean and standard deviation. For training, we use data augmentation by adding scan reflections with respect to the sagittal plane.

3.2 Performance on BraTS2017 Training and Validation Sets

Evaluation of the results is performed merging the predicted labels into three classes: enhancing tumor ET (label 1), whole tumor WT (labels 1, 2, 4), and tumor core TC (labels 1, 4), using Dice score, Hausdorff distance, Sensitivity and Specificity. Preliminary results for the BraTS 2017 Training dataset have been obtained by hold-out using 70% of the data for training and the remaining 30% for development purposes, such as early stopping or to tune some hyperparameter. In addition to that, the performance on the BraTS 2017 Validation set, reported on the challenge's leaderboard[1], is also presented in Tables 1 and 2.

In Table 1 we show Dice and Hausdorff metrics. We achieve rather high performance on the Dice metric for the whole tumor (WT) region, but low values for enhancing tumor (ET) and tumor core (TC) regions, compared to state-of-the-art. Using the BraTS Validation set, we are able to compare to other participants in the challenge. In the case of Dice-WT, our method is very close to the results obtained by the top performing methods while, again, our method achieves rather low Dice-ET and Dice-TC metrics. Hausdorff distances are higher than the best performing algorithms, being specially high for the whole-tumor region, probably indicating some outlier predictions that increase the metric.

Table 1. Results for BraTS 2017 data. Dice and Hausdorff metrics are reported.

	Dice			Hausdorff		
	ET	WT	TC	ET	WT	TC
Development set	0.671	0.869	0.685	7.145	6.410	9.584
Validation set	0.714	0.877	0.637	5.434	8.343	11.173

Even though specificity is not very informative for imbalanced classes, results from Table 2 show that we are able to properly represent background, probably due to the use of masks in the predictions. More interestingly, sensitivity shows that ET and TC regions might be underrepresented in our predicted segmentations. This results guide us to future improvements trying to overcome that behavior.

---

[1] https://www.cbica.upenn.edu/BraTS17/lboardValidation.html.

Table 2. Results for BraTS 2017 data. Sensitivity and specificity are reported.

	Sensitivity			Specificity		
	ET	WT	TC	ET	WT	TC
Development set	0.735	0.851	0.664	0.998	0.994	0.997
Validation set	0.723	0.879	0.619	0.998	0.994	0.998

These results can be further analyzed and confirmed with Train/Development curves in Fig. 4, which mostly indicate the generalization power of the method by analyzing the bias/variance trade-off. We clearly see that from epoch 18 (iteration 3600) we start overfitting the tumor core metric (Fig. 4.b) while the other regions are either slowly gaining insignificant improvements (Fig. 4.a, whole tumor) or not improving at all (Fig. 4.c, enhancing core). However the development loss is still improving due to the cross-entropy term.

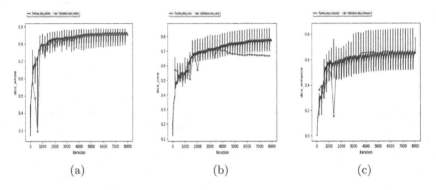

(a)   (b)   (c)

Fig. 4. Evaluation of metrics of interest during training in training (blue) and development (red) sets. Metrics: dice whole tumor (a), dice tumor core (b) and dice enhancing tumor (c) (Color figure online)

3.3   Visual Analysis

Figure 5 shows two subjects among the quantitatively better (first row) and poorer (second row) results. In both cases, it can be visually appreciated that our method correctly segments the whole tumor region. For the subject shown in Fig. 5.a, the system is able to properly capture all tumor regions, meaning that the first network is able to correctly localize the tumor and the second network is able to capture differences between tumor regions. On the other hand, in Fig. 5.b, we show a case where even though the tumor is correctly localized by the first network, the second isn't able to properly detect different tumor subregions. We see that edema (ED - label 2) is overrepresented in our segmentation in detriment of smaller classes: GD-enhancing tumor (ET - label 4) and the necrotic and non-enhancing tumor (NCR/NET - label 1). This effect can also be inferred from lower values in ET and TC dice coefficients.

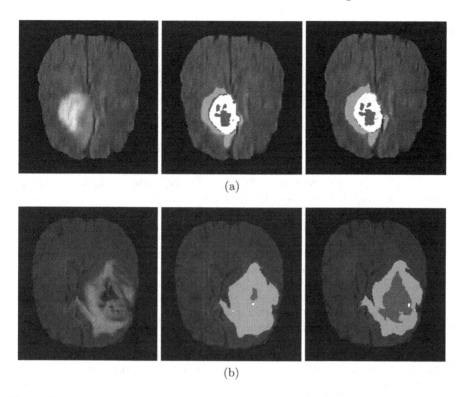

(a)

(b)

Fig. 5. Segmentation results of two subjects: (a) TCIA 479 (b) TCIA 109. From left to right we show the FLAIR sequence, followed by Prediction and GT tumor segmentation. We distinguish intra-tumoral regions by color-code: enhancing tumor (white), peritumoral edema (orange) and necrotic and non-enhancing tumor (red). (Color figure online)

4 Conclusions

In this paper we introduce a cascaded V-Net architecture that uses masks to focus training on relevant parts of the brain. We use it to solve the class imbalance problem inherent to brain tumor segmentation. We use a two-step process that (i) localizes the brain tumor area and (ii) distinguishes between different tumor regions, ignoring all other background voxels. This scheme allows to perform dense-training on MR images. We finally show results on BraTS 2017 Training and Validation sets, showing that while the results obtained for the WT segmentation are competitive with other participants' algorithms, we are not able to properly capture the less common regions (TC or ET). When trying to avoid patch-wise sampling strategies and make use of dense-training scheme, smaller classes are not well detected even using ROI masks, meaning that more weight should be placed when learning those classes. As a future work we will explore how to up-weight small tumor regions in the learning procedure.

References

1. Menze, B.H., Jakab, A., et al.: The multimodal brain tumor image segmentation benchmark (BRATS). IEEE Trans. Med. Imaging **34**(10), 1993–2024 (2015)
2. Gooya, A., Pohl, K.M., Bilello, M., Biros, G., Davatzikos, C.: Joint segmentation and deformable registration of brain scans guided by a tumor growth model. In: Fichtinger, G., Martel, A., Peters, T. (eds.) MICCAI 2011. LNCS, vol. 6892, pp. 532–540. Springer, Heidelberg (2011). https://doi.org/10.1007/978-3-642-23629-7_65
3. Zikic, D., et al.: Decision forests for tissue-specific segmentation of high-grade gliomas in multi-channel MR. In: Ayache, N., Delingette, H., Golland, P., Mori, K. (eds.) MICCAI 2012. LNCS, vol. 7512, pp. 369–376. Springer, Heidelberg (2012). https://doi.org/10.1007/978-3-642-33454-2_46
4. Parisot, S., Duffau, H., Chemouny, S., Paragios, N.: Joint tumor segmentation and dense deformable registration of brain MR images. In: Ayache, N., Delingette, H., Golland, P., Mori, K. (eds.) MICCAI 2012. LNCS, vol. 7511, pp. 651–658. Springer, Heidelberg (2012). https://doi.org/10.1007/978-3-642-33418-4_80
5. Maier, O., Wilms, M., Handels, H.: Image features for brain lesion segmentation using random forests. In: Crimi, A., Menze, B., Maier, O., Reyes, M., Handels, H. (eds.) BrainLes 2015. LNCS, vol. 9556, pp. 119–130. Springer, Cham (2016). https://doi.org/10.1007/978-3-319-30858-6_11
6. Tustison, N., Shrinidhi, K., Wintermark, M., et al.: Optimal symmetric multimodal templates and concatenated random forests for supervised brain tumor segmentation (simplified) with ANTsR. Neuroinformatics **13**, 209–225 (2015)
7. Pereira, S., Pinto, A., Alves, V., Silva, C.A.: Deep convolutional neural networks for the segmentation of gliomas in multi-sequence MRI. In: Crimi, A., Menze, B., Maier, O., Reyes, M., Handels, H. (eds.) BrainLes 2015. LNCS, vol. 9556, pp. 131–143. Springer, Cham (2016). https://doi.org/10.1007/978-3-319-30858-6_12
8. Havaei, M., Davy, A., et al.: Brain tumor segmentation with deep neural networks. Med. Image Anal. **35**, 18–31 (2016)
9. Kamnitsas, K., Ledig, C., Newcombe, V., et al.: Efficient multi-scale 3D CNN with fully connected CRF for accurate brain lesion segmentation. Med. Image Anal. **36**, 61–78 (2017)
10. Kamnitsas, K., et al.: DeepMedic for brain tumor segmentation. In: Crimi, A., Menze, B., Maier, O., Reyes, M., Winzeck, S., Handels, H. (eds.) MICCAI 2016. LNCS, vol. 10154, pp. 138–149. Springer, Cham (2016). https://doi.org/10.1007/978-3-319-55524-9_14
11. Long, J., Shelhamer, E., Darrel, T.: Fully convolutional networks for semantic segmentation. In: CVPR, Boston, USA (2015)
12. Ronneberger, O., Fischer, P., Brox, T.: U-Net: convolutional networks for biomedical image segmentation. In: Navab, N., Hornegger, J., Wells, W.M., Frangi, A.F. (eds.) MICCAI 2015. LNCS, vol. 9351, pp. 234–241. Springer, Cham (2015). https://doi.org/10.1007/978-3-319-24574-4_28
13. Milletari, F., Navab, N., Ahmadi, S.-A.: V-Net: fully convolutional neural networks for volumetric medical image segmentation. In: 2016 Fourth International Conference on 3D Vision (3DV). IEEE (2016)
14. Casamitjana, A., Puch, S., Aduriz, A., Vilaplana, V.: 3D convolutional neural networks for brain tumor segmentation: a comparison of multi-resolution architectures. In: Crimi, A., Menze, B., Maier, O., Reyes, M., Winzeck, S., Handels, H. (eds.) MICCAI 2016. LNCS, vol. 10154, pp. 150–161. Springer, Cham (2016). https://doi.org/10.1007/978-3-319-55524-9_15

15. Bakas, S., Akbari, H., Sotiras, A., Bilello, M., Rozycki, M., Kirby, J.S., Freymann, J.B., Farahani, K., Davatzikos, C.: Advancing the cancer genome atlas glioma MRI collections with expert segmentation labels and radiomic features. Nat. Sci. Data **4**, 170117 (2017)
16. Bakas, S., Akbari, H., Sotiras, A., Bilello, M., Rozycki, M., Kirby, J., Freymann, J., Farahani, K., Davatzikos, C.: Segmentation labels and radiomic features for the pre-operative scans of the TCGA-GBM collection. The Cancer Imaging Archive (2017). https://doi.org/10.7937/K9/TCIA.2017.KLXWJJ1Q
17. Bakas, S., Akbari, H., Sotiras, A., Bilello, M., Rozycki, M., Kirby, J., Freymann, J., Farahani, K., Davatzikos, C.: Segmentation labels and radiomic features for the pre-operative scans of the TCGA-LGG collection. The Cancer Imaging Archive (2017). https://doi.org/10.7937/K9/TCIA.2017.GJQ7R0EF
18. He, K., Zhang, X., Ren, S., Sun, J.: Identity mappings in deep residual networks. In: Leibe, B., Matas, J., Sebe, N., Welling, M. (eds.) ECCV 2016. LNCS, vol. 9908, pp. 630–645. Springer, Cham (2016). https://doi.org/10.1007/978-3-319-46493-0_38

Brain Tumor Segmentation Using a 3D FCN with Multi-scale Loss

Andrew Jesson$^{(\boxtimes)}$ and Tal Arbel$^{(\boxtimes)}$

McGill University, Montreal, Qc, Canada
{ajesson,arbel}@cim.mcgill.ca,
http://www.cim.mcgill.ca/~arbel

Abstract. In this work, we use a 3D Fully Connected Network (FCN) architecture for brain tumor segmentation. Our method includes a multi-scale loss function on predictions given at each resolution of the FCN. Using this approach, the higher resolution features can be combined with the initial segmentation at a lower resolution so that the FCN models context in both the image and label domains. The model is trained using a multi-scale loss function and a curriculum on sample weights is employed to address class imbalance. We achieved competitive results during the testing phase of the BraTS 2017 Challenge for segmentation with Dice scores of 0.710, 0.860, and 0.783 for enhancing tumor, whole tumor, and tumor core, respectively.

1 Introduction

In this paper, we present a 3D fully connected network with multi-scale loss for the segmentation of brain tumours. Our framework was submitted to the 2017 MICCAI Brain Tumor Segmentation (BraTS) Challenge [1–3,9]. The 2017 BraTS Challenge is comprised of two tasks: segmentation of high and low grade glioma in multi-channel MRI, and the prediction of patient survival time.

Brain tumor segmentation is a challenging task due, primarily, to three sources of variability across patient images: (1) Variability across size, shape, and texture of gliomas and surrounding edema, (2) variability in normal brain anatomy, and (3) variability in intensity range and contrast in qualitative MR imaging modalities. Additionally, the proportion of positive tumor classes to normal brain anatomy is very low, resulting in extreme class imbalance. Successful methods tackling this problem must then model local and global context in the raw imaging data, account for local and global interactions between classes, and address the difficulties arising from class imbalance.

Popular approaches to brain tumour segmentation include probabilistic graphical models [9,11], classical machine learning [9], and deep learning [4,6].

This work was supported by a Canadian Natural Science and Engineering Research Council Collaborative Research and Development Grant (CRDPJ 505357-16) and Synaptive Medical. We gratefully acknowledge the support of NVIDIA Corporation for the donation of the Titan X Pascal GPU used for this research.

Probabilistic graphical models address the challenges by modelling the statistical distributions of image intensities and textures over the tumor classes, while potentially also incorporating atlas derived spatial prior probability maps for normal brain structures [11]. Incorporation of pixel and structure level Markov Random Field (MRF) modelling has also been used to capture local and global interactions between classes [11]. Machine learning techniques capture local and global context using features derived from hand crafted filters, which are then used as input to Random Forrest or Support Vector Machine models for pixel wise classification [9].

Deep learning approaches to brain tumor segmentation have been explored, through the use of Fully Convolutional Networks (FCNs) [8] or UNets [10]. Fully Convolutional Networks have shown to be effective solutions for semantic segmentation in both natural [8] and medical images [4,6,10]. This is due to their ability to learn and combine meaningful multi-scale features for pixel classification. Furthermore, these models do not generally require extensive data preprocessing to give state of the art results [6]. In this manner, FCNs address the problem of modelling context in the imaging domain as well as, indirectly, the problems arising from image intensity and contrast variability in MRI. One limitation of FCNs is that they do not explicitly model context in the label domain. This limitation has been addressed by cascading an FCN with a graphical model such as a CRF [6]. This approach has been shown to improve the results of FCNs applied to the problem of stroke lesion segmentation [6], but generally requires a two stage model. Incorporating both an FCN and a CRF into a single, end-to-end model is still an open research area.

In this work, we present a 3D FCN architecture for brain tumor segmentation. Our method includes a multi-scale loss function on predictions given at each resolution of the FCN. In this way, the higher resolution features can be combined with the initial segmentation at a lower resolution so that the FCN models context in both the image and label domains. The model is trained using a multi-scale loss function and a curriculum on sample weights is employed to address class imbalance. We achieved competitive results during the testing phase for segmentation with Dice scores of 0.710, 0.860, and 0.783 for enhancing tumor, whole tumor, and tumor core, respectively.

2 Method

We now describe the FCN framework for brain tumour segmentation. The choice of method is informed by its capacity to address the four major challenges in brain tumor segmentation, namely: modelling context in the image domain, modelling context in the label domain, addressing the qualitative nature of MRI, and addressing the class imbalance persistent in medical imaging tasks.

We address the issue of modelling context in both the image domain and label domain by introducing prediction layers with softmax non-linearity at each spatial resolution of the FCN. These intermediate prediction layers are enforced to represent label domain information by introducing loss objectives with respect to down-sampled truth segmentation images. The intermediate predictions are

then concatenated with corresponding feature maps from the upstream path of
the FCN. Additional convolutional layers in the downstream path of the FCN
are then able to extract features representing context in the joint image and
label domains.

Fully Convolutional Networks are trained "online," which allows for the
employment of a learning curriculum to address the class imbalance problem
[5]. Here we use pixel-wise sample weighting so that each training example will
contribute to the loss based on the frequency of occurrence for its class. This
forces the model to learn features for under represented classes that otherwise
would have little influence on the objective function. The class weights are then
decayed at each training iteration until all samples are equally weighted.

2.1 Model Architecture

The model architecture is shown in Fig. 1. White boxes indicate model inputs,
here a multi-channel MR image. Red boxes indicate model outputs. In this case
confidence maps for each class to be segmented. Blue boxes indicate feature
maps. Feature maps are extracted using learned 3D convolution operations. Each
box contains the number of features and size of feature map if applicable. Arrows
indicate operations. The color code for each operation is shown in the figure.

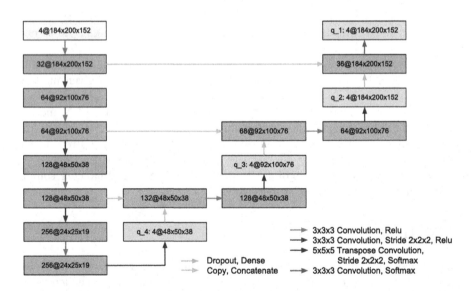

Fig. 1. Architecture of model.

2.2 Loss Function

Here we describe the objective functions that are optimized during training.
Let a given training data set have N pixels, truth segmentation distributions
$\mathbf{p} = \{p_1...p_M\}$ at M resolutions for K classes. Further, let the model produce

segmentation maps $\mathbf{q} = \{q_1...q_M\}$ at M resolutions. Finally to each segmentation class corresponds a weight w_k and the regression target has a corresponding weight w_t The objective function for segmentation when using categorical cross entropy is then:

$$\mathcal{L}_S = -\sum_{i=1}^{M}\sum_{j=1}^{N}\sum_{l=1}^{K} w_k \times p_{i,j,k} \times \ln(q_{i,j,k}). \tag{1}$$

2.3 Curriculum Sample Weighting

The sample weights, $\mathbf{w} = \{w_1...w_K\}$ and w_t are decayed over each epoch n according to the following curriculum:

$$w_\star(n) = \frac{1}{f_\star} \times r^n + 1, \tag{2}$$

where $f_\star$ is the frequency of occurrence of a given target over the training set and r is a rate parameter on $(0, 1)$. Notice that the weights converge to 1 as the number of epochs grows large ensuring that all samples receive an equal weight at the later training stages.

3 Experiments and Results

3.1 Data

BraTS 2017 Training Set. The BraTS 2017 training data set is comprised of 210 high-grade and 75 low-grade glioma patient data sets. Each data set contains a T1, T1 post contrast (T1c), T2, and FLAIR MR image, along with an expert tumor segmentation. Each brain tumor is segmented into 3 classes: edema, necrotic/non-enhancing core, and enhancing tumor core. Survival time in days and age in years is provided for 164 of the high-grade data sets [1–3,9].

BraTS 2017 Validation Set. The BraTS 2017 validation data set is comprised of 46 patient data sets. Each data set contains a T1, T1 post contrast (T1c), T2, and FLAIR MR image. No expert tumor segmentation masks are provided and the grade of each glioma is not specified [1–3,9].

BraTS 2017 Testing Set. The BraTS 2017 testing data set is comprised of 146 patient data sets. Each data set contains a T1, T1 post contrast (T1c), T2, and FLAIR MR image. No expert tumor segmentation masks are provided and the grade of each glioma is not specified [1–3,9].

3.2   Pre-processing

The challenge MRI data have been skull stripped and co-registered by the organizers [1–3,9]. We have done minimal additional preprocessing. Namely, we standardize the intensities of each image using the mean and standard deviation over the masked region of a given MR image, and the images are cropped to $184 \times 200 \times 152$.

3.3   5-Fold Cross Validation

We employ 5-fold cross validation on the training set for hyper-parameter optimization. The BraTS 2017 training set is randomly split into five folds with 57 patient data sets each. For each test fold a model is trained on three and validated on one of the remaining folds.

Parameters. We optimize the loss function in Eq. 1 using Adam [7] with a learning rate of 0.0002 and batch size of 1. The decay rate r in Eq. 2 is set to 0.95. The initial weights in Eq. 2 are set to $[1, 210, 90, 280]$ based on the inverse pixel-wise frequency of occurrence in the training set for background, tumor core, edema, and enhancing tumor, respectively. We regularize the model using data augmentation, where at each training iteration a random affine transformation is applied to the image, segmentation mask, and sample weights. Random rotation and shear angles in degrees are drawn independently from a unit normal distribution. Random scales for each spatial dimension are drawn independently from $\mathcal{N}\left(1, \left(\frac{1}{15}\right)^2\right)$. Images are also randomly flipped left to right. Truth segmentation images are then linearly down-sampled to the resolutions shown in Fig. 1 for the intermediate prediction loss functions.

Learning Curves. Figure 2 shows an example of the evolution of the dice scores for tumor core, enhancing tumor, and whole tumor for one of the 5-fold cross

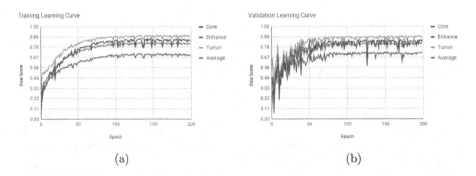

(a)   (b)

Fig. 2. Tracking dice scores during training. In these two plots we show the training curves for one of the five cross-validation experiments. Figure 2a shows the dice scores for training. Figure 2b shows the dice scores for validation.

validation experiments. We see that the curriculum results in stable training and that the model does not overfit.

3.4   Quantitative Results

Tables 1 and 2 show the results for the challenge metrics on the training and validation data sets, respectively. A visual comparison of these results between the training and validation sets is shown in Fig. 3. We can see consistent performance on both the training and validation data, which indicates that this model generalizes well to unseen examples. Table 3 shows the challenge testing set results. These are comparable to those for training and validation. Notice a large difference between the Hausdorf distance metrics between the testing and validation sets. Given the large discrepancy between the median and mean values on the testing set, it is likely that this is due to a few cases only.

Table 1. Challenge Metric Statistics: 5-Fold Cross-Validation on BraTS 2017 Training Set. Results are specified for enhancing tumor (ET), whole tumor (WT), and tumor core (TC)

	Dice			Sensitivity			Specificity			Hausdorf-95		
	ET	WT	TC	ET	WT	TC	ET	WT	TC	ET	WT	TC
Mean	0.682	0.886	0.789	0.750	0.878	0.782	0.997	0.994	0.996	6.58	7.11	8.11
StdDev	0.285	0.077	0.213	0.248	0.114	0.222	0.003	0.006	0.007	10.3	10.5	10.4
Median	0.789	0.909	0.877	0.847	0.916	0.868	0.998	0.996	0.998	2.83	3.61	4.12
25quantile	0.638	0.865	0.734	0.678	0.845	0.710	0.997	0.993	0.997	2.00	2.24	2.24
75quantile	0.863	0.937	0.923	0.915	0.953	0.924	0.999	0.998	0.999	5.66	6.71	9.38

Table 2. Challenge Metric Statistics: BraTS 2017 Validation Set. Results are specified for enhancing tumor (ET), whole tumor (WT), and tumor core (TC)

	Dice			Sensitivity			Specificity			Hausdorf-95		
	ET	WT	TC	ET	WT	TC	ET	WT	TC	ET	WT	TC
Mean	0.713	0.899	0.751	0.732	0.904	0.720	0.998	0.995	0.998	6.98	4.16	8.65
StdDev	0.291	0.070	0.240	0.288	0.102	0.259	0.003	0.004	0.003	12.1	3.37	9.35
Median	0.844	0.908	0.820	0.834	0.939	0.839	0.999	0.996	0.999	3.00	3.08	5.65
25quantile	0.650	0.891	0.685	0.676	0.902	0.558	0.998	0.992	0.998	2.00	2.24	2.24
75quantile	0.891	0.947	0.935	0.905	0.962	0.924	0.999	0.998	0.999	4.24	5.26	11.7

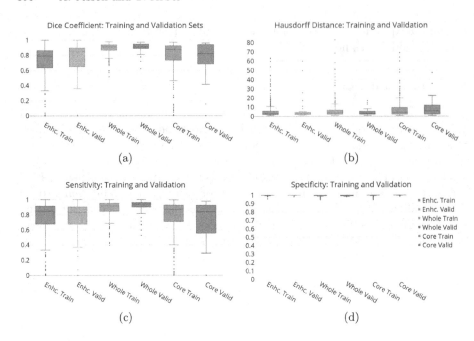

Fig. 3. Box plots of challenge metrics for the BraTS 2017 Training and BraTS 2017 Validation data sets. Results are shown in pairs for each data set and are given for enhancing tumor (enhc.), whole tumor, and tumor core.

Table 3. Challenge Metric Statistics: BraTS 2017 Testing Set. Results are specified for enhancing tumor (ET), whole tumor (WT), and tumor core (TC)

	Dice			Hausdorf-95		
	ET	WT	TC	ET	WT	TC
Mean	0.710	0.860	0.783	27.8	6.33	16.7
StdDev	0.274	0.159	0.243	89.5	9.44	60.7
Median	0.794	0.910	0.888	2.24	3.16	3.61
25quantile	0.667	0.851	0.760	1.73	2.24	2.24
75quantile	0.883	0.940	0.929	4.79	5.31	8.94

3.5   Qualitative Results

Figure 4 shows example segmentation masks on predicted high-grade test cases from the 5-fold cross validation experiment. Figure 5 shows example segmentation masks on predicted low-grade test cases from the 5-fold cross validation experiment. In both cases we see segmentation results consistent with the provided ground truth images. Furthermore, we see that the model has learned to

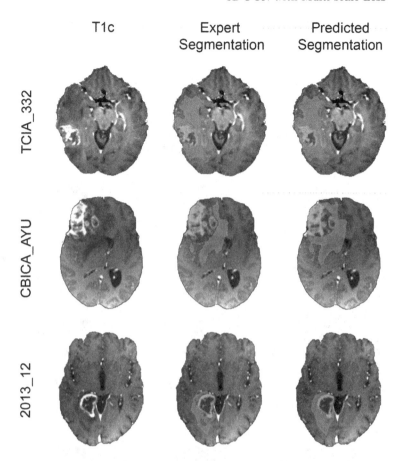

Fig. 4. Examples of high-grade glioma segmentation results for BraTS 2017 Training Data [1–3,9] 5-fold cross-validation experiment. Segmentation images are overlaid on preprocessed T1c image. Each row is an axial slice taken from a different patient. The green label is edema, the red label is non-enhancing or necrotic tumor core, and the yellow label is enhancing tumor core. (Color figure online)

model context well by noticing that normal enhancements in the T1c images are not predicted as enhancing tumor. This holds even when those enhancements are adjacent to the predicted tumor.

Figure 6 shows example segmentation masks on predicted cases from the BraTS 2017 validation data. No ground truth masks are provided with this data. It appears as though each prediction is reasonable.

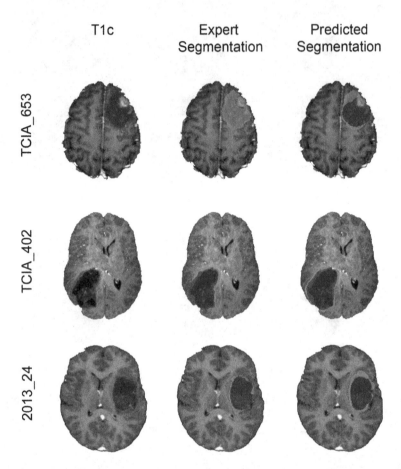

Fig. 5. Examples of low-grade glioma segmentation results for BraTS 2017 Training Data [1–3,9] 5-fold cross-validation experiment. Segmentation images are overlaid on preprocessed T1c images. Each row is an axial slice taken from different patients. The green label is edema, the red label is non-enhancing or necrotic tumor core, and the yellow label is enhancing tumor core. (Color figure online)

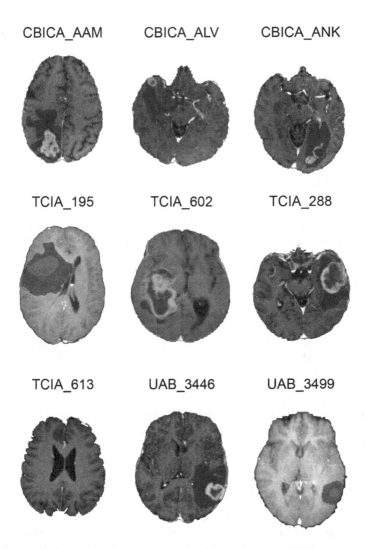

Fig. 6. Examples of segmentation results from BraTS 2017 Validation Data [1–3,9]. Segmentation images are overlaid on unprocessed T1c images. Each image is an axial slice taken from different patients. The green label is edema, the red label is non-enhancing or necrotic tumor core, and the yellow label is enhancing tumor core. (Color figure online)

4   Conclusion

In this work, we showed how a multi-task, 3D FCN architecture can be successfully developed for the context of brain tumor segmentation. Our multi-scale network combines higher resolution features with the lower level segmentation results, permitting the FCN to model context in both the image and label domains. This architecture includes a multi-scale loss function on classifications given at each resolution of the segmentation FCN. The model is trained using a curriculum on sample weights to address class imbalance, showing competitive results for brain tumor segmentation.

References

1. Bakas, S., Akbari, H., et al.: Segmentation labels and radiomic features for the pre-operative scans of the TCGA-GBM collection. https://doi.org/10.7937/K9/TCIA.2017.KLXWJJ1Q (2017)
2. Bakas, S., Akbari, H., et al.: Segmentation labels and radiomic features for the pre-operative scans of the TCGA-GBM collection. https://doi.org/10.7937/K9/TCIA.2017.GJQ7R0EF (2017)
3. Bakas, S., Akbari, H., et al.: Advancing the cancer genome atlas glioma MRI collections with expert segmentation labels and radiomic features. Nat. Sci. Data **4**, 170117 (2017)
4. Havaei, M., Davy, A., et al.: Brain tumor segmentation with deep neural networks. Med. Image Anal. **35**, 18–31 (2017)
5. Jesson, A., Guizard, N., Ghalehjegh, S.H., Goblot, D., Soudan, F., Chapados, N.: CASED: curriculum adaptive sampling for extreme data imbalance. In: Descoteaux, M., Maier-Hein, L., Franz, A., Jannin, P., Collins, D.L., Duchesne, S. (eds.) MICCAI 2017. LNCS, vol. 10435, pp. 639–646. Springer, Cham (2017). https://doi.org/10.1007/978-3-319-66179-7_73
6. Kamnitsas, K., Ledig, C., et al.: Efficient multi-scale 3D CNN with fully connected CRF for accurate brain lesion segmentation. Med. Image Anal. **36**, 61–78 (2017)
7. Kingma, D., Ba, J.: Adam: a method for stochastic optimization. arXiv preprint arXiv:1412.6980 (2014)
8. Long, J., Shelhamer, E., et al.: Fully convolutional networks for semantic segmentation. In: Proceedings of CVPR, pp. 3431–3440 (2015)
9. Menze, B.H., Jakab, A., et al.: The multimodal brain tumor image segmentation benchmark (BRATS). Trans. MI **34**(10), 1993–2024 (2015)
10. Ronneberger, O., Fischer, P., Brox, T.: U-Net: convolutional networks for biomedical image segmentation. In: Navab, N., Hornegger, J., Wells, W.M., Frangi, A.F. (eds.) MICCAI 2015. LNCS, vol. 9351, pp. 234–241. Springer, Cham (2015). https://doi.org/10.1007/978-3-319-24574-4_28
11. Subbanna, N.K., Precup, D., Collins, D.L., Arbel, T.: Hierarchical probabilistic gabor and MRF segmentation of brain tumours in MRI volumes. In: Mori, K., Sakuma, I., Sato, Y., Barillot, C., Navab, N. (eds.) MICCAI 2013. LNCS, vol. 8149, pp. 751–758. Springer, Heidelberg (2013). https://doi.org/10.1007/978-3-642-40811-3_94

Brain Tumor Segmentation Using a Multi-path CNN Based Method

Sara Sedlar[⊠]

22 000 Sremska, Mitrovica, Serbia
https://github.com/Sara04/BRATS

Abstract. In this paper an automatic brain tumor segmentation approach based on a multi-path Convolutional Neural Network (CNN) is presented. Proposition of the method was motivated by the success of multi-
path CNNs, *DeepMedic*[1] and the method presented in [2], where the
local and contextual pieces of information for segmentation were obtained
from multi-scale regions. In addition to that, the method exploits the fact
that very often tumor introduces high asymmetry to the brain. In order
to help model in distinguishing between brain lesions and healthy brain
structures such as sulci, gyri and ventricles, the model is provided with
spatial information, as well. The model's training and hyper-parameter
tuning were performed on the BraTS 2017 training dataset, model's validation was done on the BraTS 2017 validation dataset and the final
results are reported on the BraTS 2017 testing dataset. The average Dice
scores obtained on the testing dataset are 0.6049, 0.8436 and 0.6938 for
enhancing tumor, whole tumor and tumor core, respectively.

Keywords: Brain tumor · Tumor segmentation · CNN segmentation

1 Introduction

In a large number of epidemiology reviews, gathered statistics on cancer incidence and mortality, covering varying periods of previous few decades, were
published [3–23]. Due to increasing availability of imaging medical devices and
improvement of medical care, the statistics on central nervous system (CNS)
tumor incidence and mortality are nowadays available worldwide [9–23]. However, given the geographical region and period they are covering, some of those
results should be taken with reservation. Percentages of estimated brain and
other CNS cancer incidence and mortality, with respect to all cancers, in 2012
for the world's adult population were 1.8% and 2.3%, respectively [8]. In children and adolescents, those tumors are among leading cancer related diseases
[19–23]. The most common histological type of primary malignant brain tumors
is glioma (which can also affect other parts of CNS) [9–11,19].

During the last few decades, in addition to the constant improvement of
magnetic resonance imaging (MRI) techniques and development of new imaging modalities [24–30], a significant effort was put in the domain of automatic

brain image analysis. Due to very pessimistic survival rates of patients with gliomas [10] and complexity of its evaluation and treatment, this field of brain tumor analysis attracted lots of attention in medical community, among scientists and engineers.

Tumor segmentation is an important step in the evaluation of tumor's state and its monitoring. In addition, it opens a possibility of tumor's future behavior prediction. All the information about tumor's current state and its changes over time are crucial for a successful therapy and surgery planning. As manual tumor segmentation is time consuming and it is prone to the intra and inter rater variability [31], automatic tumor analysis is in demand.

To address this challenge, Multimodal Brain Tumor Image Segmentation (BraTS) Benchmark has been successfully organized in conjunction with Medical Image Computing and Computer Assisted Interventions (MICCAI) Conference since 2012 [32]. By providing multi-modal MRI datasets [32–35] and evaluation platform, this benchmark enabled researchers world wide to train, evaluate and compare their automatic and semi-automatic brain tumor segmentation methods in a fair manner.

In the last two decades, a great number of generative and discriminative methods for brain tumor segmentation was proposed, either as help to manual segmentation or in combination with manual detection (semi-automatic) or as fully automatic tool.

The most prominent generative approaches rely on atlas based segmentation. In the method presented in [36], Parzen windows were used for the estimation of probability density functions (PDEs) of healthy and tumorous (abnormal) brain regions and spatial priors of healthy brain atlas together with intensity features were used for the estimation of posterior probabilities in an iterative manner. Contrary to the [36], in [37], PDEs were estimated using Gaussian Mixture Model, a parametric model. In addition, the proposed segmentation model incorporated prior on tumor's shape using convolutional restricted Boltzmann machines. Generative channel-specific approach presented in [38] addressed the issue of different boundary appearance in different MRI modalities and for modeling of tumor's state it used latent probabilistic atlas whose parameters were iteratively estimated using expectation-maximization (EM) algorithm. An approach proposed in [39] relied on incorporation of information about tumor's growth that imitate biophysical processes occurring in the tumorous tissue and using EM algorithm iteratively estimated the parameters of tumor's growth model and posterior probabilities of tumor's substructures.

One quite popular group of discriminative algorithms for brain tumor segmentation was based on first order texture features (mean, variance, skewness, kurtosis, etc.) and hand-crafted descriptors in combination with classifiers such as Support Vector Machine (SVM) and random forests [40–44]. Another group of methods that attracted attention of engineers is group of active contour models [45–47]. In the last few years, a large percentage of the proposed discriminative methods is based on deep learning approaches [1,2,48–51]. In [48], a small multimodal voxel-wise 2D CNN model that achieved promising results on HGG cases was proposed. Instead of voxel-wise prediction, in [49], they proposed a CNN method that classifies input local multi-modal patches into one of the classes of a created label patch dictionary. In addition to being very efficient, this method performs local spatial regularization, as well. The methods that exploit both local and contextual pieces of information via multi-path CNNs were proposed in [1,2]. The latest deep learning architecture that has demonstrated high potential in the domain of biomedical image segmentation is U-Net convolutional network [52]. In addition to the information extraction from multiple scales, it is trained to perform dense inference, what, as in [49], contributes to the spatial regularization and high time efficiency. The successful employment of U-nets in brain tumor segmentation was demonstrated in [50,51].

The reminder of this article is structured as follow. Information about databases and their usage in the experiments is provided in the Sect. 2. Detailed description of the segmentation method is given in the Sect. 3. Section 4 contains implementation details. The final results and analyses of the model's inputs' contributions are presented in the Sect. 5. Conclusions and future work are given in the Sect. 6.

2 Database

Data provided for the BraTS Challenge 2017 was composed of training, validation and test datasets. The training dataset contains MRI data for 285 subjects, 210 with high grade glioma (HGG) and 75 with low grade glioma (LGG). Number of patients in the validation and test datasets are 46 and 146, respectively, without information on tumor's grade. For each subject, four MRI modalities are provided, namely T1-weighted (T1), post-contrast T1-weighted (T1ce), T2-weighted (T2) and T2 Fluid Attenuated Inversion Recovery (FLAIR). In addition, for the training dataset ground truths for four classes are given, namely necrotic and non-enhancing tumor (NCR and NET, label 1), peritumoral edema (ED, label 2), enhancing tumor (ET, label4) and everything else (label 0). All scans are provided in a pre-processed form, where the pre-processing was composed of co-registration to the same anatomical template, interpolation to the same resolution and skull-stripping [33].

In the experiments presented in this paper, 80% of the training dataset (168 HGG and 60 LGG cases) was used for the multi-path CNN's core training, while 20% (42 HGG and 15 LGG cases) was used for tuning of CNN hyper-parameters and post-processing. Algorithm was verified on the validation dataset, and the real world scenario results are reported on the test dataset.

3 Method

Proposition of the method was motivated by the success of multi-path CNNs, *DeepMedic*[1] and the method presented in [2], where the local and contextual pieces of information for segmentation were obtained from multi-scale patches centered around voxel that is being examined. The patches are extracted from each of the available MRI modalities. As suggested in [1,2], given a voxel, the large patches provide information about the voxel's broader context, while the local region patches contain information about close neighborhood's details. In addition to the information extracted from the local and broader voxel's neighborhood, the model exploits the information about brain's asymmetry, that is very often produced by tumor. To achieve this, for a given voxel, apart from the mentioned multi-scale patches, model is provided with the large patches extracted around the voxel at the position mirrored with respect to the sagittal plane. In order to help model in distinguishing between brain lesions and healthy brain structures such as sulci, gyri and ventricles, spatial information is fed to the model, as well. Spatial information of a voxel is represented as its position along sagittal, axial and coronal axes with respect to the brain's center. In the Fig. 1, extraction of local and large region patches (contextual, symmetry and spatial pieces of information) in multi-path CNN's toolchain is illustrated. One path takes as input local patches of four MRI modalities (illustrated with green color in the Fig. 1). Set of patches fed to the other path is composed of contextual and mirrored patches of four MRI modalities and three distance map patches (illustrated with red color in the Fig. 1).

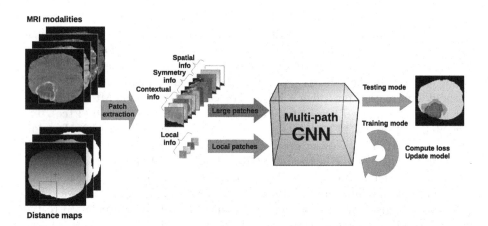

Fig. 1. Illustration of the local and large region patches in multi-path CNN's toolchain (Color figure online)

3.1   Pre-processing

Each scan is pre-processed as follows. All non-zero voxels of a scan are normalized by subtraction of mean value and division by standard deviation value of all non-zero scan's voxels. After that, in order to reduce the effect of model's over-fitting during CNN training phase, voxels are clipped to predefined bounds.

3.2 Model's Architecture

For each of the two paths, first part of the sub-model is composed of three convolutional layers. Each convolutional layer is followed by Rectified Linear Unit (ReLU) activation and along large region path, it is followed by max-pool operation. After the convolutional layers, at each path, there are two fully-connected (FC) layers with ReLU at the output. Since those FC layers contain large number of trainable parameters and with that, they are prone to over-fitting during the training phase, drop-out regularization was used [53] to address this issue. At the end, local and contextual feature vectors are merged by simple concatenation and are further processed by two additional small FC layers. First one followed by ReLU and the second one by Soft-max function in order to obtain class probabilities as the model's output. Entire model is illustrated in the Fig. 2.

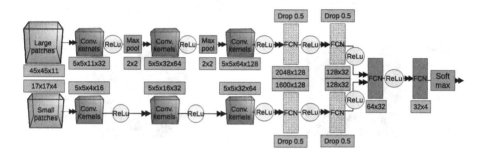

Fig. 2. Illustration of the multi-path CNN architecture

3.3 Model's Training

Since the segmentation task is very challenging within tumor (between different tumor stadiums) and within tumor's proximity, during training phase it is split into two (tumorous vs. non-tumorous) and four class segmentation problems (non-tumorous in tumor's proximity vs. NCR & NET vs. ED vs. ET), as illustrated in the Fig. 3. Motivation for this training approach is helping model to learn relevant features, or in other words avoiding learning features for classification into four classes if classification into two classes is simpler and enough. In order to achieve this, in each training iteration two batches are fed to the model. One containing patches extracted around voxels belonging to the four classes and the other one with patches from tumorous and non-tumorous classes, in both cases with equal class occurrences within a batch. Final loss function is represented as a linear combination of the two log-losses (Eq. 1).

$$loss = \alpha \cdot \frac{1}{N_2} \cdot \sum_{i=1}^{N_2} \sum_{c=1}^{2} z_{i,c}^{gt} \cdot \log q_{i,c} + \beta \cdot \frac{1}{N_4} \cdot \sum_{i=1}^{N_4} \sum_{c=1}^{4} y_{i,c}^{gt} \cdot \log p_{i,c} \qquad (1)$$

where N_2 and N_4 are the numbers of samples in the batches, $z_{i,c}^{gt}$ and $y_{i,c}^{gt}$ binary ground truth labels of the sample i with respect to the class c (where 1 indicates belonging to the class c and 0 not belonging), $q_{i,c}$ and $p_{i,c}$ output probabilities of the sample i belonging to the class c, for two and four class segmentation problems, respectively.

Regions of the MRI volumes that belong to the head's exterior were not considered neither during the training, nor during the model's test mode.

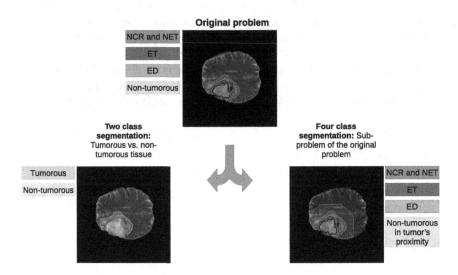

Fig. 3. Illustration of the segmentation problem split during the training mode

In addition to the drop-out [53], *DisturbLabel* regularization on loss layer was applied [54]. According to this approach, for a certain percentage of randomly selected training samples from a batch, ground truth labels were set to the values randomly selected from set of all labels.

3.4   Post-processing

Final segmentation probabilities are post-processed by thresholding, analysis of connected components and by applying mathematical morphological 3D binary closing operator [55].

4   Implementation Details

The algorithm implementation was done in Python programming language. For the basic operations, such as data reading and writing, pre- and post-processing, meta-data computations, batch extractions, NiBabel [56], scipy [57] and numpy [58] libraries were used. Segmentation model was created and trained with tensorflow [59]. The hardware employed was composed of nVidia's GeForce GTX 980 Ti (6 GB) GPU and Intel Core i7-6700K CPU @ 4.00 GHz (32 GB).

Training lasted approximately 20 h and segmentation of MRI scans for one patient lasts around 5.7 min. Total model's size is 3.6 MB.

Each volume was pre-processed with mean-std normalization (non-zero voxels) and clipped in range of $[-2.0, 2.0]$. Size of the large region (contextual, mirrored and distance map) patches is 45×45 and of local ones 17×17.

Size of the convolutional kernels was 5×5, and all convolutional and FC weights were initialized using Xavier initialization [60].

Training data was augmented by volume mirroring, jittering of MRI modality patches with values drawn from a normal distribution with standard deviation of 0.2 and by random shifting of mirrored patches within axial plane by $n <= 5$ pixels.

During the first phase of the training ($iteration <= 9000$) in each iteration 5 subjects were selected, and for each class 50 samples were extracted (both for two and four class segmentation problems). Learning rate was 10^{-4}. In the second phase ($9000 < iteration <= 10500$) number of subjects was increased to 10, while the number of samples was decreased to 25 per class. In the last, third phase ($10500 < iteration <= 13000$) learning rate was decreased to 10^{-5}. During entire training process, *drop-out* [53] probability of four FC layers (see Fig. 2) was 0.5. Percentages in *DisturbLabel* [54] regularization were 20% and 40% for two and four class segmentation problems, respectively. Weights α and β used to compute final loss were 0.25 and 0.75. Adam optimization algorithm was used to calculate weight updates [61].

In order to facilitate training process some meta-data were computed before training such as normalization parameters, brain masks and tumor distance maps.

In the post-processing stage, all the voxels that are classified as tumorous were examined according to the two and four class segmentation problems. If their probability of being tumorous or being part of one of the tumor's stadiums is below 0.915 and 0.4, respectively, they are re-classified as healthy. Once the volume is thresholded according to those criteria, connected components were analyzed. If their size is below 3000 voxels, they are re-classified as healthy. At the end, mathematical morphological closing 3D binary operator with cubic structuring element of size $3 \times 3 \times 3$ was applied.

5   Results and Analyses

In the Table 1, results obtained on BraTS 2017 training subset, validation and testing datasets, with described tumor segmentation approach, are compared in terms of average Dice scores (DSs) and average 95% Hausdorff distances (95% HDs) for the enhancing tumor (ET), tumor core (TC; union of NCR&NET and ET) and whole tumor (WT; union of NCR&NET, ET and ED). As it can be seen, the average DSs of training subset and validation dataset are consistent, while there is a difference in 95% HDs for the ET and TC. This difference might indicate over-tuning of hyper-parameters to the training subset. The average DSs obtained on the testing dataset are 3.4% and 1.9% lower for WT and TC with respect to the validation dataset and the average 95% HD for WT is slightly better. However, the average DS for ET is significantly worse (7.3%), as well as the average 95% HDs for ET and TC. Since all the hyper-parameter tunings were performed on the training subset and validation data was submitted just for verification, parameters' over-fitting to the validation dataset could be excluded from the reasons of this performance drop. In the Table 1, comparison between HGG and LGG training cases is available, as well. It can be noticed, that segmentation for LGG cases is significantly poorer for ET and with that for TC, as well. So, if the testing dataset contains greater percentage of LGG cases, than there is in the training and validation sets, this might be one of the reasons for the lower test performance. Another cause could be low generalization power of the model in case of data recorded with "unseen" MRI scanners or in the case of some difficult segmentation cases.

Table 1. Average DSs and 95% HDs for BraTS 2017 training subset, validation and test datasets

Dataset	Average DS			Average 95% HD		
	ET	WT	TC	ET	WT	TC
Training (57 cases)	0.6712	0.8586	0.7250	8.8823	11.2789	10.9890
Training (HGG, 42 cases)	0.7831	0.8474	0.7897	6.2443	11.0780	10.5023
Training (LGG, 15 cases)	0.3578	0.8898	0.5441	19.9621	11.8415	12.3517
Validation	0.6781	0.8774	0.7129	12.7491	11.0131	14.0002
Testing	0.6049	0.8436	0.6938	67.3361	9.9270	33.0524

In the Figs. 4 and 6 segmentation of several slices of HGG and LGG cases, respectively, is illustrated on T1ce modality, where the corresponding cases are selected from the training subset as the best ones according to the DS and 95% HD ranks. In the Figs. 5 and 7 the examples of slices are provided for the worst HGG and LGG cases. In the Figs. 4 and 6, we can see that the segmentation can be quite successful, independent on lesion's position and size, however Figs. 5 and 7 indicate that it is still challenging in the situations when the lesion is mostly composed of edema and when it is very rugged.

Table 2. Average DSs and 95% HDs for a subset of BraTS 2017 training dataset, obtained with multi-path CNN without post-processing

Input	Average DS			Average 95% HD		
	ET	WT	TC	ET	WT	TC
Training (57 cases)	0.6261	0.7510	0.6870	27.3364	36.9105	30.0112
Training (HGG, 42 cases)	0.7304	0.7336	0.7423	24.3643	36.1690	32.4710
Training (LGG, 15 cases)	0.3340	0.7995	0.5323	39.8196	38.9867	23.1235

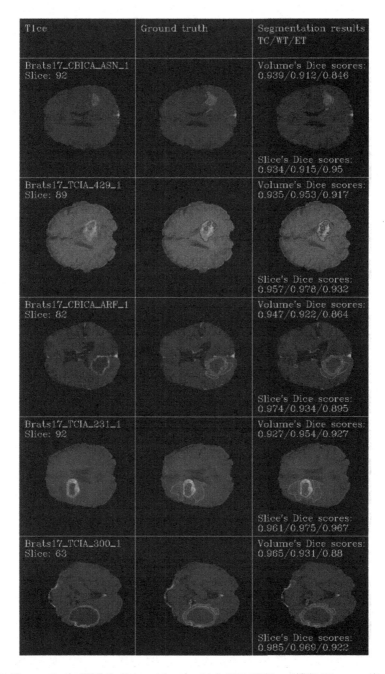

Fig. 4. Illustration of HGG slices with very high ET, WT and TC Dice scores. Corresponding cases are selected as the best ones according to the DS and 95% HD ranks. They belong to the subset of BraTS 2017 training data used for validation during CNN training process and for tuning of post-processing parameters. ***Red*** - NCR&NET, ***Blue*** - ET, ***Green*** - ED (Color figure online)

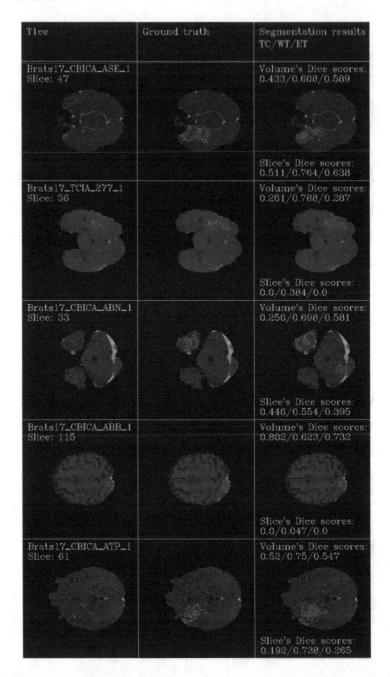

Fig. 5. Illustration of HGG slices with very low ET, WT and TC Dice scores. Corresponding cases are selected as the worst ones according to the DS and 95% HD ranks. They belong to the subset of BraTS 2017 training data used for validation during CNN training process and for tuning of post-processing parameters. *Red* - NCR&NET, *Blue* - ET, *Green* - ED (Color figure online)

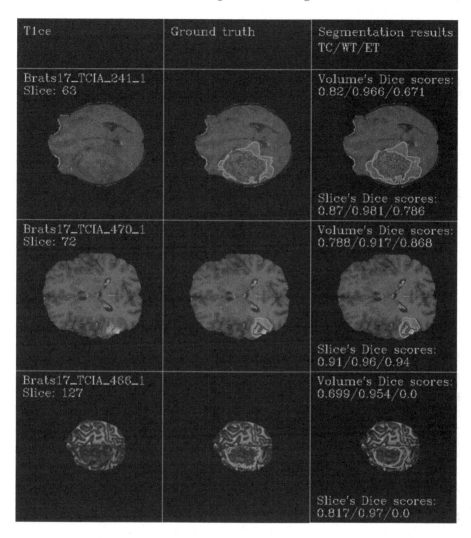

Fig. 6. Illustration of LGG slices with very high ET, WT and TC Dice scores. Corresponding cases are selected as the best ones according to the DS and 95% HD ranks. They belong to the subset of BraTS 2017 training data used for validation during CNN training process and for tuning of post-processing parameters. **Red** - NCR&NET, **Blue** - ET, **Green** - ED (Color figure online)

Results without post-processing. In the Table 2, results are provided for the tumor segmentation without post-processing. By comparing the average 95% HDs with the results from the Table 1, it is clear that post-processing removes significant amount of false positives. While for the HGG cases, it significantly improves scores for all tumor's stadiums, in case of LGG tumors, this difference is noticeable only for the tumor's edema. In the Table 3, confusion matrix

414   S. Sedlar

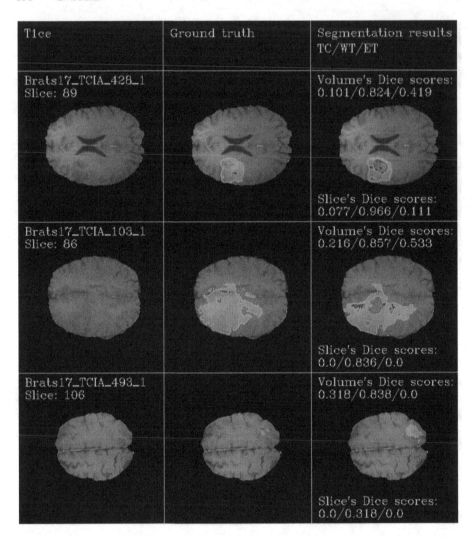

Fig. 7. Illustration of LGG slices with very low ET, WT and TC Dice scores. Corresponding cases are selected as the worst ones according to the DS and 95% HD ranks. They belong to the subset of BraTS 2017 training data used for validation during CNN training process and for tuning of post-processing parameters. *Red* - NCR&NET, *Blue* - ET, *Green* - ED (Color figure online)

and positive predictive values (PPV) are provided for the segmentation without post-processing. For the computation of all confusion matrices and PPVs in the paper only brain region is considered (not head's exterior). It can be noticed that the misclassification of tumorous tissue mostly occurs between different tumor's substructures and that the falsely classified non-tumorous regions are mostly classified as tumor's edema.

Table 3. Confusion matrix and PPVs for a subset of BraTS 2017 training dataset, obtained with multi-path CNN without post-processing

Input	Training			
Labels	0	1	2	4
0	97.23%	0.20%	2.38%	0.19%
1	1.28%	71.88%	14.54%	12.31%
2	5.05%	9.27%	82.06%	3.62%
4	1.03%	10.91%	6.20%	81.86%
PPV	99.79%	45.80%	48.09%	63.13%

5.1 Model's Inputs' Influences on Segmentation Performance

In order to analyze impact of different input's segments on the segmentation performance, parts of the input were set to Gaussian noise and the obtained results, in terms of confusion matrices, PPVs, average DSs and 95% HDs, are compared. For the sake of comparisons of the algorithm's core - multi-path CNN, post-processing stage was excluded. As the contextual patches (four MRI modalities with contextual information) are in the greatest extent responsible for the segmentation, their exclusion from the input leads to meaningless results (most of the DSs are zero).

Influence of local, mirrored and distance map patches. In the Tables 4, 5 and 6, the results are given for the experiments where the local, mirrored (symmetry) and distance map (spatial) patches were completely replaced by Gaussian noise with corresponding standard deviation and clipping. By comparing those results with ones from the Tables 2 and 3, it can be noticed that the local patches are crucial for the differentiation between NCR&NET and ET regions. In addition, they improve classification of ED. On the other side, although they help in segmentation refinement, from 95% HDs and DS of WT we can notice that they introduce lots of false positives, since some of the non-tumorous brain regions locally appear as tumorous tissue. Mirrored patches (symmetry information)

Table 4. Average DSs and 95% HDs for subset of BraTS 2017 training dataset obtained with multi-path CNN without post-processing for randomized mirrored, distance map and local patches

Input	Average DS			Average 95% HD		
	ET	WT	TC	ET	WT	TC
Local random	0.15297	0.82904	0.68564	17.3063	21.6618	22.4765
Mirrored random	0.6049	0.7289	0.6538	35.4015	46.3884	39.9674
Distance random	0.5919	0.6941	0.6467	40.6840	49.1731	47.6039

Table 5. Confusion matrix and PPVs for subset of BraTS 2017 training dataset obtained with multi-path CNN without post-processing for randomized local patches

Input	Local random			
Labels	0	1	2	4
0	99.09%	0.24%	0.62%	0.05%
1	4.15%	82.91%	9.63%	3.31%
2	23.00%	14.61%	59.73%	2.67%
4	4.39%	78.52%	5.37%	11.71%
PPV	99.06%	32.12%	67.86%	40.14%

contribute to the segmentation by decreasing false positives and misclassification of NCR&NET tissues. Distance map patches (spatial information) help by reducing misclassification of non-tumorous tissue.

Influence of different MRI modalities. In the Tables 7, 8 and 9, the results are given for the experiments where the T1, T2, T1ce and FLAIR patches (contextual, local and mirrored) were completely replaced by Gaussian noise with corresponding standard deviation and clipping. In another words, contextual, local and symmetry pieces of information, carried by a given modality, were removed. By comparing those results with ones from the Tables 2 and 3, we can notice that T1 modality reduces misclassification of non-tumorous and tumor's edema tissue into NCR&NET and ET classes. Modality T2 is important for differentiation between NCR&NET and ED and it decreases misclassification of ET regions into non-tumorous and ED regions. On the other side, it is responsible in a great extent for false positives. T1ce modality is crucial for segmentation within tumor, but it also introduces non negligible amount of false positives. Modality FLAIR is the most important one, as it is responsible for differentiation between non-tumorous and tumorous tissue (decrease of false negatives). This is mostly notable in a great misclassification of ED into non-tumorous tissue.

Table 6. Confusion matrices and PPVs for subset of BraTS 2017 training dataset obtained with multi-path CNN without post-processing for randomized mirrored and distance map patches

Input	Mirrored random				Distance random			
Labels	0	1	2	4	0	1	2	4
0	97.13%	0.25%	2.39%	0.22%	96.39%	0.32%	3.03%	0.27%
1	1.81%	66.97%	18.48%	12.74%	1.32%	70.84%	15.35%	12.48%
2	6.90%	7.17%	82.39%	3.54%	4.80%	8.93%	82.60%	3.66%
4	1.72%	9.35%	7.10%	81.83%	1.04%	10.32%	6.72%	81.93%
PPV	99.72%	42.94%	48.09%	60.06%	99.78%	41.29%	43.69%	58.01%

Table 7. Average DSs and 95% HDs for subset of BraTS 2017 training dataset obtained with multi-path CNN without post-processing for randomized T1, T2, T1ce and FLAIR patches

Input	Average DS			Average 95% HD		
	ET	WT	TC	ET	WT	TC
T1 random	0.5589	0.7513	0.6090	37.5792	39.5442	43.0214
T2 random	0.6441	0.8143	0.6490	16.8292	25.8263	22.5274
T1ce random	0.0940	0.8049	0.3993	19.8874	32.4408	20.7515
Flair random	0.5449	0.5323	0.5391	22.6974	25.8509	31.2994

Table 8. Confusion matrices and PPVs for subset of BraTS 2017 training dataset obtained with multi-path CNN without post-processing for randomized T1 and T2 patches

Input	T1 random				T2 random			
Labels	0	1	2	4	0	1	2	4
0	97.32%	0.48%	1.83%	0.38%	98.81%	0.15%	0.95%	0.08%
1	1.45%	70.47%	14.99%	13.09%	6.17%	54.17%	30.82%	8.85%
2	6.69%	13.02%	75.81%	4.48%	15.17%	5.29%	77.87%	1.67%
4	1.29%	11.84%	6.48%	80.38%	5.37%	9.95%	12.76%	71.92%
PPV	99.72%	37.52%	50.97%	53.82%	99.18%	42.52%	59.85%	73.71%

Table 9. Confusion matrices and PPVs for subset of BraTS 2017 training dataset obtained with multi-path CNN without post-processing for randomized T1ce and FLAIR patches

Input	T1ce random				Flair random			
Labels	0	1	2	4	0	1	2	4
0	98.22%	0.12%	1.58%	0.07%	99.51%	0.32%	0.09%	0.09%
1	3.05%	33.84%	47.04%	16.08%	30.42%	53.43%	3.82%	12.33%
2	8.32%	8.02%	77.84%	5.81%	71.30%	14.65%	11.69%	2.36%
4	3.38%	24.24%	62.53%	9.85%	30.02%	6.54%	1.73%	61.71%
PPV	99.62%	33.94%	47.16%	19.24%	96.88%	36.62%	61.77%	62.89%

6   Conclusions and Future Work

In this paper an approach for multi-modal brain tumor segmentation, motivated by the success of multi-path CNNs [1,2] in the previous BraTS challenges, was investigated. In addition to the contextual and local information, model was provided with spatial and information about brain's asymmetry. In order help model to learn more relevant features, the original segmentation problem was split into two and four class segmentation tasks. Although the results on training and validation subsets seemed promising, the ones obtained on testing dataset showed that generalization power of the model should be higher, especially in the case of enhancing tumor. Also, it was shown that there is a large gap in within tumor segmentation between HGG and LGG cases.

In the analysis of model's inputs' impacts on the segmentation outcome, it was shown that the model relays on contextual patches in the greatest extent, while the local patches were used for the segmentation refinement between different tumor's stadiums. Spatial and information about brain's symmetry mostly contributed by reducing false positives. Experiments demonstrated that the most informative MRI modalities for this model are T1ce and FLAIR, T1ce for the segmentation within tumor and FLAIR for the differentiation between non-tumorous and tumorous tissue.

In the future work, each stage of the segmentation tool-chain will be addressed. Different contributions of MRI modalities might indicate that each modality requires different pre-processing and that mean-std normalization with clipping removed some information important for the segmentation. Also, means of spatial and symmetry information's embedding will be further investigated. Furthermore, there is a plenty of room for experimenting with more complex and efficient CNN architectures, as well as with more appropriate loss functions for the segmentation problem. Post-processing stage can be improved by integration of relative spatial information between tumor's substructures.

References

1. Kamnitsas, K., Ledig, C., Newcombe, V.F., Simpson, J.P., Kane, A.D., Menon, D.K., Rueckert, D., Glocker, B.: Efficient multi-scale 3D CNN with fully connected CRF for accurate brain lesion segmentation. Med. Image Anal. **36**, 61–78 (2017)
2. Havaei, M., Davy, A., Warde-Farley, D., Biard, A., Courville, A., Bengio, Y., Pal, C., Jodoin, P.M., Larochelle, H.: Brain tumor segmentation with deep neural networks. Med. Image Anal. **35**, 18–31 (2017)
3. Ferlay, J., Steliarova-Foucher, E., Lortet-Tieulent, J., Rosso, S., Coebergh, J.W.W., Comber, H., Forman, D., Bray, F.: Cancer incidence and mortality patterns in europe: Estimates for 40 countries in 2012. Eur. J. Cancer **49**(6), 1374–1403 (2013). https://doi.org/10.1016/j.ejca.2012.12.027
4. Ward, E., DeSantis, C., Robbins, A., Kohler, B., Jemal, A.: Childhood and adolescent cancer statistics, 2014. CA Cancer J. Clin. **64**(2), 83–103 (2014)
5. Siegel, R.L., Miller, K.D., Jemal, A.: Cancer statistics, 2016. CA Cancer J. Clin. **66**(1), 7–30 (2016)
6. Chen, W., Zheng, R., Baade, P.D., Zhang, S., Zeng, H., Bray, F., Jemal, A., Yu, X.Q., He, J.: Cancer statistics in china, 2015. CA Cancer J. Clin. **66**(2), 115–132 (2016)
7. Miller, K.D., Siegel, R.L., Lin, C.C., Mariotto, A.B., Kramer, J.L., Rowland, J.H., Stein, K.D., Alteri, R., Jemal, A.: Cancer treatment and survivorship statistics, 2016. CA Cancer J. Clin. **66**(4), 271–289 (2016)

8. Ferlay, J., Soerjomataram, I., Dikshit, R., Eser, S., Mathers, C., Rebelo, M., Parkin, D.M., Forman, D., Bray, F.: Cancer incidence and mortality worldwide: sources, methods and major patterns in globocan 2012. Int. J. Cancer 136(5) (2015)
9. Pieros, M., Sierra, M.S., Izarzugaza, M.I., Forman, D.: Descriptive epidemiology of brain and central nervous system cancers in central and south america. Cancer Epidemiol. 44(suppl. 1), S141–S149 (2016). http://www.sciencedirect.com/science/article/pii/S1877782116300479, Supplement: Cancer in Central and South America
10. Ostrom, Q.T., Bauchet, L., Davis, F.G., Deltour, I., Fisher, J.L., Langer, C.E., Pekmezci, M., Schwartzbaum, J.A., Turner, M.C., Walsh, K.M., et al.: The epidemiology of glioma in adults: a state of the science review. Neuro-oncology 16(7), 896–913 (2014)
11. Schwartzbaum, J.A., Fisher, J.L., Aldape, K.D., Wrensch, M.: Epidemiology and molecular pathology of glioma. Nat. Rev. Neurol. 2(9), 494 (2006)
12. Jazayeri, S.B., Rahimi-Movaghar, V., Shokraneh, F., Saadat, S., Ramezani, R.: Epidemiology of primary CNS tumors in Iran: a systematic. Asian Pac. J. Cancer Prev. 14(6), 3979–3985 (2013)
13. Deltour, I., Johansen, C., Auvinen, A., Feychting, M., Klaeboe, L., Schüz, J.: Time trends in brain tumor incidence rates in Denmark, Finland, Norway, and Sweden, 1974–2003. J. Natl. Cancer Inst. 101(24), 1721–1724 (2009)
14. Trabelsi, S., Brahim, D.H.B., Ladib, M., Mama, N., Harrabi, I., Tlili, K., Yacoubi, M.T., Krifa, H., Hmissa, S., Saad, A., et al.: Glioma epidemiology in the central tunisian population. Asian Pac. J. Cancer Prev. 15(20), 8753–8757 (2014)
15. Bondy, M.L., Scheurer, M.E., Malmer, B., Barnholtz-Sloan, J.S., Davis, F.G., Il'Yasova, D., Kruchko, C., McCarthy, B.J., Rajaraman, P., Schwartzbaum, J.A., et al.: Brain tumor epidemiology: consensus from the brain tumor epidemiology consortium. Cancer 113(S7), 1953–1968 (2008)
16. Dobes, M., Shadbolt, B., Khurana, V.G., Jain, S., Smith, S.F., Smee, R., Dexter, M., Cook, R.: A multicenter study of primary brain tumor incidence in Australia (2000–2008). Neuro-oncology 13(7), 783–790 (2011)
17. de Robles, P., Fiest, K.M., Frolkis, A.D., Pringsheim, T., Atta, C., St. Germaine-Smith, C., Day, L., Lam, D., Jette, N.: The worldwide incidence and prevalence of primary brain tumors: a systematic review and meta-analysis. Neuro-oncology 17(6), 776–783 (2014)
18. Crocetti, E., Trama, A., Stiller, C., Caldarella, A., Soffietti, R., Jaal, J., Weber, D.C., Ricardi, U., Slowinski, J., Brandes, A., et al.: Epidemiology of glial and non-glial brain tumours in Europe. Eur. J. Cancer 48(10), 1532–1542 (2012)
19. Gittleman, H.R., Ostrom, Q.T., Rouse, C.D., Dowling, J.A., De Blank, P.M., Kruchko, C.A., Elder, J.B., Rosenfeld, S.S., Selman, W.R., Sloan, A.E., et al.: Trends in central nervous system tumor incidence relative to other common cancers in adults, adolescents, and children in the United States, 2000 to 2010. Cancer 121(1), 102–112 (2015)
20. Lee, C.H., Jung, K.W., Yoo, H., Park, S., Lee, S.H.: Epidemiology of primary brain and central nervous system tumors in Korea. J. Korean Neurosurg. Soc. 48(2), 145–152 (2010)
21. Ostrom, Q.T., De Blank, P.M., Kruchko, C., Petersen, C.M., Liao, P., Finlay, J.L., Stearns, D.S., Wolff, J.E., Wolinsky, Y., Letterio, J.J., et al.: Alex's lemonade stand foundation infant and childhood primary brain and central nervous system tumors diagnosed in the United States in 2007–2011. Neuro-oncology 16(suppl-10), x1–x36 (2014)

22. Papathoma, P., Thomopoulos, T.P., Karalexi, M.A., Ryzhov, A., Zborovskaya, A., Dimitrova, N., Zivkovic, S., Eser, S., Antunes, L., Sekerija, M., et al.: Childhood central nervous system tumours: incidence and time trends in 13 Southern and Eastern European cancer registries. Eur. J. Cancer **51**(11), 1444–1455 (2015)

23. Johnson, K.J., Cullen, J., Barnholtz-Sloan, J.S., Ostrom, Q.T., Langer, C.E., Turner, M.C., McKean-Cowdin, R., Fisher, J.L., Lupo, P.J., Partap, S., et al.: Childhood brain tumor epidemiology: a brain tumor epidemiology consortium review. Cancer Epidemiol. Prevent. Biomarkers, pp. cebp-0207 (2014)

24. van der Kolk, A.G., Hendrikse, J., Zwanenburg, J.J., Visser, F., Luijten, P.R.: Clinical applications of 7T MRI in the brain. Eur. J. Radiol. **82**(5), 708–718 (2013)

25. Pope, W.B., Young, J.R., Ellingson, B.M.: Advances in MRI assessment of gliomas and response to anti-vegf therapy. Curr. Neurol. Neurosci. Rep. **11**(3), 336–344 (2011)

26. Wu, D., Zhang, J.: Recent progress in magnetic resonance imaging of the embryonic and neonatal mouse brain. Front. Neuroanat. **10**, 1–8 (2016)

27. Koretsky, A.P.: New developments in magnetic resonance imaging of the brain. NeuroRx **1**(1), 155–164 (2004)

28. Mabray, M.C., Barajas, R.F., Cha, S.: Modern brain tumor imaging. Brain Tumor Res. Treat. **3**(1), 8–23 (2015)

29. Duyn, J.H.: Study of brain anatomy with high-field mri: recent progress. Magn. Reson. Imaging **28**(8), 1210–1215 (2010)

30. Villanueva-Meyer, J.E., Mabray, M.C., Cha, S.: Current clinical brain tumor imaging. Neurosurgery **81**(3), 397–415 (2017)

31. Mazzara, G.P., Velthuizen, R.P., Pearlman, J.L., Greenberg, H.M., Wagner, H.: Brain tumor target volume determination for radiation treatment planning through automated MRI segmentation. Int. J. Radiat. Oncol. Biol. Phys. **59**(1), 300–312 (2004)

32. Menze, B.H., Jakab, A., Bauer, S., Kalpathy-Cramer, J., Farahani, K., Kirby, J., Burren, Y., Porz, N., Slotboom, J., Wiest, R., et al.: The multimodal brain tumor image segmentation benchmark (brats). IEEE Trans. Med. Imaging **34**(10), 1993–2024 (2015)

33. Bakas, S., Akbari, H., Sotiras, A., Bilello, M., Rozycki, M., Kirby, J.S., Freymann, J.B., Farahani, K., Davatzikos, C.: Advancing the cancer genome atlas glioma MRI collections with expert segmentation labels and radiomic features. Sci. Data **4**, 170117 (2017)

34. Bakas, S., Akbari, H., Sotiras, A., Bilello, M., Rozycki, M., Kirby, J., Freymann, J., Farahani, K., Davatzikos, C.: Segmentation labels and radiomic features for the pre-operative scans of the TCGA-GBM collection. Cancer Imaging Arch. (2017)

35. Bakas, S., Akbari, H., Sotiras, A., Bilello, M., Rozycki, M., Kirby, J., Freymann, J., Farahani, K., Davatzikos, C.: Segmentation labels and radiomic features for the pre-operative scans of the TCGA-LGG collection. Cancer Imaging Arch. (2017)

36. Prastawa, M., Bullitt, E., Ho, S., Gerig, G.: A brain tumor segmentation framework based on outlier detection. Med. Image Anal. **8**(3), 275–283 (2004)

37. Agn, M., Puonti, O., Rosenschöld, P.M., Law, I., Van Leemput, K.: Brain tumor segmentation using a generative model with an RBM prior on tumor shape. In: Crimi, A., Menze, B., Maier, O., Reyes, M., Handels, H. (eds.) BrainLes 2015. LNCS, vol. 9556, pp. 168–180. Springer, Cham (2016). https://doi.org/10.1007/978-3-319-30858-6_15

38. Menze, B.H., van Leemput, K., Lashkari, D., Weber, M.-A., Ayache, N., Golland, P.: A generative model for brain tumor segmentation in multi-modal images. In: Jiang, T., Navab, N., Pluim, J.P.W., Viergever, M.A. (eds.) MICCAI 2010. LNCS, vol. 6362, pp. 151–159. Springer, Heidelberg (2010). https://doi.org/10.1007/978-3-642-15745-5_19

39. Gooya, A., Pohl, K.M., Bilello, M., Cirillo, L., Biros, G., Melhem, E.R., Davatzikos, C.: Glistr: glioma image segmentation and registration. IEEE Trans. Med. Imaging **31**(10), 1941–1954 (2012)

40. Bauer, S., Nolte, L.-P., Reyes, M.: Fully automatic segmentation of brain tumor images using support vector machine classification in combination with hierarchical conditional random field regularization. In: Fichtinger, G., Martel, A., Peters, T. (eds.) MICCAI 2011. LNCS, vol. 6893, pp. 354–361. Springer, Heidelberg (2011). https://doi.org/10.1007/978-3-642-23626-6_44

41. Zhang, N., Ruan, S., Lebonvallet, S., Liao, Q., Zhu, Y.: Kernel feature selection to fuse multi-spectral MRI images for brain tumor segmentation. Comput. Vis. Image Underst. **115**(2), 256–269 (2011)

42. Geremia, E., Menze, B.H., Ayache, N., et al.: Spatial decision forests for glioma segmentation in multi-channel MR images. In: MICCAI Challenge on Multimodal Brain Tumor Segmentation, vol. 34 (2012)

43. Zikic, D., Glocker, B., Konukoglu, E., Criminisi, A., Demiralp, C., Shotton, J., Thomas, O.M., Das, T., Jena, R., Price, S.J.: Decision forests for tissue-specific segmentation of high-grade gliomas in multi-channel MR. In: Ayache, N., Delingette, H., Golland, P., Mori, K. (eds.) MICCAI 2012. LNCS, vol. 7512, pp. 369–376. Springer, Heidelberg (2012). https://doi.org/10.1007/978-3-642-33454-2_46

44. Goetz, M., Weber, C., Bloecher, J., Stieltjes, B., Meinzer, H.P., Maier-Hein, K.: Extremely randomized trees based brain tumor segmentation. In: Proceeding of BRATS challenge-MICCAI, pp. 006–011 (2014)

45. Ho, S., Bullitt, E., Gerig, G.: Level-set evolution with region competition: automatic 3-D segmentation of brain tumors. In: Proceedings of 16th International Conference on Pattern Recognition, vol. 1, pp. 532–535. IEEE (2002)

46. Wang, T., Cheng, I., Basu, A., et al.: Fluid vector flow and applications in brain tumor segmentation. IEEE Trans. Biomed. Eng. **56**(3), 781–789 (2009)

47. Hamamci, A., Kucuk, N., Karaman, K., Engin, K., Unal, G.: Tumor-cut: segmentation of brain tumors on contrast enhanced MR images for radiosurgery applications. IEEE Trans. Med. Imaging **31**(3), 790–804 (2012)

48. Zikic, D., Ioannou, Y., Brown, M., Criminisi, A.: Segmentation of brain tumor tissues with convolutional neural networks. In: Proceedings MICCAI-BRATS, pp. 36–39 (2014)

49. Dvorak, P., Menze, B.H.: Local structure prediction with convolutional neural networks for multimodal brain tumor segmentation. In: MCV@ MICCAI, pp. 59–71 (2015)

50. Dong, H., Yang, G., Liu, F., Mo, Y., Guo, Y.: Automatic brain tumor detection and segmentation using u-net based fully convolutional networks. arXiv preprint arXiv:1705.03820 (2017)

51. Beers, A., Chang, K., Brown, J., Sartor, E., Mammen, C., Gerstner, E., Rosen, B., Kalpathy-Cramer, J.: Sequential 3D u-nets for biologically-informed brain tumor segmentation. arXiv preprint arXiv:1709.02967 (2017)

52. Ronneberger, O., Fischer, P., Brox, T.: U-Net: convolutional networks for biomedical image segmentation. In: Navab, N., Hornegger, J., Wells, W.M., Frangi, A.F. (eds.) MICCAI 2015. LNCS, vol. 9351, pp. 234–241. Springer, Cham (2015). https://doi.org/10.1007/978-3-319-24574-4_28

53. Srivastava, N., Hinton, G.E., Krizhevsky, A., Sutskever, I., Salakhutdinov, R.: Dropout: a simple way to prevent neural networks from overfitting. J. Mach. Learn. Res. **15**(1), 1929–1958 (2014)

54. Xie, L., Wang, J., Wei, Z., Wang, M., Tian, Q.: Disturblabel: regularizing CNN on the loss layer. In: Proceedings of the IEEE Conference on Computer Vision and Pattern Recognition, pp. 4753–4762 (2016)

55. Haralick, R.M., Sternberg, S.R., Zhuang, X.: Image analysis using mathematical morphology. IEEE Trans. Pattern Anal. Mach. Intell. **4**, 532–550 (1987)

56. Brett, M., Hanke, M., Cipollini, B., Côté, M.A., Markiewicz, C., Gerhard, S., Larson, E., Lee, G.R., Halchenko, Y., Kastman, E., et al.: nibabel: 2.1. 0. Zenodo (2016)

57. Jones, E., Oliphant, T., Peterson, P.: {SciPy}: open source scientific tools for {Python} (2014)

58. van der Walt, S., Colbert, S.C., Varoquaux, G.: The numpy array: a structure for efficient numerical computation. Comput. Sci. Eng. **13**(2), 22–30 (2011)

59. Abadi, M., Agarwal, A., Barham, P., Brevdo, E., Chen, Z., Citro, C., Corrado, G.S., Davis, A., Dean, J., Devin, M., et al.: Tensorflow: large-scale machine learning on heterogeneous distributed systems. arXiv preprint arXiv:1603.04467 (2016)

60. Glorot, X., Bengio, Y.: Understanding the difficulty of training deep feedforward neural networks. In: Proceedings of the Thirteenth International Conference on Artificial Intelligence and Statistics, pp. 249–256 (2010)

61. Kingma, D., Ba, J.: Adam: A method for stochastic optimization. arXiv preprint arXiv:1412.6980 (2014)

3D Deep Neural Network-Based Brain Tumor Segmentation Using Multimodality Magnetic Resonance Sequences

Yan Hu[1] and Yong Xia[1,2(✉)]

[1] Shaanxi Key Lab of Speech Image Information Processing (SAIIP),
School of Computer Science and Engineering,
Northwestern Polytechnical University,
Xi'an 710072, People's Republic of China
[2] Centre for Multidisciplinary Convergence Computing (CMCC),
School of Computer Science and Engineering,
Northwestern Polytechnical University,
Xi'an 710072, People's Republic of China
yxia@nwpu.edu.cn

Abstract. Brain tumor segmentation plays a pivotal role in clinical practice and research settings. In this paper, we propose a 3D deep neural network-based algorithm for joint brain tumor detection and intra-tumor structure segmentation, including necrosis, edema, non-enhancing and enhancing tumor, using multimodal magnetic resonance imaging sequences. An ensemble of cascaded U-Nets is designed to detect the tumor and a deep convolutional neural network is constructed for patch-based intra-tumor structure segmentation. This algorithm has been evaluated on the BraTS 2017 Challenge dataset and achieved Dice similarity coefficients of 0.81, 0.69 and 0.55 in the segmentation of whole tumor, core tumor and enhancing tumor, respectively. Our results suggest that the proposed algorithm has promising performance in automated brain tumor segmentation.

Keywords: Brain tumor segmentation · Deep learning
Cascaded U-Nets · Deep convolutional neural network
Magnetic Resonance Imaging (MRI)

1 Introduction

Brain malignancies, primarily gliomas, occur in around 250,000 people a year globally, and are second only to acute lymphoblastic leukemia as the most common form of cancer in children younger than 15 [1]. Despite considerable research efforts devoted to this disease, diagnosis, treatment plan and follow-up, evaluation of brain tumors, in which accurate delineation of the tumor volume is an essential step, remains a major challenges in both clinical and research practices.

© Springer International Publishing AG, part of Springer Nature 2018
A. Crimi et al. (Eds.): BrainLes 2017, LNCS 10670, pp. 423–434, 2018.
https://doi.org/10.1007/978-3-319-75238-9_36

Brain tumor segmentation is usually performed manually by medical professionals on magnetic resonance (MR) scans, since MR imaging can provide high spatial resolution of the brain anatomy and unique contrast between soft tissues. Such manual segmentation, however, requires a high degree of skills and concentration, and is time-consuming, expensive and prone to operator bias. Computer-aided brain tumor segmentation would overcome those issues and provide medical professionals an unprecedented tool for efficient and reliable analysis, visualization and interpretation of brain tumors. A number of automated brain tumor segmentation algorithms have been proposed in the literature, which are mostly based on either generative models or discriminative models.

Generative model-based methods usually incorporate the domain-specific prior knowledge, such as the tumor appearance [2–4] and tumor growth [5], into the segmentation process. Cordier et al. [3] built a probabilistic model on tissue types to delineateregions of interest enclosing high-probability tumor volumes. Agn et al. [2] characterized normal brain tissue with the spatial atlas prior and a Gaussian mixture model (GMM), and described the shape of both tumor core and complete tumor with the convolutional restricted Boltzmann machines. Gooya et al. [5] registered patients scans to healthy individuals' probabilistic atlas, into which a tumor growth model is incorporated, to locate brain tumors.

Discriminative model-based methods directly learn the characteristics of different tissue regions from manually annotated training images. Various visual features, which describe the texture and shape of tumors, have been extracted from brain MR scans, and many classifiers, such as the support vector machine (SVM) [6] and random forest [7,8], have shown their proven performance in brain tumor segmentation. Recently, deep learning techniques have achieved enormous success in semantic image segmentation. Convolutional neural networks (CNNs), which learn the representation and discrimination of images simultaneously in a unified model and avoid the hand-crafted feature extraction and engineering, have been applied to brain tumor segmentation in MR images. Havaei et al. [9] designed a TwoPathCNN to process each input image patch with both a shallow network and a deep network. Pereira et al. [10] used an 11-layer CNN for high grade gliomas (HGG) segmentation and a 9-layer CNN for low grade gliomas (LGG) segmentation. Zhao et al. [11] proposed a three-convolutional-pathway network, in which the input patches for three pathways have a size of 48×48, 28×28 and 12×12, respectively, and concatenated these three outputs for classification. Their study shows that multiscale CNNs have better performance than single scale ones. Similarly, Kamnitsas et al. [12] created a two-pathway network, one for normal resolution patches and the other for low resolution patches. To achieve stable and smooth segmentation, the Markov random field (MRF) model has been used to regularize the results with the local information provided by neighboring voxels [12,13]. Different from these patch-based methods where the patch size has to be determined empirically, end-to-end deep neural networks directly segment the entire brain MR image. Dong et al. [14] developed a U-Net based deep CNN, which use a "soft" Dice metric as the loss function, and applied it to the segmentation of both LGG and HGG. Pereira et al. [15] employed a

U-Net to locate the brain tumor and then crop a fixed size patch around the tumor as the input of another U-Net for intra-tumor structure segmentation.

In this paper, we propose a 3D deep neural network-based algorithm for joint detection of brain tumors and segmentation of intra-tumor structures, including necrosis, edema, non-enhancing and enhancing tumor, using multimodality MR scans. At the detection stage, an ensemble of cascaded U-Nets is constructed to learn the pathological presentation and location of each brain tumor using each group of three adjacent MR slices of all modalities. At the segmentation stage, each voxel within the detected tumor is further assigned to one of four intra-tumor structures by using a patch-based deep CNN. The proposed algorithm has been evaluated on the BraTS 2017 Challenge dataset [16].

2   Dataset

The BraTS 2017 Challenge dataset comprises 285 training subjects, 46 validation subjects and 146 test subjects. For each subject, there are four MRI sequences, including the T1, T1c, T2 and FLAIR. All images were rigidly aligned with the T1c and skull stripped. The resolution was guaranteed to be coherent among all MRI sequences and patients by interpolation of the sequences to the voxel size of $1 \times 1 \times 1 \, mm^3$. All studies have been segmented manually, by one to four raters, and their annotations were approved by experienced neuro-radiologists. The segmentation ground truth identifies four types of intra-tumoral structures: (a) necrosis, (b) edema, (c) non-enhancing and (d) enhancing tumor [17–19]. Ground truth annotations have been made manually by experts for validation set and test set, but were kept private for the evaluation. Two example brain MR slices with the segmentation ground truth are shown in Fig. 1.

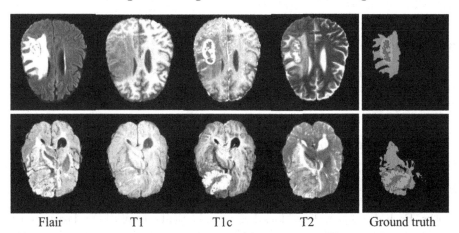

| Flair | T1 | T1c | T2 | Ground truth |

Fig. 1. Two example brain MR slices from a HGG case (top row) and a LGG case (bottom row), together with the segmentation ground truth: edema (green), non-enhancing (blue), necrosis (red), enhancing core (yellow), background and normal tissues (black). (Color figure online)

3   Method

The proposed algorithm consists of two major modules: cascaded U-Net-based brain tumor detection and deep CNN-based intra-tumor structure segmentation. A diagram that summarizes this algorithm is shown in Fig. 2.

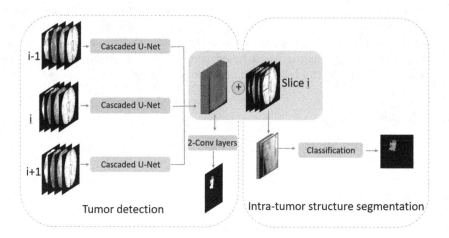

Fig. 2. Diagram of the proposed algorithm. Image representation of tree adjacent slices are learnt by three cascaded U-Net models, and they are concatenated and further processed by two convolutional layers to detect tumor region. The original image (T1, T1c, T2 and FLAIR) and the feature maps generated by three cascaded U-Net models are concatenated as new image in intra-tumor structure segmentation. Patches are cropped within tumor region detected for classification model.

3.1   Pre-processing

The ground truth is relabled into six classes, including four intra-tumoral structures, normal tissues and background. And all modalities are linearly normalized to the range 0–255.

3.2   Tumor Detection

The key component of our brain tumor detection module is a cascaded U-Net model, which consists of two U-Nets with different scales [21].

The first U-Net contains four down-sampling blocks and three up-sampling blocks. Each down-sampling block has two identical convolutional layers and a 2×2 max pooling layer. In each convolutional layer, the kernel size is 3×3, the stride is 1, and the activation function is the rectified linear unit (ReLU). The numbers of kernels in four blocks are 64, 128, 256 and 512, respectively. These down-sampling blocks convert each 224×224 input image patch into a 14×14 feature map. Similarly, each upsampling block has a deconvolutional layer, in which the kernel size is 4 × 4 and the stride is 2, and two convolutional layers with the same parameters as their counterparts in the corresponding down-sampling block. In each up-sampling block, the output of the deconvolutional layer is concatenated with the same-size output of the convolutional layers in a down-sampling block, before it is inputted to the convolutional layer. As a result, three up-sampling blocks enlarge each 14 × 14 feature map to a 112 × 112 one.

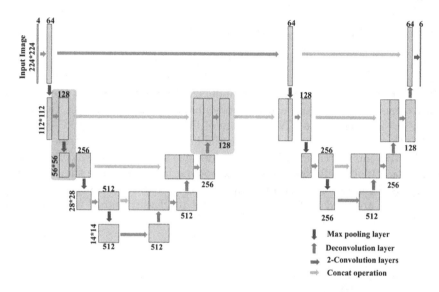

Fig. 3. Architecture of the cascaded U-Net

The second level U-Net is similar to the first one, except for containing three downsampling blocks and three up-sampling blocks. To cascade these two U-Nets, the output of the convolutional layer in first U-Net's first down-sampling block is used as the input of the second U-Net's first down-sampling block, and in the meantime the output of first U-Net is concatenated to the input of second U-Net's second down-sampling block.

The architecture of this cascaded U-Net model is shown in Fig. 3, where each arrow represents two convolutional layers, a deconvolutional layer or a pooling layer, and each rectangular represents a set of feature maps with the number and size of feature maps shown around.

The input of each cascaded U-Net is a 224 × 224 × 4 image patch, which is extracted from the center of each corresponding slice in the T1, T1c, T2 and Flair sequences. Since the brain tumor appears only on some slices, we empirically select 70% of positive patches (with tumor) and 30% of negative patches (without tumor) to train the tumor detection module.

As shown in Fig. 2, we have another two cascaded U-Net models to process the upward and downward slices, simultaneously. The image representation of tree adjacent slices learned by three cascaded U-Net models are concatenated and further processed by two convolutional layers, each of which contains six kernels of size 3 × 3 and uses a liner activation function. The 224 × 224 × 6 output of the last convolutional layer gives the probability of each voxel belonging to necrosis, edema, non-enhancing tumor, enhancing tumor, normal tissues and background.

3.3   Intra-tumor Structure Segmentation

Although the tumor detection module classified voxels into six classes, the obtained intra-tumor structures are less reliable. Therefore, we construct a deep CNN, which is based on the VGG-16 model [22], to further segment the detected brain tumor into necrosis, edema, non-enhancing and enhancing tumor. As shown in Fig. 4, this deep CNN consists of five convolutional blocks, each containing three convolutional layers with the kernel size of 3 × 3, stride of 1 and ReLU activation function, except for the first block, which has two convolutional layers. Each block is followed by a max pooling layer to reduce the size of feature maps. Then two convolutional layers with 1024 and six kernels of size 1 × 1, respectively, are used as fully connect layers to classify tumor voxel into four intra-tumor structures, normal tissues and background.

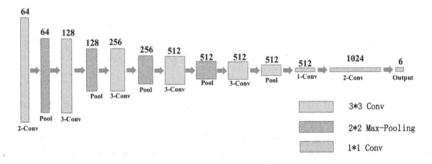

Fig. 4. Architecture of the Intra-tumor structure segmentation network

The intra-tumor structure segmentation is performed via patch-based voxel classification. First, we concatenate the original four-component image (T1, T1c, T2 and FLAIR) with the feature maps generated by three cascaded U-Net models, and thus produce a 22-component image for segmentation. As the red bounding box shown in Fig. 2, we extract 45 × 45 × 22 image patch centered on the four intra-tumoral structures, normal tissues and background from randomly selected slices as the training data for classification model. However, we only extract the same size image patch centered on voxel inside the detected brain tumor as the input of the constructed deep CNN and then assign the predicted class label to that voxel.

It should be noted that, we use the cross entropy as the loss function, adaptive moment estimator (Adam) as an optimizer with learning rate 0.0001 for both tumor detection and intra-tumor segmentation networks. These two models are trained seperately with batch size 16 in detection and 256 in intra-tumor segmentation, and hyperparameters are initialized by using a pretrained VGG-16 model when the layers are the same, otherwise, initialized randomly.

4   Experiments and Results

We evaluated the proposed brain tumor segmentation algorithm on the BraTS 2017 Challenge database. Following the request of the challenge [20], four intra-tumor structures have been grouped into three mutually inclusive tumor regions: (a) whole tumor, (b) enhancing tumor, and (c) core tumor that includes the necrosis, enhancing tumor and non-enhancing tumor.

Example slices from four Flair sequences and T1c sequences in the training dataset, together with the segmentation results and ground truth, are shown in Fig. 5. The Dice similarity coefficients for whole tumor, core tumor and enhancing tumor were shown in Table 1.

The segmentation performance of our algorithm on both validation and testing datasets can be quantitatively assessed by the average Dice similarity coefficient and Hausdorff distance, which are calculated through the challenge online evaluation system. Tables 2 and 3 give the quantitative performance of our algorithm on 46 validation and 146 testing unseen cases, respectively. It shows that our proposed algorithm produces a promising segmentation while our model faces a generation problem because new data may differ significantly in validation and testing datasets.

Table 1. Performance of the proposed algorithm on four cases shown in Fig. 5.

Evaluation	Dice similarity		
	Whole tumor	Core tumor	Enhancing tumor
Slice 1	0.82	0.81	0.74
Slice 2	0.93	0.68	0.69
Slice 3	0.97	0.95	0.92
Slice 4	0.90	0.90	0.91

Since three cascaded U-Nets and a deep CNN are used, our algorithm has a high computational complexity. It takes about twelve hours to train this algorithm (Intel Xeon 2.10 GHz CPU, NVIDIA GTX 1080 Ti GPU, 32 GB RAM).

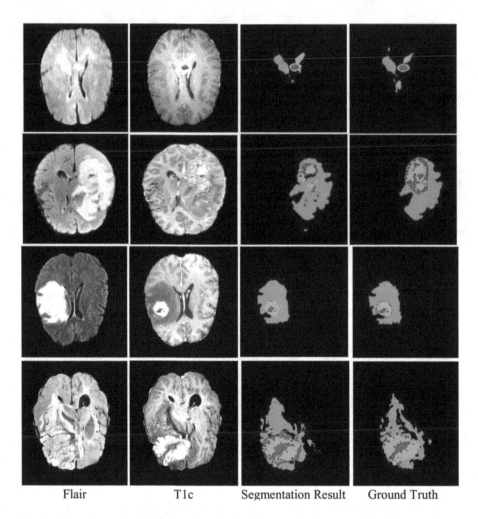

| Flair | T1c | Segmentation Result | Ground Truth |

Fig. 5. Four slices in the BraTS 2017 training dataset (1–3 are HGG and 4 is LGG), the corresponding segmentation results and ground truth: edema (green), non-enhancing (blue), necrosis (red), enhancing core (yellow) (Color figure online)

Table 2. Performance of the proposed algorithm on BraTS 2017 validation database

Evaluation	Dice similarity			Hausdorff distance		
	Enhancing tumor	Whole tumor	Core tumor	Enhancing tumor	Whole tumor	Core tumor
Mean	0.65	0.85	0.70	17.98	25.24	21.45
StdDev	0.29	0.09	0.24	30.23	29.48	25.91
Median	0.79	0.87	0.78	2.64	5.83	10.82
25quantile	0.52	0.81	0.57	1.80	3.46	3.84
75quantile	0.86	0.92	0.89	15.82	52.71	26.52

Table 3. Performance of the proposed algorithm on BraTS 2017 testing database

Evaluation	Dice similarity			Hausdorff distance		
	Enhancing tumor	Whole tumor	Core tumor	Enhancing tumor	Whole tumor	Core Tumor
Mean	0.55	0.81	0.69	64.42	24.25	31.53
StdDev	0.32	0.17	0.29	132.02	30.25	80.44
Median	0.71	0.88	0.82	3.53	7.14	6.71
25quantile	0.32	0.78	0.57	2.23	3.74	3.04
75quantile	0.79	0.91	0.90	18.64	39.35	13.45

However, it costs only about 2 to 3 min to segment the brain tumor in one mul-timodality MR study, including about thirty seconds for tumor detection and about two minutes for intra-tumor structure segmentation on average.

5 Discussion

5.1 U-Net vs Cascaded U-Net

To demonstrate the performance improvement resulted from using the cascaded U-Net, we trained another algorithm that is almost identical to the proposed one except for using the traditional U-Net on the BraTS 2017 training dataset and tested it on the validation dataset. The segmentation results obtained by applying this algorithm and the proposed one to four validation studies were shown in Fig. 6. Table 4 gives the performance of both algorithms in whole tumor segmentation measured by the average Dice similarity coefficient and sensitivity. It reveals that using the cascaded U-Net is able to improve the performance of brain tumor detection substantially than using the traditional U-Net.

Table 4. Performance of whole tumor detection on BraTS 2017 validation dataset

Methods	Dice similarity			Sensitity		
	Enhancing tumor	Whole tumor	Core tumor	Enhancing tumor	Whole tumor	Core Tumor
Using U-Net	0.55	0.79	0.69	0.80	0.81	0.75
Using cascaded U-Net	0.61	0.85	0.67	0.65	0.83	0.79

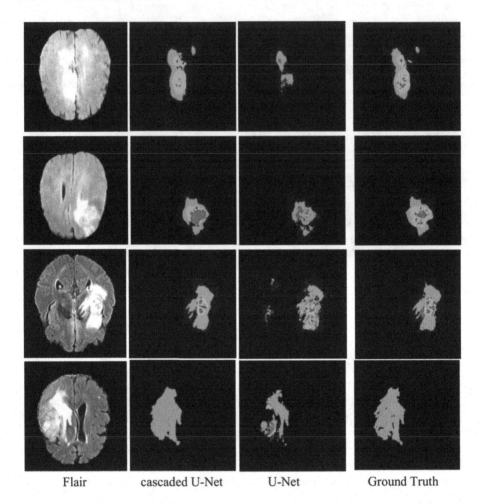

Flair   cascaded U-Net   U-Net   Ground Truth

Fig. 6. Four example slices in the BraTS 2017 training dataset with Flair sequences, the corresponding segmentation results obtained by applying the algorithm with traditional U-Net and the proposed algorithm and the ground truth.

6   Conclusion

In this paper, we propose a 3D deep neural network-based algorithm for joint detection of brain tumors and segmentation of intra-tumor structures, including necrosis, edema, non-enhancing and enhancing tumor, using multimodality MR sequences. This algorithm has been evaluated on the BraTS 2017 Challenge dataset and achieved a Dice similarity coefficient of 0.81, 0.69 and 0.55 for the segmentation of whole tumor, core tumor and enhancing tumor, respectively. Similar to other machine learning algorithms, our deep models face generation problems when new data differing significantly, thus there is a decrease in performance on testing and validation set. It would be worth researching on this problem.

Additionally, class distribution is imblanced in this task while deep models learn better on class balance data, we plan to further investigated class imblance.

Acknowledgement. This work was supported in part by the National Natural Science Foundation of China under Grants 61771397 and 61471297. We appreciate the efforts devoted by BraTS Challenge organizers to collect and share the data for comparing brain tumor segmentation algorithms for multimodality MR sequences.

References

1. Mcguire, S.: World cancer report 2014. Geneva, Switzerland: world health organization, international agency for research on cancer, WHO Press, 2015. Adva. Nutr. **7**, 418–419 (2016)
2. Agn, M., Puonti, O., Rosenschöld, P.M., Law, I., Van Leemput, K.: Brain tumor segmentation using a generative model with an RBM prior on tumor shape. In: Crimi, A., Menze, B., Maier, O., Reyes, M., Handels, H. (eds.) BrainLes 2015. LNCS, vol. 9556, pp. 168–180. Springer, Cham (2016). https://doi.org/10.1007/978-3-319-30858-6_15
3. Cordier, N., Delingette, H., Ayache, N.: A patch-based approach for the segmentation of pathologies: application to glioma labelling. IEEE Trans. Med. Imaging **35**, 1066–1076 (2016)
4. Cobzas, D., Birkbeck, N., Schmidt, M.W., Jagersand, M., Murtha, A.: 3D variational brain tumor segmentation using a high dimensional feature set. In: International Conference on Computer Vision, pp. 1–8 (2007)
5. Gooya, A., Pohl, K.M., Bilello, M., Cirillo, L., Biros, G., Melhem, E.R., Davatzikos, C.: GLISTR: glioma image segmentation and registration. IEEE Trans. Med. Imaging **31**, 1941–1954 (2012)
6. Bauer, S., Nolte, L.-P., Reyes, M.: Fully automatic segmentation of brain tumor images using support vector machine classification in combination with hierarchical conditional random field regularization. In: Fichtinger, G., Martel, A., Peters, T. (eds.) MICCAI 2011. LNCS, vol. 6893, pp. 354–361. Springer, Heidelberg (2011). https://doi.org/10.1007/978-3-642-23626-6_44
7. Zikic, D., et al.: Decision forests for tissue-specific segmentation of high-grade gliomas in multi-channel MR. In: Ayache, N., Delingette, H., Golland, P., Mori, K. (eds.) MICCAI 2012. LNCS, vol. 7512, pp. 369–376. Springer, Heidelberg (2012). https://doi.org/10.1007/978-3-642-33454-2_46
8. Tustison, N.J., Shrinidhi, K.L., Wintermark, M., Durst, C.R., Kandel, B.M., Gee, J.C., Grossman, M.C., Avants, B.B.: Optimal symmetric multimodal templates and concatenated random forests for supervised brain tumor segmentation (simplified) with ANTsR. Neuroinformatics **13**, 209–225 (2015)
9. Havaei, M., Davy, A., Wardefarley, D., Biard, A., Courville, A.C., Bengio, Y., Pal, C., Jodoin, P., Larochelle, H.: Brain tumor segmentation with deep neural networks. Med. Image Anal. **35**, 18–31 (2017)
10. Pereira, S., Pinto, A., Alves, V., Silva, C.A.: Brain tumor segmentation using convolutional neural networks in MRI images. IEEE Trans. Med. Imaging **35**, 1240–1251 (2016)
11. Zhao, L.Y., Jia, K.B.: Multiscale CNNs for brain tumor segmentation and diagnosis. Comput. Math. Methods Med. **2016**, 1–7 (2016)

12. Konstantinos, K., Enzo, F., Sarah, P., Cristian, L., Aditya, N., Antonio, C., Daniel, R., Glocker, B.: DeepMedic on brain tumor segmentation. In: Crimi, A., Menze, B., Maier, O., Reyes, M., Winzeck, S., Handels, H. (eds.) BrainLes 2016. LNCS, vol. 10154, pp. 138–149. Springer, Cham (2016)

13. Zhao, X., Wu, Y., Song, G., Li, Z., Fan, Y., Zhang, Y.: Brain tumor segmentation using a fully convolutional neural network with conditional random fields. In: Crimi, A., Menze, B., Maier, O., Reyes, M., Winzeck, S., Handels, H. (eds.) BrainLes 2016, vol. 10154, pp. 75–87. Springer, Cham (2016). https://doi.org/10.1007/978-3-319-55524-9_8

14. Dong, H., Yang, G., Liu, F., Mo, Y., Guo Y.: Automatic brain tumor detection and segmentation using U-Net based fully convolutional networks. In: MIUA (2017)

15. Pereira, S., Oliveira, A., Alves, V., Silva, C.: On hierarchical brain tumor segmentation in MRI using fully convolutional neural networks: a preliminary study. In: 2017 IEEE 5th Portuguese Meeting on Bioengineering

16. BraTS 2017 Image Repository. http://www.med.upenn.edu/sbia/brats2017/data.html

17. Bakas, S., Akbari, H., Sotiras, A., Bilello, M., Rozycki, M., Kirby, J.S., Freymann, J.B., Farahani, K., Davatzikos, C.: Advancing the cancer genome Atlas glioma MRI collections with expert segmentation labels and radiomic features. Sci. Data 4 (2017). https://doi.org/10.1038/sdata.2017.117

18. Bakas, S., Akbari, H., Sotiras, A., Bilello, M., Rozycki, M., Kirby, J., Freymann, J., Farahani, K., Davatzikos, C.: Segmentation labels and radiomic features for the preoperative scans of the TCGA-GBM collection. The Cancer Imaging Archive (2017). https://doi.org/10.7937/K9/TCIA.2017.KLXWJJ1Q

19. Bakas, S., Akbari, H., Sotiras, A., Bilello, M., Rozycki, M., Kirby, J., Freymann, J., Farahani, K., Davatzikos, C.: Segmentation labels and radiomic features for the preoperative scans of the TCGA-LGG collection. The Cancer Imaging Archive (2017). https://doi.org/10.7937/K9/TCIA.2017.GJQ7R0EF

20. Menze, B.H., Jakab, A., Bauer, S., Kalpathy-Cramer, J., Farahani, K., Kirby, J., Burren, Y., Porz, N., Slotboom, J., Wiest, R., Lanczi, L., Gerstner, E., Weber, M.A., Arbel, T., Avants, B.B., Ayache, N., Buendia, P., Collins, D.L., Cordier, N., Corso, J.J., Criminisi, A., Das, T., Delingette, H., Demiralp, Ç., Durst, C.R., Dojat, M., Doyle, S., Festa, J., Forbes, F., Geremia, E., Glocker, B., Golland, P., Guo, X., Hamamci, A., Iftekharuddin, K.M., Jena, R., John, N.M., Konukoglu, E., Lashkari, D., Mariz, J.A., Meier, R., Pereira, S., Precup, D., Price, S.J., Raviv, T.R., Reza, S.M., Ryan, M., Sarikaya, D., Schwartz, L., Shin, H.C., Shotton, J., Silva, C.A., Sousa, N., Subbanna, N.K., Szekely, G., Taylor, T.J., Thomas, O.M., Tustison, N.J., Unal, G., Vasseur, F., Wintermark, M., Ye, D.H., Zhao, L., Zhao, B., Zikic, D., Prastawa, M., Reyes, M., Van Leemput, K.: The multimodal brain tumor image segmentation benchmark (BRATS). IEEE Trans. Med. Imaging 34(10), 1993–2024 (2015)

21. Ronneberger, O., Fischer, P., Brox, T.: U-Net: convolutional networks for biomedical image segmentation. In: International Conference on Medical Image Computing and Computer-Assisted Intervention, pp. 234–241 (2015)

22. Simonyan K., Zisserman A.: Very deep convolutional networks for large-scale image recognition. arXiv:1409.1556 (2014)

Automated Brain Tumor Segmentation on Magnetic Resonance Images and Patient's Overall Survival Prediction Using Support Vector Machines

Alexander F. I. Osman[(✉)] [iD]

Radiation Oncology Department, American University of Beirut Medical Center,
Beirut 1107 2020, Riad El-Solh, Lebanon
alexanderfadul@yahoo.com

Abstract. This study is aimed to develop two algorithms for glioma tumor segmentation and patient's overall survival (OS) prediction with machine learning approaches. The segmentation algorithm is fully automated to accurately and efficiently delineate the whole tumor on a magnetic resonance imaging (MRI) scan for radiotherapy treatment planning. The survival algorithm predicts the OS for glioblastoma multiforme (GBM) patients based on regression and classification principles. Multi-institutional BRATS'2017 data of MRI scans from 477 patients with high-grade and lower-grade glioma (HGG/LGG) used in this study. Clinical patient survival data of 291 glioblastoma multiforme (GBM) were available in the provided data. Support vector machines (SVMs) were used to develop both algorithms. The segmentation chain comprises pre-processing with a goal of noise removal, feature extraction of the image intensity, segmentation process using a non-linear classifier with 'Gaussian' kernel, and post-processing to enhance the segmentation morphology. The OS prediction algorithm sequence involves two steps; extraction of patient's age, and segmented tumor's size and its location features; prediction process using a non-linear classifier and a linear regression model with 'Gaussian' kernels. The algorithms were trained, validated and tested on BRATS'2017's training, validation, and testing datasets. Average Dice for the whole tumor segmentation obtained on the validation and testing datasets is 0.53 ± 0.31 (median 0.60) which indicates the consistency of the proposed algorithm on the new "unseen" data. For OS prediction, the mean accuracy is 0.49 for the validation dataset and 0.35 for the testing dataset based on regression principle; whereas an overall accuracy of 1.00 achieved in classification into short, medium, and long-survivor classes for a designed validation dataset. The computational time for the automated segmentation algorithm took approximately 3 min. In its present form, the segmentation tool is fully automated, fast, and provides a reasonable segmentation accuracy on the multi-institutional dataset.

Keywords: Brain tumors · MRI · Image segmentation · SVM
Glioma overall survival

© Springer International Publishing AG, part of Springer Nature 2018
A. Crimi et al. (Eds.): BrainLes 2017, LNCS 10670, pp. 435–449, 2018.
https://doi.org/10.1007/978-3-319-75238-9_37

1 Introduction

Glioma tumors are the most common primary brain malignancies [1]. They tend to have different degrees of aggressiveness, variable prognosis, and various heterogeneous histological sub-regions (i.e. peritumoral edema, necrotic core, enhancing tumor core, and non-enhancing tumor core) [1]. Glioma tumors are broadly classified into high-grade and lower-grade. High-grade glioma (HGG) tumors are invasive tumors that aggressively grow in a relatively short period of time leading to the patient's death. Glioblastoma multiforme (GBM) is the most common and aggressive HGG (grade IV) tumor with a median survival rate of two years or less and requires immediate treatment [2, 3]. Low-grade glioma (LGG) tumors, on the other hand, are slow-growing with a life expectancy of several years.

External beam radiation therapy is a treatment option for patients with glioma tumor. Tumor delineation represents an essential step in the patient's radiation therapy chain, and the patient's treatment quality deeply relies on accurate tumor delineation. Multimodal magnetic resonance imaging (MRI) scans are used in the process of delineating glioma tumor structures, where they offer soft tissue contrast superior to that of computed tomography (CT) images "The tumor volumes are usually drawn on CT slices acquired during the patient's treatment simulation, MRI studies are required for image registration/fusion. CT–MR image registration or fusion combines the accurate volume definition from MR with the electron density information available from CT. The MR data set is superimposed on the CT data set through a series of translations, rotations, and scaling. This process allows the visualization of both studies side by side in the same imaging plane even if the patient has been scanned in a completely different treatment position." [4]. The Glioma delineation process is also crucial in adaptive radiation therapy (ART), where tumor volume shrinkages in response to the radiation during the patient's treatment course. Consequently, new delineation is required as a result to develop a new patient's treatment plan. The tumor delineation process is usually done manually by radiologists as well as it involves a considerable amount of time and effort. Additionally, for a given tumor delineation task, there are significant variations among the radiation oncologists themselves in contouring the tumor.

Therefore, introducing the image processing routines and state-of-the-art machine learning algorithms that can computationally delineate glioma tumors in multimodal MRI scans could have the potential in the improvement of diagnosis, treatment planning, and follow-up of individual patients. It could serve as a supportive tool for radiotherapy planning or replace the conventional segmentation methods. It would be remarkably useful for standardizing the segmentation process and significantly expediting clinic workflow. However, developing an automatic or semi-automatic algorithm for brain tumor segmentation is technically challenging. For example, one reason is that lesion areas are only defined through intensity changes that are relative to encompassing normal tissue. And, even manual segmentations by expert raters show significant variations when intensity gradients between adjacent structures are smooth or obscured by/with artifacts. Another reason is that glioma tumors and its sub-structures vary considerably among patients in its appearance and shape, localization, and size.

In the literature [5–36], many algorithms have been developed using different approaches (generative and discriminative models) for computational segmentation of brain tumors in MR images. Over the past few years, discriminative probabilistic methods [37, 38] that rely on a random forest classifier and convolutional neural networks [18, 19, 39] have shown as the most successful methods for segmentation of brain tumors. Fussing segmentations from different algorithms have shown indications for better performance than the best individual algorithm applied to the same task [40]. Ensemble learning [41] fits well when a set of predictors that are unbiased but with high variability in the individual prediction. It is expected more anticipated to provide a better solution in the next future due to its concept of averaging over multiple predictors which reduce variance and, hence, decreases the prediction error. It has been shown that it is hard to compare the most of these different segmentation strategies that have been reported since the authors' datasets differ so widely. In this direction, recently few community-wide efforts [40, 42] have focused on brain tumor segmentation algorithms. They have made available multimodal MRI datasets and established validation frameworks that have used as a benchmark for the evaluation of different segmentation algorithms for brain tumors. This year (2017), the multimodal brain tumor segmentation (BRATS'2017) challenge [40, 43–45] is making available a large "standard" dataset with accompanying delineations of the relevant tumor sub-regions, and patient's overall survival data.

Nowadays, as most of the proposed algorithms based on neural networks, we believe that it is interesting to see the potentials of other methods such as support vector machines (SVMs) for glioma segmentation [26, 46] which has not widely explored among the other methods. In this paper, we propose approaches for glioma tumor segmentation and patient's overall survival based on support vector machine methods. The first method offers an algorithm for automated whole tumor segmentation on an MRI scan via sophisticated non-linear pattern classification methods. The segmentation process consists of four stages. At first, the volumetric MR data pre-processed with a goal of noise removal. Next, the relevant features extracted. Subsequently, a non-linear SVM classifier with 'Gaussian' kernel implemented to the fed features to train the classifier. And lastly, the generated segmentation labels post-processed to enhance the produced segmentation. The second method offers patient's overall survival prediction from the segmented tumor and patient's age data via the linear regression and non-linear pattern classification methods to obtain better-estimated information of the patient's expected survival characterization. The OS prediction process consists of two steps of both, regression or classification. Step one involves features extraction. The extracted features include patient's age, tumor size, and tumor location. Step two involves OS prediction. Initially, these features accompanied by the 'ground truth' patient's survival data are used to train a non-linear SVM classifier and a linear SVM regression model, both with 'Gaussian' kernel. Then, the trained models are used to predict the OS for new 'unseen' data, into classes such as short (<6 months), medium (6 to 18 months), or long (>18 months) survivors; or estimating a single value.

2 Materials and Methods

2.1 Dataset

Clinical pre-operative multimodal MRI scans from 477 HGG/LGG patients with 291 available GBM patient's OS data used in this study provided by BRATS'2017 challenge [40, 43–45]. The provided MRI scans were clinically-acquired in a routine way in multi-institutions using different scanners and various protocols.

For the segmentation task, the given images grouped into training, validation, and testing datasets. Out of 477 patients' MRI data, 285 (60%) provided as a training dataset, 46 (10%) as validation dataset, and 146 (30%) as testing dataset. Training dataset supplied with their ground truth segmentation labels of various glioma sub-regions. The manually segmented labels performed by experts following the same annotation protocol, and their annotations revised and approved by board-certified neuroradiologists. Annotation labels included were the gadolinium (GD) enhancing tumor (ET), the peritumoral edema (ED) – whole tumor (WT), and the necrotic and non-enhancing tumor (NCR/NET) – tumor core (TC). Each patient multimodal imaging data consisted of four MRI modalities (Fig. 1) namely; (a) T1-weighted (T1), (b) post-contrast/gadolinium T1c-weighted (T1-GD), (c) T2-weighted (T2), and (d) T2-Flair (Fluid Attenuated Inversion Recovery). They were co-registered with aligning the volumes of the four MRI modalities to the same anatomical template, and interpolated to the same resolution of $1 \times 1 \times 1$ mm^3 and skull-stripped to correlate all four images for each patient.

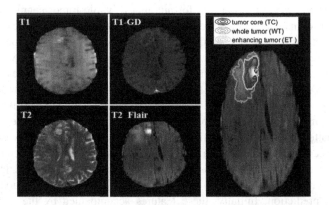

Fig. 1. Shown is an example of a segmentation training dataset (one patient). Four MRI modalities (Left) namely; T1-weighted (T1), T1-weighted with gadolinium contrast (T1-GD), T2 –weighted (T2), and T2-weighted Flair (T2-Flair) with manually segmented annotations (right) of glioma tumor sub-structures (ground truth segmentation labels).

The provided clinical OS data and the patient's age data included with correspondences to the pseudo-identifiers of the GBM/HGG imaging data. Out of 291 included patients' data, 163 (60%) were given as training data, 33 (10%) as validation data, and 95 (30%) as testing data. Only training data were provided with their clinical ground truth OS data.

2.2 Feature Extraction

The image intensity feature used in the proposed segmentation algorithm. Pixel values in the MR images were normalized to the maximum global intensity value in the three-dimensional (3D) MRI data. Thresholding performed on the pixels. We used a fixed threshold of 30% (pixel values higher than the threshold considered). We found that this proposed threshold value appropriate for the provided multi-institutions MRI data. The assumption of using a fixed threshold value supports our fully automated idea but has limitations as well (not optimal for the segmentation where MRI signals that produce the image intensities vary for different patients/scanners/protocols). The 3D matrix of the thresholded image intensities transformed to a vector. Standardized scaling of the fracture data by the weighted feature mean and standard deviation will be performed later when fed into the classifier for segmentation.

Features used for the proposed OS prediction algorithm were patient's age, tumor size estimated as the total number of pixels in the segmented tumor volume, and tumor location roughly estimated from the tumor's center of mass coordinates (X, Y, and Z pixel coordinates). Similarly, feature scaling will be performed later when they fed into the classifier and the regression model. These features were handled independently with no correlation between them. For the class prediction, patient's age feature alone was considered. We found that the accuracy of the class prediction (short, medium, and long survivors) were optimal with solely patient's age feature.

2.3 Support Vector Machines

Support vector machines [41, 47–49] are discriminative machine learning methods can be used for classification and regression problems.

For a calcification problem, the SVM classifier searches for an optimal hyperplane that separates the data into two classes with the maximum-margin, which makes it a superior choice for classification tasks. In a situation of non-separating classes, SVMs can use a soft margin [47] by adding slack variables ξ_j and a penalty parameter C to get a minimal number of errors. The objective is to solve the SVM optimization problem

$$\min_{\beta,b,\xi}\left(\|\beta\|^2 + C\sum_j \xi_j \right), \tag{1}$$

subject to

$$y_j f(x_j) \geq 1 - \xi_j, \ and \ \xi_j \geq 0, \tag{2}$$

for all $j = 1, \ldots, n$, and for a positive scalar C. The vector β contains the coefficients that define an orthogonal vector to the hyperplane, b is the hyperplane offset or the bias term, and the root of $f(x)$ for particular coefficients defines a hyperplane, and x_j, y_j are an observation pair or data points. SVM Kernels [50] may be implemented for non-simple hyperplane examples for a class of functions $G(x_1, x_2)$ with the property that there is a linear space S and a function φ mapping x to S such that

$$G(x_1, x_2) = \ <\varphi(x_1), \varphi(x_2) >, \tag{3}$$

where the dot product takes place in the space S. Special properties of the decision surface ensure high generalization ability of the learning machine.

SVM regression, a nonparametric technique, relies on kernel functions [50]. The soft-margin minimization can be solved using common quadratic programming techniques. Including slack variables, similar to the soft margin concept in SVM classification, the SVM regression objective function of an optimization problem is to minimize

$$J(\beta) = \beta' \beta + C \sum_{n=1}^{N} \left(\xi_n + \xi_n^* \right), \tag{4}$$

subject to

$$\forall n : y_n - \left(x_n' \beta + b \right) \leq \varepsilon + \xi_n, \left(x_n' \beta + b \right) - y_n \leq \varepsilon + \xi_n^*, \xi_n^* \geq 0, \xi_n \geq 0, \tag{5}$$

where, constant C is the box constraint, a positive numeric value that controls the penalty imposed on observations that lie outside the epsilon margin (ε) and helps to prevent overfitting (regularization). This value determines the trade-off between the flatness of $f(x)$ and the amount up to which deviations larger than ε have tolerated. It has been shown that it is computationally expensive to use quadratic programming algorithms. Alternatively, sequential minimal optimization (SMO) method [51] may be used which speeds up the computation and overcomes the running out of memory problem.

2.4   Automated Segmentation and OS Prediction Algorithms

We summarize here the concepts of the two proposed methods, segmentation framework, and OS prediction, using the SVM approach. First, we illustrate a fully automated algorithm to generate segmentation labels of the whole tumor (edema structure) using one MRI modality, T2-FLAIR. Although the segmentation task in the competition aimed to produce the entire tumor sub-structure labels (enhancing tumor, whole tumor, and the tumor core), the proposed method implemented to generate the segmentation just to the whole tumor. Then, we give a detailed description of the OS prediction method based on classification and regression principles. This algorithm uses the segmentation results produced by the segmentation algorithm and the patient's clinical data to predict the overall survival of GBM patients with regression (estimating a single value) or classes (short, medium, or long survivors).

Segmentation Algorithm. In this method, the segmentation process consists of four stages. *At first*, the volumetric MR data go through pre-processing. The goal of the pre-processing is to remove the noise in the data. Denoising process performed on the volumetric MRI data by employing a 3D median filter. *Next*, the processed data undergo features selection and extraction during this stage ("Feature Extraction" section). Image intensity is only feature used for segmentation in the proposed method. The denoised image data normalized to the global maxima in the volumetric image data, and a thresholding technique with an adequate constant value (30% has shown to be appropriate) applied. The volumetric data are transformed into a vector and prepared to feed the classifier. *Subsequently*, the imaging data undergo core segmentation through a non-linear SVM classifier. The classifier returns a full trained SVM classification model (trained using the training data with 'ground truth'). To train the classifier, the image intensity feature data accompanied with the 'ground truth' segmentation data fed into the classifier. The features scaled by the weighted feature mean and standard deviation. A radial basis function 'Gaussian' kernel [50], which showed the best results amongst the kernels for the classification understudy during the training phase, used with an appropriate scaling factor (the default box constraint value for the classification set as the interquartile range of response variable divided by 1.349). SMO method [51], which is relatively fast, used for objective-function minimization with the minimum estimated cross-validation loss. Once the classification process completed, the algorithm checked whether it successfully converged or not. To produce the segmentation labels for new 'unseen' data, a prediction function [52] used to return the predicted segmentation labels using the trained SVM classifier. *And finally*, the produced segmentation labels undergo post-processing. The core step in the post-processing stage is to perform morphological analysis and enhance the produced segmentation. Morphological image analysis [53] filters employed to improve the produced segmentation. A first filter to suppress light segmented regions connected to border pixels using 4-connectivity. A second filter creates a diamond-shaped structuring element using 5 pixels distance from the structuring element origin to the points of the diamond. A third filter performs morphological closing on the segmented region returning the second filter. And a fourth filter fills holes in the segmented region.

OS Prediction Algorithm. The OS prediction process consists of two steps for regression or classification. *Step one* involves feature excretion. The features include patient's age, tumor size, and tumor location, and they are directly estimated as shown in the "Feature Extraction" section. They combined independently and fed into the classifier and the regression model. For the class prediction, patient's age feature alone used. *Step two* involves OS prediction. In this step, initially, these features accompanied by the 'ground truth' OS data and fed into a non-linear SVM classifier and a linear SVM regression model to train the models. Features scaled by the weighted feature mean and standard deviation. In both models, a radial basis function kernel [50] with

Segmentation algorithm workflow   OS algorithm workflow

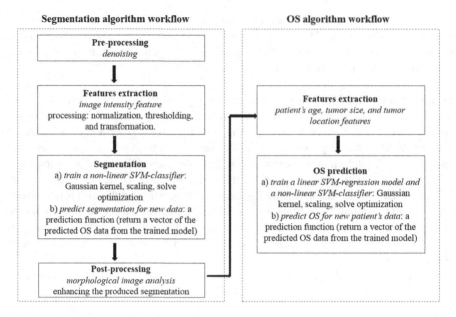

Fig. 2. Illustration of the segmentation and overall survival prediction chains for the two proposed methods.

adequate scaling and SMO [51] method used as similarly as in the proposed segmentation method. Then, a prediction function [52] used to return a vector of the predicted classes and regression for the new 'unseen' data using the trained SVM classifier and regression model, respectively (Fig. 2).

2.5 Performance Evaluation

To evaluate the performance of the segmentation and OS prediction (regression) proposed algorithms, BRATS'2017 validation and testing datasets were used for this purpose. For the OS class prediction algorithm, validation was performed using a hold-out data (n = 16) with "ground truth" from the BRATS'2017 training data. The segmentation and the OS predicted results of the two algorithms were benchmarked using BRAT'2017 challenge evaluation system. Dice score and accuracy measures were used as performance measure for the segmentation and OS prediction, respectively.

3   Results

The predicted glioma segmentation results and the OS predictions on the BRATS'2017 validation and testing datasets summarized in this section. The produced segmentation labels for the whole tumor with the developed algorithm are shown in Fig. 3. The figure shows the performance of the proposed segmentation method qualitatively.

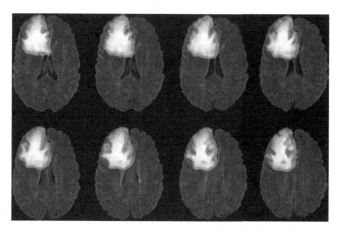

Fig. 3. An example of predicted segmentation labels (whole tumor) on a T2-Flair MRI scan (8 axial views) of one validation dataset with our automated algorithm.

The quantitative measures of the segmentation algorithm performance in the BRATS'2017 challenge presented in Table 1. Average Dice score for the whole tumor segmentation obtained on the validation and testing datasets is 0.53 ± 0.30, which indicates the consistency of the proposed algorithm on the "unseen" data. The average median is 0.60, and the average 75th percentile is 0.81 on the validation and testing datasets. The latter means that 75% of the evaluated segmentations with Dice score 0.81 or less.

Table 1. Evaluation results of the proposed method in the BRATS'2017 challenge for the whole tumor (WT) segmentation on 46 validation and 146 testing datasets.

	Validation phase	Testing phase
	Dice WT	Dice WT
Mean	0.533	0.528
STD	0.299	0.317
Median	0.613	0.583
25 quantile	0.231	0.229
75 quantile	0.798	0.827

The survival predicted results for regression and class prediction with the proposed prediction algorithms are shown in Fig. 4. The figure shows the regions of the predicted classes and the regression fit of the OS.

In Fig. 4 (*Left*), the constructed regions are well separating the OS classes with borders. The regression fit of the OS data (Fig. 4 (*Right*)) seems reasonable with a few features used for prediction. The evaluation results of the survival prediction on the validation and testing datasets listed in Table 2. For the OS regression, the main accuracy decreased in the testing dataset, which probably explained as an overfitting issue.

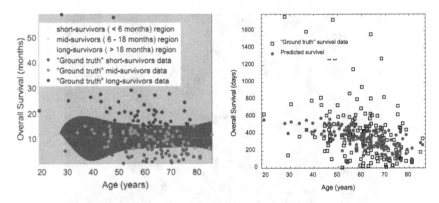

Fig. 4. The plots of the OS class predicted regions (*Left*) and the OS fit (*Right*) results during the training phase with 'ground truth' data.

Table 2. Evaluation results of the proposed method in the BRATS'2017 challenge for OS prediction on 33 validation and 95 testing data.

	Valuation phase	Testing phase
	Accuracy	Accuracy
Regression	0.49	0.35
Classification[a]	1.00[b]	–

[a]Classification principle is not evaluated by the BRATS'2017 challenge.
[b]Indicates the overall class prediction accuracy as well as the individual accuracy in prediction into short, medium, and long survivors.

In class prediction, a mean accuracy of 1.00 was achieved based on short, medium, and long-survivor OS class predictions on a designed validation dataset. The overall accuracy is 1.00 in predicting the classes which indicate that the model is perfect. The computational time for the automated segmentation algorithm took approximately 3 min where a few seconds needed for the OS prediction algorithm.

4   Discussion

Two tasks of glioma brain tumor segmentation and patient's overall survival predictions using BRATS'2017 datasets were successfully implemented in this work using the support vector machine methods. The reason behind choosing SVM is a superior algorithm for classification tasks. Its concept based on searching for a maximum-margin distance between the hyperplane and the closest examples (group data).

One feature, image intensity, was used in the proposed segmentation algorithm. We assumed that it is the most prominent feature. We could not include more features in this study, although we believe that the more features considered the most likely better accuracy achieved. The quantitative evaluation measure of the proposed segmentation algorithm on the BRATS'2017 validation and testing datasets showed an accuracy of 0.53 (Dice score of 0.53 on both datasets). We consider this accuracy is reasonable for our segmentation algorithm which could be associated with some factors. For instance, we used a single feature for the segmentation process. Another factor is that we did not propose a way to deal with the multi-institution imaging data acquired using different scanners with large variations. The predicted segmentation results of our algorithm need to be much improved to provide higher segmentation accuracy. A possible approach to improve its accuracy is (a) standardizing image intensities of imaging modalities/scanners and patient images with methods that proposed by Nyul et al. [54] which could significantly reduce the effect of the patients/modalities variations and improve the predicted segmentation. A second approach (b) is including more representative input features. Above all, the segmentation model achieved similar levels of performance on the validation and testing datasets, even though the latter contains data from different sources, indicating the robustness of the method.

Prediction of patient's overall survival using the segmented tumor in combination with patient's age and tumor radiomic features could serve as a survival-predictor and provide an informative clue about the patient's treatment outcome. Among the extracted features for OS prediction (three features with equal weights for regression, and one feature with full weight for class prediction), patient's age parameter was found to be the most relevant feature in the prediction of the patient's survival. The quantitative evaluation measure of the proposed OS algorithm on the BRATS'2017 validation and testing datasets showed a drop in accuracy from 0.49 to 0.35 when the algorithm implanted on new 'unseen' data. This decrease in accuracy could be explained as an overfitting issue. For the class prediction model, which is not evaluated by the BRATS'2017, the model showed a perfect class prediction (overall accuracy is 1.00) with no mistake made in the classification. We would like to stress that the classification model evaluated using a lower number of data, therefore validating and testing it on more data is required to establish higher confidence. Considering more appropriate radiomic features that capture phenotypic differences between tumors ("personalized") could provide a better regressive prediction of GBM patient's overall survival.

5 Conclusions

We developed two algorithms for glioma tumor segmentation on MR images and patient's overall survival prediction based on SVM learning algorithms. The segmentation and OS prediction algorithms were trained, validated, and tested using the BRATS'2017 challenge datasets. In its current form, the segmentation tool is fully automated, fast, and provides a reasonable accuracy on multi-institutional data. The OS prediction algorithm showed perfect accuracy in class prediction and reasonable accuracy in regressive prediction. Further improving the segmentation algorithm could provide a robust, accurate, and cost-effective supplement tool to the conventional methods. Similarly, considering more appropriate radiomic features that capture phenotypic differences between tumors ("personalized") could provide a better regressive prediction of GBM patient's overall survival. Even though the accuracy of the proposed segmentation algorithm underperformed the recently established BRATS baseline, it showed a robust consistency on the new "unseen" data. A set of different algorithms combined with an ensemble learning approach would certainly be ideal for this task.

References

1. Holland, E.C.: Progenitor cells and glioma formation. Curr. Opin. Neurol. **14**(6), 683–688 (2001)
2. Ohgaki, H., Kleihues, P.: Population-based studies on incidence, survival rates, and genetic alterations in astrocytic and oligodendroglial gliomas. J. Neuropathol. Exp. Neurol. **64**(6), 479–489 (2005)
3. Louis, D.N., Ohgaki, H., Wiestler, O.D., Cavanee, W.K.: WHO Classification of Tumours of the Central Nervous System, 4th edn. WHO/IARC, Lyon (2007)
4. Podgorsak, E.B.: Radiation Oncology Physics: A Handbook for Teachers and Students. International Atomic Energy Agency, Vienna (2005)
5. Angelini, E.D., Clatz, O., Mandonnet, E., et al.: Glioma dynamics and computational models: a review of segmentation, registration, and in silico growth algorithms and their clinical applications. Curr. Med. Imaging Rev. **3**(4), 262–276 (2007)
6. Bauer, S., Wiest, R., Nolte, L.P., Reyes, M.: A survey of MRI-based medical image analysis for brain tumor studies. Phys. Med. Biol. **58**(13), R97–R129 (2013)
7. Kaus, M.R., Warfield, S.K., Nabavi, A., Chatzidakis, E., Black, P.M., Jolesz, F.A., Kikinis, R.: Segmentation of meningiomas and low grade gliomas in MRI. In: Taylor, C., Colchester, A. (eds.) MICCAI 1999. LNCS, vol. 1679, pp. 1–10. Springer, Heidelberg (1999). https://doi.org/10.1007/10704282_1
8. Bach Cuadra, M., De Craene, M., Duay, V., et al.: Dense deformation field estimation for atlas-based segmentation of pathological MR brain images. Comput. Methods Programs Biomed. **84**(2–3), 66–75 (2006)
9. Weizman, L., Ben Sira, L., Joskowicz, L., et al.: Automatic segmentation, internal classification, and follow-up of optic pathway gliomas in MRI. Med. Image Anal. **16**(1), 177–188 (2012)
10. Fletcher-Heath, L.M., Hall, L.O., Goldgof, D.B., Murtagh, F.R.: Automatic segmentation of non-enhancing brain tumors in magnetic resonance images. Artif. Intell. Med. **21**(1–3), 43–63 (2001)
11. Prastawa, M., Bullitt, E., Ho, S., Gerig, G.: A brain tumor segmentation framework based on outlier detection. Med. Image Anal. **8**(3), 275–283 (2004)
12. Pohl, K.M., Fisher, J., Levitt, J.J., Shenton, M.E., Kikinis, R., Grimson, W.E.L., Wells, W. M.: A unifying approach to registration, segmentation, and intensity correction. In: Duncan, J.S., Gerig, G. (eds.) MICCAI 2005. LNCS, vol. 3749, pp. 310–318. Springer, Heidelberg (2005). https://doi.org/10.1007/11566465_39
13. Kaster, F.O., Menze, B.H., Weber, M.-A., Hamprecht, F.A.: Comparative validation of graphical models for learning tumor segmentations from noisy manual annotations. In: Menze, B., Langs, G., Tu, Z., Criminisi, A. (eds.) MCV 2010. LNCS, vol. 6533, pp. 74–85. Springer, Heidelberg (2011). https://doi.org/10.1007/978-3-642-18421-5_8
14. Fischl, B., Salat, D.H., Busa, E., et al.: Whole brain segmentation: automated labeling of neuroanatomical structures in the human brain. Neuron **33**(3), 341–355 (2002)
15. Ashburner, J., Friston, K.J.: Unified segmentation. Neuroimage **26**(3), 839–851 (2005)

16. Zacharaki, E.I., Shen, D., Lee, S.K., Davatzikos, C.: ORBIT: a multiresolution framework for deformable registration of brain tumor images. IEEE Trans. Med. Imaging **27**(8), 1003–1017 (2008)
17. Cuadra, M.B., Pollo, C., Bardera, A., et al.: Atlas-based segmentation of pathological brain MR images using a model of lesion growth. IEEE Trans. Med. Imaging **23**(10), 1301–1314 (2004)
18. Pereira, S., Pinto, A., Alves, V., Silva, C.A.: Brain tumor segmentation using convolutional neural networks in MRI images. IEEE Trans. Med. Imaging **35**(5), 1240–1251 (2016)
19. Kamnitsas, K., Ledig, C., Newcombe, V.F., et al.: Efficient multi-scale 3D CNN with fully connected CRF for accurate brain lesion segmentation. Med. Image Anal. **36**, 61–78 (2017)
20. Fedorov, A., Beichel, R., Kalpathy-Cramer, J., et al.: 3D Slicer as an image computing platform for the Quantitative Imaging Network. Magn. Reson. Imaging **30**(9), 1323–1341 (2012)
21. Jiang, J., Wu, Y., Huang, M., et al.: 3D brain tumor segmentation in multimodal MR images based on learning population- and patient-specific feature sets. Comput. Med. Imaging Graph. **37**(7–8), 512–521 (2013)
22. Zhuge, Y., Krauze, A.V., Ning, H., et al.: Brain tumor segmentation using holistically nested neural networks in MRI images. Med. Phys. **44**(10), 5234–5243 (2017)
23. Li, Y., Jia, F., Qin, J.: Brain tumor segmentation from multimodal magnetic resonance images via sparse representation. Artif. Intell. Med. **73**, 1–13 (2016)
24. Hou, L., Samaras, D., Kurc, T., et al.: Patch-based convolutional neural network for whole slide tissue image classification. In: Proceedings of the IEEE Conference on Computer Vision and Pattern Recognition, pp. 2424–2433. IEEE (2010)
25. Shelhamer, E., Long, J., Darrell, T.: Fully convolutional networks for semantic segmentation. IEEE Trans. Pattern Anal. Mach. Intell. **39**(4), 640–651 (2017)
26. Bauer, S., Nolte, L.-P., Reyes, M.: Fully automatic segmentation of brain tumor images using support vector machine classification in combination with hierarchical conditional random field regularization. In: Fichtinger, G., Martel, A., Peters, T. (eds.) MICCAI 2011. LNCS, vol. 6893, pp. 354–361. Springer, Heidelberg (2011). https://doi.org/10.1007/978-3-642-23626-6_44
27. Tustison, N.J., Shrinidhi, K.L., Wintermark, M., et al.: Optimal symmetric multimodal templates and concatenated random forests for supervised brain tumor segmentation (simplified) with ANTsR. Neuroinformatics **13**(2), 209–225 (2015)
28. Havaei, M., Jodoin, P.-M., Larochelle, H.: Efficient interactive brain tumor segmentation as within-brain kNN classification. In: 22nd International Conference on Pattern Recognition 2014, pp. 556–561. IEEE (2014)
29. Gooya, A., Pohl, K.M., Bilello, M., et al.: GLISTR: glioma image segmentation and registration. IEEE Trans. Med. Imaging **31**(10), 1941–1954 (2012)
30. Parisot, S., Duffau, H., Chemouny, S., Paragios, N.: Joint tumor segmentation and dense deformable registration of brain MR images. In: Ayache, N., Delingette, H., Golland, P., Mori, K. (eds.) MICCAI 2012. LNCS, vol. 7511, pp. 651–658. Springer, Heidelberg (2012). https://doi.org/10.1007/978-3-642-33418-4_80
31. Wels, M., Carneiro, G., Aplas, A., Huber, M., Hornegger, J., Comaniciu, D.: A discriminative model-constrained graph cuts approach to fully automated pediatric brain tumor segmentation in 3-D MRI. In: Metaxas, D., Axel, L., Fichtinger, G., Székely, G. (eds.) MICCAI 2008. LNCS, vol. 5241, pp. 67–75. Springer, Heidelberg (2008). https://doi.org/10.1007/978-3-540-85988-8_9

32. Bauer, S., Nolte, L.-P., Reyes, M.: Fully automatic segmentation of brain tumor images using support vector machine classification in combination with hierarchical conditional random field regularization. In: Fichtinger, G., Martel, A., Peters, T. (eds.) MICCAI 2011. LNCS, vol. 6893, pp. 354–361. Springer, Heidelberg (2011). https://doi.org/10.1007/978-3-642-23626-6_44

33. Wu, W., Chen, A.Y., Zhao, L., Corso, J.J.: Brain tumor detection and segmentation in a CRF (conditional random fields) framework with pixel-pairwise affinity and superpixel-level features. Int. J. Comput. Assist. Radiol. Surg. **9**(2), 241–253 (2014)

34. Rios Velazquez, E., Meier, R., Dunn Jr., W.D., et al.: Fully automatic GBM segmentation in the TCGA-GBM dataset: prognosis and correlation with VASARI features. Sci. Rep. **5**, 1–10 (2015)

35. Riklin-Raviv, T., Van Leemput, K., Menze, B.H., et al.: Segmentation of image ensembles via latent atlases. Med. Image Anal. **14**, 654–665 (2010)

36. Corso, J.J., Sharon, E., Dube, S., et al.: Efficient multilevel brain tumor segmentation with integrated Bayesian model classification. IEEE Trans. Med. Imaging **27**(5), 629–640 (2008)

37. Zikic, D., Glocker, B., et al.: Decision forests for tissue-specific segmentation of high-grade gliomas in multi-channel MR. In: Ayache, N., Delingette, H., Golland, P., Mori, K. (eds.) MICCAI 2012. LNCS, vol. 7512, pp. 369–376. Springer, Heidelberg (2012). https://doi.org/10.1007/978-3-642-33454-2_46

38. Le Folgoc, L., Nori, A.V., Ancha, S., Criminisi, A.: Lifted auto-context forests for brain tumour segmentation. In: Alessandro, C., et al. (eds.) BrainLes 2016. LNCS, vol. 10154, pp. 171–183. Springer, Heidelberg (2016)

39. Urban, G., Bendszus, M., Hamprecht, F., Kleesiek, J.: Multi-modal brain tumor segmentation using deep convolutional neural networks. In: MICCAI-BraTS 2014, pp. 31–35 (2014)

40. Menze, B.H., Jakab, A., Bauer, S., et al.: The multimodal brain tumor image segmentation benchmark (BRATS). IEEE Trans. Med. Imaging **34**(10), 1993–2024 (2015)

41. Hastie, T., Tibshirani, R., Friedman, J.: The Elements of Statistical Learning, 2nd edn. Springer, New York (2009). https://doi.org/10.1007/978-0-387-84858-7

42. Archip, N., Jolesz, F.A., Warfield, S.K.: A validation framework for brain tumor segmentation. Acad. Radiol. **14**(10), 1242–1251 (2007)

43. Bakas, S., Akbari, H., Sotiras, A., et al.: Advancing the Cancer Genome Atlas glioma MRI collections with expert segmentation labels and radiomic features. Nat. Sci. Data **4**, 170117 (2017)

44. Bakas, S., Akbari, H., Sotiras, A., et al.: Segmentation labels and radiomic features for the pre-operative scans of the TCGA-GBM collection. Cancer Imaging Arch. (2017). https://doi.org/10.7937/K9/TCIA.2017.KLXWJJ1Q

45. Bakas, S., Akbari, H., Sotiras, A., et al.: Segmentation labels and radiomic features for the pre-operative scans of the TCGA-LGG collection. Cancer Imaging Arch. (2017). https://doi.org/10.7937/K9/TCIA.2017.GJQ7R0EF

46. Verma, R., Zacharaki, E.I., Ou, Y., et al.: Multiparametric tissue characterization of brain neoplasms and their recurrence using pattern classification of MR images. Acad. Radiol. **15**(8), 966–977 (2008)

47. Cortes, C., Vapnik, V.: Support-vector networks. Mach. Learn. **20**(3), 273–297 (1995)

48. Christianini, N., Shawe-Taylor, J.: An Introduction to Support Vector Machines and Other Kernel-Based Learning Methods, 1st edn. Cambridge University Press, Cambridge (2000)

49. Fan, R.-E., Chen, P.-H., Lin, C.-J.: Working set selection using second order information for training support vector machines. J. Mach. Learn. Res. **6**, 1889–1918 (2005)

50. Schoelkopf, B., Smola, A.: Learning with Kernels: Support Vector Machines, Regularization, Optimization, and Beyond. MIT Press, Cambridge (2002)

51. Platt, J.: Sequential minimal optimization: a fast algorithm for training support vector machines. Technical report MSR-TR-98-14 (1999)
52. Platt, J.: Probabilistic outputs for support vector machines and comparisons to regularized likelihood methods. In: Smola, A.J., Bartlett, P., Schoelkopf, B., Schuurmans, D. (eds.) Advances in Large Margin Classifiers 1999, pp. 61–74. MIT Press (2000)
53. Soille, P.: Morphological Image Analysis: Principles and Applications, pp. 164–165. Springer, Heidelberg (1999). https://doi.org/10.1007/978-3-662-05088-0
54. Nyul, L.G., Udupa, J.K., Zhang, X.: New variants of a method of MRI scale standardization. IEEE Trans. Med. Imaging **19**(2), 143–150 (2000)

Ensembles of Multiple Models and Architectures for Robust Brain Tumour Segmentation

K. Kamnitsas$^{(\boxtimes)}$ ⓘ, W. Bai, E. Ferrante, S. McDonagh, M. Sinclair,
N. Pawlowski, M. Rajchl, M. Lee, B. Kainz, D. Rueckert, and B. Glocker

Biomedical Image Analysis Group, Imperial College London, London, UK
konstantinos.kamnitsas12@imperial.ac.uk

Abstract. Deep learning approaches such as convolutional neural nets have consistently outperformed previous methods on challenging tasks such as dense, semantic segmentation. However, the various proposed networks perform differently, with behaviour largely influenced by architectural choices and training settings. This paper explores Ensembles of Multiple Models and Architectures (EMMA) for robust performance through aggregation of predictions from a wide range of methods. The approach reduces the influence of the meta-parameters of individual models and the risk of overfitting the configuration to a particular database. EMMA can be seen as an unbiased, generic deep learning model which is shown to yield excellent performance, winning the first position in the BRATS 2017 competition among 50+ participating teams.

1 Introduction

Brain tumours are among the most fatal types of cancer [1]. Out of tumours that originally develop in the brain, gliomas are the most frequent [2]. They arise from glioma cells and, depending on their aggressiveness, they are broadly categorized into high and low grade gliomas [3]. High grade gliomas (HGG) develop rapidly and aggressively, forming abnormal vessels and often a necrotic core, accompanied by surrounding oedema and swelling [2]. They are malignant, with high mortality and average survival rate of less than two years even after treatment [3]. Low grade gliomas (LGG) can be benign or malignant, grow slower, but they may recur and evolve to HGG, thus their treatment is warranted. For treatment, patients undergo radiotherapy, chemotherapy and surgery [1].

Firstly for diagnosis and monitoring the tumour's progression, then for treatment planning and afterwards for assessing the effect of treatment, various neuro-imaging protocols are employed. Magnetic resonance imaging (MRI) is widely used in both clinical routine and research studies. It facilitates tumour analysis by allowing estimation of extent, location and investigation of its subcomponents [2]. This however requires accurate delineation of the tumour, which proves challenging due

---

W. Bai, E. Ferrante, S. McDonagh and M. Sinclair—Equal contribution, in alphabetical order.

ⓒ Springer International Publishing AG, part of Springer Nature 2018
A. Crimi et al. (Eds.): BrainLes 2017, LNCS 10670, pp. 450–462, 2018.
https://doi.org/10.1007/978-3-319-75238-9_38

to its complex structure and appearance, the 3D nature of the MR images and the multiple MR sequences that need to be consulted in parallel for informed judgement. These factors make manual delineation time-consuming and subject to inter- and intra-rater variability [4].

Automatic segmentation systems aim at providing an objective and scalable solution. Representative early works are the atlas-based outlier detection method [5] and the joint segmentation-registration framework, often guided by a tumour growth model [6–8]. The past few years saw rapid developments of machine learning methods, with Random Forests being among the most successful [9,10]. More recently, convolutional neural networks (CNN) have gained popularity by exhibiting very promising results for segmentation of brain tumours [11–13].

A variety of CNN architectures have been proposed, each presenting different strengths and weaknesses. Additionally, networks have a vast number of meta parameters. The multiple configuration choices for a system influence not only performance but also its behaviour (Fig. 1). For instance, different models may perform better with different types of pre-processing. Consequently, when investigating their behaviour on a given task, findings can be biased. Finally, a configuration highly optimized on a given database may be an over-fit, and not generalise to other data or tasks.

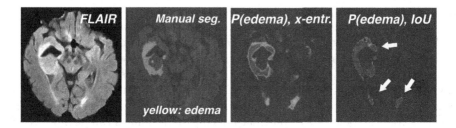

Fig. 1. Left to right: FLAIR; manual annotation of a BRATS'17 subject, where yellow depicts oedema surrounding tumour core; confidence of a CNN predicting oedema, trained with cross-entropy or IoU loss. Although overall performance is similar, training with IoU (or Dice, not shown) loss alters the CNN's behaviour, which tends to output only highly confident predictions, even when false.

In this work we push towards constructing a more *reliable* and *objective* deep learning model. We bring together a variety of CNN architectures, configured and trained in diverse ways in order to introduce high variance between them. By combining them, we construct an *Ensemble of Multiple Models and Architectures* (EMMA), with the aim of *averaging away* the variance and with it model- and configuration-specific behaviours. Our approach leads to: (1) a system robust to unpredictable failures of independent components, (2) enables objective analysis with a generic deep learning model of unbiased behaviour, (3) introduces the new perspective of *ensembling for objectiveness*. This is in contrast to common ensembles, where a single model is trained with small variations such as initial seeds, which renders the ensemble biased by the main architectural choices. As a first milestone in this endeavour, we evaluated EMMA in the Brain Tumour Segmentation (BRATS) challenge 2017. Our method won the first position in the final testing stage among 50+ competing teams. This indicates the reliability of the approach and paves the way for its use in further analysis.

2   Background: Model Bias, Variance and Ensembling

Feedforward neural networks have been shown capable of approximating any function [14]. They are thus models with zero bias, possible of no systematic error. However they are not a panacea. If left unregularized they can overfit noise in the training data, which leads to mistakes when they are called to generalise. Coupled with the stochasticity of the optimization process and the multiple local minima, this leads to unpredictable inconsistent errors between different instances. This constitutes models with high variance. Regularization reduces the variance but increases the bias, as expressed in the bias/variance dilemma [15]. Regularization can be explicit, such as weight decay that prevents networks from learning rare noisy patterns, or implicit, such as the local connectivity of CNN kernels, which however does not allow the model to learn patterns larger than the its receptive field. Architectural and configuration choices thus introduce bias, altering the behaviour of a network.

One route to address the bias/variance dilemma is ensembling. By combining multiple models, ensembling seeks to create a higher performing model with low variance. The most popular combination rule is averaging, which is not sensitive to inconsistent errors of the singletons [16]. Commonly, instances of a network trained with different initial weights or from multiple final local minima are ensembled, with the majority correcting irregular errors. Intuitively, only inconsistent errors can be averaged out. Lack of consistent failures can be interpreted as statistical independency. Thus methods for de-correlating the instances have been developed. The most popular is *bagging* [17], commonly used for random forests. It uses bootstrap sampling to learn less correlated instances from different subsets of the data.

The above works often discuss ensembling as a means of increasing performance. [18] approached high variance from the scope of *unreliability*. They discussed ensembling as a type of N-version programming, which advocates reliability through redundancy. When producing N-versions of a program, versions may fail independently but through majority voting they behave as a reliable system. They formalize intuitive requirements for reliability: (a) the target function to be covered by the ensemble and (b) the majority to be correct. This in turn advocates diversity, independence and overall quality of the components.

Biomedical applications are reliability-critical and high variance would deter the use of neural networks. For this reason we set off to investigate robustness of diverse ensembles. Diverting from the above works, we introduce another perspective of ensembling: creating an objective, configuration-invariant model to facilitate objective analysis.

3   Ensembles of Multiple Models and Architectures

A variety of CNN architectures has shown promising results in recent literature. Regarding the architectures, they commonly differ in depth, number of filters and how they process multi-scale context among others. Such architectural choices bias the model behaviour. For instance, models with large receptive fields may show improved localisation capabilities but can be less sensitive to fine texture than models emphasizing local information. Strategies to handle class imbalance is another performance relevant parameter. Common strategies are training with class-weighted sampling or class-weighted cross entropy. As analysed in [13], these methods strongly influence the sensitivity of the model to each class. Furthermore, the choice of the loss function impacts results. For example, we observed that networks trained to optimize Intersection over Union (IoU), Dice or similar losses [19] tend to give worse confidence estimations than when trained with cross entropy (Fig. 1). Finally, the setting of hyper-parameters for the optimization can strongly affect performance. It is often observed by practitioners that the choice of the optimizer and its configuration, for instance the learning rate schedule, can make the difference between bad and good segmentation.

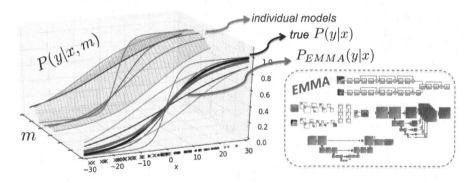

Fig. 2. Our ensemble of diverse networks, EMMA (red), averages out the bias infused by individual model configurations m, to approximate more reliably the true posterior (black), while being robust to suboptimal configurations. Posteriors on the left were obtained from multiple perceptrons, trained to classify clusters centred on 10 and −10 as a toy example, with different losses, regularizations and noise in the training labels. Their ensemble provides reliable estimates. (Color figure online)

The sensitivity to such meta-parameters is a greater problem than merely a time-consuming manual optimization of configurations:

- A configuration setting optimized on one set of training data may be overfitting them and not perform well on unseen data or another task. This can be viewed as another source of high model variance (Sect. 2).
- By biasing the behaviour of the model, it also biases the findings of any analysis performed with it.

We now formalize the problem and our perspective of ensembling as a solution as follows. Given training data X with labels Y, we need to learn the generating process $P(y|x)$. This is commonly approximated by a model $P(y|x; \theta_m, m)$, which has trainable parameters θ_m that are learnt via an optimization process that minimizes:

$$\theta_m = \min_{\theta_m} d(P(Y|X; \theta_m, m), P(Y|X)) \tag{1}$$

where d is a distance (defined by the type of loss) computed at the points given by the training data, while m represents the choice of the meta-parameters. It is commonly neglected although it conditions (biases) the learnt estimator. To take it into account, we instead define m as a stochastic variable over the space of meta-parameter configurations, with a corresponding prior $P(m)$. In order to learn a model of $P(y|x)$ unbiased by m, we marginalize out its effect:

$$P(y|x) = \sum_m P(y, m|x) = \sum_m P(y|x, m)P(m)$$

$$\approx \sum_{\forall m \in E} P(y|x; \theta_m, m) \frac{1}{|E|} = P_{EMMA}(y|x) \tag{2}$$

Here E is the set of models within the ensemble. The prior $P(m)$ is considered uniform over a subspace of m that is covered by the models in E and zero elsewhere. Note we have arrived at the standard ensembling with averaging, by considering that each individual model $P(y|x; \theta_m, m)$ approximates a conditional $P(y|x, m)$ on m, and the true posterior is approximated by the ensemble which marginalizes away effects of m. Note that the case of a single model configured by m can be derived from the above, by setting a dirac prior $P(m) = \delta(m)$. Thus the ensemble relaxes a pre-existing neglected strong prior.

The above formulation presents averaging ensembles from a new perspective: The marginalization over a subspace of the joint $P(y|x, m)$ offers generalisation, regularising the (manual) optimization process of m from falling into minima where $P(Y|X, m)$ overfits $P(Y|X)$ on the given training data (Y, X) (Fig. 2). Moreover, the process leads to a more objective approximation of $P(y|x)$ where the biasing effect of m has been marginalized out. The exposed limitations agree with the requirements for ensembling mentioned in Sect. 2: we need to restrict the subspace of m into an area of relatively high quality models and we need to cover it with a relatively small number of models, thus diversity is key.

In the remainder of this section we describe the main properties of the models used to construct the collection E of EMMA, which cover various contemporary architectures, configured and trained under different settings[1].

3.1 DeepMedic

Model description: We include two DeepMedics in EMMA. The main architecture, originally presented in [13,20], is a fully 3D, multi-scale CNN, designed

---

[1] Implementation and configuration details considered less important for this work were omitted to avoid cluttering the manuscript.

with a focus on efficient processing of 3D images. For this it employs parallel pathways, with the secondary taking as input down-sampled context, thus avoiding to convolve large volumes at full resolution to remain computationally cheap. Although originally developed for segmenting brain lesions, it was found promising on diverse tasks, such as segmentation of placenta [21], making it a good component for a robust ensemble. The first of the two models we used is the residual version previously employed in BRATS 2016 [22], depicted in Fig. 3. The second is a wider variant, with double the number of filters at each layer.

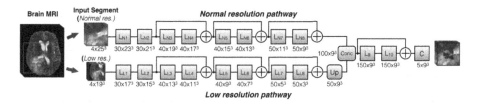

Fig. 3. We used two DeepMedics [13] in our experiments. The smaller of the two is depicted, where the number of feature maps and their dimension at every layer are depicted in the format ($Number \times Size$). The second model used in the ensemble is wider, with double the number of feature maps at every layer. All kernels and feature maps are 3D, even though not depicted for simplicity.

Configuration: The models are trained by extracting multi-scale image segments with a 50% probability centred on healthy tissue and 50% probability on tumour as proposed in [13]. The wider variant is trained on larger inputs, of width 34 and 22 for the two scales respectively. Both are trained with cross-entropy loss. All other meta-parameters were adopted from the original configuration.

3.2 FCN

Model description: We integrate three 3D FCNs [23] in EMMA. A schematic of the first architecture is depicted in Fig. 4. The second FCN is constructed larger, replacing each convolutional layer with a residual block with two convolutions. The third is also residual-based, but with one less down-sampling step. All layers use batch normalisation, ReLUs and zero-padding.

Training details: We draw training patches of width 64 for the first and 80 voxels for the residual-based FCNs, with an equal probability from each label. They were trained using Adam. The first was trained to optimize the IoU loss [19] while the Dice was used similarly for the other two. The trained models are then applied fully convolutionally on whole volumes for inference.

3.3 U-Net

Model description: We employ two 3D versions of the U-Net architecture [24] in our ensemble. The main elements of the first architecture are depicted in Fig. 5.

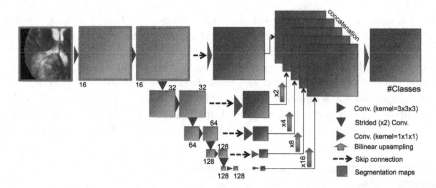

Fig. 4. Schematic of one of the FCN architecture used in EMMA. Shown are number of feature maps per layer. All kernels and feature maps are 3D, even though not depicted for simplicity.

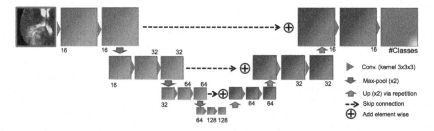

Fig. 5. Schematic of an adapted Unet used in our experiments. Depicted are number of feature maps per layer. All kernels and feature maps are 3D, even though not depicted for simplicity.

In this version we follow the strategy suggested in [25] to reduce model complexity, where skip connections are implemented via summations of the signals in the up-sampling part of the network, instead of the concatenation originally used. The second architecture is similar but concatenates the skip connections and uses strided convolutions instead of max pooling. All layers use batch normalisation, ReLUs and zero-padding.

Training Details: The U-Nets were trained with input patches of size $64 \times 64 \times 64$. The patches were sampled only from within the brain, with equal probability being centred around a voxel from each of the four labels. They were trained minimizing cross entropy via AdaDelta and Adam respectively, with different optimization, regularization and augmentation meta-parameters. The trained models are then applied fully convolutionally on whole volumes for inference.

3.4   Ensembling

The above models are all trained completely separately. At testing time, each model segments individually an unseen image and outputs its class-confidence maps. The models are then ensembled into EMMA, according to Eq. 2. For this, the ensemble's confidence maps for each class are created by calculating for each voxel the average class confidence of the individual models. The final segmentation is made by assigning to each voxel the class with the highest confidence.

3.5   Implementation Details

The original implementation of DeepMedic was used for the corresponding two models, available on https://biomedia.doc.ic.ac.uk/software/deepmedic/. The FCNs were implemented using DLTK, a deep learning library with a focus on medical imaging applications that allowed quick implementation and experimentation (https://github.com/DLTK/DLTK). Finally, an adaptation of the Unet will be released on https://gitlab.com/eferrante.

4   Evaluation

4.1   Material

Our system was evaluated on the data from the Brain Tumour Segmentation Challenge 2017 (BRATS) [4,26–28]. The training set consists of 210 cases with high grade glioma (HGG) and 75 cases with low grade glioma (LGG), for which manual segmentations are provided. The segmentations include the following tumour tissue labels: (1) necrotic core and non enhancing tumour, (2) oedema, (4) enhancing core. Label 3 is not used. The validation set consists of 46 cases, both HGG and LGG but the grade is not revealed. Reference segmentations for the validation set are hidden and evaluation is carried out via an online system that allows multiple submissions. In the testing phase of the competition, a test set of 146 cases is provided to the teams, and the teams have a 48 hours window for a single submission to the system. For evaluation, the 3 predicted labels are merged into different sets of whole tumour (all labels), the core (labels 1,4) and the enhancing tumour (label 4). For each subject, four MRI sequences are available, FLAIR, T1, T1 contrast enhanced (T1ce) and T2. The datasets are pre-processed by the organisers and provided as skull-stripped, registered to a common space and resampled to isotropic $1\,\text{mm}^3$ resolution. Dimensions of each volume are $240 \times 240 \times 155$.

4.2   Ensembling Multiple Pre-processing Methods

We experimented with three different versions of intensity normalisation as pre-processing: (1) Z-score normalisation of each modality of each case individually, with the mean and stdev of the brain intensities. (2) Bias field correction followed by (1). (3) Bias field correction, followed by piece-wise linear normalisation [29], followed by (1). Preliminary comparisons were inconclusive. We instead chose to average away the normalisation's effect with EMMA. For each of the seven networks in Sect. 3, three instances were trained, each on data processed with different normalisation. They were applied to correspondingly processed images for inference and all results were averaged in EMMA (Fig. 6).

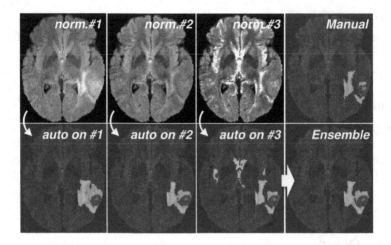

Fig. 6. Results are affected by normalization. To make a system robust to this factor, we introduce in EMMA models trained on differently normalized data.

4.3   Post-processing

The segmentations from EMMA were finally post-processed by removing secondary connected-components smaller than 250 voxels.

4.4   Results

We provide the results that EMMA achieved on the validation and testing set of the BRATS'17 challenge[2] on Table 1. Our system won the competition by achieving the overall best performance in the testing phase, based on Dice score (DSC) and Haussdorf distance. We also show results achieved on the validation set by the teams that ranked in the next two positions at the testing stage.

Table 1. Performance of EMMA on the validation and test sets of BRATS 2017 (submission id biomedia1). Our system achieved the top segmentation performance in the testing stage of the competition. For comparison we show the performance on validation set of the teams that ranked in the next two position. Performance of other teams in the testing stage is not available to us.

	DSC			Sensitivity			Hausdorff_95			#submits
	Enh.	Whole	Core	Enh.	Whole	Core	Enh.	Whole	Core	
EMMA (val)	73.8	90.1	79.7	78.3	89.5	76.2	4.50	4.23	6.56	2
UCL-TIG (val)	78.6	90.5	83.8	77.1	91.5	82.2	3.28	3.89	6.48	21
MIC_DKFZ (val)	73.2	89.6	79.7	79.0	89.6	78.1	4.55	6.97	9.48	2
EMMA (test)	72.9	88.6	78.5	–	–	–	36.0	5.01	23.1	1

[2] Leaderboard: https://www.cbica.upenn.edu/BraTS17/lboardValidation.html.

No testing-phase metrics are available to us for these methods. We note that EMMA achieves similar levels of performance on validation and test sets, even though the latter contains data from different sources, indicating the robustness of the method. In comparison, competing methods were very good fits for the validation set, but did not manage to retain the same levels on the testing set. This emphasizes the importance of research towards robust and reliable systems.

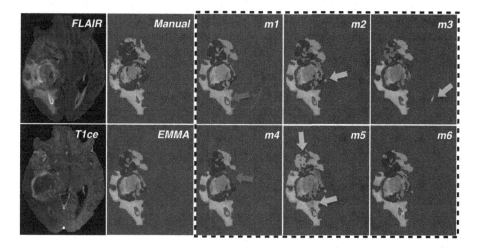

Fig. 7. FLAIR, T1ce and manual annotation of a case in the training set, along with automatic segmentation from preliminary version of EMMA consisting of six models. Green arrows point inconsistent mistakes by the individual models that are corrected by ensembling, while red arrows show consistent mistakes. (Color figure online)

5   Conclusion

Neural networks have been proven very potent, yet imperfect estimators, often making unpredictable errors. Biomedical applications are reliability-critical however. For this reason we first concentrate on improving robustness. Towards this goal we introduced EMMA, an ensemble of widely varying CNNs. By combining a heterogeneous collection of networks we construct a model that is insensitive to independent failures of CNN components and thus generalises well (Fig. 7). We also introduced the new perspective of ensembling for objectiveness. Biased behaviour, introduced by configuration choices, is marginalised out via ensembling, making EMMA a model more fit for objective analysis. Even though the individual networks in this work have straight-forward architectures and were not optimized for the task, EMMA won first place in the final testing stage of the BRATS 2017 challenge among 50+ teams, indicating strong generalisation.

By being robust to suboptimal configurations of its components, EMMA may offer re-usability on different tasks, which we aim to explore in the future. EMMA may also prove useful for unbiased investigation of factors such as sensitivity of CNNs to different sources of domain shift that affect large-scale studies [30]. Finally, EMMA's uncertainty could serve as a more objective measure of what type of tumours are most challenging to learn.

Computational requirements of ensembles increase with their size. Inference time is commonly of interest. Conveniently, EMMA's models can be parallelised. If multiple GPUs are not available, parallelisation on CPUs may also be practical. As an indication, segmentation of a brain scan with DeepMedic takes five minutes on a single CPU thread. Thus parallelising EMMA's components on different threads allows practical inference times for various applications on modern workstations and CPU cluster. Where computational and storage requirements need to be minimal, knowledge distillation offers an attractive solution [31].

Acknowledgements. This work is supported by the EPSRC (EP/N023668/1, EP/N024494/1 and EP/P001009/1) and partially funded under the 7th Framework Programme by the European Commission (CENTER-TBI: https://www.center-tbi. eu/). KK is supported by the President's PhD Scholarship of Imperial College London. EF is beneficiary of an AXA Research Fund postdoctoral grant. NP is supported by Microsoft Research through its PhD Scholarship Programme and the EPSRC Centre for Doctoral Training in High Performance Embedded and Distributed Systems (HiPEDS, Grant Reference EP/L016796/1). We gratefully acknowledge the support of NVIDIA with the donation of GPUs for our research.

References

1. DeAngelis, L.M.: Brain tumors. N. Engl. J. Med. **344**(2), 114–123 (2001)
2. Bauer, S., Wiest, R., Nolte, L.P., Reyes, M.: A survey of MRI-based medical image analysis for brain tumor studies. Phys. Med. Biol. **58**(13), R97 (2013)
3. Louis, D., et al.: The 2016 world health organization classification of tumors of the central nervous system: a summary. Acta Neuropathol. **131**(6), 803–820 (2016)
4. Menze, B.H., Jakab, A., Bauer, S., Kalpathy-Cramer, J., Farahani, K., Kirby, J., Burren, Y., Porz, N., Slotboom, J., Wiest, R., et al.: The multimodal brain tumor image segmentation benchmark (BRATS). IEEE TMI **34**(10), 1993–2024 (2015)
5. Prastawa, M., Bullitt, E., Ho, S., Gerig, G.: A brain tumor segmentation framework based on outlier detection. Med. Image Anal. **8**(3), 275–283 (2004)
6. Gooya, A., Pohl, K.M., Bilello, M., Biros, G., Davatzikos, C.: Joint segmentation and deformable registration of brain scans guided by a tumor growth model. In: Fichtinger, G., Martel, A., Peters, T. (eds.) MICCAI 2011. LNCS, vol. 6892, pp. 532–540. Springer, Heidelberg (2011). https://doi.org/10.1007/978-3-642-23629-7_65
7. Parisot, S., Duffau, H., Chemouny, S., Paragios, N.: Joint tumor segmentation and dense deformable registration of brain MR images. In: Ayache, N., Delingette, H., Golland, P., Mori, K. (eds.) MICCAI 2012. LNCS, vol. 7511, pp. 651–658. Springer, Heidelberg (2012). https://doi.org/10.1007/978-3-642-33418-4_80
8. Bakas, S., et al.: GLISTRboost: combining multimodal MRI segmentation, registration, and biophysical tumor growth modeling with gradient boosting machines for glioma segmentation. In: Crimi, A., Menze, B., Maier, O., Reyes, M., Handels, H. (eds.) BrainLes 2015. LNCS, vol. 9556, pp. 144–155. Springer, Cham (2016). https://doi.org/10.1007/978-3-319-30858-6_13

9. Zikic, D., et al.: Decision forests for tissue-specific segmentation of high-grade gliomas in multi-channel MR. In: Ayache, N., Delingette, H., Golland, P., Mori, K. (eds.) MICCAI 2012. LNCS, vol. 7512, pp. 369–376. Springer, Heidelberg (2012). https://doi.org/10.1007/978-3-642-33454-2_46

10. Le Folgoc, L., Nori, A.V., Ancha, S., Criminisi, A.: Lifted auto-context forests for brain tumour segmentation. In: Crimi, A., Menze, B., Maier, O., Reyes, M., Winzeck, S., Handels, H. (eds.) BrainLes 2016. LNCS, vol. 10154, pp. 171–183. Springer, Cham (2016). https://doi.org/10.1007/978-3-319-55524-9_17

11. Urban, G., Bendszus, M., Hamprecht, F., Kleesiek, J.: Multi-modal brain tumor segmentation using deep convolutional neural networks. In: BRATS-MICCAI (2014)

12. Pereira, S., Pinto, A., Alves, V., Silva, C.A.: Brain tumor segmentation using convolutional neural networks in MRI images. IEEE TMI **35**(5), 1240–1251 (2016)

13. Kamnitsas, K., Ledig, C., Newcombe, V.F., Simpson, J.P., Kane, A.D., Menon, D.K., Rueckert, D., Glocker, B.: Efficient multi-scale 3D CNN with fully connected CRF for accurate brain lesion segmentation. Med. Image Anal. **36**, 61–78 (2017)

14. Hornik, K., Stinchcombe, M., White, H.: Multilayer feedforward networks are universal approximators. Neural Netw. **2**(5), 359–366 (1989)

15. Geman, S., Bienenstock, E., Doursat, R.: Neural networks and the bias/variance dilemma. Neural Netw. **4**(1), 1–58 (2008)

16. Kittler, J., Hatef, M., Duin, R.P., Matas, J.: On combining classifiers. IEEE Trans. Pattern Anal. Mach. Intell. **20**(3), 226–239 (1998)

17. Breiman, L.: Bagging predictors. Mach. Learn. **24**(2), 123–140 (1996)

18. Sharkey, A.J., Sharkey, N.E.: Combining diverse neural nets. Knowl. Eng. Rev. **12**(3), 231–247 (1997)

19. Nowozin, S.: Optimal decisions from probabilistic models: the intersection-over-union case. In: CVPR, pp. 548–555 (2014)

20. Kamnitsas, K., Chen, L., Ledig, C., Rueckert, D., Glocker, B.: Multi-scale 3D convolutional neural networks for lesion segmentation in brain MRI. In: Proceedings of ISLES-MICCAI (2015)

21. Alansary, A., et al.: Fast fully automatic segmentation of the human placenta from motion corrupted MRI. In: Ourselin, S., Joskowicz, L., Sabuncu, M.R., Unal, G., Wells, W. (eds.) MICCAI 2016. LNCS, vol. 9901, pp. 589–597. Springer, Cham (2016). https://doi.org/10.1007/978-3-319-46723-8_68

22. Kamnitsas, K., Ferrante, E., Parisot, S., Ledig, C., Nori, A.V., Criminisi, A., Rueckert, D., Glocker, B.: DeepMedic for brain tumor segmentation. In: Crimi, A., Menze, B., Maier, O., Reyes, M., Winzeck, S., Handels, H. (eds.) BrainLes 2016. LNCS, vol. 10154, pp. 138–149. Springer, Cham (2016). https://doi.org/10.1007/978-3-319-55524-9_14

23. Long, J., et al.: Fully convolutional networks for semantic segmentation. In: CVPR, pp. 3431–3440 (2015)

24. Ronneberger, O., Fischer, P., Brox, T.: U-Net: convolutional networks for biomedical image segmentation. In: Navab, N., Hornegger, J., Wells, W.M., Frangi, A.F. (eds.) MICCAI 2015. LNCS, vol. 9351, pp. 234–241. Springer, Cham (2015). https://doi.org/10.1007/978-3-319-24574-4_28

25. Guerrero, R., Qin, C., Oktay, O., Bowles, C., Chen, L., Joules, R., Wolz, R., Valdes-Hernandez, M., et al.: White matter hyperintensity and stroke lesion segmentation and differentiation using convolutional neural networks. arXiv:1706.00935 (2017)

26. Bakas, S., Akbari, H., Sotiras, A., Bilello, M., Rozycki, M., Kirby, J., Freymann, J., Farahani, K., Davatzikos, C.: Advancing the cancer genome atlas glioma MRI collections with expert segmentation labels and radiomic features. Nat. Sci. Data **4**, 170117 (2017)
27. Bakas, S., Akbari, H., Sotiras, A., Bilello, M., Rozycki, M., Kirby, J., Freymann, J., Farahani, K., Davatzikos, C.: Segmentation labels and radiomic features for the pre-operative scans of the TCGA-GBM collection. The Cancer Imaging Archive (2017)
28. Bakas, S., Akbari, H., Sotiras, A., Bilello, M., Rozycki, M., Kirby, J., Freymann, J., Farahani, K., Davatzikos, C.: Segmentation labels and radiomic features for the pre-operative scans of the TCGA-LGG collection. The Cancer Imaging Archive (2017)
29. Nyúl, L.G., Udupa, J.K., Zhang, X.: New variants of a method of MRI scale standardization. IEEE TMI **19**(2), 143–150 (2000)
30. Kamnitsas, K., et al.: Unsupervised domain adaptation in brain lesion segmentation with adversarial networks. In: Niethammer, M., Styner, M., Aylward, S., Zhu, H., Oguz, I., Yap, P.-T., Shen, D. (eds.) IPMI 2017. LNCS, vol. 10265, pp. 597–609. Springer, Cham (2017). https://doi.org/10.1007/978-3-319-59050-9_47
31. Bucilu, C., Caruana, R., Niculescu-Mizil, A.: Model compression. In: Knowledge Discovery and Data Mining, pp. 535–541. ACM (2006)

Tumor Segmentation from Multimodal MRI Using Random Forest with Superpixel and Tensor Based Feature Extraction

H. N. Bharath[1,2(✉)], S. Colleman[3], D. M. Sima[1,2], and S. Van Huffel[1,2]

[1] Department of Electrical Engineering (ESAT), STADIUS Center for Dynamical Systems, Signal Processing and Data Analytics, KU Leuven, Leuven, Belgium
Bharath.HalandurNagaraja@esat.kuleuven.be
[2] Imec, Leuven, Belgium
[3] Department of Electrical Engineering (ESAT), KU Leuven, Leuven, Belgium

Abstract. Identification and localization of brain tumor tissues plays an important role in diagnosis and treatment planning of gliomas. A fully automated superpixel wise two-stage tumor tissue segmentation algorithm using random forest is proposed in this paper. First stage is used to identify total tumor and the second stage to segment sub-regions. Features for random forest classifier are extracted by constructing a tensor from multimodal MRI data and applying multi-linear singular value decomposition. The proposed method is tested on BRATS 2017 validation and test dataset. The first stage model has a Dice score of 83% for the whole tumor on the validation dataset. The total model achieves a performance of 77%, 50% and 61% Dice scores for whole tumor, enhancing tumor and tumor core, respectively on the test dataset.

Keywords: Superpixel · Multilinear singular value decomposition
Random forest · MRI · Tumor segmentation

1 Introduction

Accurate characterisation and localization of tissue types plays a key role in brain tumor diagnosis and treatment planning. Neuro-imaging methods in particular magnetic resonance imaging (MRI) provide anatomical and pathophysiological information about brain tumors and aid in diagnosis, treatment planning and follow-up of patients. Manual segmentation of tumor tissue is a tedious and time consuming job, it also suffers from inter and intra-rater variability. An automated brain tumor segmentation algorithm will help to overcome those problems. However, automation of brain tumor tissue segmentation is a difficult problem and often fails when applied on MRI images from different centres/scanners.

Superpixels are gaining popularity in image segmentation algorithms, and have also been used in the context of brain tumor segmentation from MRI [1]. Performing superpixel-level image segmentation offers certain advantages over pixel-level segmentation like spatial smoothness, capturing image redundancy

© Springer International Publishing AG, part of Springer Nature 2018
A. Crimi et al. (Eds.): BrainLes 2017, LNCS 10670, pp. 463–473, 2018.
https://doi.org/10.1007/978-3-319-75238-9_39

and reducing computational complexity [1,2]. Recently, tensor decompositions such as the canonical polyadic decomposition and the multilinear singular value decomposition (MLSVD) [3] have been used to extract features from high-dimensional data to use in classification algorithms [4]. MLSVD is the generalization of the matrix singular value decomposition, where the tensor is decomposed into a "all-orthogonal" core tensor multiplied by orthogonal factor matrices along each mode [5]. The factor matrices contain orthonormal bases for their respective modes. Multimodal MRI consisting of T2, T1, T1+contrast and FLAIR imaging after co-registration and re-sampling to the same resolution, can be naturally represented as a 3-D tensor. In this paper we develop a fully automatic tumor tissue segmentation algorithm using a random forest classifier, where both superpixel-level image segmentation and tensor decomposition methods are combined to extract features for the classifier.

2   Method

2.1   Preprocessing

First, each individual 3D image is scaled to the range: 0–1. Next, intensities are normalized by applying histogram equalization. A reference histogram is generated by selecting 10 random images from the training set and extracting a histogram from the combined image. Histogram equalization is applied separately to different modalities. Background is removed from each slice using Ostu's image threshold method [6].

2.2   Feature Extraction

The MR images are divided into smaller patches which are better aligned with intensity edges, called superpixels [7]. The superpixels are generated from each slice from one of the modalities as shown in Fig. 1. The tissue assignment is done on superpixel-level instead of individual pixel, which helps to reduce computational cost and improve spatial smoothness [1].

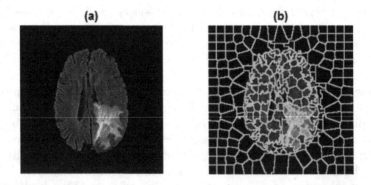

Fig. 1. (a) One slice of the FLAIR image. (b) Generated superpixels for the slice in (a).

Different features extracted from each superpixel are explained below

- Feature1: Mean intensity values of all the 4 modalities and 6 difference images (e.g.: abs(T1-T2)) over each superpixel.
- Feature2: Entropy and standard deviation over each superpixel.
- Feature3: A 3-D tensor is constructed for each superpixel, where the frontal slices are the covariance matrix of pixel-level features and the third mode is the modality and the difference images of the modalities. Pixel-level features consist of mean, median, standard deviation and entropy over a 5×5 window. Features are extracted by applying a rank-2 truncated multilinear singular value decomposition (MLSVD) on the 3D Tensor as shown in Fig. 2.
- Feature4: A 4-D tensor is constructed for each superpixel where the first two modes are 5×5 image patches with the main voxel at the centre, third mode consists of image patches from all four modalities (T1, T2, T1C and FLAIR) and patches from six difference images of the modalities (abs(T1-T2), abs(T1-T1C), abs(T1-FLAIR), abs(T1C-T2), abs(T1C-FLAIR), abs(T2-FLAIR)) and the fourth mode consists of voxels within the superpixel. Again MLSVD is used for feature extraction. Only the mode-1, mode-2, mode-3 and the core tensor are used as feature.
- Feature5: A 3-D tensor is constructed for each superpixel, where the first mode is the pixels from 5×5 image patches with the main voxel at the centre, the second mode is the modality and the difference images (e.g.: abs(T1-T2)) of the modalities and the third mode consists of the voxels within the superpixel. Again, features are extracted by applying rank-2 MLSVD. Only the mode-1, mode-2 and core tensor are used as feature.

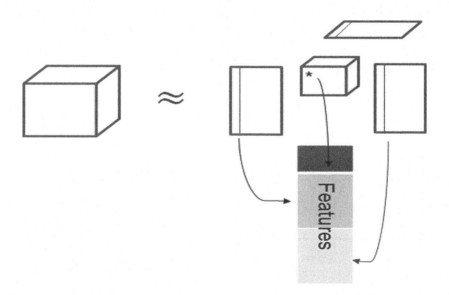

Fig. 2. Truncated multilinear singular value decomposition and feature extraction.

- Feature6: For each superpixel a covariance matrix is estimated from the intensity values of all the modalities and the difference images. Covariance matrix plus two dominant eigenvectors and eigenvalues are used as features.
- Feature7: Local spectral histograms which are texture descriptors based on local distribution of filter responses [8] are estimated for all 4 modalities and 6 difference images. A 3D tensor is constructed for each superpixel, where the first mode includes local spectral histograms, second mode is the modality and the difference images of the modalities and the third mode consists of the voxels within the superpixel. Features are extracted by applying rank-2 MLSVD. Only the mode-1, mode-2 and core tensor are used as feature. The mean of the local spectral histograms over the superpixel are also used along with the MLSVD features.

2.3   Training and Tissue Segmentation

Tumor tissue segmentation was performed using a two-stage classifier. In the first stage a binary classification was performed on the superpixels to segment tumor and non-tumor regions. In the second-stage a multi-class classification was performed on the superpixels which are inside the estimated tumor region to segment enhancing tumor (ET), edema (ED), necrotic and non-enhancing tumor (NCR/NET) and healthy tissue. The two-stage operation is demonstrated in Fig. 3. For both stages a random forest classifier was used.

First Stage: In the first stage, superpixels are obtained from FLAIR because the total tumor is brighter in this modality. The feature set for this stage consists of Feature1, Feature2, Feature3 and Feature4. The dataset is divided in three groups, and random forest classifiers with 100 trees are trained from each group.

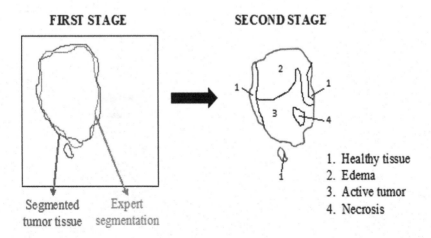

Fig. 3. Demonstration of whole tumor segmentation in first stage and sub-tissue segmentation in second stage.

The prediction is result from majority voting of the classifiers learned from three data groups. For each model training is done iteratively, where a class balanced subset from the respective group is used for initial training. Next the trained model is tested on the remaining data from the respective group, the data that are classified wrongly are added to the initial subset and trained again with 100 tree random forest binary classifier. After the first stage classification at superpixel level, image filling and continuity-based denoising developed by [9] is performed on the whole tumor segmentation before going to the second stage.

Second Stage: In the second stage, superpixels are obtained from T1+contrast imaging modality because the enhancing tumor is brighter in this modality. Feature1, Feature5, Feature6 and Feature7 are used as features in this stage. Random forest classifiers with 250 trees are trained using a iterative method. Initially, 60 patients are randomly selected from the dataset for training and the trained model is tested on the remaining subset of the database. Next, the patients which resulted in low Dice scores are included in the training set and a new model is trained. This is continued until all the patients in the dataset are used. Initially, the training is started with balanced data. The list of all features with its corresponding dimension and the stage where they are used is shown Table 1.

Table 1. Features used in stage one and stage two along with there corresponding dimension.

	Feature1	Feature2	Feature3	Feature4	Feature5	Feature6	Feature7
Dimension	10	20	36	48	78	122	196
Stage One	✓	✓	✓	✓	X	X	X
Stage Two	✓	X	X	X	✓	✓	✓

3   Results and Discussion

3.1   First Stage: Whole Tumor Segmentation

A first stage model with three classifiers was trained using the BRATS 2017 training database [10–13] containing 210 HGG and 75 LGG patients. The performance of the trained model in segmenting the whole tumor is tested on the validation dataset of BRATS 2017 challenge. Average Dice score and sensitivity obtained from the trained first stage model over 46 HGG patients are shown in Table 2. The boxplots of the Dice scores and sensitivity are shown in Fig. 4.

Table 2. Mean, standard deviation, median 25 quantile and 75 quantile of Dice score and sensitivity for whole tumor (WT) over 46 patients using only first stage model.

	Dice WT	Sensitivity WT
Mean	0.8330	0.8574
Std	0.1186	0.1318
Median	0.8673	0.9024
25 quantile	0.8298	0.8114
75 quantile	0.9084	0.9415

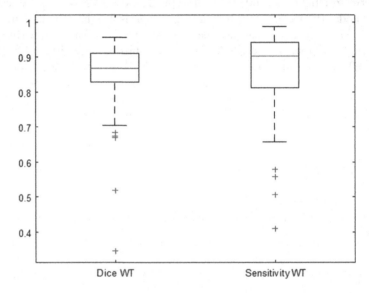

Fig. 4. Boxplots of Dice scores and sensitivity for whole tumor (WT) obtained from first stage model on BRATS 2017 validation dataset of 46 patients.

3.2   High Grade Glioma

The BRATS 2017 high grade glioma database [10–13] containing 210 patients is split into training set (70%) and test set (30%). A first stage model with a single classifier plus the second stage model is trained using only HGG and the trained model is tested on 63 HGG patients. Figure 5 shows the segmentation of tumor tissue for two different slices. We can observe from the figure that the enhancing tumor and edema region are segmented properly. However the NCR/NET region is not identified properly.

   The boxplot of the Dice scores is shown in Fig. 6 and the average Dice score and sensitivity obtained from the trained model for 63 HGG patients are shown in Table 3. From the boxplot, we can observe that the algorithm performs well on most of the patients. However there are still some patients where the algorithm fails to segment properly.

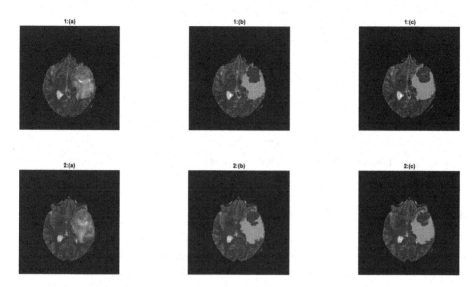

Fig. 5. Segmentation results on two slices 1–2. (a) T2 image of one slice, (b) Estimated segmentation (c) Expert segmentation. Green-Edema, Brown-enhancing tumor and Blue-Necrosis. (Color figure online)

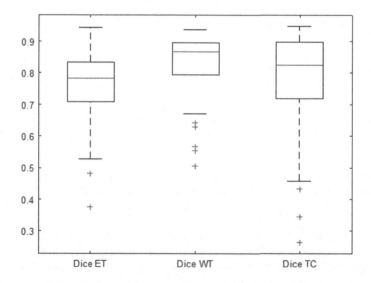

Fig. 6. Boxplots of Dice scores for enhancing tumor (ET), whole tumor (WT) and tumor core (TC) on BRATS 2017 training dataset of 63 patients.

Table 3. Mean, standard deviation, median 25 quantile and 75 quantile of Dice score and sensitivity for enhancing tumor (ET), whole tumor (WT) and tumor core (TC) over 63 HGG patients.

	Dice ET	Dice WT	Dice TC	Sensitivity ET	Sensitivity WT	Sensitivity TC
Mean	0.761	0.833	0.783	0.855	0.815	0.777
Std	0.106	0.096	0.147	0.126	0.090	0.191
Median	0.783	0.867	0.824	0.886	0.837	0.826
25 quantile	0.708	0.795	0.723	0.820	0.769	0.721
75 quantile	0.833	0.895	0.898	0.941	0.884	0.908

3.3   Validation and Test Dataset Results

The trained model consisting of both first and second stage is also tested on the BRATS 2017 validation dataset [10–13]. The results are shown in Fig. 7 and Table 4. The performance is worse when compared to only HGG case.

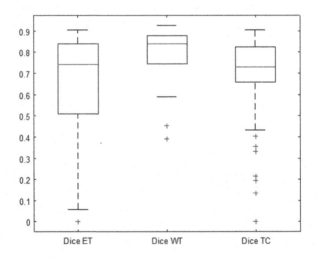

Fig. 7. Boxplots of Dice scores for enhancing tumor (ET), whole tumor (WT) and tumor core (TC) on BRATS 2017 validation dataset of 46 patients.

This algorithm does not identify necrotic and non-enhancing tumor (NCR/NET) tissue properly, it results in bad performance for LGG patients where NCR/NET tissue is larger than enhancing tumor in most cases. Also, when there is no enhancing tumor in patients, the algorithm identifies it falsely in some superpixels. This results in Dice score of zero for enhancing tumor, which can be seen from the boxplot in Fig. 7. Post-processing methods to remove such false positives may improve the average performance.

Table 4. Mean, standard deviation, median 25 quantile and 75 quantile of Dice score and sensitivity for enhancing tumor (ET), whole tumor (WT) and tumor core (TC) over 46 validation dataset.

	Dice ET	Dice WT	Dice TC	Sensitivity ET	Sensitivity WT	Sensitivity TC
Mean	0.6125	0.7928	0.6734	0.6971	0.8320	0.6763
Std	0.3013	0.1217	0.2215	0.2347	0.1221	0.2297
Median	0.7419	0.8410	0.7291	0.7683	0.8614	0.6921
25 quantile	0.5240	0.7441	0.6607	0.6365	0.8053	0.5961
75 quantile	0.8383	0.8788	0.8213	0.8468	0.9169	0.8482

Finally the complete algorithm is applied on BRATS 2017 test dataset consisting of 146 patients. The average results are shown in Table 5.

Table 5. Mean, standard deviation, median 25 quantile and 75 quantile of Dice score and Hausdorff95 for enhancing tumor (ET), whole tumor (WT) and tumor core (TC) over test dataset of 146 patients.

	Dice ET	Dice WT	Dice TC	Hausdorff95 ET	Hausdorff95 WT	Hausdorff95 TC
Mean	0.5032	0.7701	0.6105	71.27	31.33	38.90
Std	0.3054	0.1871	0.2954	132.94	30.61	84.13
Median	0.6376	0.8400	0.7416	6.56	14.56	9.56
25 quantile	0.2137	0.7202	0.4597	3.70	4.69	6.48
75 quantile	0.7447	0.8902	0.8358	39.46	54.40	29.73

4   Conclusion

In this paper, we developed a fully automated algorithm for brain tumor segmentation from multimodal MRI data. Superpixels and a tensor based feature extraction algorithm is proposed to be used with a two-stage random forest classifier for segmenting tumor tissue. The superpixels are restricted to 2-D slices because of the different resolution in the third dimension. In future work, the 2-D superpixels can be directly extended to 3D provided the difference in resolution is considered when constructing superpixels. The performance of the algorithm is comparable to the state-of-the-art methods when applied only to HGG patients. However, its performance deteriorates when tested on the BRATS 2017 validation and test database, which contains both low grade glioma (LGG) and HGG patients. The proposed superpixel method has good performance in segmenting the whole tumor using only the first stage model on the BRATS 2017 validation set. However, this method does not perform well in segmenting the sub-regions, specifically the NCR/NET region. We assume that the features may not be discriminant enough to separate the NCR/NET region from others (mainly normal). In future work, identification of the NCR/NET region can be improved by using texture based features like Gabor and applying feature selection for selecting dominant and removing redundant features. Therefore, the proposed method is more suited to segment the whole tumor and not good in identifying sub-regions, especially in LGG patients.

Acknowledgment. This research was supported by: Flemish Government FWO project G.0869.12N (Tumor imaging), G.0830.14N (Block term decompositions); IWT IM 135005; imec funds 2017; imec ICON project: ICON HBC.2016.0167, 'SeizeIT', #316679 and ERC Advanced Grant. The research leading to these results has received funding from the European Research Council under the European Union's Seventh Framework Programme (FP7/2007-2013)/ERC Advanced Grant: BIOTENSORS (no 339804). This paper reflects only the author's views and the Union is not liable for any use that may be made of the contained information.

References

1. Wu, W., Chen, A.Y., Zhao, L., Corso, J.J.: Brain tumor detection and segmentation in a CRF (conditional random fields) framework with pixel-pairwise affinity and superpixel-level features. Int. J. Comput. Assist. Radiol. Surg. **9**(2), 241–253 (2014)
2. Jia, S., Zhang, C.: Fast and robust image segmentation using an superpixel based FCM algorithm. In: 2014 IEEE International Conference on Image Processing (ICIP). IEEE (2014)
3. Sidiropoulos, N.D., De Lathauwer, L., Fu, X., Huang, K., Papalexakis, E.E., Faloutsos, C.: Tensor decomposition for signal processing and machine learning. IEEE Trans. Signal Process. **65**(13), 3551–3582 (2017)
4. Fargeas, A., Albera, L., Kachenoura, A., Dréan, G., Ospina, J.D., Coloigner, J., Lafond, C., Delobel, J.B., De Crevoisier, R., Acosta, O.: On feature extraction and classification in prostate cancer radiotherapy using tensor decompositions. Med. Eng. Phys. **37**(1), 126–131 (2015)
5. De Lathauwer, L., De Moor, B., Vandewalle, J.: A multilinear singular value decomposition. SIAM J. Matrix Anal. Appl. **21**(4), 1253–1278 (2000)
6. Otsu, N.: A threshold selection method from gray-level histograms. IEEE Trans. Syst. Man. Cybern. **9**(1), 62–66 (1979)
7. Achanta, R., Shaji, A., Smith, K., Lucchi, A., Fua, P., Süsstrunk, S.: SLIC superpixels compared to state-of-the-art superpixel methods. IEEE Trans. Pattern Anal. Mach. Intell. **34**(11), 2274–2282 (2012)
8. Liu, X., Wang, D.: A spectral histogram model for texton modeling and texture discrimination. Vis. Res. **42**(23), 2617–2634 (2002)
9. Wu, W., Chen, A.Y.C., Zhao, L., Corso, J.J.: Brain tumor detection and segmentation in a CRF (conditional random fields) framework with pixel-pairwise affinity and superpixel-level features. Int. J. Comput. Assist. Radiol. Surg. **9**(2), 241–253 (2014)

10. Menze, B.H., Jakab, A., Bauer, S., Kalpathy-Cramer, J., Farahani, K., Kirby, J., Burren, Y., Porz, N., Slotboom, J., Wiest, R., Lanczi, L., Gerstner, E., Weber, M.A., Arbel, T., Avants, B.B., Ayache, N., Buendia, P., Collins, D.L., Cordier, N., Corso, J.J., Criminisi, A., Das, T., Delingette, H., Demiralp, C., Durst, C.R., Dojat, M., Doyle, S., Festa, J., Forbes, F., Geremia, E., Glocker, B., Golland, P., Guo, X., Hamamci, A., Iftekharuddin, K.M., Jena, R., John, N.M., Konukoglu, E., Lashkari, D., Mariz, J.A., Meier, R., Pereira, S., Precup, D., Price, S.J., Raviv, T.R., Reza, S.M., Ryan, M., Sarikaya, D., Schwartz, L., Shin, H.C., Shotton, J., Silva, C.A., Sousa, N., Subbanna, N.K., Szekely, G., Taylor, T.J., Thomas, O.M., Tustison, N.J., Unal, G., Vasseur, F., Wintermark, M., Ye, D.H., Zhao, L., Zhao, B., Zikic, D., Prastawa, M., Reyes, M., Van Leemput, K.: The multimodal brain tumor image segmentation benchmark (BRATS). IEEE Trans. Med. Imaging **34**(10), 1993–2024 (2015)
11. Bakas, S., Akbari, H., Sotiras, A., Bilello, M., Rozycki, M., Kirby, J.S., Freymann, J.B., Farahani, K., Davatzikos, C.: Advancing the cancer genome atlas glioma MRI collections with expert segmentation labels and radiomic features. Nat. Sci. Data **4**, 170117 (2017)
12. Bakas, S., Akbari, H., Sotiras, A., Bilello, M., Rozycki, M., Kirby, J., Freymann, J., Farahani, K., Davatzikos, C.: Segmentation labels and radiomic features for the pre-operative scans of the TCGA-GBM collection. The Cancer Imaging Archive (2017). https://doi.org/10.7937/K9/TCIA.2017.KLXWJJ1Q
13. Bakas, S., Akbari, H., Sotiras, A., Bilello, M., Rozycki, M., Kirby, J., Freymann, J., Farahani, K., Davatzikos, C.: Segmentation labels and radiomic features for the pre-operative scans of the TCGA-LGG collection. The Cancer Imaging Archive (2017). https://doi.org/0.7937/K9/TCIA.2017.GJQ7R0EF

Towards Uncertainty-Assisted Brain Tumor Segmentation and Survival Prediction

Alain Jungo[1](✉)(iD), Richard McKinley[2], Raphael Meier[1], Urspeter Knecht[2],
Luis Vera[3], Julián Pérez-Beteta[3], David Molina-García[3],
Víctor M. Pérez-García[3], Roland Wiest[2], and Mauricio Reyes[1]

[1] Institute for Surgical Technology and Biomechanics,
University of Bern, Bern, Switzerland
`alain.jungo@istb.unibe.ch`
[2] Support Center for Advanced Neuroimaging,
Institute for Diagnostic and Interventional Neuroradiology,
University Hospital Inselspital and University of Bern, Bern, Switzerland
[3] Mathematical Oncology Laboratory, Universidad de Castilla-La Mancha,
Ciudad Real, Spain

Abstract. Uncertainty measures of medical image analysis technologies, such as deep learning, are expected to facilitate their clinical acceptance and synergies with human expertise. Therefore, we propose a full-resolution residual convolutional neural network (FRRN) for brain tumor segmentation and examine the principle of Monte Carlo (MC) Dropout for uncertainty quantification by focusing on the Dropout position and rate. We further feed the resulting brain tumor segmentation into a survival prediction model, which is built on age and a subset of 26 image-derived geometrical features such as volume, volume ratios, surface, surface irregularity and statistics of the enhancing tumor rim width. The results show comparable segmentation performance between MC Dropout models and a standard weight scaling Dropout model. A qualitative evaluation further suggests that informative uncertainty can be obtained by applying MC Dropout after each convolution layer. For survival prediction, results suggest only using few features besides age. In the BraTS17 challenge, our method achieved the 2nd place in the survival task and completed the segmentation task in the 3rd best-performing cluster of statistically different approaches.

Keywords: Deep learning · Brain tumor segmentation
Uncertainty estimation · Survival prediction

1 Introduction

Over the past years, large improvements could be observed in brain tumor segmentation. This is partly due to the adoption of the fast-evolving deep learning approaches from the field of computer vision. An even more important reason for the recent advances is the availability of public datasets and online

© Springer International Publishing AG, part of Springer Nature 2018
A. Crimi et al. (Eds.): BrainLes 2017, LNCS 10670, pp. 474–485, 2018.
https://doi.org/10.1007/978-3-319-75238-9_40

benchmarks [15]. This progress has later guided research to focus on optimizing model architectures for achieving high segmentation performance. However, as the robustness of these systems still requires expert monitoring of results, clinical applications such as radiological and high-throughput data analysis would benefit greatly from additional uncertainty information along with a good segmentation performance. Information on the segmentation uncertainty can first leverage the trust of users on such automated segmentation systems, but it could be also used to e.g. guide an operator in making manual corrections to the automatic segmentation results. In this work, we thus focus on the largely unexplored aspect of quantifying model uncertainty in the context of brain tumor segmentation. Existing work of uncertainty in brain tumor segmentation includes a perturbation-based approach for conditional random fields [1,14] and a level set-based method defined via a Gaussian Process [13]. The limitations of these techniques are their lack of transferability to neural networks and their restriction to quantify uncertainty of a specific model only.

The segmentation of brain tumor compartments can be part of a radiomic process, where features are extracted from the segmented tumor and used in subsequent data mining [9]. A particularly important radiomic application is the survival prediction [20], where imaging features are used within a radiomics workflow to predict patient survival. Typically, features are handcrafted and include regional gray-level features (e.g., first- and second-order statistics) and morphological features (e.g., surface and volume [18]). In addition to imaging features, clinical features such as age or extent of resection may also be considered [5]. Geometrical features such as tumor surface irregularity or enhancing tumor heterogeneity have been reported as predictive biomarkers for patient survival [6,12,16]. However, these studies rely on manual or semi-automatic delineation of the tumor compartments.

The aim of this work is twofold. First, to explore uncertainty estimation in deep learning-based methods for brain tumor segmentation, and second, to predict survival from age and image-derived geometrical features of a segmented tumor shape. Therefore, as a baseline for the segmentation task, we adopt the a full-resolution residual network (FRRN) [17] architecture. Then, we incorporate the idea of Monte Carlo (MC) Dropout [8] to obtain model uncertainty. In an experiment, we examine the impact of different MC Dropout position strategies and compare the performance to the standard weight scaling Dropout [19]. For the survival prediction task, we use the resulting fully-automated segmentations to determine geometrical features and to build a predictive model thereof.

2   Methods

In this section, we present details of the approach subdivided for segmentation and survival prediction.

2.1   Segmentation

First, we present the employed convolutional neural network architecture. Second, we focus on the method used to quantify segmentation uncertainty.

FRRN Architecture. The adopted full-resolution residual network (FRRN) [17] is based on two streams; a residual stream and a pooling stream. The first one is responsible for maintaining a residual path between the network input and output. This has been shown to improve the gradient flow and thus training [10]. Moreover, the residual stream allows the network to carry information at full image resolution required for precise segmentation of the image details [17]. The second stream reduces the resolution by pooling operations before returning to original resolution by upsampling. Due to the reduced resolution, the filters on the pooling stream can capture contextual information. An important aspect of the architecture are the connections between pooling and residual streams. This enables the network to simultaneously combine both global and local image information [17].

We propose a full-resolution residual network architecture with four max-pooling/upsampling steps. The input consists of slices of all four image sequences (T1-weighted, T1-weighted post-contrast, T2-weighted, Fluid attenuation inversion recovery (FLAIR)), which we define as $I = [I_{T1}, I_{T1c}, I_{T2}, I_{FLAIR}] \in \mathbb{R}^{m \times n \times 4}$ where m and n are the in-plane resolution. The output is defined to be a segmentation mask for the corresponding input slice I, which contains the labels of the tumor compartments (edema, enhancing tumor and necrosis together with non-enhancing tumor) and the background, i.e. $C = \{0, 1, 2, 4\}$. For each input I, the network determines the posterior probability distribution $p(Y \mid I)$ where $Y \in C^{m \times n}$. Although the prediction is performed slice-wise, the formulation can be extended to subject volumes with $\mathbf{I} \in \mathbb{R}^{l \times m \times n \times 4}$ and $\mathbf{Y} \in C^{l \times m \times n}$ (l being the slices).

The architecture of the network is depicted in Fig. 1. Figure 2 shows a detailed view of the residual units (RU) and full-resolution residual units (FRRU). Due to the anisotropy in the image resolution of the original data, we consider the slices from all three planes (axial (a), coronal (c) and sagittal (s)) by rotating the input volumes $\mathbf{I}$ to $\mathbf{I}_a, \mathbf{I}_c$ and $\mathbf{I}_s$ during training and testing. This results in three predictions $p(\mathbf{Y}_a \mid \mathbf{I}_a)$, $p(\mathbf{Y}_c \mid \mathbf{I}_c)$, $p(\mathbf{Y}_s \mid \mathbf{I}_s)$ per subject. In order to combine them, the three outputs are averaged to $p(\mathbf{Y} \mid \mathbf{I}) = 1/3 \sum_{j \in \{a,c,s\}} p'(\mathbf{Y}_j \mid \mathbf{I}_j)$ where p' denotes the posterior probabilities in the space of $\mathbf{I}$, before determining the maximizing class $\hat{y} = \arg\max_{c \in C} p(y = c \mid I)$ for each voxel. Together with the volume-wise intensity normalization ($\mu = 0$, $\sigma = 1$), this combined prediction on all image planes had the largest impact on our validation set performance.

Uncertainty Estimation. As presented by Gal and Ghahramani [8], Dropout regularization can be interpreted as an approximation for Bayesian inference over the weights of the network. A fully Bayesian network requires applying Dropout after each convolution layer. Kendall et al. [11] showed that applying Dropout at

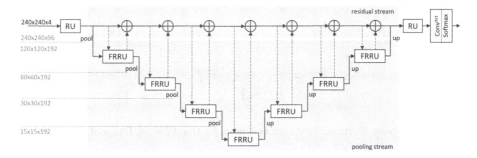

Fig. 1. Full-resolution residual network with four pooling steps. Dashed lines represent the exchange connections between the residual and pooling streams.

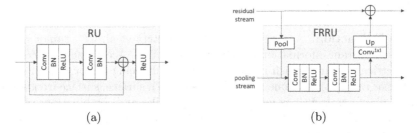

(a)   (b)

Fig. 2. Detailed view of the units of the architecture in Fig. 1. (a) The residual unit (RU) including its residual connection (BN: Batch normalization, ReLU: Rectified Linear Unit). (b) The full-resolution residual unit (FRRU) where *pool* and *up* adapt to the pooling and residual stream, respectively. The 1×1 convolution aligns the number of feature channels among the streams. Unless specified differently, the convolution kernels are of size 3×3.

key positions of the network can be sufficient for semantic segmentation, and that it additionally favors training convergence. Following this observation, we select the positions after each pooling layer and before each upsampling operations as well as the position before and after the latter residual unit as key Dropout positions (Fig. 3). Hereinafter, these positions will be referred to as *core* and *end* Dropout positions.

The Dropouts are applied during training and test time. At test time, the Dropouts produce randomly sampled networks, which can be viewed as Monte Carlo samples over the posterior distribution $p(\mathbf{W} \mid \mathcal{I}, \mathcal{Y})$ of the model weights $\mathbf{W}$ (with subject dataset $\mathcal{I}$ and corresponding label set $\mathcal{Y}$). K network samples are used to produce one prediction with uncertainty estimation. The classification of one voxel is determined by the average of posterior probabilities $p(y \mid I) = \sum_{c \in \mathcal{C}} \left(\frac{1}{K} \sum_{k=1}^{K} p(y_k = c \mid I) \right)$ over K predictions. As described by Gal [7], the class uncertainty can be computed with the approximated predictive entropy $H \approx -\sum_{c \in \mathcal{C}} \left(\frac{1}{K} \sum_{k=1}^{K} p(y_k = c \mid I) \right) \log \left(\frac{1}{K} \sum_{k=1}^{K} p(y_k = c \mid I) \right)$.

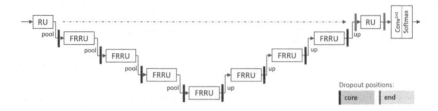

Fig. 3. Dropout positions *core* and *end* used for the different Dropout strategies.

2.2 Survival Prediction

Once the tumor compartments are segmented they serve as input for the overall survival prediction. Subsequent paragraphs elucidate the steps to build the survival prediction regression model.

Feature Extraction. As presented by Pérez-Beteta et al. [16], tumor geometry holds important information for survival prediction. Accordingly, we consider 26 geometrical features which include volumes (enhancing tumor (V_{ce}), necrosis (V_n), tumor core (V_c)), volume ratios (e.g., $\frac{V_c}{V_{ce}}$, $\frac{V_c}{V_n}$), surface, surface irregularity, maximal diameter as well as median, mean, quartiles and combinations of quartiles of the enhancing tumor rim width. In addition to the geometrical features, the subject's age is included.

Feature Selection. This step identifies the most important features before creating a prognostic model. We performed filtering with extensive cross-validation processes on the training set based on several information measurements (e.g. Gini impurity, variance reduction with respect to target attribute). It revealed that four seems to be the optimal number of features for our set. The four selected features are (listed according to their importance):

1. Age
2. Tumor core (enhancing tumor and necrotic tissue) surface
3. Surface irregularity (surface compared to sphere with equal volume)
4. 1st quartile of contrast-enhancing rim width

Survival Model. With the four selected features, we train a fully connected neural network with one hidden layer and linear activation function. Other prediction models such as SVM with RBF kernels, sparse grid or combinations of them were investigated but resulted in inferior performance.

3   Experiments and Results

In this section, we first focus on the segmentation performance of several MC Dropout models compared to a traditional Dropout model before we perform a qualitative evaluation of the obtained uncertainties. In a second experiment, we are interested in the survival prediction performance.

3.1   Segmentation

In order to examine MC Dropout, we compare four MC Dropout and one standard weight scaling (WS) Dropout [19] strategies. WS Dropout at the *core* positions is applied with a Dropout rate $p = 0.5$ (WSCore05). The four MC Dropout strategies are: Dropout at *core* positions with $p = 0.5$ (MCCore05) and with $p = 0.75$ (MCCore075), Dropout at *end* positions with $p = 0.5$ (MCEnd05) and Dropout after every convolution layer with $p = 0.5$ (MCFull05).

According to Kendall et al. [11] a minimum of approximately $K = 6$ Dropout Monte Carlo samples are required to improve segmentation performance (on the CamVid dataset) compared to an architecture where the Dropout weights are averaged during testing. For the MC Dropout models, we use a rather large $K = 20$. The reason is that compared to Kendall et al. [11], we are not only interested in an improved segmentation performance but also in exploiting the uncertainty comprised in the K predictions.

Table 1. Quantitative results of the comparison between the Dropout strategies WSCore05, MCCore05, MCCore075, MCEnd05, MCFull05 on the BraTS17 validation dataset (reported as mean ± standard deviation). Bold numbers highlight the best result for a given metric and tumor region (ET: enhancing tumor, WT: whole tumor, TC: tumor core).

	Model	ET	WT	TC
Dice	WSCore05	0.749 (±0.277)	**0.901** (±0.086)	**0.790** (±0.239)
	MCCore05	**0.756** (±0.275)	0.898 (±0.093)	0.775 (±0.245)
	MCCore075	0.730 (±0.290)	0.896 (±0.103)	0.776 (±0.243)
	MCEnd05	0.738 (±0.284)	0.894 (±0.114)	0.785 (±0.240)
	MCFull05	0.734 (±0.299)	0.884 (±0.141)	0.768 (±0.257)
Sensitivity	WSCore05	**0.800** (±0.273)	**0.900** (±0.130)	**0.760** (±0.263)
	MCCore05	0.775 (±0.273)	0.884 (±0.139)	0.721 (±0.270)
	MCCore075	0.783 (±0.263)	0.894 (±0.146)	0.740 (±0.267)
	MCEnd05	0.783 (±0.262)	0.882 (±0.154)	0.744 (±0.264)
	MCFull05	0.759 (±0.299)	0.857 (±0.177)	0.724 (±0.281)
Specificity	WSCore05	0.998 (±0.005)	0.995 (±0.004)	0.998 (±0.003)
	MCCore05	0.998 (±0.003)	0.996 (±0.005)	**0.999** (±0.003)
	MCCore075	0.998 (±0.005)	0.995 (±0.004)	0.998 (±0.003)
	MCEnd05	0.998 (±0.003)	0.996 (±0.004)	0.998 (±0.003)
	MCFull05	0.998 (±0.004)	**0.997** (±0.003)	0.998 (±0.004)
Hausdorff95 (mm)	WSCore05	5.379 (±10.068)	5.409 (±9.710)	**7.487** (±8.935)
	MCCore05	5.025 (±10.098)	5.255 (±10.129)	8.842 (±15.023)
	MCCore075	5.425 (±9.812)	4.319 (±5.122)	8.909 (±14.292)
	MCEnd05	**4.671** (±9.600)	**4.059** (±4.349)	7.924 (±14.616)
	MCFull05	4.695 (±9.243)	4.216 (±4.166)	7.582 (±8.710)

The comparison of the approaches was performed on the 46 subjects of BraTS17 validation dataset [2–4,15]. All five models were trained on 265 randomly selected training subjects out of the 285 subjects available in the BraTS17 training dataset [2–4,15]. The remaining 20 training subjects were used for validation during training and model selection. Table 1 lists a summary of the achieved results for the five methods. Additionally, the distribution of the obtained Dice coefficients and Hausdorff (95th percentile) distances are presented in Fig. 4.

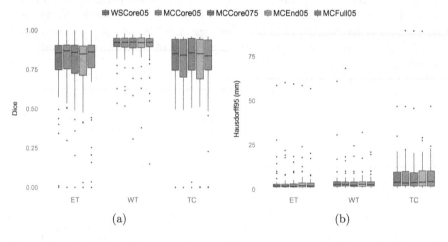

Fig. 4. Boxplots for the Dice coefficient (a) and Hausdorff (95th percentile) distance (b) for the different Dropout strategies; weight scaling Dropout at *core* positions with Dropout rate $p = 0.5$ (WSCore05), Monte Carlo (MC) Dropout at *core* positions with $p = 0.5$ (MCCore05) and $p = 0.75$ (MCCore075), MC Dropout at *end* positions with $p = 0.5$ (MCEnd05) and MC Dropout after each convolution layer with $p = 0.5$ (MCFull05).

On the BraTS17 challenge dataset [2–4,15] with 146 subjects, the proposed method achieved the 7th rank in the segmentation task (results listed in Table 2). Furthermore, the method ranked third with regards to statistical differences among the approaches.

Table 2. BraTS17 challenge dataset results obtained by the WSCore05 model (reported as mean ± standard deviation, ET: enhancing tumor, WT: whole tumor, TC: tumor core).

	ET	WT	TC
Dice	0.670 (±0.312)	0.874 (±0.121)	0.736 (±0.304)
Hausdorff95(mm)	54.791 (±127.862)	8.825 (±15.550)	31.332 (±89.496)

As an additional output, the presented models produce uncertainty maps. A qualitative result is shown in Fig. 5 which depicts an exemplary case of an uncertainty map for each model along with the obtained segmentation. In contrast to the models with MC Dropout, the model applying weight scaling Dropout (WSCore05) does not perform Monte Carlo sampling. In this case, we determine the uncertainty through the entropy of the posterior probability distribution $H = - \sum_{c \in C} p(y = c \mid I) \log p(y = c \mid I)$ for every voxel.

3.2 Survival Prediction

The evaluation of the survival prediction model was performed on the BraTS17 survival validation dataset [2–4, 15], which is a subset (33 out of 46 subjects) of the segmentation validation dataset. For this subset, the subject's age is provided with the data and is used as input for the prediction along with the computed segmentation results. Table 3 lists the results on the validation dataset (top row).

In the BraTS17 challenge, the presented model achieved the 2nd place in the survival task. The results achieved on the 95 subjects of the challenge dataset [2–4, 15] are presented in the bottom row of Table 3.

Table 3. Quantitative results of the survival prediction on the BraTS17 validation and challenge datasets.

Dataset	Accuracy	MSE	Median SE	Std SE
Validation	0.424	$245.7 \cdot 10^3$	$562.8 \cdot 10^3$	$540.7 \cdot 10^3$
Challenge	0.568	$213.0 \cdot 10^3$	$28.1 \cdot 10^3$	$662.6 \cdot 10^3$

4   Discussion

The evaluation of the validation dataset results in Table 1 reveals that the segmentation performance of all five models (WSCore05, MCCore05, MCCore075, MCEnd05, MCFull05) is comparable. Nevertheless, the best overall performance is achieved by the model with weight scaling Dropout (WSCore05). This is rather surprising since Kendall et al. [11] as well as Gal and Ghahramani [8] found that MC Dropout, besides providing uncertainty, can also improve the segmentation performance. Since the BraTS challenge evaluation aims at achieving a high segmentation performance, we used the WSCore05 model for the segmentation and survival task at the BraTS17 challenge. Furthermore, Fig. 4 shows that the five models with different Dropout strategies are as well comparable in terms of variation of Dice coefficient and Hausdorff distance (95th percentile). However, in contrast to the average results in Table 1, the median and interquartile range of the MCFull05 model are close to the WSCore05 distribution. This difference can be explained by the rather high amount of outliers in the Dice coefficient variation of the MCFull05 model. Table 2 lists the results achieved on the BraTS17

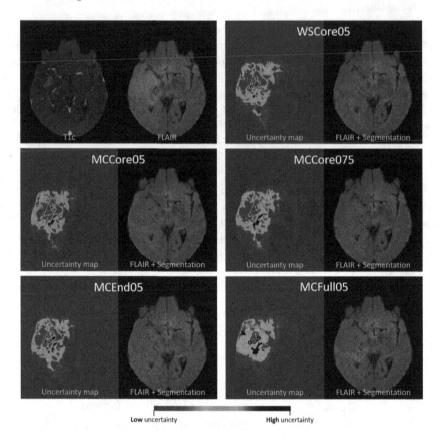

Fig. 5. Uncertainty maps next to FLAIR slices with the segmentation overlaid for each Dropout strategy. The corresponding subject is CBICA_ATW_1 from the BraTS17 validation dataset. As a reference, the raw T1-weighted post-contrast and FLAIR sequences are depicted in the top left.

challenge dataset. Compared to the validation dataset results, the metrics are inferior for all three tumor regions. Reasons might be (a) the performed model selection according to validation dataset results, (b) the difference of the validation dataset and challenge dataset size and (c) a validation dataset that is possibly closer to the training dataset distribution than the challenge dataset.

The qualitative results of the produced uncertainty maps in Fig. 5 highlight that the resulting uncertainty maps of the MC Dropout models MCCore05, MCCore075 and MCEnd05 are visually not distinctively more informative than the entropy determined by the weight scaling model WSCore05 (without MC samples). This problem might come from the rather complex models we use; we could observe that even with a small number of MC samples, the MC Dropout models achieved good segmentation performances (close to the ones shown). It seems that the large complexity allows the models to compensate for the dropped weights and thus minimize the variance in the K MC samples. In contrast to the aforementioned MC Dropout models, the uncertainty produced by the MCFull05 seems to appear more informative. It shows uncertainty where the other models do not (e.g. most parts of the edema), and has increased uncertainty in regions where the other models are uncertain as well. One reason for the more informative uncertainty estimation might be that a fully Bayesian neural network is applied in MCFull05.

The results obtained for the survival prediction on the BraTS validation dataset (Table 3, top row) are not among the best-performing, when comparing it to the results yielding the 2nd place (Table 3, bottom row) in the challenge. We hypothesize that this difference is due to the rather small validation dataset size ($n = 33$) which might bias the outcomes. Moreover, the likewise small training dataset size could lead to overfitting when using a large number of features. Since our model uses only four features, the chance to overfit is greatly reduced. The avoidance of fine-tuning towards the validation dataset could also play a role in the discrepancy of the results. Furthermore, irregularity of tumor shape turned out to be one of the most predictive features for patient survival which confirms previous findings in literature [6, 12, 16].

In a next step, we plan to incorporate the generated uncertainty maps into the survival prediction pipeline in order to enhance prediction performance.

5   Conclusion

In conclusion, the results show that the presented models with weight scaling and Monte Carlo Dropout strategies achieve a good segmentation performance and that the visually most informative uncertainty can be obtained by a fully Bayesian neural network (MC Dropout after each convolution layer). First evidence suggests that there might be a trade-off between model complexity and model uncertainty. We could further observe that age and other geometrical features play an important role in survival prediction. Additionally, results in survival prediction indicate a potential prevention of overfitting due to the usage of a small number of features.

Acknowledgments. This work was supported by the Swiss National Foundation by grant number 169607, the Swiss Cancer League project MANAGE KFS-3979-08-2016, the Spanish Ministerio de Economía y Competitividad/FEDER by grant number MTM2015-71200-R, and the James S. Mc. Donnell Foundation 21st Century Science Initiative in Mathematical and Complex Systems Approaches for Brain Cancer [Special Initiative Collaborative – Planning Grant 220020420 and Collaborative award 220020450].

References

1. Alberts, E., Rempfler, M., Alber, G., Huber, T., Kirschke, J., Zimmer, C., Menze, B.H.: Uncertainty quantification in brain tumor segmentation using CRFs and random perturbation models. In: Proceedings - International Symposium on Biomedical Imaging, vol. 2016 June, pp. 428–431. IEEE, April 2016

2. Bakas, S., Akbari, H., Sotiras, A., Bilello, M., Rozycki, M., Kirby, J.S., Freymann, J.B., Farahani, K., Davatzikos, C.: Advancing the cancer genome atlas glioma MRI collections with expert segmentation labels and radiomic features. Nat. Sci. Data **4**, 170117 (2017)

3. Bakas, S., Akbari, H., Sotiras, A., Bilello, M., Rozycki, M., Kirby, J.S., Freymann, J.B., Farahani, K., Davatzikos, C.: Segmentation labels and radiomic features for the pre-operative scans of the TCGA-LGG collection. The Cancer Imaging Archive, January 2017. https://wiki.cancerimagingarchive.net/display/DOI/Segmentation+Labels+and+Radiomic+Features+for+the+Pre-operative+Scans+of+the+TCGA-LGG+collection

4. Bakas, S., Akbari, H., Sotiras, A., Bilello, M., Rozycki, M., Kirby, J.S., Freymann, J.B., Farahani, K., Davatzikos, C.: Segmentation labels and radiomic features for the pre-operative scans of the TCGA-GBM collection. The Cancer Imaging Archive, January 2017. https://wiki.cancerimagingarchive.net/display/DOI/Segmentation+Labels+and+Radiomic+Features+for+the+Pre-operative+Scans+of+the+TCGA-GBM+collection;jsessionid=C2BE9FB8F9D5532DCA9E5CD294787DBC

5. Cui, Y., Tha, K.K., Terasaka, S., Yamaguchi, S., Wang, J., Kudo, K., Xing, L., Shirato, H., Li, R.: Prognostic imaging biomarkers in glioblastoma: development and independent validation on the basis of multiregion and quantitative analysis of MR images. Radiology **278**(2), 546–553 (2016)

6. Czarnek, N., Clark, K., Peters, K.B., Mazurowski, M.A.: Algorithmic three-dimensional analysis of tumor shape in MRI improves prognosis of survival in glioblastoma: a multi-institutional study. J. Neurooncol. **132**(1), 55–62 (2017)

7. Gal, Y.: Uncertainty in Deep Learning. Ph.D. thesis, University of Cambridge (2016)

8. Gal, Y., Ghahramani, Z.: Bayesian convolutional neural networks with Bernoulli approximate variational inference, June 2015. http://arxiv.org/abs/1506.02158

9. Gillies, R.J., Kinahan, P.E., Hricak, H.: Radiomics: images are more than pictures, they are data. Radiology **278**(2), 563–577 (2016)

10. He, K., Zhang, X., Ren, S., Sun, J.: Deep residual learning for image recognition. In: 2016 IEEE Conference on Computer Vision and Pattern Recognition (CVPR), pp. 770–778 (2016)

11. Kendall, A., Badrinarayanan, V., Cipolla, R.: Bayesian SegNet: model uncertainty in deep convolutional encoder-decoder architectures for scene understanding. In: Proceedings of the British Machine Vision Conference (BMVC) (2017)

12. Kickingereder, P., Neuberger, U., Bonekamp, D., Piechotta, P.L., Götz, M., Wick, A., Sill, M., Kratz, A., Shinohara, R.T., Jones, D.T.W., Radbruch, A., Muschelli, J., Unterberg, A., Debus, J., Schlemmer, H.P., Herold-Mende, C., Pfister, S., von Deimling, A., Wick, W., Capper, D., Maier-Hein, K.H., Bendszus, M.: Radiomic subtyping improves disease stratification beyond key molecular, clinical and standard imaging characteristics in patients with glioblastoma. Neuro-Oncology, nox188 (2017)

13. Lê, M., Unkelbach, J., Ayache, N., Delingette, H.: GPSSI: gaussian process for sampling segmentations of images. In: Navab, N., Hornegger, J., Wells, W.M., Frangi, A.F. (eds.) MICCAI 2015. LNCS, vol. 9351, pp. 38–46. Springer, Cham (2015). https://doi.org/10.1007/978-3-319-24574-4_5

14. Meier, R., Knecht, U., Jungo, A., Wiest, R., Reyes, M.: Perturb-and-MPM: quantifying segmentation uncertainty in dense multi-label CRFs, March 2017. http://arxiv.org/abs/1703.00312

15. Menze, B., Jakab, A., Bauer, S., Kalpathy-Cramer, J., Farahani, K., Kirby, J., Burren, Y., Porz, N., Slotboom, J., Wiest, R., Lanczi, L., Gerstner, E., Weber, M.A., Arbel, T., Avants, B., Ayache, N., Buendia, P., Collins, L., Cordier, N., Corso, J., Criminisi, A., Das, T., Delingette, H., Demiralp, C., Durst, C., Dojat, M., Doyle, S., Festa, J., Forbes, F., Geremia, E., Glocker, B., Golland, P., Guo, X., Hamamci, A., Iftekharuddin, K., Jena, R., John, N., Konukoglu, E., Lashkari, D., Antonio Mariz, J., Meier, R., Pereira, S., Precup, D., Price, S.J., Riklin-Raviv, T., Reza, S., Ryan, M., Schwartz, L., Shin, H.C., Shotton, J., Silva, C., Sousa, N., Subbanna, N., Szekely, G., Taylor, T., Thomas, O., Tustison, N., Unal, G., Vasseur, F., Wintermark, M., Hye Ye, D., Zhao, L., Zhao, B., Zikic, D., Prastawa, M., Reyes, M., Van Leemput, K.: The multimodal brain tumor image segmentation benchmark (BRATS). IEEE Trans. Med. Imaging **34**, 33 (2014)

16. Pérez-Beteta, J., Martínez-González, A., Molina, D., Amo-Salas, M., Luque, B., Arregui, E., Calvo, M., Borrás, J.M., López, C., Claramonte, M., Barcia, J.A., Iglesias, L., Avecillas, J., Albillo, D., Navarro, M., Villanueva, J.M., Paniagua, J.C., Martino, J., Velásquez, C., Asenjo, B., Benavides, M., Herruzo, I., Delgado, M.D.C., del Valle, A., Falkov, A., Schucht, P., Arana, E., Pérez-Romasanta, L., Pérez-García, V.M.: Glioblastoma: does the pre-treatment geometry matter? a postcontrast T1 MRI-based study. Eur. Radiol. **27**(3), 1096–1104 (2017)

17. Pohlen, T., Hermans, A., Mathias, M., Leibe, B.: Full-resolution residual networks for semantic segmentation in street scenes. In: 2017 IEEE Conference on Computer Vision and Pattern Recognition (CVPR) (2017)

18. Velazquez, R.E., Meier, R., Dunn, W.D., Alexander, B., Wiest, R., Bauer, S., Gutman, D.A., Reyes, M., Aerts, H.J.W.L.: Fully automatic GBM segmentation in the TCGA-GBM dataset: prognosis and correlation with VASARI features. Scientific reports 5, 16822, November 2015

19. Srivastava, N., Hinton, G., Krizhevsky, A., Sutskever, I., Salakhutdinov, R.: Dropout: a simple way to prevent neural networks from overfitting. J. Mach. Learn. Res. **15**, 1929–1958 (2014)

20. Yip, S.S.F., Aerts, H.J.W.L.: Applications and limitations of radiomics. Phy. Med. Biol. **61**(13), R150–R166 (2016)

Ischemic Stroke Lesion Image Segmentation

WMH Segmentation Challenge:
A Texture-Based Classification Approach

Mariana Bento[1,2,3](✉) (iD), Roberto de Souza[1,3], Roberto Lotufo[3],
Richard Frayne[1,2], and Letícia Rittner[3]

[1] Radiology and Clinical Neuroscience, Hotchkiss Brain Institute,
University of Calgary, Calgary, AB, Canada
mariana.pinheirobent@ucalgary.ca
[2] Calgary Image Processing and Analysis Centre, Foothills Medical Centre,
Calgary, AB, Canada
[3] School of Electrical and Computer Engineering, University of Campinas,
Campinas, SP, Brazil

Abstract. This Grand Challenge at MICCAI 2017 aims to directly compare methods for the automatic segmentation of White Matter Hyperintensities (WMH) of presumed vascular origin. Our method automatically segment WMH by using texture-based classification of pixels within the brain white matter. It uses no *a priori* information about the WMH size, contrast or location. The main goal is to compute the probability of each pixel being normal or WMH tissue, by generating a probability map. Based on this probability map, we can automatically segment the WMHs.

Keywords: White matter hyperintensity · MR imaging
Texture features · Segmentation

1 Introduction

Brain tissue abnormalities on magnetic resonance (MR) scans are commonly observed with many neurological and psychiatric conditions, and are often used as biomarkers of disease presence and progression [25]. MR is the most suitable diagnostic imaging modality to detect brain abnormalities because of the excellent image contrast between normal and abnormal tissues [36].

However, MR image quality is dependent on acquisition parameters, magnetic field, patient motion during scanning, and vendor specificities, among other factors. All of these factors become challenging, particularly when conducting large, multi-center studies.

These challenges in brain MR image analysis have stimulated the development of computer-assisted diagnosis (CAD) techniques that aim to improve disease diagnosis [15]. Machine learning-based approaches have been focusing on the study of WMH, reducing the analysis subjectivity and making it more

© Springer International Publishing AG, part of Springer Nature 2018
A. Crimi et al. (Eds.): BrainLes 2017, LNCS 10670, pp. 489–500, 2018.
https://doi.org/10.1007/978-3-319-75238-9_41

robust and agile [2,6]. This quantitative evaluation of WMH may aid specialists achieve accurate diagnosis and proper evaluation of patient progression over time through cross-sectional and longitudinal studies.

These automatic methods to quantitatively evaluate WMH may be categorized in two main groups. The first one includes the methods that aim to detect/segment WMHs by verifying if a given subject presents lesions, and if so locate and delineate them [5,7,8,10,12,20,23,28,29,33]. These methods often combine image processing and machine learning techniques, such as texture analysis, region-based segmentation, morphological operators; pattern recognition classifier and deep learning algorithms. Besides, some of them use a priori information about the WMH to perform their tasks, such as their intensity, possible round shape and location.

The second category includes methods that aim to characterize WMHs, to classify/cluster lesions according to some feature (shape, location, volume, etiology) [1,16,17,19,32,39], or to track these characteristics over time in longitudinal studies [4,18,21,24,34].

The majority of these related methods are performed with limited, homogeneous datasets and have not provided a robustness assessment for large, heterogeneous, multi-center datasets. Further, these machine learning-based methods generally present usability issues, requiring multiple images modalities and tuning of many parameters, limiting their wide-spread usability.

Contributions: Our main goal is to automatically segment WMH by combining textures descriptors, classifiers and morphological operators using MR imaging. We evaluate the method on a large, heterogeneous and multicenter dataset as part of the WMH segmentation challenge[1]. The challenge allows the benchmarking by directly comparing the achieved results with related methods.

Paper Organization: Sect. 2 describes the MR dataset. Section 3 details the proposed method. Section 4 presents our results and compares their performance against other methods. Section 5 summarizes our conclusions.

2   MR Dataset

Experiments were conducted using the data assembled for the WMH segmentation challenge on the Brain Lesion Workshop of the 20th International Conference on Medical Image Computing and Computer Assisted Intervention (MICCAI-17).

The challenge made available a training set containing images from 60 patients acquired in three different institutes (Table 1), presenting varying shape and contrast (Fig. 1). The testing data contains images of 110 patients from the same three institutes as the training data, acquired using five different scanners (3T Philips Achieva, 3T Siemens TrioTim, 3T GE Signa HDxt, 3T Philips Ingenuity, 1.5T GE Signa HDxt) (Table 2).

---

[1] http://wmh.isi.uu.nl/.

Table 1. Training dataset description: institute, scanner, amount of patients, slices per image and slice dimensions.

Institute	Scanner	#Patients	#Slices per image	Slice dimensions
UMC Utrecht	3T Philips Achieva	20	48	240 × 240
NUHS Singapore	3T Siemens TrioTim	20	48	232 × 256
VU Amsterdam	3T GE Signa HDxt	20	83	132 × 256

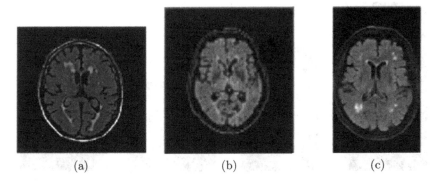

(a)   (b)   (c)

Fig. 1. Training data samples varying shape and contrast according to the acquisition center: (a) UMC Utrecht; (b) NUHS Singapore; (c) VU Amsterdam.

Table 2. Testing dataset description: institute, scanner and amount of patients.

Institute	Scanner	#Patients
UMC Utrecht	3T Philips Achieva	30
NUHS Singapore	3T Siemens TrioTim	30
VU Amsterdam	3T GE Signa HDxt	30
VU Amsterdam	3T Philips Ingenuity	10
VU Amsterdam	1.5T GE Signa HDxt	10

3   Method

The proposed method is performed on a slice-by-slice basis and has four key steps (outlined in Fig. 2).

Pre-processing aim to standardize the images to perform the pixel-based feature extraction: (1a) crops the image to just fit the brain, (1b) resizes it to 200 x 200 (on a per slice basis) using a bicubic interpolation, (1c) segments the white matter, and 1d) normalizes image intensities to the range [0, 255] (Fig. 3).

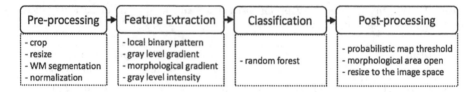

Fig. 2. Method overview: pre-processing and feature extraction, are followed by the probabilistic random forest classification and post-processing (Steps 1 to 4).

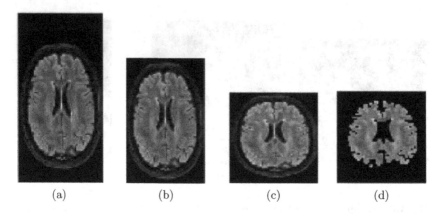

Fig. 3. Pre-processing step (Step 1 in Fig. 2): (a) original FLAIR image; (b) cropped image; (c) resized (200×200) image; (d) mask containing only white matter.

The white matter segmentation is automatically performed by using a max-tree structure [30]. The max-tree node corresponding to the connected component with largest rectangularity ratio, *i.e.*, volume of the object divided by the volume of its bounding-box, is selected as being the most appropriate white-matter segmentation. Only nodes with volumes ranging between 200 ml and 500 ml are considered.

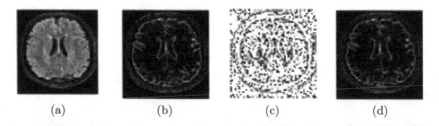

Fig. 4. Feature extraction (Step 2 in Fig. 2) on a pixel-by-pixel basis showing intensity values in: (a) original FLAIR image; (b) local binary pattern; (c) structural gradient; (d) morphological gradient images.

Feature extraction aims to compute discriminant features from the given MR slices [3]. First, (2a) the local binary pattern (LBP) [9], and both (2b) gray level convolutional-based and (2c) morphological gradients are computed for each slice (Fig. 4). Then for each pixel within the white matter, a feature vector is computed containing (2d) the intensity value of that pixel in the following images: T1, FLAIR, next most anterior FLAIR slice, next most posterior FLAIR slice, LBP, gradient, morphological gradient; and the mean white matter intensity (to provide overall information about the slice). A total of eight features are extracted for each pixel within the white matter. These features aim to represent relevant information about the WMH, such as high intensity in the FLAIR MR image, continuity in several MR slices and texture.

Classification aims to train and test a model to distinguish normal from WMH pixels. The training data is used to train a probabilistic random forest classifier [26]. This classifier was selected for presenting desire characteristics such as low complexity, not time-consuming on the training nor testing phases and limit amount of parameters to be set. The output of this classifier is a probabilistic map, containing the probability that each pixel is WMH. Images within the testing dataset are then tested using this classifier.

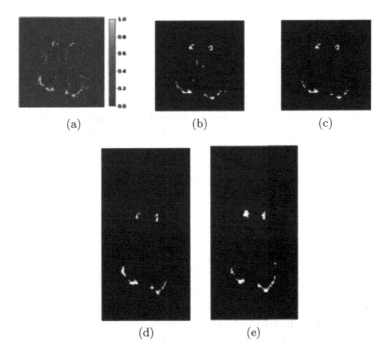

Fig. 5. Post-processing step (Step 4 in Fig. 2): (a) WMH probability map; (b) threshold probabilistic map; (c) morphological area opening; (d) final result after resizing to the original image space; (e) reference segmentation for comparison purposes.

Post-processing: The WMH segmentation is achieved after post-processing (Step 4). First (4a) the WMH probabilistic map is thresholded using a grid-searching technique [26]. After the probability map thresholding (≥ 0.7 - optimal parameter in the training set), the resulting connected components serve as regions of interest (ROIs) (*i.e.*, they contain pixels with high probability of being WMH). Then, (4b) a morphological area opening operator is applied to the three dimensional ROIs to remove noise and other MR artifacts (*i.e.*, ROIs of < 10 pixels are removed). This post-processing limits the method to only detect WMH larger than 10 pixels. The resulting segmentation is (4c) resized back to the original image space, giving the final WMH segmentation result (Fig. 5).

3.1   Development Environment

All codes were developed by using python code, an image processing [11,37,38] and machine learning [26] libraries and auxiliary functions developed in our research group using a Mac Pro 2.7 GHz 12-Core Intel Zeon E5, 64 GB DDR3 memory. No GPUs were used to perform the experiments.

In order to participate in the WMH segmentation challenge, the testing code and trained classifier were distributed in a Docker container [22] shared with the organizers.

4   Results and Discussion

The achieved WMH segmentation results were evaluated by considering several metrics [35]: Dice coefficient, Hausdorff distance (modified, 95th percentile), average volume difference (AVD, expressed as a percentage), sensitivity for individual lesions (Recall, expressed as a percentage) and F1-score for individual lesions. The individual lesions were defined as being a 3D connected component [31].

Each individual metric was averaged over all testing scans. In the challenge, for each metric, the participating teams were sorted from best receiving rank of 0 to worst, receiving rank of 1. Thus, all teams were ranked in (0,1) relative to their performance by each metric. In order to achieve the overall and final rank, the five individual ranks were averaged. Our team (text-class) was ranked in the 18th position (Table 3).

Even though the proposed method did not performed as well as the top methods, some characteristics may be highlighted. The method is based on only 8 features extracted from pixels using 2D slices. This low complexity in understanding and reproducing the proposed method may be valuable in some applications. Besides, since handcrafted texture features were used, it is possible to characterize and evaluate which features are the most relevant ones to accomplish the proposed task.

The proposed method also did not use deep learning techniques, such as U-Nets convolutional networks [27]. This deep network have been often used in medical imaging segmentation problems. They requires a large amount of

Table 3. Final overall and individual ranks for the WMH segmentation challenge for the twenty participant teams. Our method, called text-class, was ranked in the 18th position with a final rank of 0.5725.

	Team	RANK	Dice	Hausdorff	AVD	Recall	F1
1	sysu-media	0.0076	0.80	6.30	21.88	0.84	0.76
2	cian	0.0366	0.78	6.82	21.72	0.83	0.70
3	nlp-logix	0.0485	0.77	7.16	18.37	0.73	0.78
4	nic-vicorob	0.0735	0.77	8.28	28.54	0.75	0.71
5	k2	0.1368	0.77	9.79	19.08	0.59	0.70
6	lrde	0.1635	0.73	14.57	21.71	0.63	0.67
7	misp	0.1659	0.72	14.88	21.36	0.63	0.68
8	ipmi-bern	0.2498	0.69	9.72	19.92	0.44	0.57
9	nih-cidi	0.2697	0.68	12.82	196.38	0.59	0.54
10	scan	0.2762	0.63	14.34	34.67	0.55	0.51
11	achilles	0.2962	0.63	11.82	24.41	0.45	0.52
12	skkumedneuro	0.3492	0.58	19.02	58.54	0.47	0.51
13	tignet	0.3802	0.59	21.58	86.22	0.46	0.45
14	tig	0.3858	0.60	17.86	34.34	0.38	0.42
15	knight	0.4159	0.70	17.03	39.99	0.25	0.35
16	upc-dlmi	0.4337	0.53	27.01	208.49	0.57	0.42
17	nist	0.4747	0.53	15.91	109.98	0.37	0.25
18	**text-class**	0.5725	0.50	28.33	146.64	0.27	0.29
19	neuro.ml	0.5960	0.51	37.36	614.05	0.71	0.21
20	hadi	0.8886	0.23	52.02	828.61	0.58	0.11

annotated training samples. When a large amount of data is not available, data augmentation techniques could be used to enhance the limited number of annotated samples and so as other techniques, such as transfer learning.

The usage of these networks improves the segmentation results in medical imaging problems, but its limited understanding, mainly in the deepest layers does not allow a fully description of the segmentation method (*i.e.*, what features are the most relevant to segment a specific structure or abnormalities like a WMH). Methods that combine handcrafted and convolutional features have been used to take advantage of the best characteristics of these different approaches: improving segmentation results with a better understanding of the method operation and performance, and results meaning [13]. Unlike many other imaging applications, a full understanding and characterization of a given image processing and/or machine learning technique is required when dealing with medical imaging. This knowledge allows correlations to be performed between MR imaging findings with clinical information and longitudinal studies [10, 14, 24, 35].

Our proposed method presented reasonable/fair results using only limited amount of resources (*e.g.*, not using GPUs) and does not require a large amount of parameters to be set, such as U-nets with 3×3 convolutional layers, that requires $7,846,081$ parameters to be learned. Thus, our texture-based classification method may be used in applications with limited amount of resources, to have a straightforward and fast result (around 90 s per volume in the experiment machine) about the WMH burden in a give patient.

Another relevant characteristic of the proposed method is its generalizability, because similar Dice coefficients were achieved in the training (0.59) and testing sets (0.52) when considering only the testing samples acquired in the same scanners as the training ones.

The method presented better results when testing images acquired in the same scanners as the training samples. The lowest rates were achieved when the method was evaluated in images acquired in a 1.5 T scanner (Table 4). This result was expected since we are using an intensity- and pixel-based technique.

Table 4. Final overall and individual ranks (per scanner) for the presented method in the WMH segmentation challenge.

Testing set	Dice	Hausdorff	AVD	Recall (Sensitivity)	F1
UMC Utrecht	0.60	18.33	43.78	0.30	0.36
NUHS Singapore	0.52	25.21	103.85	0.20	0.21
VU GE 3 T	0.43	31.86	162.28	0.31	0.30
VU GE 1.5 T	0.35	50.80	507.13	0.27	0.28
VU Philips	0.45	33.51	176.20	0.28	0.27
Weighted average	0.50	28.23	146.64	0.27	0.29

In the challenge, an exploratory comparison of the metrics on a subject-by-subject basis by using box-plot (Fig. 6) was performed. This data makes possible an evaluation not only the mean metric values but also their variabilities (*e.g.*, first-to-third quartile range) within the testing set. The worst mean scores were achieved for the testing images acquired with the VU GE 1.5 T scanner, but also the largest variability, illustrating our method's limitation when processing images acquired by using another field strength.

A possible improvement to this approach is to combine the proposed handcrafted features with convolutional features by using transfer learning techniques [13]. Experiments using this combined set of features may be used to verify if handcrafted and convolutional features are redundant or complementary, giving as a result a robust and discriminant set of features.

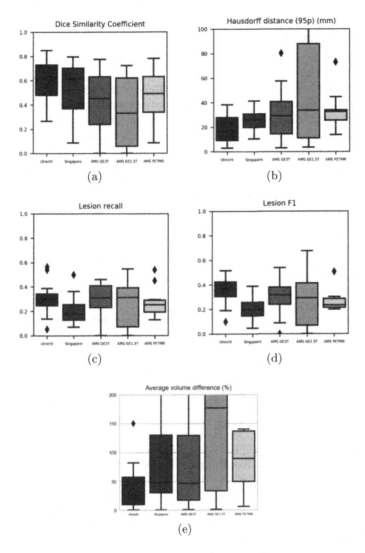

Fig. 6. Box plot of different metrics in the testing set: (a) Dice coefficient; (b) Hausdorff distance; (c) Recall (Sensitivity); (d) F1 and (e) AVD. Larger variability may be observed in the AMS GE1.5T subset.

5   Conclusions

This paper presented a method to automatically segment WMH using a texture-based classification approach on 2D MR images. It combines texture features with probabilistic classifiers to distinguish normal from WMH pixels. The proposed method does not consider *a priori* information about the WMHs, such as location, size and shape.

Our solution is generalizable obtaining similar results in the training and testing sets. Highlights include that the proposed method does not require parameter-setting, or large computational power. It has a low computational time (around 90 s to run a testing volume).

This proposed WMH segmentation method was directly compared with related methods through the WMH segmentation challenge, achieving the 18th position in the final ranking. In future works, the method is going to be improved by combining the handcrafted texture features with convolutional ones.

Acknowledgments. The authors would like to thank Hotchkiss Brain Institute; CAPES process PVE 88881.062158/2014-01; FAPESP processes 2012/21826-1 CEPID2013/07559-3 for providing financial support.

References

1. Appenzeller, S., Vasconcelos Faria, A., Li, L.M., Costallat, L.T., Cendes, F.: Quantitativemagnetic resonance imaging analyses and clinical significance of hyperintense white matter lesions in systemic lupus erythematosus patients. Ann. Neurol. **64**(6), 635–643 (2008)
2. Bento, M., Rittner, L., Lotufo, R.: Texture descriptors and pattern recognition classifiers based analysis of white matter hyperintensity in MR images. In: Proceedings of Workshop of Theses and Dissertations in SIBGRAPI 2013 (XXVI Conference on Graphics, Patterns and Images) (2013)
3. Bento, M., Sym, Y., Frayne, R., Lotufo, R., Rittner, L.: Probabilistic segmentation of brain white matter lesions using texture-based classification. In: Karray, F., Campilho, A., Cheriet, F. (eds.) ICIAR 2017. LNCS, vol. 10317, pp. 71–78. Springer, Cham (2017). https://doi.org/10.1007/978-3-319-59876-5_9
4. Calabrese, M., Rocca, M., Atzori, M., Mattisi, I., Bernardi, V., Favaretto, A., Barachino, L., Romualdi, C., Rinaldi, L., Perini, P., Gallo, P., Filippi, M.: Cortical lesions in primary progressive multiple sclerosis: a 2-year longitudinal MR study. Neurology **72**(15), 1330–1336 (2009)
5. Chen, L., Bentley, P., Rueckert, D.: A novel framework for sub-acute stroke lesion segmentation based on random forest. In: Proceedings of Brainlesion: Glioma, Multiple Sclerosis, Stroke and Traumatic Brain Injuries: First International Workshop, Brainles 2015, Held in Conjunction with MICCAI 2015 (2015)
6. Despotovic, I., Goossens, B., Philips, W.: MRI segmentation of the human brain: challenges, methods, and applications. Comput. Math. Methods Med. **2015**(1), 1–23 (2015)
7. Feng, C., Zhao, D., Huang, M.: Segmentation of Ischemic stroke lesions in multispectral MR images using weighting suppressed FCM and three phase level set. In: Crimi, A., Menze, B., Maier, O., Reyes, M., Handels, H. (eds.) BrainLes 2015. LNCS, vol. 9556, pp. 233–245. Springer, Cham (2016). https://doi.org/10.1007/978-3-319-30858-6_20
8. Griffanti, L., Zamboni, G., Khan, A., Li, L., Bonifacio, G., Sundaresan, V., Schulz, U., Kuker, W., Battaglini, M., Rothwell, P., Jenkinson, M.: BIANCA (Brain Intensity Abnormality Classification Algorithm): a new tool for automated segmentation of white matter hyperintensities. NeuroImage **141**, 191–205 (2016)
9. He, D.C., Wang, L.: Texture unit, texture spectrum, and texture analysis. IEEE Trans. Geosci. Remote Sens. **28**(1), 509–512 (1990)

10. Ithapu, V., Singh, V., Lindner, C., Austin, B., Hinrichs, C., Carlsson, C., Bendlin, B., Johnson, S.: Extracting and summarizing white matter hyperintensities using supervised segmentation methods in Alzheimer's disease risk and aging studies. Hum. Brain Mapping **35**(1), 4219–4235 (2014)
11. Jones, E., Oliphant, T., Peterson, P., et al.: SciPy: open source scientific tools for Python (2001). http://www.scipy.org/
12. Kamnitsas, K., Chen, L., Ledig, C., Rueckert, D., Glocker, B.: Multi-scale 3D convolutional neural networks for lesion segmentation in brain MRI. In: Proceedings of Brainlesion: Glioma, Multiple Sclerosis, Stroke and Traumatic Brain Injuries: First International Workshop, Brainles 2015, Held in Conjunction with MICCAI 2015 (2015)
13. Kashif, M., Raza, S., Sirinukunwattana, K., Arif, M., Rajpoot, N.: Handcrafted features with convolutional neural networks for detection of tumor cells in histology images. In: Proceedings of IEEE 13th International Symposium on Biomedical Imaging (2016)
14. Kloppenborg, R., Nederkoorn, P., Geerlings, M., Berg, E.: Presence and progression of white matter hyperintensities and cognition: a meta-analysis. Neurology **82**(1), 2127–2138 (2014)
15. Lao, Z., Shen, D., Liu, D., Jawad, A.F., Melhem, E.R., Launer, L.J., Bryan, R.N., Davatzikos, C.: Computer-assisted segmentation of white matter lesions in 3D MR images, using support vector machine. Acad. Radiol. **15**(3), 300–313 (2008)
16. Lapa, A., Bento, M., Rittner, L., Ruocco, H., Castellano, G., Damasceno, B., Costallat, L., Lotufo, R., Cendes, F., Appenzeller, S.: Support vector machines classification of texture parameters of white matter lesions in childhood-onset systemic lupus erythematosus. Possible mechanism to distinguish between demyelination and ischemia. Ann. Rheum. Dis. **71**(269) (2013)
17. Leite, M., Gobbi, D., Salluzi, M., Frayne, R., Lotufo, R., Rittner, L.: 3D texture-based classification applied on brain white matter lesions on MR images. In: Proceedings Volume 9785: Medical Imaging 2016: Computer-Aided Diagnosis SPIE (2016)
18. Leite, M., Lapa, A., Appenzeller, S., Lotufo, R., Rittner, L.: A new approach for longitudinal study of white matter lesion based on texture variation. In: Proceedings of XXV Congresso Brasileiro de Engenharia Biomédica (2016)
19. Leite, M., Rittner, L., Appenzeller, S., Ruocco, H., Lotufo, R.: Etiology-based classification of brain white matter hyperintensity on magnetic resonance imaging. J. Med. Imaging **2**(1), 014002-1–014002-10 (2015)
20. Loizou, C., Petroudi, S., Seimenis, I., Seimenis, I., Pantziaris, M.: Pattichis: quantitative texture analysis of brain white matter lesions derived from T2-weighted MR images in MS patients with clinically isolated syndrome. Neuroradiology **42**(2), 99–114 (2015)
21. Loizou, C., Seimenis, I., Seimenis, I., Pantziaris, M., Kasparis, T., Kyriacou, E., Pattichis, C.: Texture image analysis of normal appearing white matter areas in clinically isolated syndrome that evolved in demyelinating lesions in subsequent MRI scans: multiple sclerosis disease evolution. In: Proceedings of the 10th IEEE International Conference on Information Technology and Applications in Biomedicine (2010)
22. Merkel, D.: Docker: lightweight Linux containers for consistent development and deployment. Linux J. **2014**(239) (2014). Article No. 2
23. Mortazavi, D., Kouzani, A., Soltanian, H.: Segmentation of multiple sclerosis lesions in MR images: a review. Neuroradiology **54**(4), 299–320 (2012)

24. Nourbakhsh, B., Nunan-Saah, J., Maghzi, A., Julian, L., Spain, R., Jin, C., Lazar, A., Pelletier, D., Waubant, E.: Longitudinal associations between MRI and cognitive changes in very early MS. Multiple Sclerosis Relat. Disord. **5**(1), 47–52 (2016)
25. Oppedal, K., Eftestol, T., Engan, K., Beyer, M., Aarsland, D.: Classifying dementia using local binary patterns from different regions in magnetic resonance images. Int. J. Biomed. Imaging **2015**, 1–14 (2015)
26. Pedregosa, F., Varoquaux, G., Gramfort, A., Michel, V., Thirion, B., Grisel, O., Blondel, M., Prettenhofer, P., Weiss, R., Dubourg, V., Vanderplas, J., Passos, A., Cournapeau, D., Brucher, M., Perrot, M., Duchesnay, E.: Scikit-learn: machine learning in Python. J. Mach. Learn. Res. **12**(1), 2825–2830 (2011)
27. Ronneberger, O., Fischer, P., Brox, T.: U-Net: convolutional networks for biomedical image segmentation. In: Navab, N., Hornegger, J., Wells, W.M., Frangi, A.F. (eds.) MICCAI 2015. LNCS, vol. 9351, pp. 234–241. Springer, Cham (2015). https://doi.org/10.1007/978-3-319-24574-4_28
28. Roura, E., Oliver, A., Cabezas, M., Valverde, S., Pareto, D., Vilanova, J., Ramió-Torrentà, L., Rovira, A., Lladó, X.: A toolbox for multiple sclerosis lesion segmentation. Neuroradiology **57**(10), 1031–1043 (2015)
29. Roura, E., Sarbu, N., Oliver, A., Valverde, S., González-Villà, S., Cervera, R., Bargalló, N., Lladó, X.: Automated detection of lupus white matter lesions in MRI. Front. Neuroinformatics **10**(33), 1–11 (2016)
30. Salembier, P., Oliveras, A., Garrido, L.: Antiextensive connected operators for image and sequence processing. IEEE Trans. Image Process. **7**(4), 555–570 (1998)
31. Samet, H., Tamminen, M.: Efficient component labeling of images of arbitrary dimension represented by linear bintrees. IEEE Trans. Pattern Anal. Mach. Intell. **10**(4), 579 (1988)
32. Stankiewicz, J., Glanz, B., Healy, B., Arora, A., Neema, M., Benedict, R., Guss, Z., Tauhid, S., Buckle, G., Houtchens, M., Khoury, S., Weiner, H., Guttmann, C., Bakshi, R.: Brain MRI lesion load at 1.5T and 3T vs. clinical status in multiple sclerosis. J. Neuroimaging **21**(2), 1–15 (2011)
33. Steenwijk, M., Pouwels, P., Daams, M., Dalen, J., Caan, M., Richard, E., Barkhof, F., Vrenken, H.: Accurate white matter lesion segmentation by k nearest neighbor classification with tissue type priors (kNN-TTPs). NeuroImage Clin. **3**, 462–469 (2013)
34. Sudre, C., Cardoso, M., Ourselin, S.: Longitudinal segmentation of age-related white matter hyperintensities. Med. Image Anal. **38**, 50–64 (2017)
35. Taha, A., Hanbury, A.: Metrics for evaluating 3D medical image segmentation: analysis, selection, and tool. BMC Med. Imaging **15**(29), 1–29 (2015)
36. Vernooij, M., Ikram, M., Tanghe, H., Vincent, A., Hofman, A., Krestin, G., Niessen, W., Breteler, M., van der Lugt, A.: Incidental findings on brain MRI in the general population. New England J. Med. **357**(18), 1821–1828 (2007)
37. Walt, S., Colbert, S., Varoquaux, G.: The NumPy array: a structure for efficient numerical computation. Comput. Sci. Eng. **13**, 22–30 (2011)
38. van der Walt, S., Schönberger, J.L., Nunez-Iglesias, J., Boulogne, F., Warner, J.D., Yager, N., Gouillart, E., Yu, T.: The scikit-image contributors: Scikit-image: image processing in Python. Peer J. Bioinform. Software Tools Collect. **2**, e453 (2014)
39. Zhang, Y.: MRI texture analysis in multiple sclerosis. Int. J. Biomed. Imaging **2012**, 1–7 (2012). Article ID 762804

White Matter Hyperintensities Segmentation in a Few Seconds Using Fully Convolutional Network and Transfer Learning

Yongchao Xu[1,2,3], Thierry Géraud[1(✉)] ⓘ, Élodie Puybareau[1], Isabelle Bloch[2], and Joseph Chazalon[1,4]

[1] EPITA Research and Development Laboratory (LRDE),
Le Kremlin-Bicêtre, France
thierry.geraud@lrde.epita.fr
[2] LTCI, Télécom ParisTech, Université Paris-Saclay, Palaiseau, France
[3] Huazhong University of Science and Technology, Wuhan, China
[4] Université de La Rochelle, La Rochelle, France

Abstract. In this paper, we propose a fast automatic method that segments white matter hyperintensities (WMH) in 3D brain MR images, using a fully convolutional network (FCN) and transfer learning. This FCN is the Visual Geometry Group neural network (VGG for short) pre-trained on ImageNet for natural image classification, and fine tuned with the training dataset of the MICCAI WMH Challenge. We consider three images for each slice of the volume to segment: the T1 slice, the FLAIR slice, and the result of a morphological operator that emphasizes small bright structures. These three 2D images are assembled to form a 2D color image, that inputs the FCN to obtain the 2D segmentation of the corresponding slice. We process all slices, and stack the results to form the 3D output segmentation. With such a technique, the segmentation of WMH on a 3D brain volume takes about 10 s including pre-processing. Our technique was ranked 6-th over 20 participants at the MICCAI WMH Challenge.

Keywords: 3D brain MRI · Lesion segmentation
White matter hyperintensities · Mathematical morphology
Fully convolutional network

1 Introduction

1.1 Context

This work has been done in the context of the MICCAI WMH Challenge[1]. The aim was to provide a fully automated pipeline for the segmentation of White Matter Hyperintensities (WMH) of vascular origin. WMH are the consequences

---

[1] http://wmh.isi.uu.nl.

© Springer International Publishing AG, part of Springer Nature 2018
A. Crimi et al. (Eds.): BrainLes 2017, LNCS 10670, pp. 501–514, 2018.
https://doi.org/10.1007/978-3-319-75238-9_42

Table 1. Overview of the challenge database.

Hospital	Scanner	Number of training images	Number of test images
UMC Utrecht	3T Philips Achieva	20	30
NUHS Singapore	3T Siemens TrioTim	20	30
VU Amsterdam (AMS)	3T GE Signa HDxt	20	30
	3T Philips Ingenuity	0	10
	1.5T GE Signa HDxt	0	10

of small vessel diseases and are visible on brain MR images [24]. Small vessel diseases are involved in cerebrovascular diseases and are a cause of cognitive decline and functional loss during ageing [16]. Studies of WMH parameters (volume, shape, etc.) can hence be a key for diagnosis and follow-up for patients under treatment for dementia and neurodegenerative diseases.

The visual analysis of images to detect WMH is a difficult process and automated methods could helpfully assist diagnosis [1]. However, the evaluation and comparison of automated WMH segmentation techniques remain difficult because of the diversity of datasets and evaluation criteria [1]. The aim of the MICCAI WMH Challenge was to compare automated WMH segmentation techniques. This comparison yields a ranking of the techniques applied on data acquired from different scanner platforms (different origins, different resolutions, etc.). Data used during the challenge originated from three hospitals and five different scanners as shown in Table 1. A training set of 60 scans was provided by the organizer and the testing set of 110 scans remained secret.

1.2 Related Work

WMH segmentation has always been challenging, and it appears to be really complicated to obtain a reliable fully automated method [1,4]. Indeed, a Dice similarity coefficient will be considered as good if it is higher than 0.7 [1]. The problem of WMH segmentation can be considered with several approaches. The FLAIR modality seems to be one of the best for this kind of segmentation: it is possible to segment the hyperintensities with an optimal FLAIR intensity threshold based on the analysis of histograms as described by Jack et al. [7]. Some methods rely on random Markov fields, either using FLAIR [9] or some other modality [21]. In [15], morphological operators and max-tree representations are used to segment the WMH in newborn T2 brain images, but this method is not fully automated. As machine learning really improved the results of some segmentation tasks, some new methods emerged using supervised machine learning procedures or unsupervised approaches. In [5] WMH segmentation is performed using CNN with anatomical location information, and in [6] using transfer learning with a domain adaptation and patches, reaching a Dice score of 0.76. The authors suggested the idea to replace their CNN network with a FCN one, for example U-Net [17]. In a previous work published in the International Conference on Image

Processing (ICIP) in 2017 [25], 3D brain MR volumes were segmented using fully convolutional network (FCN) and transfer learning. The network used for transfer learning is VGG (Visual Geometry Group) [22], pre-trained on the ImageNet dataset. It takes as input a 2D color image that is here a *3D-like* image, composed of 3 consecutive slices of the 3D volume (see Fig. 1). This method uses only one modality, and reaches good results for brain segmentation.

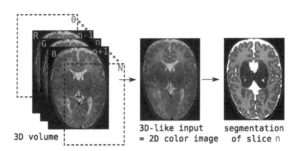

Fig. 1. Illustration of 3D-like color image and associated segmentation used in [25].

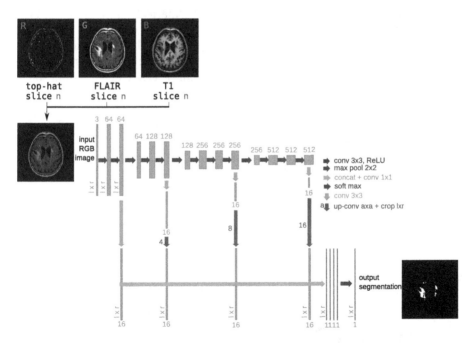

Fig. 2. Architecture of the proposed network. We fine tune it and combine linearly fine to coarse feature maps of the pre-trained VGG network [22]. Note that each color image (**Input**) is built from the slice n of the T1 and FLAIR sequences, and from a pre-processing result. (Color figure online)

For this challenge, we extended this previous work on brain MRI segmentation [25], leveraging the power of a fully convolutional network pre-trained on a large dataset and later fine-tuned on the training set of the challenge. The main contributions include:

1. a preprocessing technique based on mathematical morphology which enhances small lesions to improve their segmentation;
2. a merging technique which enables the input of several modalities (T1, FLAIR and custom preprocessing) in the segmentation chain for each slice.

An overview of the proposed method is given in Fig. 2. The method is fully automatic, and uses both T1 and FLAIR sequences. The details of the whole pipeline are given hereafter. This method is really fast as about 10 s are needed to process a complete scan volume, and also efficient: we reached the 6th place during the MICCAI WMH Challenge.

2   Method Description

2.1   Forewords on Mathematical Morphology

Whereas the most popular operators of mathematical morphology (MM) rely on structuring elements, the class of "connected operators" does not necessarily [11,20]. This class is very interesting because those operators do not shift object contours (they cannot create some new contours, they just suppress some existing ones). Some connected operators can be easily defined from some

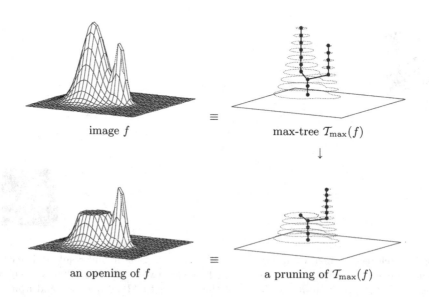

$$\text{image } f \quad \equiv \quad \text{max-tree } \mathcal{T}_{\max}(f)$$

$$\downarrow$$

$$\text{an opening of } f \quad \equiv \quad \text{a pruning of } \mathcal{T}_{\max}(f)$$

Fig. 3. A morphological connected operator (here an opening) based on a tree-based image representation.

tree-based representations of a gray-level image [8,18,19]; such image representations express the inclusion of the connected components obtained by thresholding the image. Note that computing, storing, and processing such a component tree is very efficient [2,14]. In the following, we rely on the *max-tree* representation, denoted by $\mathcal{T}_{\max}$, obtained by upper thresholding. Such a tree is displayed in Fig. 3 (top right). If we prune this tree, such as in Fig. 3 (bottom right), we can reconstruct the function depicted in Fig. 3 (bottom left). In the following, we filter out any component of the max-tree which size (or area, i.e., number of pixels) is below a threshold N, which leads to an *area opening* [23]. In all our experiments, we set N to 25 pixels.

In Fig. 4(b), such an operator was applied on the image of Fig. 4(a). In this result, some small bright components are removed, without the rest of the image being modified (it is a connected operator); let us also note that this operator has the ability to filter out low-contrasted objects in the same way as it does with high-contrasted ones. The removed components correspond to small spots of white matter intensities. The residue of this filtering step, i.e., the result minus the input, is called an *area top-hat*; it is depicted in Fig. 4(c).

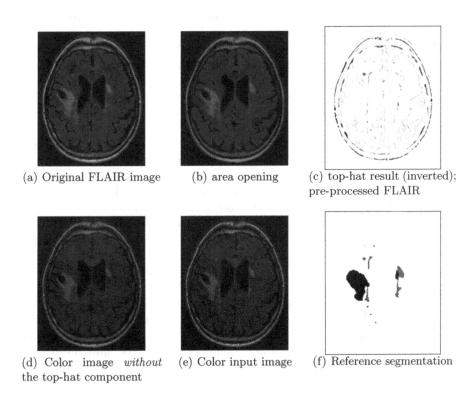

(a) Original FLAIR image   (b) area opening   (c) top-hat result (inverted); pre-processed FLAIR

(d) Color image *without* the top-hat component   (e) Color input image   (f) Reference segmentation

Fig. 4. Illustration of the top-hat procedure.

2.2   Pre-processing

We use the bias field corrected FLAIR image and the bias field corrected T1 image aligned with FLAIR. The main issue with WMH segmentation is the segmentation of small lesions. An idea to help the network find the lesions is to enhance them.

We first perform a requantization of voxel intensity values on 8 bits. The FLAIR slices are filtered using a morphological operator (an area opening), so that small lesions are filtered out, and we compute the residue (difference between the original FLAIR image and the filtered one); in this final image, called "pre-procesed FLAIR" in the following and illustrated in Fig. 4(c), small lesions are particularly visible and large ones do not appear.

2.3   Deep FCN for WMH Segmentation

Fully convolutional network (FCN) and transfer learning have proved their efficiency for natural image segmentation [12]. In a previous paper [25], we proposed to rely on this method to segment 3D brain MR images, although those images are very different from natural images. As it was a succes, we adapted it to WMH segmentation. We rely on the 16 layers VGG network [22], which was pre-trained on millions of natural images of ImageNet for image classification [10]. For our application, we keep only the 4 stages of convolutional parts called *"base network"* and discard the fully connected layers at the end of VGG network. This base network is mainly composed of convolutional layers: $z_i = w_i \times x + b_i$, Rectified Linear Unit (ReLU) layers for non linear activation function: $f(z_i) = \max(0, z_i)$, and max pooling layers between two successive stages, where x is the input of each convolutional layer, w_i is the convolution parameter, and b_i is the bias term. The three max pooling layers divide the base network into four stages of fine to coarse feature maps. Inspired by the work in [12,13], we add specialized convolutional layers (with a 3×3 kernel size) with K (e.g. $K = 16$) feature maps after the convolutional layers at the end of each stage. All the specialized layers are then rescaled to the original image size, and concatenated together. We add a last convolutional layer with kernel size 1×1 at the end. This last layer combines linearly the fine to coarse feature maps in the concatenated specialized layers, and provides the final segmentation result. The proposed network architecture is schematized in Fig. 2.

The architecture described above is very similar to the one used in [13] for retinal image analysis, where the retinal images are already 2D color images. For our application, the question amounts to how to prepare appropriate inputs given that a brain MR image is a 3D volume. To get RGB input images, we propose to use 2D slices from different modalities. Precisely, to form an input artificial color image for the pre-trained network to segment the nth slice, we use the slice n of FLAIR, of the T1 and of the pre-processed FLAIR as the three different color channels of a 2D color image. The green, blue and red channels thus carry different information; note that the match "particular information/chosen channel" does not matter for the network at end, except that this match has to remain always the same in the learning and testing stages. This process is depicted in Fig. 2 (left). Each 2D color image thus forms a representation of a part (a slice of FLAIR and T1) of the MR volume. Using such a 2D representation avoids the expensive computational and memory requirements of fully 3D FCN.

For the training phase, we use the multinomial logistic loss function for a one-of-many classification task, passing real-valued predictions through a softmax to get a probability distribution over classes. During training, we use the classical data augmentation strategy by scaling and rotating. Each channel of the training images is then centered (we subtract 127 to values to ensure input value are within the $[-127, 127]$ range). We fine tune the network for the first 50k iterations using a learning rate of 10^{-8}, and the last 100k with a smaller learning rate of 10^{-9}. We rely on stochastic gradient descent to minimize the loss function with a momentum of 0.99 for the first 50k iterations and 0.999 for the next 100k, and a weight decay of 0.0005. The loss function is averaged over 20 images.

At test time, after having pre-processed the 3D volume (requantization), we prepare the set of 2D color images. Then we subtract 127 for each channel, and pass every image through the network.

We run the train and test phases on a GPU card: NVIDIA GeForce GTX 1080 Ti, having 11Go. The training phase lasts 4 hours while the testing one lasts less than 10 s per volume. The 4 h of the learning remains reasonable, and the network can be learned again if scans from new machines are provided. It could be useful, especially if the new scans are different (resolution, contrast, etc.).

The output of the network for one slice during the inference phase is a 2D segmented slice. After processing all the slices of the volume, all the segmented slices are stacked to recover a 3D volume with the same shape as the initial volume, and containing only the segmented lesions.

Last, let us remark that, in the case of small lesions, the use of multi-modality can be an important key. Indeed, the small lesions are not present on a lot of slices, thus limiting the interest of 3D representations. The use of combination of T1 and FLAIR images for one slice gives more information for lesion detection. As the proportion of small lesions is small compared to the total number of pixels, every information that can be discriminant for lesion detection is important.

3   Experiments and Results

This section presents the experiments and results obtained, during the development of our method first (using the training dataset), and then the results of the challenge. The metrics used to evaluate the results are:

- Dice Similarity Coefficient,
- Hausdorff distance (modified, 95th percentile, in mm) [3],
- Average volume difference (in percentage),
- Sensitivity for individual lesions, or recall (in percentage),
- F1-score for individual lesions: $2PR/(P+R)$, where P and R are respectively the precision and the recall.

3.1   Development Phase

In this part, we used the 60 scans from the training set of the challenge to validate and tune our approach. Those scans were acquired in three hospitals using three scanners from different vendors (see Table 1).

Training. We trained our model on 30 scans (10 from each hospital), randomly chosen. The model was trained using the parameters described in the previous section.

Testing. We tested on the 30 remaining scans. We measured 4 parameters using the code provided by the organizers: the dice coefficient, the average volume distance (AVD), the sensitivity for individual lesion detection and the F1-score for individual lesions. The results are shown in Table 2, line 3.

Table 2. Quantitative comparison of the influence of the top-hat on the pre-competition dataset. We submitted the 2D with top-hap method for the challenge. *In this table and in the following ones, ↑ (resp. ↓) means that a higher (resp. lower) value is better.*

Type	Dice ↑	AVD ↓	Lesion detection↑	F1 score ↑
3D-like	0.72	23.90	0.38	0.46
2D w/o top-hat	0.72	28.24	0.39	0.48
2D with top-hat	0.75	22.63	0.61	0.63

An illustration of our segmentation results, with a qualitative comparison to the reference segmentation, can be found in Fig. 5. False negatives and false positives are very reduced.

Validation of the top-hat 2D choice. To evaluate the influence of the top-hat and the 2D input on our results, we trained and tested with and without the top-hat on 2D images (the last channel was replaced by the same slice from T1) and we tested the 3D-like approach from our previous work [25]. Results are shown in Table 2. The results of the 3D-like approach and of the 2D approach *without* top-hat are quite similar. The lesion detection is a little bit better for the 2D combination, but this is not significant. The 3D information is hence not relevant for this application. The 2D approach including the top hat image slightly improved the Dice and the AVD, but the best improvement is for the lesion detection. On this dataset, the measurement of the sensitivity for individual lesion raised from 0.38% or 0.39% to 0.61% thanks to the 2D top-hat procedure. The small lesions enhancement indeed helped the detection of lesions.

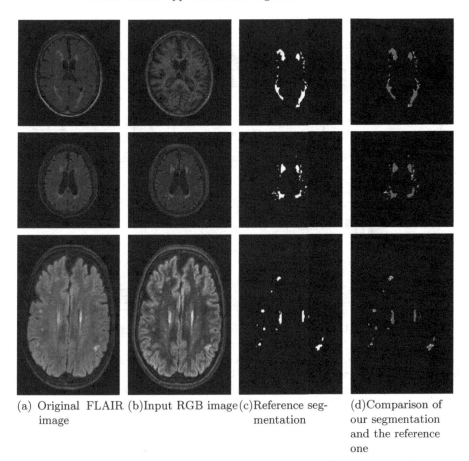

(a) Original FLAIR image   (b)Input RGB image   (c)Reference segmentation   (d)Comparison of our segmentation and the reference one

Fig. 5. Example of results on each database. Note that the input images are different as they come from different hospitals. From top to bottom: Utrecht, Singapore, and Amsterdam. The intersection between the reference segmentation and our result is depicted in yellow; the green pixels (false negatives) are in the reference segmentation but not in our segmentation; the red ones (false positives) are in our segmentation but not in the reference one. (Color figure online)

3.2   Challenge Results

The testing dataset of the MICCAI WMH Challenge remained secret. It was composed of 110 scans of patients from three hospitals and five different scanners from three vendors (see Table 1).

The metrics used for the evaluation are the five metrics described at the beginning of this section. The rank is included between 0 (best result) and 1 (worst result). It is computed by the organizers of the challenge as follows: the teams are sorted from best to worst for each metric. The best team will be ranked 0 and the worst team 1. The other teams are ranked between 0 and 1 relative to

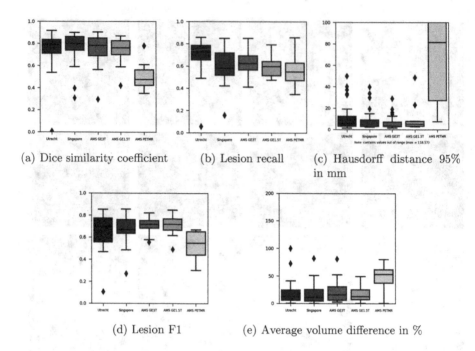

(a) Dice similarity coefficient   (b) Lesion recall   (c) Hausdorff distance 95% in mm

(d) Lesion F1   (e) Average volume difference in %

Fig. 6. Box plot for each metric depending on the origin of the scans; UMC Utrecht in dark blue, NUHS Singapore in green, and VU Amsterdam (AMS): 3T GE Signa HDxt in brown, 3T Philips Ingenuity in pink, and 1.5T GE Signa HDxt in light blue. (Color figure online)

their performance within the range of that metric. The final rank is the average of the 5 metric ranks. Table 3 shows the results of our method for the challenge.

Our best performance is for the AVD where we have a really good rank as shown in Tables 3 and 4, while our worst score is for the lesion detection. Based on these measurements, we can conclude that our method still misses some lesions but that the ones it detects are close to the reference segmentation. We were ranked 0.164 on the overall average and reached the 6th place of the challenge. The top methods of the challenge also use deep learning for the segmentation. They mainly use patches of images instead of whole images. About the architecture used, it is interesting to notice that the winner of this challenge uses a U-Net architecture with pre-processing and post-processing steps.

The analysis of the results against each data source reveals that our method performs poorly on data acquired with the Philips scanner, for which no training data were available and test images remained secret, preventing us from investigating further. We can also note that while no training data were available for the GE 1.5T, our method still performs well on such data. The box plots (Fig. 6) show the inhomogeneities of these results. Despite this, our method appears quite stable among the different acquisition devices.

Table 3. Results of our method on the challenge dataset. The five first lines are the results for each metric of each pool of data. The sixth line is the weighted average of each metric. The last line corresponds to the rank for each metric.

Origin	Dice ↑	H95 ↓	AVD ↓	Recall ↑	F1 ↑
UMC Utrecht	0.74	11.22	19.07	0.70	0.66
NUHS Singapore	0.77	8.28	17.64	0.61	0.68
AMS GE 3T	0.75	6.75	21.91	0.62	0.71
AMS GE 1.5T	0.73	10.94	16.66	0.60	0.71
AMS Philips 3T	0.50	70.27	46.33	0.57	0.53
Weighted average	0.73	14.54	21.71	0.63	0.67
Rank [0 . . . 1] ↓	0.122	0.180	0.004	0.352	0.159

Table 4. Competition results, sorted with respect to the AVD metric.

Team	Rank ↓	DSC ↑	H95 ↓	AVD ↓	Recall ↑	F1 ↑
nlp_logix	0.0485	0.77	7.16	18.37	0.73	0.78
k2	0.1368	0.77	9.79	19.08	0.59	0.70
ipmi-bern	0.2498	0.69	9.72	19.92	0.44	0.57
misp	0.1659	0.72	14.88	21.36	0.63	0.68
lrde	0.1635	0.73	14.54	**21.71**	0.63	0.67
cian	0.0366	0.78	6.82	21.72	0.83	0.70
sysu_media	0.0076	0.80	6.30	21.88	0.84	0.76
achilles	0.2962	0.63	11.82	24.41	0.45	0.52
nic-vicorob	0.0735	0.77	8.28	28.54	0.75	0.71
tig	0.3858	0.60	17.86	34.34	0.38	0.42
scan	0.2762	0.63	14.34	34.67	0.55	0.51
knight	0.4159	0.70	17.03	39.99	0.25	0.35
skkumedneuro	0.3492	0.58	19.02	58.54	0.47	0.51
tignet	0.3802	0.59	21.58	86.22	0.46	0.45
nist	0.4747	0.53	15.91	109.98	0.37	0.25
text_class	0.5725	0.50	28.23	146.64	0.27	0.29
nih_cidi	0.2697	0.68	12.82	196.38	0.59	0.54
upc_dlmi	0.4337	0.53	27.01	208.49	0.57	0.42
neuro.ml	0.5960	0.51	37.36	614.05	0.71	0.21
hadi	0.8886	0.23	52.02	828.61	0.58	0.11

4   Conclusion

In the context of the MICCAI WMH Challenge, we developed a fast, robust and automated method that segments white matter hyperintensities (WMH) in 3D brain MR images. It is an extension of a method we proposed for brain MRI segmentation. It uses fully convolutional network (FCN) and transfer learning to segment the lesions. It takes as input 2D color images (3 channels), corresponding to a slice of a 3D volume. The two first channels are composed of a combination of FLAIR and T1 slices. To improve the detection of the lesions, the last channel is a modified FLAIR slice where the small hyperintensities are enhanced by a top-hat procedure. The FCN is the VGG network for natural image classification, pre-trained on ImageNet database. We fine tuned it on the training dataset of the challenge. When all slices are processed, the results are stacked to reconstruct the resulting 3D segmented volume. During the development phase, we validated the benefits of the 2D pre-processed images with small lesions enhancement over the 2D images containing only T1 and FLAIR slices, and also over a 3D-like image as in [25]. With such a technique, the complete segmentation of WMH on a 3D brain volume takes about 10 s. During the challenge, the organizers ran our method on their database composed of 5 different sets. Our results are quite stable over acquisition methods except for the Philips scanner, thus exhibiting the reliability of our method. Finally, we achieved a top score on the AVD metric with a rank of 0.004 (best is 0, worst is 1) for an AVD value of 21.71. Our overall score is 0.164 (average of the 5 metrics used for the challenge), leading us to the 6th place. With our method, we could consider other applications for other purposes such as the TUPAC16 MICCAI Grand Challenge (Tumor Proliferation Assessment Challenge 2016) which aims to predict the tumor proliferation score for breast cancer, or the Multimodal Brain Tumor Segmentation Challenge (BraTS) which focuses on the prediction of patient overall survival from the study of brain lesions.

Acknowledgments. The authors want to thank the organizers of the White Matter Hyperintensities Segmentation Challenge at MICCAI 2017, and the reviewers for their valuable comments.

References

1. Caligiuri, M.E., Perrotta, P., Augimeri, A., Rocca, F., Quattrone, A., Cherubini, A.: Automatic detection of white matter hyperintensities in healthy aging and pathology using magnetic resonance imaging: a review. Neuroinformatics **13**(3), 261–276 (2015)
2. Carlinet, E., Géraud, T.: A comparative review of component tree computation algorithms. IEEE Trans. Image Process. **23**(9), 3885–3895 (2014)
3. Dubuisson, M.P., Jain, A.K.: A modified Hausdorff distance for object matching. In: Proceedings of the 12th International Conference on Pattern Recognition, vol. 1, pp. 566–568. IEEE (1994)
4. García-Lorenzo, D., Francis, S., Narayanan, S., Arnold, D.L., Collins, D.L.: Review of automatic segmentation methods of multiple sclerosis white matter lesions on conventional magnetic resonance imaging. Med. Image Anal. **17**(1), 1–18 (2013)
5. Ghafoorian, M., Karssemeijer, N., Heskes, T., van Uden, I.W., Sanchez, C.I., Litjens, G., de Leeuw, F.E., van Ginneken, B., Marchiori, E., Platel, B.: Location sensitive deep convolutional neural networks for segmentation of white matter hyperintensities. Sci. Rep. **7**, 5110 (2017)

6. Ghafoorian, M., Mehrtash, A., Kapur, T., Karssemeijer, N., Marchiori, E., Pesteie, M., Guttmann, C.R.G., de Leeuw, F.-E., Tempany, C.M., van Ginneken, B., Fedorov, A., Abolmaesumi, P., Platel, B., Wells, W.M.: Transfer learning for domain adaptation in MRI: application in brain lesion segmentation. In: Descoteaux, M., Maier-Hein, L., Franz, A., Jannin, P., Collins, D.L., Duchesne, S. (eds.) MICCAI 2017, Part III. LNCS, vol. 10435, pp. 516–524. Springer, Cham (2017). https://doi.org/10.1007/978-3-319-66179-7_59

7. Jack, C.R., O'Brien, P.C., Rettman, D.W., Shiung, M.M., Xu, Y., Muthupillai, R., Manduca, A., Avula, R., Erickson, B.J.: FLAIR histogram segmentation for measurement of leukoaraiosis volume. J. Magn. Reson. Imaging 14(6), 668–676 (2001)

8. Jones, R.: Component trees for image filtering and segmentation. In: Coyle, E. (ed.) Proceedings of the IEEE Workshop on Nonlinear Signal and Image Processing, Mackinac Island (1997)

9. Khayati, R., Vafadust, M., Towhidkhah, F., Nabavi, M.: Fully automatic segmentation of multiple sclerosis lesions in brain MR FLAIR images using adaptive mixtures method and Markov random field model. Comput. Biol. Med. 38(3), 379–390 (2008)

10. Krizhevsky, A., Sutskever, I., Hinton, G.E.: Imagenet classification with deep convolutional neural networks. In: Advances in Neural Information Processing Systems, pp. 1097–1105 (2012)

11. Lazzara, G., Géraud, T., Levillain, R.: Planting, growing and pruning trees: Connected filters applied to document image analysis. In: Proceedings of the 11th IAPR International Workshop on Document Analysis Systems (DAS), Tours, France, pp. 36–40 (2014)

12. Long, J., Shelhamer, E., Darrell, T.: Fully convolutional networks for semantic segmentation. In: Proceedings of IEEE International Conference on Computer Vision and Pattern Recognition, pp. 3431–3440 (2015)

13. Maninis, K.-K., Pont-Tuset, J., Arbeláez, P., Van Gool, L.: Deep retinal image understanding. In: Ourselin, S., Joskowicz, L., Sabuncu, M.R., Unal, G., Wells, W. (eds.) MICCAI 2016, Part II. LNCS, vol. 9901, pp. 140–148. Springer, Cham (2016). https://doi.org/10.1007/978-3-319-46723-8_17

14. Meijster, A., Wilkinson, M.H.F.: A comparison of algorithms for connected set openings and closings. IEEE Trans. Pattern Anal. Mach. Intell. 24(4), 484–494 (2002)

15. Morel, B., Xu, Y., Virzi, A., Géraud, T., Adamsbaum, C., Bloch, I.: A challenging issue: detection of white matter hyperintensities on neonatal brain MRI. In: Proceedings of the Annual International Conference of the IEEE Engineering in Medicine and Biology Society (EMBC), pp. 93–96 (2016)

16. Pantoni, L.: Cerebral small vessel disease: from pathogenesis and clinical characteristics to therapeutic challenges. Lancet Neurol. 9(7), 689–701 (2010)

17. Ronneberger, O., Fischer, P., Brox, T.: U-Net: convolutional networks for biomedical image segmentation. In: Navab, N., Hornegger, J., Wells, W.M., Frangi, A.F. (eds.) MICCAI 2015, Part III. LNCS, vol. 9351, pp. 234–241. Springer, Cham (2015). https://doi.org/10.1007/978-3-319-24574-4_28

18. Salembier, P., Oliveras, A., Garrido, L.: Antiextensive connected operators for image and sequence processing. IEEE Trans. Image Process. 7(4), 555–570 (1998)

19. Salembier, P., Serra, J.: Flat zones filtering, connected operators and filters by reconstruction. IEEE Trans. Image Process. 3(8), 1153–1160 (1995)

20. Salembier, P., Wilkinson, M.H.: Connected operators. IEEE Signal Process. Mag. 26(6), 136–157 (2009)

21. Schwarz, C., Fletcher, E., DeCarli, C., Carmichael, O.: Fully-automated white matter hyperintensity detection with anatomical prior knowledge and without FLAIR. Inf. Process. Med. Imaging **21**, 239–251 (2009)
22. Simonyan, K., Zisserman, A.: Very deep convolutional networks for large-scale image recognition. CoRR abs/1409.1556 (2014)
23. Vincent, L.: Grayscale area openings and closings, their efficient implementation and applications. In: Proceedings of the EURASIP 1st Workshop on Mathematical Morphology and its Applications to Signal Processing, Barcelona, Spain, pp. 22–27, May 1993
24. Wardlaw, J.M., Smith, E.E., Biessels, G.J., Cordonnier, C., Fazekas, F., Frayne, R., Lindley, R.I., O'Brien, J.T., Barkhof, F., Benavente, O.R., et al.: Neuroimaging standards for research into small vessel disease and its contribution to ageing and neurodegeneration. Lancet Neurol. **12**(8), 822–838 (2013)
25. Xu, Y., Géraud, T., Bloch, I.: From neonatal to adult brain MR image segmentation in a few seconds using 3D-like fully convolutional network and transfer learning. In: Proceedings of the 23rd IEEE International Conference on Image Processing (ICIP), Beijing, China pp. 4417–4421, September 2017. http://www.lrde.epita.fr/~theo/papers/geraud.2017.icip.pdf

Author Index

Printed in the United States
By Bookmasters